Contents

Orthopedic Manual Therapy

An Evidence-Based Approach

Second Edition

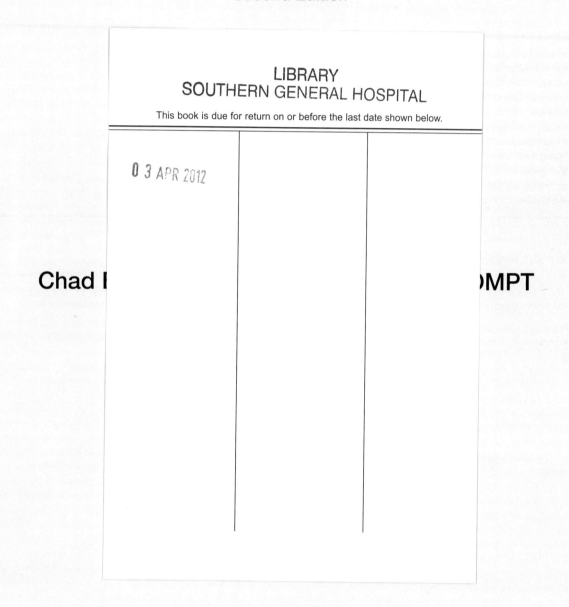

Chad   OMPT

Pearson

Boston   Columbus   Indianapolis   New York   San Francisco   Upper Saddle River
Amsterdam   Cape Town   Dubai   London   Madrid   Milan   Munich   Paris   Montreal   Toronto
Delhi   Mexico City   Sao Paulo   Sydney   Hong Kong   Seoul   Singapore   Taipei   Tokyo

Library of Congress Cataloging-in-Publication Data

Cook, Chad.
  Orthopedic manual therapy : an evidence based approach / Chad E. Cook. —
2nd ed.
     p. ; cm.
  Includes bibliographical references and index.
  ISBN-13: 978-0-13-802173-3
  ISBN-10: 0-13-802173-2
  1. Manipulation (Therapeutics) 2. Orthopedics. 3. Medicine, Physical.
I. Title.
  [DNLM: 1. Manipulation, Orthopedic—methods. WB 535]
  RM724.C66 2012
  615.8'2—dc22
                          2010040563

Notice:
The author and the publisher of this volume have taken care that the information and technical recommendations contained herein are based on research and expert consultation and are accurate and compatible with the standards generally accepted at the time of publication. Nevertheless, as new information becomes available, changes in clinical and technical practices become necessary. The reader is advised to carefully consult manufacturers' instructions and information material for all supplies and equipment before use and to consult with a health care professional as necessary. This advice is especially important when using new supplies or equipment for clinical purposes. The author and publisher disclaim all responsibility for any liability, loss, injury, or damage incurred as a consequence, directly or indirectly, of the use and application of any of the contents of this volume.

Publisher: Julie Levin Alexander
Assistant to Publisher: Regina Bruno
Editor-in-Chief: Mark Cohen
Executive Editor: John Goucher
Associate Editor: Melissa Kerian
Assistant Editor: Nicole Ragonese
Editorial Assistant: Rosalie Hawley
Media Editor: Amy Peltier
Media Product Manager: Lorena Cerisano
Managing Production Editor: Patrick Walsh
Production Liaison: Christina Zingone

Production Editor: Patty Donovan, Laserwords, Maine
Manufacturing Manager: Ilene Sanford
Manufacturing Buyer: Alan Fischer
Design Director: Jayne Conte
Art Director: Suzanne Behnke
Director of Marketing: David Gesell
Executive Marketing Manager: Katrin Beacom
Marketing Specialist: Michael Sirinides
Composition: Laserwords, India
Printer/Binder: Courier/Kendallville
Cover Printer: Lehigh-Phoenix Color/Hagerstown

10 9 8 7 6 5 4 3 2 1

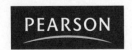

www.pearsonhighered.com

ISBN-10 0-13-802173-2
ISBN-13 978-0-13-802173-3

Foreword

As a clinician who first practiced physical therapy in the early 1990s, I feel certain that I shared a belief of many others; that there was mainstream musculoskeletal physical therapy, and then there was "manual therapy." Manual therapy was practiced by the apprentices of a handful of trailblazing gurus, each of whom taught their followers special techniques that could cure a patient with the skillful laying on of the hands. Many perceived that the skill set of these practitioners was closer to magic than science. In the early phases of manual therapy, most of the practitioners did little to dispel this conception.

Fortunately for manual therapy (and physical therapy), those gurus influenced a group of inquisitive physical therapists that would fuel an explosion of research that has added to a bourgeoning bolus of science to the art of manual therapy. One of these physical therapists is Dr. Chad Cook, who is a voracious consumer and producer of the science of manual therapy. A component of this production was the first edition of *Orthopedic Manual Therapy: An Evidence-Based Approach.*

The first edition took the science of manual therapy and presented that science in an eclectic format, which was both easily digestible and clinically applicable. This book debunked many of the myths associated with the manual therapy examination and intervention, such as treating the spine based on coupled motion and the necessity of moving joints based on a convex/concave rule, while steadfastly supporting other constructs with a scientific basis such as centralization or classification. Based on the national and international success of the book, the approach has been a needed and welcome approach.

Never one to rest on success, Dr. Cook has created an almost wholesale revision. As the evidence for manual therapy has changed and grown so have the teachings and practice of the editor. Included are mobilization with movement techniques and a more detailed section on outcomes for each body region. The book includes two new chapters on nervous system mobilization and soft tissue mobilization. Despite these inclusions, the second edition is a more efficient yet a more comprehensive presentation of manual therapy for every practitioner. The consistency of the presentation of assessment and intervention procedures, not to mention the decreased heft of the book, makes this version of *Orthopedic Manual Therapy* more user friendly for professors, clinicians, and students. This is the one text on manual therapy that all should have in their collection.

Eric Hegedus, PT, DPT, MHSc, OCS
Associate Professor, Duke University

Foreword

Acquiring knowledge and developing clinical competency are two of the greatest challenges facing orthopedic manual therapists. Knowledge provides the solid foundation for evidence-enhanced practice and increasingly establishes the parameters that define the scope of orthopedic physical therapy. Clinical competency requires the succinct synthesis of anatomy, physiology, and current research to serve as a framework for the utilization and development of appropriate evaluation and treatment techniques.

An orthopedic manual therapist cannot be complacent in the pursuit of knowledge. Regardless of the therapist's governing regulations, all orthopedic manual therapists must function as a direct access practitioner in the sense of competency and responsibility. The rapidly evolving discipline of manual therapy dictates the aggressive pursuit of updated knowledge and skills. The second edition of *Orthopedic Manual Therapy: An Evidence-Based Approach* effectively presents the foundations of patient management, sound clinical reasoning, reflective practice, and problem solving, which assists in the management of the unique challenge presented by each patient. Our patients require and deserve our ongoing commitment to excellence and development of our knowledge of human behavior and function to achieve optimum resolutions.

Dr. Cook's comprehensive, regional approach to the body allows the practicing therapist to synthesize current research, didactic knowledge, and clinical expertise in one resource. Chapters 1–4 provide detailed information pertaining to orthopedic manual therapy assessment, evaluation, treatment, and contraindications. This carefully organized preamble to the regional technique section is necessary reading for all physical therapists, regardless of one's area of specialty or experience. A therapist's ability to recognize and appropriately address the orthopedic issues with any patient requires a knowledge base supported by a comprehensive understanding of anatomy, pathology, and applicable research. The following 12 chapters offer an in-depth, regional insight into the prevalence of musculoskeletal conditions supported by the relevant anatomy, biomechanics, clinical examination protocols, treatment techniques, and outcomes. Within this section, research and scientific knowledge specific to each region are analyzed and correlated to support the tests, techniques, and clinical reasoning presented. Each chapter provides the reader with an extensive bibliography to facilitate further investigation and underscore the supporting evidence.

A major strength of the text is the extensive and comprehensive technique section, which is representative of a wide variety of manual therapy philosophies. This integrated approach allows the therapist to compare and investigate the most appropriate method of intervention for each patient, rather than being directed into one specific system or viewpoint. In addition, over 700 color pictures supplement this section, facilitating a more efficient understanding and application of the techniques presented.

The first edition of *Orthopedic Manual Therapy* immediately became required reading for our Functional Manual Therapy Fellowship program in 2007. This text has provided the fellows in training with a comprehensive resource for information that guides the appropriate evaluation, testing, and treatment of each patient, in addition to being the primary resource in studying for their examinations. I eagerly anticipate the release of the expanded and enhanced version, bringing to our profession an up-to-date synopsis of relevant research and techniques for all orthopedic patient populations. I am confident the second edition of *Orthopedic Manual Therapy: An Evidence-Based Approach* will continue to augment the advanced training of not only Manual Therapy Fellows and Residents, but all physical therapists dedicated to excellence in clinical management and patient care. I am honored to write a Foreword to such a high-quality and important text.

Gregory S. Johnson, PT
Co-Founder, Institute of Physical Art, Inc.
President, Johnson and Johnson Physical Therapy, Inc.
Vice Chairman, Functional Manual Therapy Foundation
Program Director, FMT Fellowship
Program Administrator, FMT Orthopedic Residency
Secretary, FMT Certification Board
Associate Professor, Touro College

Preface

It is with great pleasure that I present the second edition of *Orthopedic Manual Therapy: An Evidence-Based Approach*. As is appropriate for any text espousing evidence-based elements, I have updated and expanded accordingly. As I mentioned in the preface to the first edition,[1] literature describing and measuring "evidence-based" care has grown significantly over the last decade.[2] The core components of evidence-based concepts were developed in the 1970s and 1980s with the application of epidemiological principles of patient care.[3,4] These epidemiological principles advocate that using evidence-based care allows clinicians to apply the current best evidence from research to the clinical care of the individual patient.[3,5] The overwhelming collective evidence is daunting and the ability of one textbook to capture all aspects is simply unattainable.

But it's not as if we haven't tried. The second edition has enlisted the assistance of a number of new collaborators, including Christopher Fiander, Amy Cook, Megan Donaldson, and Roy Coronado. Ken Learman has contributed an additional chapter and Bob Fleming has returned to update the knee chapter. In addition, two new chapters have been added to expand the material within the textbook. A neurodynamics chapter (Chapter 15) and a soft tissue mobilization chapter (Chapter 16) should improve the comprehensiveness of the text, which now covers all elements of manual therapy. Chapters 5–16 each have two or three dedicated patient cases and we've included videos of selected techniques to improve the understanding and carryover to the clinic. Visit www.myhealthprofessionskit.com to view these videos. To further improve the textbook's ease of application in a clinical setting, we've placed the anatomy and arthrological elements (with new illustrations) online at www.myhealthprofessionskit.com.

The most notable difference from the first edition is the further emphasis on clinical decision making. Different models of decision making are discussed as are clinical decision-making aids such as clinical prediction rules, within- and between-session findings, and a brief discussion on classification. Gone from the second edition is the level of detail on special tests, which isn't truly germane to the care provided by a manual therapist. In its place are the presentations of more home exercise activities for carryover of care and mobilization with movement techniques to further broaden the scope of the text.

What remains a bastion of this text is its emphasis on the debunking of myths and its polarizing discussion on weaknesses of certain manual therapy approaches. The text still exposes faulty philosophies, theories, and other clinical provisos that are advocated and does so for the sake of simplicity. Good manual therapy (provided with the appropriate motor training) should not be so complex that all clinicians can't use it. And if I'm wrong in my take of the evidence, then I do so in the spirit of simplicity and clinical utility for all therapists.

Chad E. Cook
Professor and Chair, Walsh University

References

1. Cook C. *Orthopedic manual therapy: An evidence-based approach.* Upper Saddle River, NJ; Prentice Hall: 2007.
2. Cohen AM, Stavri PZ, Hersh WR. A categorization and analysis of the criticisms of evidence based medicine. *Int J Med Informatics.* 2004;73:35–43.
3. Sackett DL. The fall of clinical research and the rise of clinical practice research. *Clin Invest Med.* 2000;23:331–333.
4. Buetow MA, Kenealy T. Evidence based medicine: the need for new definition. *J Evaluation Clin Pract.* 2000; 6:85–92.
5. Sackett DL, Strauss SE, Richardson WS, Rosenberg W, Haynes RB. Evidence-based medicine. In: *How to practice and teach EBM.* Edinburgh; Churchill Livingstone: 2000.

Acknowledgments

I'd like to acknowledge the following individuals who have significantly impacted the material within this textbook:

Jean-Michel Brismee: A great clinician, but an even better person.

Amy, Zach, Jaeger, and Simon Cook: "Dad, quit checking your emails!"

Bob Fleming and Ken Learman: Solid friends and collaborators.

Eric Hegedus: You are making progress, Sisyphus!

John Medeiros and the people involved with the *Journal of Manual and Manipulative Therapy:* A gentlemanly leader of an unpretentious journal.

Chris Showalter and my friends at MAPS: Toga! Toga!

Phillip Sizer, Jr.: The man never sleeps!

Special thanks to Steve Houghton who created the majority of the tables for the Anatomy and Biomechanics sections of each chapter.

My former students from Duke University: Intellectual juggernauts.

Geoff Maitland, Gregory Grieve, Bob Sprague, Bob Elvey, and the numerous other manual therapy pioneers that have created the framework in which manual therapy stands: We are riding your wave—and it's a BIG one.

Contributors

Amy Cook, PT, MS
Contract Physical Therapist
North Canton, Ohio

Rogelio Coronado, PT, MS, FAAOMPT
PhD Student
Department of Rehabilitative Sciences
University of Florida
Gainesville, Florida

Megan Donaldson, PT, PhD, FAAOMPT
Assistant Professor
Department of Physical Therapy
Walsh University
North Canton, Ohio

Christopher Fiander, DPT, OCS
Senior Physical Therapist
Department of Physical Therapy and Occupational Therapy
Duke University
Durham, North Carolina

Robert Fleming, Jr., PT, DPT, MS, OCS, FAAOMPT
Rehabilitation Services Manager
Ellis Hospital
Schenectady, New York

Ken Learman, MPT, PhD, OCS, FAAOMPT
Associate Professor
Department of Physical Therapy
Youngstown State University
Youngstown, Ohio

Reviewers

Second Edition

Dr. Jason A. Craig, MCSP, DPhil, PT
Marymount University
Arlington, Virginia

Michelle Dolphin, PT, DPT, MS, OCS
SUNY Upstate Medical University
Syracuse, New York

Megan Donaldson, PT, PhD
Walsh University
North Canton, Ohio

Marcia Epler, PhD, PT, ATC
Lebanon Valley College
Annville, Pennsylvania

Lisa T. Hoglund, PT, PhD, OCS, CertMDT
University of the Sciences in Philadelphia
Philadelphia, Pennsylvania

John Leard, EdD, PT, ATC
University of Hartford
West Hartford, Connecticut

Marcia Miller Spoto, PT, DC, OCS
Nazareth College
Rochester, New York

Clare Safran-Norton, PhD, MS, MS, PT, OCS
Simmons College
Boston, Massachusetts

Michael P. Reiman, PT, DPT, OCS, ATC, CSCS
Wichita State University
Wichita, Kansas

Toni S. Roddey, PT, PhD, OCS, FAAOMPT
Texas Woman's University
Houston, Texas

First Edition

Stephania Bell, MS, PT, OCS, CSCS
Kaiser Hayward Orthopedic Manual Therapy Fellowship
Union City, California

Robert E. Boyles, PT, DSc, OCS, FAAOMPT
U.S. Army–Baylor University
Fort Sam Houston, Texas

Jean-Michel Brismee, ScD, PT, OCS, FAAOMPT
Texas Tech University Health Sciences Center
Odessa, Texas

Joshua Cleland, DPT, PhD, OCS
Franklin Pierce College
Concord, New Hampshire

Evan Johnson, PT, MS, OCS, MTC
Columbia University
New York, New York

Kenneth E. Learman, MEd, PT, OCS, COMT, FAAOMPT
Youngstown State University
Youngstown, Ohio

Kevin Ramey, MS, PT
Texas Tech University Health Sciences Center
Odessa, Texas

Christopher R. Showalter, LPT, OCS, FAAOMPT
Maitland-Australian Physiotherapy Seminars
Cutchogue, New York

Andrea P. Simmons, CMT, CNMT
Medical Careers Institute
Richmond, virginia

Orthopedic Manual Therapy

Chad E. Cook

Objectives

- Define orthopedic manual therapy.
- Outline the mechanical changes associated with manual therapy intervention.
- Compare and contrast the effects of static stretching, manually assisted movements, mobilization, and manipulation.
- Outline the neurophysiological changes associated with manual therapy intervention.
- Outline the proposed psychological changes associated with manual therapy intervention.
- Compare and contrast the different methods of reporting of evidence.
- Outline the levels of evidence used to judge quality of information.

What Constitutes Orthopedic Manual Therapy?

Construct

Within the professional fields of medicine and rehabilitation, orthopedic manual therapy is best defined by the description of the application. Orthopedic manual therapy may reflect selected passive or active assistive techniques such as stretching, mobilization, manipulation, and muscle energy–related methods (Table 1.1 ■). Each application is used for the purposes of modulation of pain, reducing or eliminating soft tissue inflammation, improving contractile and noncontractile tissue repair, extensibility, and/or stability, and increasing range of motion (ROM) for

■ TABLE 1.1 Definitions of the Most Common Applications of Orthopedic Manual Therapy

Construct/Application	Definition
Passive stretching	Passive technique involving application of a tensile force to tissue in an effort to increase the extensibility of length (and resultant range of motion) of the targeted tissue.
Mobilization	Passive technique designed to restore full painless joint function by rhythmic, repetitive passive movements, well within the patient's tolerance, in voluntary and/or accessory ranges.
Manipulation	An accurately localized or globally applied single, quick, and decisive movement of small amplitude, following a careful positioning of the patient.
Muscle energy technique	A manually assisted method of stretching/mobilization where the patient actively uses his or her muscles, on request, while maintaining a targeted preposition against a distinctly executed counterforce.
Passive mobilization with an active movement	A passive technique that consists of a rhythmic, repetitive passive movement to the patient's tolerance, in voluntary and/or accessory ranges, performed concomitantly with an active movement of the patient at the same region.

facilitation of movement and return to function. Other types of "manual therapy" that make curative claims beyond those I have just outlined are outside the scope of this textbook and often offer dubious claims of mental, physical, and behavioral changes. The validity of other methods requires further study. Truly, the variations in the types of manual therapies are extraordinary, specifically when one explores the incongruent philosophical and theoretical constructs of each type.

Terminology

Simply stating that the terminology of manual therapy is inconsistent among its users may be considered the penultimate understatement. The variations in language have prompted a call for consistency[1] and the development of standardized manipulation terminology in practice.[2,3] The proposed terminology reflects descriptive language designed to homogenize how one describes an application or technique. The terms advocated are (1) rate of force application, (2) location in range of available movement, (3) direction of force, (4) target of force, (5) relative structural movement, and (6) patient position (Table 1.2 ■). In nearly all circumstances these terms are adopted by this textbook during the descriptions of each of the techniques.

The Science of Orthopedic Manual Therapy

The precise nature of why manual therapy benefits various conditions has given rise to conflicting theories and heated debate.[4] Explanations outlining the reasons why manual therapy is beneficial have ranged from the scientifically pertinent to the inexplicably strange. To date, most theories remain hypothetical, have involved investigations that were poorly designed, or were predominantly promoted by personal opinion. There are no shortages of hypotheses driven primarily by researchers and theoreticians in chiropractic, physical therapy, osteopathic, and massage-based fields. Hypotheses have included; movement of the nucleus pulposis[5,6] activation of the gate-control mechanism,[7] neurophysiological and biomechanical responses,[8,9] and resultant reductions in paraspinal muscle hypertonicity.[10,11]

The constructs behind the use of stretching, mobilization, manipulation, and muscle energy–related methods are similar and share comparable indications and contraindications for use. Most importantly, the application of each treatment method results in similar functional outcomes and comparable hypothesized effects.[12] These hypothesized effects are frequently categorized as biomechanical and neurophysiological,[8,13] with an understanding that the two effects have significant interactions that improve one another (Table 1.3 ■). Additionally, manual therapy may provide measurable psychological changes such as relaxation, decreased anxiety, or improved general well-being. The majority of this chapter is dedicated to analysis of these three areas.

Biomechanical Changes

Joint Displacement It is suggested that restricted tissue mobility may have a physiological origin within the joint segment and surrounding tissues.[14] These physiological changes are often termed a "hypomobility" during joint assessment. **Hypomobility** may lead to a lower volume of

■ TABLE 1.2 Proposed Standardized Manual Therapy Terminology

Term	Definition
Rate of force application	The rate at which the force was applied during the procedure.
Location in range of available movement	Where in the availability of range of the segment the application was applied.
Direction of force	The direction in which the force is applied.
Target of force	The location in which the therapist applied the force (e.g., level of the spine, area of the periphery).
Relative structural movement	The movement of a targeted structure in comparison to the stable structure.
Patient movement	The position of the patient during the application of the procedure.

Adapted from AAOMPT/Mintken et al.[2,3]

■ **TABLE 1.3** The Hypothesized Effects of Manual Therapy[30]

Term	Definition
	Biomechanical
Improved movement	Gains in range of motion or normalized movement patterns.
Improved position	Reduction in positional fault.
	Neurophysiological
Spinal cord	Hypoalgesia, diminished sensitivity to pain; sympathoexcitatory, changes in blood flow, heart rate, skin conductance, and skin temperature; muscle reflexogenic, decrease in hypertonicity of muscles.
Central mediated	Alterations in pain "experience" in the amygdala, periaquaductal gray, and rostral ventromedial medulla including a lessening of temporal summation; a central nervous system condition that demonstrates an increase in perception of pain to repetitive painful stimuli.
Peripheral inflammatory	Alteration of blood levels of inflammatory mediators.
	Interaction
Neurophysiological and biomechanical	The two effects function together to demonstrate catalytic gains for both.

synovial fluid within the joint cavity, which results in an increase in intra-articular pressure during movement.[14] Consequently, the distance between articular surfaces declines and reduces the lubricating properties of the joint, thus increasing irregular collagen cross-links.[15,16] Cross-links between collagen-based fibers inhibit normal connective tissue gliding, which leads to restricted joint movement[17] and corresponding range-of-motion loss and impairment. Additional contributors such as intra-articular meniscoids,[18] entrapment of a fragment of posterior annular material from the intervertebral disc,[19] and excessive spasm or **hypertonicity** of the deep intrinsic musculature[20,21] may further the impairment of joint mobility. Consequential debilitating changes include impaired strength, endurance, coordination, and alterations in the autonomic nervous system.[22]

Some evidence exists that mobilization and/or manipulation techniques solicit joint displacement.[23] In theory, this joint displacement solicits a temporary increase in the degree of displacement that is produced with force due to hysteresis effects.[24] Chiropractors suggest that when joint structures are rapidly stretched, cavitation internally occurs and an audible "pop" may be heard, resulting in increased range of motion after the cavitation.[25] What is unknown is whether the movement or the corresponding neurophysiological changes are responsible for the increased movement and whether the new range of movement is maintained over time.

The amount of movement necessary for reduction of symptoms is also unknown. Overall, most studies have either been poorly performed,[26,27] have used spines from cadavers for the experimental analysis,[28] or have reported the effect of manipulation on the spine of a canine.[29] Additionally, one well-cited study used surface markers during assessment of joint-related movements.[24] The use of surface markers is associated with a high degree of error since the measurement of skin displacement is a component of the movement. Subsequently, the findings of studies that have investigated movement using skin markers or other erroneous devices may provide misleading results.

When explaining the biological benefit of manual therapy for biomechanical improvements it is important to note that most changes reported have been short-term in nature.[30] Lasting structural changes are rarely identified (if at all) and immediate benefits are likely reflective of muscle-reflexogenic changes or neurophysiological alterations of pain. Furthermore, whether or not true positional faults are corrected is also unknown as the reliability and validity behind this concept is questionable.[30]

Summary

- Although very limited in gross amount, joint displacement does occur during manipulation and mobilization.
- Joint displacement may be associated with an audible pop.
- An audible pop is not necessary for neurophysiological changes.

Neurophysiological Changes

Spinal Cord Mechanisms   Manual therapy may have an effect on the spinal cord[30] and has been associated with hypoalgesia, which is a diminished sensitivity to pain.[31-33] The hypoalgesia is likely a consequence of segmental postsynaptic inhibition on the dorsal horn pain pathway neurons during manual therapy application. Glover et al.[34] reported a reduction of pain 15 minutes after performing a manipulation. They hypothesized that the spine manipulation altered the central processing of innocuous mechanical stimuli, which correspondingly increased the pain threshold levels. Others have found similar short-term effects with manipulation[35,36] and mobilization forces.[37,38]

Manual therapy is also associated with a **sympathoexcitatory response**,[39-42] which is a change in blood flow, heart rate, skin conductance, and skin temperature. The sympathoexcitatory response provides the benefit of modulation of pain and has a nonlocalized, nonspecific effect. Stimulation of the cervical spine has demonstrated upper extremity changes in pain response. Wright[43] outlines that hypoalgesia and sympathoexcitation are correlated, suggesting that individuals who exhibit the most change in pain perception also exhibit the most change in sympathetic nervous system function.

Manual therapy has also been associated with changes in muscle activity (muscle-reflexogenic) and motoneuron pool activity.[44] By definition, muscle-reflexogenic changes are decreases in hypertonicity of muscles. For many years, practitioners of manual therapy have purported reflexogenic benefits with selected directed manual therapy techniques[8,45-47] and have categorized these effects under spinal cord neurophysiological benefits. The thrust-like forces incurred during a manipulation[9,34-36,48-52] or repeated oscillatory forces used during nonthrust mobilization[46,48,49] are hypothesized to reduce pain through inducing reflex inhibition of spastic muscles. Muscle reflexogenic inhibition is a consequence of stimulation to the skin, muscle, and articular joint receptors.

A primary role of skin, muscle, and articular joint mechanoreceptors is to detect the presence of movement or energy input and provide the central nervous system with proprioceptive or nociceptive information. The location and the design of the mechanoreceptor outlines the role it plays in proprioception or pain response, although current evidence is conflicting on the extent of this role. Three (I–III) of the four mechanoreceptors are stimulated by muscle-length change and/or deformation, the fourth (IV) by chemical irritation and/or tension, and not all articular regions have equal representation of mechanoreceptor types.

Type I–IV mechanoreceptors have been identified in the cervical spine zygopophyseal joints. However, only Type I–III mechanoreceptors have been found in the lumbar and thoracic spine.[53] This suggests that the current mechanoreceptor system within the lumbar and thoracic spine will respond to extreme rather than midrange joint movements.[53]

Mechanoreceptors have been found in varying levels of density throughout the spine as well. There are fewer Type I–III receptors identified in the thoracic and lumbar spines, which may indicate either that the importance of the receptors is reduced in these regions or that the receptor fields are relatively large in area in these facet joints.[53] Type III and IV mechanoceptors, identified as nociceptors, have been found within the sacroiliac joint and surrounding muscular-ligamentous support structures.[54] This indicates that the mechanoreceptor system within the sacroiliac joint has a greater role in pain generation than proprioception.

There are several purported mechanisms that outline the benefit of manual therapy stimulation of joint receptors. One theory is that manual therapy techniques could potentially "reset" the reflex activity by stimulating the muscle spindles and Golgi tendon organs.[10] This theory is advocated by Korr,[55] who reported that manipulation increases joint mobility by producing a barrage of impulses stimulating Group Ia and possibly Group II afferents. Zusman[56] hypothesized related changes with mobilization following sustained or repetitive passive movements, although not all authors agree. Recently, Sung and colleagues[57] demonstrated that manipulative techniques applied at a rate of 200 milliseconds in duration lead to higher reflexogenic responses (i.e., Golgi tendon and muscle spindle discharge) than slower techniques that occur during nonthrust mobilization.

Others have suggested that muscle activity inhibition through transient reduction in alpha motor neuron activity (H reflex), a decrease in electromyographical (EMG) activity, and a reduction of excitatory Type III and IV nociceptors are all consequences of direct spinal manipulation.[58,59] Measurable alterations in EMG activity in local and distant spinal muscles[10] and depression of the **H reflex** have been documented after use of mobilization and/or manipulation methods.[59,60] Although these effects yield unknown pain inhibition responses, it is theorized that these physiological consequences may reduce the nociceptive afferent barrage to the dorsal horn.[34,35,56]

Peripheral Mechanisms   There is laboratory evidence that exercise and activity (movement) reduces the lactate concentration and reduces the pH changes within damaged tissue.[6] Manual therapy has been shown to alter blood levels of inflammatory mediators at the region of the application. During an injury, a chemical reaction occurs that produces a cascade of chemically related pain. Injury may stimulate the release of proteoglycans, metalo-matrix protease inhibitors, and other factors that trigger an autoimmune reaction and the influx of spinal cord mediators such as bradykinin, serotonin, histamines, and prostaglandins that irritate surrounding Type C nerve endings. The result is a diffuse pain that is activated during "normal" activity that usually would not stimulate pain.[61] The passive movement associated with mobilization and manipulation may change the pH structure and alter the acute inflammatory response of the area, thus resulting in decreased pain, although further study is needed for substantiation.

Central-Mediated Mechanisms   Manual therapy may affect the central and peripheral mechanisms of pain control and create neurophysiological responses and changes in pain perception.[41,62,63] **Central facilitation** occurs when the dorsal horn is hyperresponsive to afferent input.[64] This process may cause a lowering of the pain threshold and results in lower levels of pain-producing stimuli. Central facilitation may occur regionally at the injured site or in the brain's pain processing centers. Manual therapy may provide alterations in pain "experience" in the anterior cingular cortex, amygdala, and rostral ventromedial medulla, including a lessening of temporal summation, a central nervous system (CNS) condition that demonstrates an increase in perception of pain to repetitive painful stimuli.[30] Passive mobilization forces arouse descending inhibitory systems that originate in the lateral periaqueductal gray matter of the brainstem.[41]

There also appears to be a reduction of afferent nociceptive input into the CNS, thus evoking descending pain inhibitory systems[43,59] consequently resulting in hypoalgesia. The reduction of pain through descending mechanisms appears to happen by two separate pathways. The primary (rapid-onset) analgesic effect is from the dorsal periaqueductal gray (PAG) area and is sympathoexcitatory in nature.[65,66] This is a nonopioid mechanism because it is unaffected by the administration of naloxone.[67] The secondary mechanism is from the ventral PAG and is sympathoinhibitory in nature and is referred to as an opioid mechanism.[66] It is described as opioid because administration of naloxone will attenuate the effect.[67] The preceding mechanisms of pain control have been clearly linked to spinal manipulation but not as strongly linked to spinal mobilization according to Wright's review article.[43] There is moderate evidence to support that spinal manual therapy has a hypoalgesic effect specific to mechanical nociception.[39,40,68] However, the majority of studies were poorly designed or resulted in conflicting findings among authors.[8]

Other explanations have included the activation of the gate-control mechanism proposed by Melzack and Wall,[69] neural hysteresis, and release of endogenous opioids. Small-diameter nociceptors tend to open the "gate," thus facilitating perception of pain, whereas larger-diameter fibers tend to close the gate of pain. Gating pain is a mechanism in which afferent and descending pathways modulate sensory transmission by inhibitory mechanisms within the central nervous system. Some have suggested that manual therapy movements may stimulate afferent fibers in the joint, muscle, skin, and ligaments, potentially providing an effective overstimulation response, although further work is needed to confirm this theory.

Temporal Effects   The temporal effects of manual therapy procedures such as manipulation, mobilization, or muscle energy techniques, when not combined with another intervention, are short term.[59,70,71] Studies suggest a carryover effect of 20–30 minutes only. Consequently, to maximize the benefits of manual therapy, follow-up exercises that strengthen or move the patient into the newly gained range of movement may be necessary for long-term outcomes. Further investigation is needed.

Summary

- It is suggested that manual therapy demonstrates pain reduction through inhibition of nociceptors, dorsal horn, and inhibitory descending pathways of the spinal cord.
- Manual therapy may improve chemical alterations secondary to injury and CNS thresholds.
- Both manipulation and nonthrust mobilization forces have demonstrated neurophysiological changes in discriminatory analysis.
- Manual therapy may improve altered pain thresholds.
- Manual therapy, specifically nonthrust mobilization, has been shown to demonstrate a sympathoexcitatory effect.
- Sympathoexcitatory activity and hypoalgesia appear to function concurrently and are considered positive-responsive during an application of manual therapy. A primary role of skin, muscle, and articular joint receptors is to detect the presence of movement or energy input and provide the central nervous system with proprioceptive or nociceptive information.
- There are four primary articular receptors.
- There are theories dictating why reflexogenic changes occur, including stimulation of mechanoreceptors, resetting reflex responses, and the gate control theory.
- One theory is that manual therapy techniques "reset" the reflex activity by stimulating the muscle spindles and Golgi tendon organs.
- Measurable alterations in electromyographical (EMG) activity in local and distant spinal muscles and depression of the **H reflex** have been documented after use of mobilization and/or manipulation methods.

Psychological Changes

Placebo   Because orthopedic manual therapy is a mechanical intervention it is very prone to a phenomenon called the **placebo effect.** These effects are found in drugs, surgery, biofeedback, psychiatric interventions, and diagnostic tests. They include some form of sham treatment, and are not the same as an untreated controlled group.[70] The placebo effect is generally qualitative in nature (it is based on patient perception) but can lead to quantitative changes, especially if an individual's stress level is reduced.

The placebo effect is the measurable or observable after-effect target to a person or group of participants that have been given some form of expectant care. The expectation that he or she will improve is often the driving force behind any and all aspects of newfound well-being. The common fallacy associated with the placebo effect is the credit of improvement to a specific treatment, just because the improvement followed the treatment. Selected authors have suggested that manual therapy elicits a powerful, short-term placebo effect that in some respect explains the perceived benefit.[40] The ability to design a well-performed sham study using sham nonthrust mobilization or manipulation is very difficult; therefore the likelihood of an unadulterated measurement of placebo in a manual therapy study is very low. It is worth mentioning that some of the previously discussed studies found ROM changes that were significantly greater than placebo or sham care.

Patient Satisfaction and Expectation   Although it is intuitive to consider patient satisfaction is directly related to the outcome of care, it appears this concept is actually more complicated than one may expect.[72] Some studies have found a significant relationship between the two variables,[73,74] whereas others have shown only tentative or poor relationships.[72] Treatments that consist of manual therapy techniques routinely display better patient satisfaction scores than other nonmanual therapy–related methods[72,73] regardless of whether a benefit occurred during the intervention. Selected authors[72,75] suggest that meeting patient expectations is more likely associated with patient satisfaction (than pure patient outcomes), and manual therapists have a greater capacity of doing so through mechanical methods of patient care administration. Satisfaction differs from expectations because it fails to consider what the patient anticipated to gain from the form of intervention.

Williams et al.[76] report that the most desired aspect of patient expectation is an explanation of the problem and a mechanism in which to adapt to the problem. It is possible that a manual therapist has the potential to reorient patients' pain experience into a more positive framework[77] that contributes in some part to overall patient satisfaction. By nature, manual therapy provides a mechanical method of treatment that may have significant carryover to home programs and self-treatment. Additionally, by placing a mechanical identifier on a particular disorder, a reduction in esoteric aspects of pain perception and demonstration may improve the communication of symptoms from clinician to patient.

Main and Watson[78] elaborate on the failure to meet patient expectations and report that "failed treatment can have a profoundly demoralizing affect" and may become "significantly disaffected with healthcare professionals, particularly if they feel they have been misled in terms of likely benefit from treatment." This emphasizes the necessity to build a relationship of trust between the clinician and the patient and to explore common goals among the partnership. Curtis et al.[73] reported that patients who had earlier experience with manual therapy treatment demonstrated quicker recovery than subjects with no prior experience.

The likelihood of recognizing those who will "buy in" to a manual therapy treatment plan may improve the development of trust. Axen et al.[79] found that chiropractors had the capacity to predict those with good prognoses over bad prognoses based on the reaction to a first, single manual therapy treatment. This finding and the discovery in the Curtis et al.[73] study suggest that certain patients are more apt to benefit from manual therapy than others.

The Role of Psychological Covariates   Melzack and Casey[80] suggested that an individual's pain perception depends on complex neural interactions in the nervous system. The complexities include impulses generated by tissue damage that are modified both by ascending pathways to the brain and by descending pain-suppressing systems. Nonetheless, pain perception is not limited solely to physiological criteria; pain perception is conspicuously influenced by various environmental and psychological factors. Thus, perception of pain is the result of a dynamic process of perception and interpretation of a wide range of incoming stimuli. The interpretation of the stimuli dictates the description of the pain, regardless of whether the stimuli are associated with truly substantial pain-generating agents. Furthermore, it has been suggested that the risk of progressing from an acute impairment to chronic pain syndrome is unrelated to actual pain intensity[81] and is more directly related to psychosocial factors.[82]

Several psychosocial factors that have been investigated may contribute to perception and chronicity of pain. There is some evidence to support that reduction in levels of distress, pain, tension, discomfort, and mood are possible with treatments such as massage.[83] Because development of a chronic pain syndrome appears to reflect a failure to adapt to the change in condition,[82] treatment of pain exclusively may still result in a regression of the patient's status. Instead of true pain-related changes, most individuals fail to cope with the unimproved symptoms and the decrease in function. The presence of selected psychosocial factors that interfere with adaptation may promote the development of pain syndromes. These factors include the derivatives of emotion, beliefs, and coping strategies.

Emotions   Main and Watson[78] identify anxiety, fear, depression, and anger as the four emotions that best characterize the distress of those with chronic pain. Much of the patient anxiety may be traced to unmet expectations. Anxiety is often present in patients who have not received a clear explanation for the origin or cause methods to manage pain.[78]

Fear is an emotional response that stems from a belief that selected movements or interventions may damage one's present condition.[78] Fear has been associated with catastrophizing behavior and may increase patients' self-report of pain intensity.[84] Most notably, fear of movement may reduce a patient's buy-in to a particular treatment, specifically if pain is reproduced within the treatment process. Fear of movement or reinjury and subsequent hypokinesis is highly correlated with an increased pain report.[85]

Depression is more difficult to acknowledge. Main and Watson[78] suggest that it is important to distinguish between dsyphoric moods from depressive illness. Dysphoric behavior is common in patients who have experienced long-term pain but will most likely be absent of the debilitating effects of depression. Depression often leads to a learned helplessness, dependency of pharmaceuticals, and other debilitating behaviors.

The complex relationship between anger and frustration is not well understood[78] but is believed to alter judgment and may reduce the internal commitment the patient has to improving his or her own condition. Recent evidence suggests that expressive anger style is associated with elevated pain sensitivity, secondary to dysfunction within the body's antinociceptive system.[86]

Coping Strategies   During their discussion of coping strategies, DeGood et al.[87] distinguish three distinct fields of inquiry: (1) specific beliefs about pain and treatment, (2) the thought processes involved in judgment or appraisal, and (3) coping styles or strategies. Schultz et al.[88] report that effective treatment to improve coping strategies requires

accurate distinction between chronic pain and a chronic pain syndrome. Theoretically, the most effective treatments designed to improve coping strategies should incorporate both psychological and physical components and require intervention by an interdisciplinary team. Generally, early treatment of pain syndromes may improve employment-related outcomes, but even those with long-standing syndromes generally improve dramatically.[89] Improvements in coping include the use of a biopsychosocial model. A biopsychosocial model assumes an interaction between mental and physical aspects of disability, assumes that the relationship between impairment and disability is mediated by psychosocial factors, and that beliefs about illness/disability are as important as illness. Presence of a chronic pain syndrome strongly suggests that medical interventions (including surgery) may not be effective.[89] In some instances of physical improvements, separate psychological interventions may be necessary for reducing back pain incidence.[90]

Summary

- The placebo effect could potentially explain some of the pain reduction benefit associated with manual therapy.
- It is difficult to design a study in which an effective and comparable placebo sham is used during manual therapy intervention.
- Treatments that consist of manual therapy techniques routinely display better patient satisfaction scores than other nonmanual therapy–related methods.
- Manual therapists may improve the likelihood of meeting patient expectations secondary to the nature of the physical intervention.
- Failure to meet patient expectations is associated with poor patient satisfaction.
- Anxiety, fear, depression, and anger are common emotional components that may alter a manual therapist's outcome.
- A manual therapist may reduce the anxiety associated with unknown symptoms.
- Fear is commonly associated with decreased movement and trepidation of reinjury.
- Depression coexists with numerous other variables, all which can lead to poor patient outcomes.
- Anger and outcome are poorly understood, yet there does appear to be a relationship between higher report of pain and increased anger.
- Coping strategy is reportedly a reason why some disorders progress to chronic pain syndrome.
- There is little evidence to suggest that manual therapy intervention will decrease the progression to chronic pain syndrome.
- Purportedly, a biopsychosocial model should demonstrate effectiveness in treating patients with chronic pain syndrome.

Hierarchy of Evidence

This textbook advocates an evidence-based medicine (EBM) nature, thus it is imperative to recognize that evidence does come in many flavors. Evidence-based information is not solely limited to information gathered in randomized trials and meta-analyses; in fact, most manual therapy–related evidence has not been vetted to that level of detail. If no randomized clinical trial has been performed, we are empowered to gather the best available evidence and make decisions based on that information and supportive information from ours and our patients' experiences.[91]

It is worth noting that given the scenario of limited evidence, many clinicians are often derailed or mislead in their effects of using evidence-based information. This occurs partly because exploration of evidence as well as development of evidence takes significant effort, time, and rigor.[92] In some cases, clinicians who feel they are evidence based use traditional sources of information (e.g., clinical experience, opinion of colleagues, and textbooks) for clinical decision making as frequently as non-evidence-based medicine users.[92,93]

When it comes to reporting "evidence," a hierarchical structure or pyramid does exist (Figure 1.1 ■). Understanding the hierarchy improves one's ability to discriminate the magnitude of the finding toward clinical practice. The "lowest" levels of evidence[94] reflect *in vitro* or animal-based studies, as the findings may not be clinically relevant or transferable. In many cases, the *in vitro* or animal-based studies are used in the early stages of fact finding. For the findings to harbor clinical applicability, human studies are required.

Ideas, editorials, and opinions should only be used in the absence of collected data and should routinely be challenged through empirical investigation. Ideas, editorials, and opinions are presented in many ways, but each involves a personalized report of one's interpretation of findings without a systematic process of discrimination of the facts.

Case studies, case series, and case-control designs do not allow cause-and-effect relationships, therefore the findings from each should be assimilated into clinical practice with caution.[94] Case reports involve data that are collected on a single subject without using a design, allowing systematic comparison against baseline or an alternative intervention. Case-series studies involve data that are collected on a single group of patients in which no comparison group is instituted. Typically, case series are limited to study of a specific intervention.

Case-control designs involve a comparison of two groups of people: those with the disease or condition under study (cases) and a very similar group of people who do not have the disease or condition (controls). If the targeted data are identified prior to collection, the study is considered prospective. If the outcome or data are collected after exposure (recall or preexisting data), the study is retrospective. Case-control designs offer more compelling evidence than case studies, series, or editorials.

The next level of evidence involves cohort studies. Cohort studies are useful to examine "real-world" findings for interventions but suffer from the inability to control for potentially confounding variables.[94] Prospective cohorts are longitudinal studies where subgroups of patients are enrolled and research

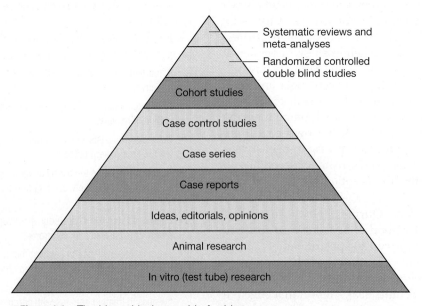

■ **Figure 1.1**   The hierarchical pyramid of evidence

questions are defined at a relevant baseline point (prior to when outcomes occur). Retrospective cohorts involve a longitudinal study where a group or groups of patients are involved in prospective data collection but the research questions (and variables) were defined retrospectively.

For individual trials, randomized controlled trials (RCT) are considered the highest level of evidence.[95] However, although strong with respect toward providing utility of a particular intervention, an RCT should demonstrate strong internal, external, and model validity. Internal validity reflects the ability of the independent variable to affect the dependent variable. If the experiment can clearly establish that the treatment causes an effect, then the experiment has internal validity. External validity reflects the ability to generalize beyond the specific study, including the ability to translate the findings to other settings, with other subject populations, and with other, but related variables. Model validity is a component within external validity, and reflects how well the study design actually models real practice settings. In essence, a model resembles the target system in some aspects while at the same time it differs in other aspects that are not considered essential. If a study design is technically correct, but differs so significantly from actual clinical practice, the study may lack external validity.

When a series of studies are available, systematic literature reviews or meta-analyses are more useful tools for assessing the effect of a particular intervention. A meta-analysis is a commonly used systematic reviewing strategy for addressing health-related scientific research[96] and involves a systematic statistical explanation of available evidence in multiple studies.[97] Meta-analyses are used for public and health-care policy decision making,[98–102] and are especially helpful in making decisions when a number of small studies

exists that lack statistical power.[102] The calculations require essential methodological elements for combining data and statistical information across sources[96–102] such as an estimate of effect size and assessment of heterogeneity of data available for comparison.[96] Meta-analyses enhance precision by improving effect estimation. Effect estimation is enhanced by providing comparisons of characteristics not involved in the original root studies and by answering questions about whether conflicting studies exist.[97] Cumulative results from the meta-analysis can display the relative change in magnitude of the effect size or empirical evidence on how the treatment effect has changed over time.[97]

RCTs are the framework of meta-analyses, although observational cohort studies have been used in the past as well. Low-quality RCTs result in poorly homogenous meta-analyses and potentially biased data for health-care clinicians.

Managing the Quantity of Information

The 5S Model   One of the most significant roadblocks to the use of evidence-based information is the shear quantity of evidence available that the clinician must consume. Success in delivering an evidence-based method relies heavily on the ability to take information and transpose it toward evidence-based health-care practice for each individual patient. Although no information is perfect and the transfer of information is often altered in methods that impact clinical decisions, recent mechanistic suggestions may improve our ability to consume the large quantities of information.

Brian Haynes suggests the use of the 5S model for organization of evidence-based information[103] (Figure 1.2 ■). The 5S model begins at the top of the hierarchy of evidence, and adds three additional steps

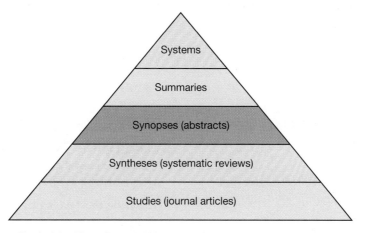

■ **Figure 1.2**   The 5S model for synthesizing and managing information[103]

■ TABLE 1.4 Methodological Guidelines Outlined by the *U.S. Clinical Practice Guidelines for Acute Low Back Problems in Adults*

Category	Description
1. Strong evidence: Level A	Includes interventions deemed either *effective* or *ineffective* with strong support in the literature as determined by consistent findings/results in several high-quality randomized controlled trials or in at least one meta-analysis.
2. Moderate evidence: Level B	Includes interventions deemed either *effective* or *ineffective* with moderate support in the literature as determined by consistent findings/results in one high-quality randomized controlled trial and one or several low-quality randomized controlled trials.
3. Limited/contradictory evidence: Level C	Includes interventions with weak or conflicting support in the literature as determined by one randomized controlled trial (high or low quality), or inconsistent findings between several randomized controlled trials.
4. No known evidence: Level D	Includes interventions that have not been sufficiently studied in the literature in terms of effectiveness and no randomized controlled trials in this area.

for information synthesis. The lowest levels (studies) reflect clinical trials and the syntheses reflect systematic literature reviews or meta-analyses. Synopses usually provide a summary of evidence from one or more articles, and may include a clinical "bottom line." Summaries draw upon the syntheses of information to formulate the best evidence regarding the information. Systems involve decision support services that match information and tests and measures from a specific patient to best-evidence practices of diagnosis and treatment.[104]

Assigning Levels of Evidence

Methodological Guidelines

There are a number of methodological guidelines for report of the quality of existing evidence. One challenge to using a methodological quality guideline is that the stratification and scoring used in the study often affects the outcome of the analyses.[105] Thus, different tools will provide different results and recommendations even during use of the same studies! Nonetheless, the use of a quality tool such as those outlined by the *U.S. Clinical Practice Guidelines for Acute Low Back Problems in Adults*[106] provides a benchmark for performance in an attempt not to over support interventions that lack validity.

The guidelines[106] (Table 1.4 ■) reflect four primary levels of evidence (Levels A, B, C, and D). Level A includes findings from a number of high-quality RCTs or at least one well-designed meta-analysis. Level B includes information from only one high-quality RCT or one or more low-quality RCTs. Level C outlines conflicting information from a number of studies. Level D indicates that the intervention has not been properly investigated. This four-level quality measure is used throughout the book to outline the evidence behind dedicated interventions.

Chapter Questions

1. Identify the three hypothesized effects of manual therapy and describe the scientific evidence that supports the suppositions.

2. Outline the different forms of neurophysiological effects of manual therapy.

3. Describe why meeting patient expectations is often considered as important as patient outcome when addressing patient satisfaction.

4. Describe the levels of evidence and the quality designations.

References

1. Flynn TW, Childs JD, Bell S, Magel JS, Rowe RH, Plock H. Manual physical therapy: We speak gibberish. *J Orthop Sports Phys Ther.* 2008;38:97–98.

2. Mintken PE, Derosa C, Little T, Smith B; for the American Academy of Orthopaedic Manual Physical Therapists. A Model for Standardizing Manipulation Terminology in Physical Therapy Practice. *J Man Manip Ther.* 2008;16(1):50–56.

3. Mintken PE, Derosa C, Little T, Smith B; for the American Academy of Orthopaedic Manual Physical Therapists. A Model for Standardizing Manipulation Terminology in Physical Therapy Practice. *J Orthop Sports Phys Ther.* 2008;38:A1–6.

4. Bourdillon J, Day E. *Spinal manipulation.* 4th ed. London; Appleton & Lange: 1987.

5. Haldeman S. The clinical basis for discussion of mechanics in manipulative therapy. In: Korr I (ed). *The neurobiologic mechanisms in manipulative therapy.* London; Plenum Press: 1978.

6. Holm S, Nachemson A. Variations in the nutrition of the canine intervertebral disc induced by motion. *Spine.* 1983;8:866–873.

7. Wyke BD. Articular neurology and manipulative therapy. In Glasgow EF, Twomey LT, (eds). *Aspects of manipulative therapy.* 2nd ed. Melbourne; Churchill Livingstone: 1985;81–96.

8. Potter L, McCarthy C, Oldham J. Physiological effects of spinal manipulation: A review of proposed theories. *Phys Ther Reviews.* 2005;10:163–170.

9. Collaca C, Keller T, Gunzberg R. Neuromechanical characterization of in vivo lumbar spinal manipulation. Part 2. Neurophysiologic response. *J Manipulative Physiol Ther.* 2003;26:579–591.

10. Herzog W, Scheele D, Conway P. Electromyographic responses of back and limb muscles associated with spinal manipulative therapy. *Spine.* 1999;24:146–153.

11. Vernon H. Qualitative review of studies of manipulation-induced hypalgesia. *J Manipulative Physiol Ther.* 2000;23:134–138.

12. Hurwitz EL, Morgenstern H, Harber P, Kominski GF, Belin TR, Yu F, Adams AH; University of California–Los Angeles. A randomized trial of medical care with and without physical therapy and chiropractic care with and without physical modalities for patients with low back pain: 6-month follow-up outcomes from the UCLA low back pain study. *Spine.* 2002;27(20):2193–2204.

13. Arkuszewski Z. (abstract). Joint blockage: A disease, a syndrome or a sign. *Man Med.* 1988;3:132–134.

14. Schollmeier G, Sarkar K, Fukuhara K, Uhthoff HK. Structural and functional changes in the canine shoulder after cessation of immobilization. *Clin Orthop.* 1996;(323):310–315.

15. Akeson WH, Amiel D, Mechanic GL, Woo SL, Harwood FL, Hamer ML. Collagen cross-linking alternations in joint contractures: Changes in reducible cross-links in periarticular connective tissue collage after nine weeks of immobilization. *Connect Tissue Res.* 1977;5(1):15–19.

16. Amiel D, Frey C, Woo SL, Harwood F, Akeson W. Value of hyaluronic acid in the prevention of contracture formation. *Clin Othop.* 1985;196:306–311.

17. Donatelli R, Owens-Burkhart H. Effects of immobilization on the extensibility of periarticular connective tissue. *J Orthop Sports Phys Ther.* 1981;3:67–72.

18. Mercer S, Bogduk N. Intra-articular inclusions of the cervical synovial joints. *Brit J Rheumatol.* 1993;32:705–710.

19. Bogduk N, Twomey LT. *Clinical anatomy of the lumbar spine.* London; Churchill Livingstone: 1997.

20. Blunt KL, Gatterman MI, Bereznick DE. Kinesiology: An essential approach toward understanding chiropractic subluxation. In Gatterman MI (ed). *Foundations of chiropractic: Subluxation.* St. Louis, MO; Mosby: 1995.

21. Norlander S, Astc-Norlander U, Nordgren B, Sahlstedt B. Mobility in the cervico-thoracic motion segment: An indicative factor of musculoskeletal neck–shoulder pain. *Scand J Rehabil Med.* 1996;28(4):183–192.

22. Wright A. Pain-relieving effects of cervical manual therapy. In: Grant R. *Physical therapy of the cervical and thoracic spine.* 3rd ed. New York; Churchill Livingston: 2002.

23. Cramer G, Tuck N, Knudsen J. et al. Effects of side-posture positioning and side-posture adjusting on the lumbar zygopophyseal joints as evaluated by magnetic resonance imaging: A before and after study with randomization. *J Manipulative Physiol Ther.* 2000;23:380–394.

24. Herzog W. *Clinical biomechanics of spinal manipulation.* London; Churchill Livingstone: 2000.

25. Mierau D, Cassidy JD, Bowen V. Manipulation and mobilization of the third metacarpophalangeal joint. *Man Med.* 1988;3:135–140.

26. Lee R, Evans J. Load-displacement time characteristics of the spine under posteroanterior mobilization. *Aust J Physiotherapy.* 1992;38:115–123.

27. Lee M, Svensson N. Effect of loading frequency on response of the spine to lumbar posteroanterior forces. *J Manipulative Physiol Ther.* 1993;16:439–446.

28. Gal JM, Herzog W, Kawchuk GN, Conway PJ, Zhang Y-T. Forces and relative vertebral movements during SMT to unembalmed post-rigor human cadavers: Peculiarities associated with joint cavitation. *J Manipulative Physiol Ther.* 1995;18:4–9.

29. Smith D, Fuhr A, Davis B. Skin accelerometer displacement and relative bone movement of adjacent vertebrae in response to chiropractic percussion thrusts. *J Manipulative Physiol Ther.* 1989;12:26–37.

30. Bialosky JE, Bishop MD, Price DD, Robinson ME, George SZ. The mechanisms of manual therapy in the treatment of musculoskeletal pain: A comprehensive model. *Man Ther.* 2009;14(5):531–538.

31. O'Leary S, Falla D, Hodges PW, Jull G, Vicenzino B. Specific therapeutic exercise of the neck induces immediate local hypoalgesia. *Clin J Pain.* 2007;8:832–839.

32. Mohammadian P, Andersen OK, Arendt-Nielsen L. Correlation between local vascular and sensory changes following tissue inflammation induced by repetitive application of topical capsaicin. *Brain Res.* 1998;792(1):1–9.

33. Bialosky JE, George SZ, Bishop MD. How spinal manipulative therapy works: Why ask why? *J Orthop Sports Phys Ther.* 2008;38(6):293–295.

34. Glover J, Morris J, Khosla T. Back pain: A randomized clinical trial of rotational manipulation of the trunk. *Br J Physiol.* 1947;150:18–22.

35. Terrett AC, Vernon H. Manipulation and pain tolerance: A controlled study of the effect of spinal manipulation on paraspinal cutaneous pain tolerance levels. *Am J Phys Med.*1984;63(5):217–225.

36. Vernon H, Dhami M, Howley T, Annett R. Spinal manipulation and beta-endorphin: A controlled study of the effect of a spinal manipulation on plasma beta-endorphin levels in normal males. *J Manipulative Physiol Ther.* 1986;9:115–123.

37. Wright A, Thurnwald P, Smith J. An evaluation of mechanical and thermal hyperalgesia in patients with lateral epicondylalgia. *Pain Clin.* 1992;5:199–282.

38. Wright A, Thurbwald P, O'Callaghan J. Hyperalgesia in tennis elbow patients. *J Musculoskel Pain.* 1994;2:83–89.

39. Zusman M. Mechanisms of musculoskeletal physiotherapy. *Phys Ther Rev.* 2004;9:39–49.

40. Sterling M, Jull G, Wright A. Cervical mobilization: Concurrent effects on pain, sympathetic nervous system activity and motor activity. *Man Ther.* 2001;6:72–81.

41. Shacklock M. Neural mobilization: A systematic review of randomized controlled trials with an analysis of therapeutic efficacy. *J Man Manip Ther.* 2008;16(1):23–24.

42. Simon R, Vicenzino B, Wright A. The influence of an anteroposterior accessory glide of the glenohumeral joint on measures of peripheral sympathetic nervous system function in the upper limb. *Man Ther.* 1997;2(1):18–23.

43. Wright A. Hypoalgesia post-manipulative therapy: A review of a potential neurophysiologic mechanism. *Man Ther.* 1995;1:1–16.

44. Bulbulian R, Burke J, Dishman JD. Spinal reflex excitability changes after lumbar spine passive flexion mobilization. *J Manipulative Physiol Ther.* 2002;25(8):526–532.

45. Haldeman S. The clinical basis for discussion of mechanisms of manipulative therapy. In: Korr I. (ed). *The neurobiologic mechanisms in manipulative therapy.* New York; Plenum Press: 1978.

46. Farfan H. The scientific basis of manipulation procedures. In: Buchanan W, Kahn M, Rodnan G, Scott J, Zvailfler N, Grahame R, (eds). *Clinics in rheumatic diseases.* London; WB Saunders: 1980.

47. Giles L. *Anatomical basis of low back pain.* Baltimore; Williams and Wilkins: 1989.

48. Randall T, Portney L, Harris B. Effects of joint mobilization on joint stiffness and active motion of the metacarpal–phalangeal joint. *J Orthop Sports Phys Ther.* 1992;16:30–36.

49. Shamus J, Shamus E, Gugel R, Brucker B, Skaruppa C. The effect of sesamoid mobilization, flexor hallucis strengthening, and gait training on reducing pain and restoring function in individuals with hallux limitus: A clinical trial. *J Orthop Sports Phys Ther.* 2004;34:368–376.

50. Raftis K, Warfield C. Spinal manipulation for back pain. *Hosp Pract.* 1989;15:89–90.

51. Denslow JS. Analyzing the osteopathic lesion. 1940. *J Am Osteopath Assoc.* 2001;101(2):99–100.

52. Sran MM. To treat or not to treat: New evidence for the effectiveness of manual therapy. *Br J Sports Med.* 2004;38(5):521–525.

53. McLain R, Pickar J. Mechanoreceptor ending in human thoracic and lumbar facet joints. *Spine.* 1998;23:168–173.

54. Sakamoto N, Yamashita T, Takebayashi T, Sekine M, Ishii S. An electrophysiologic study of mechanoreceptors in the sacroiliac joint and adjacent tissues. *Spine.* 2001;26:468–471.

55. Korr IM. Proprioceptors and somatic dysfunction. *J Amer Osteopath Assoc.* 1975;74:638–650.

56. Zusman M. Spinal manipulative therapy: Review of some proposed mechanisms and a hew hypothesis. *Australian J Physio* 1986;32:89–99.

57. Sung P, Kang YM, Pickar J. Effect of spinal manipulation duration on low threshold mechanoreceptors in lumbar paraspinal muscles. *Spine.* 2004;30:115–122.

58. Keller T, Collaca C, Guzburg R. Neuromechanical characterization of in vivo lumbar spinal manipulation. Part 1. Vertebral motion. *J Manipulative Physiol Ther.* 2003;26:567–578.

59. Dishman J, Bulbulian R. Spinal reflex attenuation associated with spinal manipulation. *Spine.* 2000; 25:2519–2525.

60. Murphy B, Dawson N, Slack J. Sacroiliac joint manipulation decreases the H-reflex. *Electromyog Clin Neurophysiol.* 1995;35:87–94.

61. Sizer PS, Matthijs O, Phelps V. Influence of age on the development of pathology. *Curr Rev Pain* 2000;4:362–373.

62. Cook C. *Orthopedic manual therapy: An evidence-based approach.* Upper Saddle River, NJ; Prentice Hall: 2006.

63. Shacklock MO. The clinical application of central pain mechanisms in manual therapy. *Aust J Physiother.* 1999;45(3):215–221.

64. Picker J. Neurophysiologic effects of spinal manipulation. *Spine J.* 2002;2:357–371.

65. Lovick TA, Li P. Integrated function of neurones in the rostral ventrolateral medulla. *Prog Brain Res.* 1989;81:223–232.

66. Lovick T. Interactions between descending pathways from the dorsal and ventrolateral periaqueductal gray matter in the rat. In: Depaulis A, Bandler R. (eds). *The midbrain periaqueductal gray matter.* New York; Plenum Press: 1991.

67. Cannon JT, Prieto GJ, Lee A, Liebeskind JC. Evidence for opioid and non-opioid forms of stimulation-produced analgesia in the rat. *Brain Res.* 1982;243(2): 315–321.

68. Vicenzino B, Paungmali A, Buratowski S, Wright A. Specific manipulative therapy treatment for chronic lateral epicondylalgia produces uniquely characteristic hypoalgesia. *Man Ther.* 2001;6:205–212.

69. Lederman E. Overview and clinical application. In: *Fundamentals of manual therapy.* London: Churchill Livingstone, 1997; 213–220.

70. Wigley R. When is a placebo effect not an effect? *Clin Med.* 2007;7:450–2.

71. Degenhardt BF, Darmani NA, Johnson JC, et al. Role of osteopathic manipulative treatment in altering pain biomarkers: A pilot study. *J Am Osteo Assoc.* 2007; 107:387–400.

72. Suter E, McMorland G, Herzog W. Short-term effects of spinal manipulation on H-reflex amplitude in healthy and symptomatic subjects. *J Manipulative Phsyiol Ther.* 2005;28:667–672.

73. Curtis P, Carey TS, Evans P, Rowane MP, Jackman A, Garrett J. Training in back care to improve outcome and patient satisfaction. Teaching old docs new tricks. *J Fam Pract.* 2000;49(9):786–792.

74. Licciardone J, Stoll S, Fulda K, et al. Osteopathic manipulative treatment for chronic low back pain: A randomized controlled trial. *Spine.* 2003;28:1355–1362.

75. Cherkin D, Deyo R, Battie M, Street J, Barlow W. A comparison of physical therapy, chiropractic manipulation, and provision of an educational booklet for the treatment of patients with low back pain. *N Engl J Med.* 1998;339(15):1021–1029.

76. Williams S, Weinman J, Dale J, Newman S. Patient expectations: What do primary care patients want from the GP and how far does meeting expectations affect patient satisfaction? *Fam Pract.* 1995;12(2):193–201.

77. Goldstein M. *Alternative health care: Medicine, miracle, or mirage?* Philadelphia; Temple University Press: 1999.

78. Main CJ, Watson PJ. Psychological aspects of pain. *Man Ther.* 1999;4(4):203–215.

79. Axen I, Rosenbaum A, Robech R, Wren T, Leboeuf-Yde C. Can patient reactions to the first chiropractic treatment predict early favorable treatment outcome in persistent low back pain? *J Manipulative Physiol Ther.* 2002;25(7):450–454.

80. Melzack R, Casey K. Sensory, motivational and central control determinants of pain. In: Kenbshalo D (ed). *The skin senses.* Springfield, MA; Charles Thomas: 1968.

81. Epping-Jordan JE, Wahlgren DR, Williams RA, et al. Transition to chronic pain in men with low back pain: Predictive relationships among pain intensity, disability, and depressive symptoms. *Health Psychol.* 1998; 17(5):421–427.

82. Haldeman S. Neck and back pain. In: Evans R. *Diagnostic testing in neurology.* Philadelphia; Saunders Group: 1999.

83. Sullivan MJ, Thibault P, Andrikonyte J, Butler H, Catchlove R, Larivière C. Psychological influences on repetition-induced summation of activity-related pain in patients with chronic low back pain. *Pain.* 2009;141(1-2):70–78.

84. Peters M, Vlaeyen J, Weber W. The joint contribution of physical pathology, pain-related fear and catastrophizing to chronic back pain disability. *Pain.* 2005; 115:45–50.

85. de Jong J, Valeyen J, Onghena P, Goosens M, Geilen Mulder M. Fear of movement/(re)injury in chronic low back pain: Education or exposure in vivo as mediator to fear reduction? *Clin J Pain.* 2005;21:9–17.

86. Bruehl S, Chung O, Burns J, Biridepalli S. The association between anger expression and chronic pain intensity: Evidence for partial mediation by endogenous opiod dysfunction. *Pain.* 2003;106:317–324.

87. DeGood D, Shutty M, Turk D, Melzack R. *Handbook of pain assessment.* New York; Guilford Press: 1992.

88. Schultz I, Crook J, Berkowitz S, et al. Biopsychosocial multivariate predictive model of occupational low back disability. *Spine.* 2002;27(23):2720–2725.

89. Jordan A, Bendix T, Nielsen H, Hansen FR, Host D, Winkel A. Intensive training, physiotherapy or manipulation for patients with chronic neck pain: A prospective, single-blinded, randomized clinical trial. *Spine.* 1998;1:23(3):311–318.

90. Alaranta H, Rytokoski U, Rissanen A, et al. Intensive physical and psychosocial training program for patients with chronic low back pain. A controlled clinical trial. *Spine.* 1994;19(12):1339–1349.

91. Sackett DL, Rosenberg WM, Gray JA, Haynes RB, Richardson WS. Evidence based medicine: What it is and what it isn't. *BMJ* 1996;312:71–72.

92. Walshe K, Ham C, Appleby J. Clinical effectiveness. Given in evidence. *Health Serv J.* 1995;105(5459):28–29.

93. McAlister FA, Graham I, Karr GW, Laupacis A. Evidence-based medicine and the practicing clinician. *J Gen Intern Med.* 1999;14(4):236–242.

94. Brighton B, Bhandari M, Tornetta P, Felson DT. Hierarchy of evidence: From case reports to randomized controlled trials. *Clin Orthop Relat Res.* 2003;(413):19–24.

95. Concato J, Shah N, Horwitz RI. Randomized, controlled trials, observational studies, and the hierarchy of research designs. *N Engl J Med.* 2000;342(25):1887–1892.

96. Stangl DK, Berry DA. Meta-analysis: Past and present challenges. In: Stangl DK, Berry DA (eds). *Meta-analysis in medicine and health policy.* New York; Marcel Dekker: 2000; 1–28.

97. Skekelle PG, Morton SG. Principles of meta-analysis. *J Rheumatol.* 2000;27(1):251–252.

98. Chalmers TC, Lau J. Changes in clinical trials mandated by the advent of meta-analysis. *Stat Med.* 1996;15(12):1263–1268; discussion 1269–1272.

99. Mosteller F, Colditz GA. Understanding research synthesis (meta-analysis). *Annu Rev Public Health.* 1996; 17:1–23.

100. Naylor CD. Meta-analysis and the meta-epidemiology of clinical research. *BMJ.* 1997;315(7109):617–619.

101. Schoenfeld PS, Loftus EV. Evidence-based medicine (EBM) in practice: Understanding tests of heterogeneity in metaanalysis. *Am J Gastroenterol.* 2005;100(6): 1221–1223.

102. Ioannidis JP, Lau L. Evidence on interventions to reduce medical errors: An overview and recommendations for future research. *J Gen Intern Med.* 2001; 16(5):325–334.

103. Haynes RB. Of studies, syntheses, synopses, summaries, and systems: The "5S" evolution of information services for evidence-based healthcare decisions. *Evid Based Med.* 2006;11(6):162–164.

104. Centre for Evidence Based Medicine. Accessed 5-14-09 at: http://www.cebm.net/

105. Juni P, Witschi A, Bloch R, Egger M. The hazards of scoring the quality of clinical trials for meta-analysis. *JAMA.* 1999;282(11):1054–1060.

106. van Tulder MW, Koes BW, Bouter LM. Conservative treatment of acute and chronic nonspecific low back pain: A systematic review of randomized controlled trials of the most common interventions. *Spine.* 1997;22(18):2128–2156.

Orthopaedic Manual Therapy Assessment

Chad E. Cook

Chapter 2

Objectives

- Compare and contrast the clinical decision-making models.
- Compare and contrast selected manual therapy backgrounds and their assessment philosophies.
- Determine if any of the philosophical elements of manual therapy are best supported by scientific evidence.
- Describe the purposes, types, and necessities of a manual therapy diagnosis.
- Describe the strengths and weaknesses of the patient response model.

Clinical Decision-Making Models

Clinical decision making is routinely viewed along a spectrum; with an assumption of being right on one end and wrong on the other. Modern decision-making models recognize that patients, environments, pathologies, and clinicians are complex, and that the complexities suggest that there is no right or wrong, mainly just variations in the correctness of our decision-making abilities.

All decision-making models are designed to provide clinicians with information that targets a **"threshold effect"** toward decision making. The threshold approach is a method of optimizing medical decision making by applying critical thinking during the solving of questions concerning directions toward treatment.[1] In essence, the threshold approach is a given set of findings or a level of findings that triggers a reaction by the health-care provider. For example, the discovery of a category 1 finding of blood in the sputum may trigger a threshold approach of referring the patient for chest radiology. A finding of recent (within 24 hours) of urinary retention may trigger a threshold effect of referral to an emergency room setting to rule out the presence of cauda equina symptoms. Threshold findings are critical clinical findings that have significant impact on the patient.

A decision that is based on the threshold approach is sometimes referred to as categorical reasoning. Categorical reasoning involves a decision that is made with minimal reservations in which a dedicated set of rules apply in the majority of clinical situations.[2] A categorical decision is based on few findings, is unambiguous, and is easy to judge regarding importance.[3] This judgment may involve a decision to reduce the negative consequences associated with the suspected disorder (e.g., cauda equina, cancer) or may have an economical or potential benefit of morbidity reduction (e.g., breast cancer screening programs). What is imperative to recognize is that threshold approach decision making (categorical decision making), which is not easy to justify based on validity of the tool, should be questioned.

There are numerous proposed models of decision making that are targeted to provide data to support obtainment of the threshold approach, although within the field of manual therapy, there are two primary models we discuss within this book[1]: hypothetical-deductive and[2] heuristic. A third model, mixed, also deserves discussion (see Table 2.1 ■).

Hypothetical-Deductive

Hypothetical-deductive decision making involves the development of a hypothesis during the clinical examination, and the refuting or acceptance of that hypothesis, which occurs during the process of the examination. Deductive reasoning argues from the general to the specific by allowing the clinician to build a case by adding findings. A decision is formulated

■ **TABLE 2.1** Clinical Decision-Making Models in Manual Therapy

Model	Description
Hypothetical-deductive	Hypothetical-deductive decision making involves the development of a hypothesis during the clinical examination, and the refuting or acceptance of that hypothesis that occurs during the process of the examination.
Heuristic	Heuristic decision making involves pattern recognition and the ability to lump useful findings into coherent groups.
Mixed	The mixed model involves decision-making elements of hypothetical-deductive, heuristic, and pathognomonic.

after accumulation and processing clinical findings and confirming or refuting preexisting hypotheses. The process is considered a bottom-up approach, as it allows *any* pertinent finding to be a qualifier during the decision-making process.

A benefit of the hypothetical-deductive model is that most examination processes tend to be comprehensive, focused, and quite extensive. Pertinent findings are rarely unexplored. Clinicians are allowed to address a number of potential options because the data captured during the examination are extensive and detailed.

There are a number of challenges with this particular model. For starters, the model assumes that all findings are essential and can equally impact the hypothesis exploration. In truth, a number of clinical findings do not provide useful information toward diagnosis or patient care management. In addition, although the hypothetical-deductive model is a logical model and can be used in a number of noncomplicated circumstances, the process is less efficient for experienced clinicians and may lead to a significant investment in refuting or confirming irrelevant hypotheses.

An element of the hypothetical-deductive model is the pathognomonic diagnosis. A **pathognomonic diagnosis** involves a decision based on a sign or symptom that is so characteristic of a disease or an outcome that the decision is made on the spot. In essence, a pathognomonic diagnosis is an immediate "threshold"-level finding prompting immediate action such as referral out or further testing. It is predicated on the assumption that all conditions are diagnosable in nature.

The pathognomonic diagnosis is a constituent of the history-taking, database analysis (patient intake forms), physical examination, and monitoring of the patient's condition during follow-up.[4] A pathognomonic diagnosis is generally considered for use in the early stages of an examination but can be used at any time, specifically if new findings are present. Discerning the meaning of each of the findings may warrant

the use of selected testing methods specifically designed to determine if the patient would benefit from additional medical consultation.

The most routine situation in which a pathognomonic diagnosis is used is during assessment of comorbidities, which may contribute or potentially harm a patient's recovery and/or function. Comorbidities such as high blood pressure, arthritis, or depression are commonly encountered in practice,[5,6] whereas other disorders such as a neurological illness, fracture, or neoplasm are less common, but represent comorbidities or "red flags" that are potentially threatening to the patient. Red flags are signs and symptoms that may tie a disorder to a serious pathology.[4,7] When combinations or singular representations of selected red flag features are encountered during an examination, a clinician may improve his or her ability to assess the risk of a serious underlying pathology.[8] Differential assessment for red flags in individual patients by a clinician involves the use of *special tests* or *standardized examinations* in order to identify individuals needing special intervention. A recent study demonstrated that < 5% of primary care physicians routinely examine for red flags during an initial screening,[9] whereas physical therapists document and screen at a much higher rate (>60%).[10]

Heuristic Decision Making (Clinical Gestalt)

Heuristic decision making, or **clinical gestalt,** is a process that assumes health-care practitioners actively organize clinical perceptions into coherent construct wholes. This implies that clinicians have the ability to indirectly make clinical decisions in absence of complete information and can generate solutions that are characterized by generalizations that allow transfer from one problem to the next. In essence, clinical gestalt is pattern recognition and is characterized as a heuristic approach to decision making.[11] At present, the literature suggests that experience does positively influence decision-making accuracy, as experienced clinicians have better pattern recognition skills.[11]

There are a number of benefits associated with heurism or gestalt. The method allows a quick global interpretation within seconds of data collection.[12] This process is considered "top down," that is, clinicians organize data in a manner that creates the most coherent, seamless perception possible.[13] Seasoned clinicians often advocate the usefulness of heuristic decision making. Arguably, without a working knowledge of gestalt principles, clinicians would be hopelessly bogged down with "bottom-up" assessments (hypothetical-deductive) of their patients, begrudgingly plowing through reams of clinical data to form a workable hypothesis. Yet despite the utility of clinical gestalt, it is important to realize that this method is not without error. For example, at present, most healthcare providers use tools for decision making that demonstrate only marginal value.[14] Most clinicians also make errors in diagnosis when faced with complex and even noncomplex cases[14] and up to 35% of these errors can cause harm to patients.[15]

Although intuitive, heuristic decision making is riddled with five tangible errors[16]: (1) the *representative heuristic* (if it's similar to something else, it must be like that); (2) the *availability heuristic* (we are more inclined to find something if it's something we are used to finding); (3) the *confirmatory bias* (looking for things in the exam to substantiate what we want to find); (4) the *illusory correlation* (linking events when there is actually no relationship); and (5) *overconfidence*. Of these five decision-making errors, overconfidence may be the most predominant. Most diagnosticians feel that they are better decision-makers than what they demonstrate in actual clinical practice.[15] In fact, the least skilled diagnosticians are also the most overconfident and most likely to make a mistake![15]

These mistakes can occur in two domains: (1) the empirical aspect (real-world observation of findings, or the data collection phase) and (2) the rational aspect (the clinical decision-making phase during which clinicians make sense of the data at hand).[17] Although both are common, the reasoning (rational) aspect is by far the most common.[17]

Mixed Model Decision Making

In reality, most decision-making models are mixed. For examination, most clinicians use a hypothetical-deductive approach to identify variables that support a pre-examination hypothesis. During the development of most clinical prediction rules (CPR), gestalt has been a driver in capturing most variables for study. Using assessment modifiers such as **probabilistic decision-making** analyses, one can assign predictive values to pertinent findings captured during a hypothetical-deductive approach. Probabilistic tools are

also useful in capturing the true value of a pathognomonic test finding. Because of the strengths and weaknesses of each area, it is advised that the manual therapy clinician use a mixed model during decision making. A careful clinician always recognizes the weaknesses of each model and compensates by using the strengths of the other.

Summary

- A threshold approach is the accumulation of information to a specified level that triggers a clinician to make a decision.
- There are two primary clinical decision-making models in manual therapy: (1) hypothetical-deductive and (2) heuristic decision making.
- Hypothetical-deductive decision making involves the development of a hypothesis during the clinical examination and the refuting or acceptance of that hypothesis that occurs during the process of the examination.
- Heuristic decision making involves pattern recognition and the ability to collate useful findings into coherent groups.
- Most true models are mixed models of decision making.

Assessment Modifiers of Decision Making

Assessment modifiers are elements that are used in any of the three decision-making models that are designed to improve the accuracy of the outcome. Assessment modifiers are not decision-making models, because each does not contain a unique decision-making characteristic and is not exclusive within one particular model. Modifiers do affect decision-making uniquely when evaluated under specific circumstances. Examples of assessment modifiers include probabilistic statistics and clinical prediction rules.

Within epidemiological literature, the two most commonly discussed assessment modifiers are **moderators** and **mediators.** While referred to as "assessment modifiers" in this textbook, moderators and mediators are actually *outcomes modifiers,* which can influence the outcome of the assessment or intervention.

Moderators and mediators are useful in explaining why some patients change and others do not. Both involve dedicated variables that influence the causality link between treatment and outcome.[18] Both are essential when considering the true effect of an intervention during an assessment of therapeutic outcome. Failure to consider moderators and mediators during observational or randomized controlled designs may lead to an overestimation or underestimation of the effect magnitude.

An outcome mediator functions to partially identify the possible mechanisms through which a treatment might achieve its effects. These mechanisms are causal links between treatment and outcome[19] in which the treatment affects the mediator and the consequence of the mediator (after exposure to the treatment) affects the targeted outcome. Mediators can positively or negatively affect an outcome by virtue of a "change" in the variable during the time frame of the intervention. To qualify as an outcome mediator, the variable of interest must (1) change during exposure to treatment, (2) be correlated with the treatment, and (3) explain all or a portion of the effect of the treatment on the desired outcome measure.

In contrast, an outcome moderator is a baseline variable that (1) precedes the treatment temporally, (2) is independent of the treatment (is not affected by the treatment), but (3) influences the outcome (e.g., Oswestry or Short Form 36) when stratified by selected values. Potential moderators may be sociodemographic variables, genotype, or baseline clinical characteristics (comorbidities) that *are not influenced* by active treatment mechanisms.

It is somewhat challenging to differentiate moderators from mediators when evaluating outcomes of a clinical trial, when designing a study, or when considering the appropriate treatment for clinical care. As discussed by Kraemer and colleagues,[19] there is ambiguity between a moderator and a mediator and in the directionality of moderation and mediation. Moderators clarify the magnitude of treatment effects through adjustment of estimates for imbalances in the group with respect to covariables.[20] Mediators establish 'how' or 'why' one variable predicts or causes an outcome variable.[19,21] Consider an example using graded exposure for low back and the effects of fear-avoidance beliefs on low back pain perceived disability.[22] One could argue that if stratified, fear avoidance could dictate change scores for specific outcomes. Higher fear-avoidance scores should relate to lower outcomes, moderate fear avoidance scores should relate to slightly better outcomes, and very low fear-avoidance scores should relate to excellent outcomes. If this is the case then fear-avoidance strata could be considered a moderator. Yet prior to determining whether fear avoidance should function as a moderator or mediator, one must examine the affect of the treatment on the moderator or mediator. Graded exposure is hypothesized to positively improve fear avoidance behavior, which in turn should improve overall outcomes.[23] When a treatment influences the variable, the variable must be considered a mediator. Figure 2.1 ■ provides a graphic example of how moderators and mediators influence outcomes.

Why is this information useful? Moderators, when stratified, assist in defining which groups are likely to benefit from a particular form of manual therapy. For example, the moderators associated with the clinical

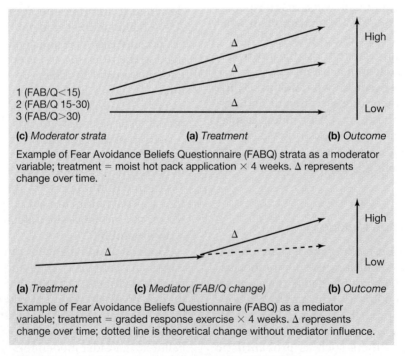

(c) *Moderator strata*   **(a)** *Treatment*   **(b)** *Outcome*

Example of Fear Avoidance Beliefs Questionnaire (FABQ) strata as a moderator variable; treatment = moist hot pack application × 4 weeks. Δ represents change over time.

(a) *Treatment*   **(c)** *Mediator (FAB/Q change)*   **(b)** *Outcome*

Example of Fear Avoidance Beliefs Questionnaire (FABQ) as a mediator variable; treatment = graded response exercise × 4 weeks. Δ represents change over time; dotted line is theoretical change without mediator influence.

■ **Figure 2.1** Graphic Example of Moderators and Mediators of Outcomes Comparison of Fear Avoidance Beliefs Questionnaire Score and Theoretical Influence on Outcome When Used as a Moderator or Mediator Variable

prediction rule for manipulation of the thoracic spine in patients with mechanical neck pain are used to predict who is likely to improve from a specific intervention. In contrast, findings such as high fear avoidance behaviors, poor coping strategies, low self-efficacy, and depression are considered mediating variables. These are considered mediators if a specific exercise approach changes the finding of the mediator (e.g., if graded exposure reduces the fear-avoidance behaviors). This information can be used to target specific interventions that can affect the mediators and subsequently improve the outcome.

Probabilistic Decision Making

Health-care providers always make decisions in the face of uncertainty.[24] Probabilistic modification is the use of a probability estimate for determining diagnosis, prognosis, or treatment of a patient and is a form of moderator. Probabilistic modification is an inductive method that uses a statistically oriented overview to determine decisions. This method of modification uses given information from the dedicated circumstance of the patient, and specific statistical laws associated with probability, to determine the occurrence of the event that is expected with high logical or inductive probability.[25] This modification suppresses many of the errors associated with heuristic decision making by allowing the strength of a giving decision-making instrument (i.e., clinical tool) to dictate outcomes, versus internal judgment.

Bayesian assessment is considered a form of probabilistic modification. Bayesian assessment is sometimes referred to as "knowledge-based decision making" and is predicated on prior estimates of probabilities, based on additional experience, and influenced by additive information. In essence, a prior estimate of a condition is fixed, and a finite set of revisionist tests and measures are performed that revise the initial probability estimate. Appropriate tests and measures significantly modify the probability estimate.

Although probability modifications provide complexity to hypothetical-deductive and heuristic decision making, the process can be simplified through the use of clinical prediction rules or decision rules. Clinical prediction rules capture selected variables that have demonstrated the ability to influence the posttest probability of a positive (or a negative) change in a patient's condition. Most are obtained by capturing conditionally independent measures that are associated toward an outcome. A high-quality clinical prediction rule allows clinicians to improve their probability of success with a diagnosis or an intervention when patient characteristics and examination findings match the identified rules.

Although modifiers such as these have shown improved outcomes over gestalt methods, it is worth noting that CPRs are only as good as the derivation/validation sequence of the study.[26,27] At present, there are a number of CPRs that have been published in the literature that are reflective of a manual therapy procedure, and the majority has exceptionally weak methodology.[27,28] Although the development of a CPR is recommended to improve outcomes, a careful and iterative process is necessary to assure clinicians we are using the proper predictive tools. In addition, CPRs are not a substitute for good clinical decision making; CPRs are a "process modifier" within the clinical decision-making sequence.

Patient Response Triggers

A **patient response trigger** is a finding within an examination that facilitates a dedicated care response, expectation of prognosis, or diagnosis, and is a form of mediator. Patient response triggers differ from pathognomonic findings because these are generally not solely associated with a negative finding. Typically, patient response triggers are gathered during a physical examination that consists of pain reproduction and reduction (using pain provocation and reduction methods). During this examination, various movements are found that alter patient report of symptoms (either improving or worsening findings). The process assumes that the clinical findings are relevant toward the outcome of the patient and ties each treatment intervention that may be unique to each particular patient.

Germane to the patient response trigger is the expectation that the patient response triggers are predictive of **within-session** (during the same session)[29] or **between-session** (after the patient returns)[30] changes during the care of that patient. Many clinicians use the within- and between-session changes to adjust their treatment dosage, intensity, and application for the optimal targeted result advocating primarily the use of within-session (immediate response) changes toward a positive long-term outcome. In truth, within- and between-session changes have been shown to be useful in predicting a positive outcome for acute lumbar spine pain, impairments, and neck pain. Surprisingly, there is little research on between-session changes, although it is arguably the more important of the two.

Classification or Clusters

Classification is a mechanism of labeling or placing a patient into a known group to target a preconceived, directed clinical approach to that patient. The process uses both probabilistic and heuristic influences, but also dwells heavily on pre-existing prognostic literature toward what benefits that patient. In most cases, classifications are developed through regression (statistical) modeling, which captures subgroups of patients who benefit from a dedicated procedure.

Treatment by classification has demonstrated a better outcome than independent clinician decision making and as a whole provides a fairly well-vetted mechanism for general treatment of patients. Combining hypothetical-deductive, patient-response findings within a classification allows a specified approach to target the most effective treatment to the patient. In Chapter 4, we discuss the use of general versus specific techniques. Specific techniques are those gathered during combined hypothetical-deductive, patient-response findings such as "pain during closing" or "pain during dorsiflexion."

Summary

- Probabilistic modification is an inductive method that uses a statistically oriented overview to determine decisions and can be used to enhance or modify any decision-making model.
- A patient response trigger is a finding within an examination that facilitates a dedicated care response, expectation of prognosis, or diagnosis.
- Classification is the process of labeling or placing a patient into a known group to target a preconceived, directed clinical approach to that patient.

Clinical Reasoning

Clinical reasoning is a thinking process to direct a clinician to take "wise" action or to take the best judged action in a specific context.[31] It is a process in which the therapist, who interacts with the patient and other appropriate parties, helps patients develop health management strategies for their condition based on the unique findings for that patient and the patient's own response to their condition.[32] Clinical reasoning is the overarching element of clinical decision making and involves processes beyond diagnosis and intervention, such as assessment and management during continued care.

As stated previously, most clinicians use a mixed model for decision making, which combines the elements of heurism and hypothetical-deductive thinking. The ability to partition, combine, or modify the decision-making components of each *is* clinical reasoning. This requires a patient-centered approach that is grounded in a biopsychosocial framework,[33] requires storing of findings that are based either on pattern recognition, probabilistic importance, or that have influenced within-session findings, and allows

adjustments toward emphasis on each category based on changes in findings or the patient's condition.

Consider the following examples. Suppose a patient seen for general low back pain provides encouraging outcomes after administration of a lumbar manipulative technique on the first visit. The manipulation technique was selected secondary to the patient's classification as a candidate for passive movement (assessment modifier) and a positive response during mobilization during the examination (hypothetical-deductive/assessment modifier–patient response). The patient's report of pain and range of motion are markedly improved (assessment modifier, between-session change) yet the patient still reports a low level of function and fear in returning to work. Heuristic influences (pattern recognition) would suggest an active approach may benefit this patient versus a purely passive approach. In addition, on the third visit, the patient reports bladder retention, bilateral leg pain, and rapid neurological changes[34] (pathognomonic findings) prompting the clinician to immediately refer the patient for diagnostic work-up. The scenario describes a mixed model where assessment modifiers alter the clinical decision-making process. The process as a "whole" is clinical reasoning.

Summary

- Clinical reasoning is a thinking process to direct a clinician to take "wise" action or to take the best judged action in a specific context.
- Clinical reasoning is the overarching act of appropriate clinical decision making and may involve any of the models of clinical decision making.

Decision Making in Manual Therapy

There are significant philosophical variations in decision making between practicing manual clinicians. The philosophical variations robustly harbor influential internal biases that affect decision making in manual therapy. Components of one's philosophy are likely affected by a number of factors, including the overwhelming amount of information that is present in the literature and the difficulty as a clinician in maintaining current understanding of that knowledge. Clinicians often use mechanisms such as continuing education programs, colleagues, or textbooks to gather "new" material, all of which have potential weaknesses.

The most dominant mechanism is one's background exposure (or experience) toward a specific manual therapy approach. Passion toward one specific approach can lead to the unwillingness to accept selected decision-making components that fall outside a philosophical construct or that are not endorsed by the "guru" or "gurus" within that particular faction. Although this aspect of clinical decision making in manual therapy has less influence on clinicians each year, the philosophical differences among backgrounds is still an overwhelming factor that restricts growth toward evidence-based manual therapy.

Manual Therapy Backgrounds

Farrell and Jensen[35] define a **manual therapy philosophical approach** as a set of general beliefs, concepts, and attitudes. They suggested that the philosophical approach dictates how a clinician performs the specific mechanics of the patient assessment process. Although most manual therapy philosophies demonstrate similarities in the examination process, variations of the role of applied anatomy, biomechanics, and the origin of structures often dictate the perspective of a particular model. Because physical therapy educators have different philosophical backgrounds, variation in the education of manual therapy in physical therapy schools is widespread.

In 1988, the most prevalent manual therapy assessment models taught in pre-licensure settings were Kaltenborn and Maitland, followed by Paris and Cyriax.[36] A more recent investigation (1997) found that the Maitland approach was emphasized the most (22%), followed by McKenzie (17%), with Paris and Osteopathic tied for third (14% each).[36] A 2004 survey by Cook and Showalter,[37] which asked practicing clinicians to identify the background they have adopted for their manual therapy assessment approach, found that the McKenzie approach was the most common assessment model with 34.7%, followed by Maitland (20.9%) and eclectic (10.6%). A follow up study that was comprised of American Physical Therapy Association (APTA), Board Certified Orthopedic Clinical Specialists (OCS), and/or Fellows of the American Academy of Orthopaedic Manual Physical Therapists (AAOMPT) also provided a report of manual therapy background.[38] The most common reported backgrounds included Maitland (24.1%), Osteopathic (19.4%), McKenzie (14.7%), Paris (12.3%), and Kaltenborn (8.2%). Because 99% of physical therapy schools teach manual therapy within the curriculum,[36] there is a significant chance that exposure to one specific philosophy occurs prior to actual clinical practice.

Studies involving clinicians in other countries have also demonstrated background preferences. The four most popular postgraduate courses attended by respondents to a survey in Northern Ireland were Maitland peripheral short courses (48.0%), Maitland spinal short courses (42.1%), McKenzie A (76.3%), and McKenzie B (65.8%).[39] Respondents indicated that 71.4% of patients with low back pain were treated with McKenzie techniques, 43.8% were treated with Maitland mobilization, and 5.9% were treated with Cyriax techniques.[39] Foster et al.[40] surveyed physiotherapists in England/Scotland and Ireland managing nonspecific low back pain, and found that 53.9% attended postgraduate Maitland vertebral mobilization classes and 53.2% attended McKenzie Part A courses. For spinal treatment, Maitland mobilizations were used by 58.9% of therapists and McKenzie techniques were used by 46.6% of therapists.[40] A survey of Canadian physiotherapists found that 67% of respondents reported using Maitland techniques and 41% reported using Cyriax techniques for cervical spine treatments.[41]

Philosophical Differences   In 1979, Cookson[42] and Cookson and Kent[43] published comparative data among four popular manual therapy philosophies for treatment of the spine and extremities, respectively. Discussion of the principle philosophies for the extremity and spinal treatment philosophies included the Cyriax, Kaltenborn, Maitland, and Mennell approaches. There were notable differences regarding the method in which each philosophy converted examination findings to treatment methods. In an overview of assessment of extremities, Cookson[42] noted that Cyriax and Kaltenborn based examination results on the presence of capsular patterns and the results of resisted testing. Both backgrounds used Cyriax's etiological philosophy for identification of guilty lesions. Cyriax's selection of treatment depended greatly on the examination findings and the classification of the impairments. For example, the selection of a physiological movement, accessory movement, or other form of treatment was dependent on the pain level, end-feel, capsular pattern, and presence of a contractile or noncontractile lesion.

For selection of specific treatment techniques, Kaltenborn extrapolated the findings of the examination toward the theoretical relationship of arthrokinematic movements. These arthrokinematic movements were based on the convex–concave rules originally developed from the work of MacConail.[44] Kaltenborn's philosophy was to divide joints into hyper- or hypomobilities and to restore movement or stabilize as needed. The philosophy for treatment of hypomobility includes mobilization methods such as traction and accessory glides, often incorporating procedures at the end ranges to target selective stiffness.

Mennell used a concept of joint dysfunction, which was based on onset, presence of trauma, and subjective findings. For treatment of joint dysfunction, the

Mennell approach used quick thrusts designed to increase range of motion upon findings of joint limitation.[45] Often, active movements followed mobilization to encourage "muscular reeducation." One notable belief was the exclusion of therapeutic movements in the presence of inflammation.

The Maitland approach targeted treatments that affected the comparable sign of the patient. The comparable sign was defined as the motion or combination of motions that reproduce the pain or stiffness of the patient. Maitland divided the oscillatory-based application into four primary grades.[43] These grades differed in force, amplitude, and objective and were ascertained during patient assessment. Maitland's treatment approach was independent of capsular patterns, arthrokinematic patterns, or other biomechanical regulations.

There were similar differences found in the philosophical treatment of the spine.[42] Of the four approaches outlined for treatment of the spine, the Maitland and Mennell approach advocated the affiliation of examination and treatment techniques. Maitland focused more on oscillatory movements for joints that were considered either hypo- or hypermobile, whereas Mennell used a series of traction and positioning techniques for pain relief. As with the peripheral analysis, the Kaltenborn spinal approach was based on biomechanical classification. Three treatment methods were used, depending on the examination findings, which ranged from mobilization to treatment procedures. Cyriax used a priori clustering of selected pathologies, but essentially maintained that the disk was the primary pathology of most spine ailments. Treatment generally consisted of generalized mobilization techniques or reduction/traction methods if radiculopathy was perceptible.[42]

A similar analysis of manual therapy philosophies was performed in 1992 by Farrell and Jensen[35] with the addition of two approaches: Osteopathic and McKenzie. Similar to the Cookson series,[42,43] Farrell and Jensen[35] reported numerous differences among the representative philosophies. For example, Cyriax's assessment system was dedicated toward his interpretation of applied anatomy and use of capsular patterns. Mennell's philosophy was oriented toward joint dysfunction-based techniques. Although the approaches advocated by Maitland, McKenzie, and Kaltenborn have many examination elements that were similar to Cyriax, Maitland assigned less credence to diagnostic or pathological labels and supports the use of re-examination to verify treatment effectiveness. McKenzie used a series of repeated movements and postural (positioning assessment) to determine the patient response during clinical examination. McKenzie assigned a classification of the spinal impairment into one of three

groups: postural, derangement, or dysfunction. The Osteopathic method emphasized the interpretation of three potential findings: a positional fault, restriction fault, and/or segmental or multisegmental impairment. Table 2.2 ■ summarizes the findings of the three articles and outlines the similarities and differences of these approaches.

Summary

- Numerous manual therapy assessment models have been taught in educational settings. The most commonly reported models are those of Maitland, McKenzie, Kaltenborn, Osteopathic, and eclectic.

- The most common continuing education courses both nationally and internationally are those provided by Maitland, McKenzie, Osteopathic, Kaltenborn, and Paris.

- The most commonly recognized manual therapy assessment approaches have notable similarities and differences. Past studies have outlined those comparisons and contrasts.

Philosophical Analysis

It is apparent that disparate manual therapy assessment philosophies exist. Upon face analysis, there appears to be three discrete assessment philosophical approaches or bases among the multiple manual therapy backgrounds. The first assessment format focuses on arthrokinematic and biomechanical principles. This **biomechanical–pathological assessment method** utilizes a priori selected biomechanical theories for assessment of abnormalities in movement and positioning then targets treatments using similar arthrokinematic principles. Treatment techniques are based on theoretical relationships between anatomical contributions and pathological presentations. Often, these relationships are extrapolated into determination of a specific pathology or diagnosis. Some approaches rely on a given pathology or diagnostic label prior to administration of treatment. For example, the presence of a movement restriction based on the findings of Cyriax's capsular pattern is often labeled adhesive capsulitis of the glenohumeral joint.[46] Assessment formats that use this process of assessment and treatment would then extrapolate the arthrological findings to related arthrological theories, most notably the convex–concave rule. Since external rotation is typically the range of motion that has the highest ratio of loss, and since the humerus is a convex structure moving on a concave gleniod fossa, a posterior to anterior glide mobilization would be considered the appropriate mobilization direction.[47]

The second method, the **patient response method,** addresses pain reproduction and reduction (using pain provocation and reduction methods) with various movements and does not rely on specific biomechanical

■ **TABLE 2.2** A Summary of the Philosophical Properties of Each Manual Therapy Theory

	Cyriax	Kaltenborn	Maitland	McKenzie	Mennell	Osteopathic
Philosophy adopts selected biomechanical and arthrological constructs	Yes	Yes	No	Yes and no	Mixed	Mixed
Approach places an emphasis on patient education	Yes	Yes	Yes	Yes	Yes	Yes
Evaluative criteria	Isolation of anatomical guilty structure	Biomechanical analysis of joint and soft tissue pathology	Identify relevant patient signs and symptoms	Interpretation whether impairment is a dysfunction, derangement, or postural syndrome	Assessment of joint dysfunction	Identification of positional fault, restriction fault, or single vs. multi-segmental findings
Key concepts	Diagnosis of soft tissue lesions and isolation of contractile vs. noncontractile components	Assessment of somatic involvement and application of biomechanical-based treatment systems	Examination and treatment methods are highly interrelated	Examination and treatment methods are highly related; selected positions may encourage certain disorders	Joint play assessment is critical	Assessment of somatic involvement; assessment focuses on the presence of asymmetry, restriction of movement, and palpation of soft tissue

models for diagnostic assessment. The patient response method assesses the response of single or repeated movements and/or positions on the patient's comparable complaint of pain or abnormality of movement. Treatment techniques are often similar to the direction and form of assessment method. The particular treatment technique is based on the movement method that reproduces the patient's pain in a way designed to yield a result that either reduces pain or increases range of motion. The direction, amplitude, force, and speed of the treatment would depend on the patient response during and after the application. For example, using the same example of adhesive capsulitis; a provocation assessment would target the movement that most reproduced the patient's symptoms in a desirable fashion. The clinician may have found that during the application of an anterior to posterior (AP) glide, the result was an improvement in external rotation and a reduction in pain, therefore validating the selection of that method.

Analogous to clinical decision making, manual therapy philosophical assessment methods are more commonly mixed than singular. Within a mixed method, both anatomical and biomechanical theories are used to initiate treatment, and variations that occur during treatment outside the rigid boundaries of biomechanical theory are often warranted. A mixed model allows identification of pertinent biomechanical findings that have prognostic influence and should drive treatment decisions.

Summary

- There appear to be three primary assessment approaches in manual therapy.
- The first approach consists of biomechanical analysis, consisting of assessments using capsular patterns, coupling motions of the spine, biomechanical movement theory, and treatment methods using convex–concave rules.
- The second approach is a patient response approach, which consists of movements and treatments based on patient report of symptom provocation and resolution.
- The third approach consists of parameters of both assessment models. This combined approach may rely more heavily on biomechanical assessment and patient response treatment, vice versa, or will use an ad hoc eclectic model.

What Is the Best Approach?

Unfortunately, there is no direct evidence to determine which assessment philosophy reigns superiorly over another. Therefore, it is inappropriate to make conclusive judgments regarding the different approaches because no direct comparisons involving patient outcome assessment are known to exist. At present, only indirect suppositions are possible. Nevertheless, there is evidence that some methods of manual therapy assessment (that are used in the hypothetical-deductive decision making model) have performed less successfully during methodological scrutiny and could result in inappropriate, inaccurate, or invalid assessment. Use of invalid measures during decision making can lead to errors and bias during the assessment process.

The Convex–Concave Rule The **convex–concave rule** is a standard of biomechanical-based assessment methods that is not universally applicable to all regions. The convex–concave theory of arthrokinematic motion was first described by MacConail.[44] This theory asserts that the joint surface geometry dictates the accessory movement pattern during physiological movement.[48] The convex–concave rule states that when a concave surface rotates about a convex surface that rolling and gliding will occur in the same direction.[49] Conversely, if a convex surface rotates on a concave surface, rolling and gliding occur in opposite directions.[49] This pattern is purported to be irrespective of muscle movement or passive contributions of surrounding structures and pathology, and is purely a product of articular geometry.[50] To some extent, there is reasonable data to support that this process is predictive in the knee and ankle.[51,52] Indeed, this model is often used to describe spinal-related movements, especially during end-range physiological activities.[53] Nonetheless, there is sizeable evidence that the shoulder fails to conform to the convex–concave guidelines. Numerous studies indicate that the glenohumeral joint does not always move as a ball and socket joint, but occasionally during pathology displays translatory-only movements.[48,54,55] Because of this, it appears that the selection of a technique that focuses on a specific direction based solely on the convex–concave rule may not yield values any better than the antagonistic direction at the shoulder.[55–57]

An additional problem is that some joints demonstrate irregularities of anatomy. The joint surfaces of C1 on C2 have been described as both convex on concave and convex on convex.[58] Often, the acromioclavicular joint demonstrates irregularity as well.[59] Because variations are so minute, it is difficult for a clinician to alter their biomechanical examination and treatment paradigm based on palpatory or observation-based findings. These irregularities may lead to variations in treatment and in theory, such as the inappropriate direction during treatment application.

Although this evidence is condemning for use at the shoulder joint and in a situation where anatomical variation is present, one additional bit of information may be just as troublesome. The assertion that a manual therapist is able to apply a selected accessory-based movement that is biomechanically designed to replicate the active physiological movement of the patient is unsupported.[60] There is no evidence that lends credibility to the doctrinaire assertion that selected accessory techniques must be applied at specific angles or planes.

Isometric Tension Testing Cyriax had three principles for examination by **selective tissue tension.** The first involved isometric contraction of contractile tissue to determine if pain or weakness were present during loading. Cyriax proposed that contractile tissues (muscle, tendon, and bony insertion) are painful during an applied isometric contraction and inert structures (capsule, ligaments, bursae) are painful during passive movement. He furthered this definition by providing subdefinitions to the findings or the provocation tests. Franklin et al.[61] found some consistencies and inconsistencies with Cyriax's theory. First, as Cyriax noted, patients with minor contractile tissue lesions did display initially unchanged passive range of motion and pain with increased resistive activity.[62] However, in contrast to Cyriax's parameters, active range did worsen over time, as did strength. This questions the parameter "strong and painful," and suggests the existence of another category, "weak and painful." Table 2.3 ■ outlines Cyriax's selective tension testing.

Cyriax's Capsular Pattern The second component of Cyriax's selective tissue tension concept is the capsular pattern. Several studies have demonstrated mixed value regarding Cyriax's definition of **capsular pattern theory.**[46,63–65] Klassbo and Harms-Ringdahl[63] and Bijl et al.[65] found poor relationship between hip range-of-motion losses secondary to osteoarthritis and evidence of a capsular pattern. Klassbo and Harms-Ringdahl[63] also investigated the modified definition of the hip capsular patterns suggested by Kaltenborn[66] that also failed to demonstrate association.

The findings in the knee are mixed. Hayes et al.[64] used a strict interpretation of the ratio of flexion to extension loss of the knee in their investigation of a capsular pattern. Using a strict definition, they found poor validity among their population of knee patients. Mitsch et al.[46] discovered variability in the capsular

■ TABLE 2.3 Potential Findings during Resisted Movement Testing[62]

Classification	Description
Strong and painless	The contractile tissue is not involved.
Strong and painful	There is a minor lesion of the contractile tissue.
Weak and painless	There may be signs of a complete rupture of the contractile tissue or it may be a disorder of the nervous system.
Weak and painful	A major lesion has occurred.
All painful	Once all sinister pathologies are ruled out the therapist should consider that the affective component may be the chief generator of pain. Additionally, this could be a gross lesion lying proximally; usually capsular and produced with joint movement is not fully restrained.
Painful on repetition	If the movement is strong and painless but hurts after several repetitions, the examiner should suspect intermittent claudication.

pattern in patients diagnosed with adhesive capsulitis of the shoulder; Bijl et al.[65] also did not find consistency. In contrast, Fritz et al.[67] found the capsular pattern to be useful and consistent. The reason why each group found differences may lie in the interpretation and patient selection. It appears that Fritz et al.,[67] Hayes et al.,[64] and Mitsch et al.[46] placed some consideration on physician diagnosis, while Bijl et al.[65] used Altmann's clinical classification criteria for arthritis. Subsequently, some conflict exists regarding a stable capsular pattern at the hip and shoulder and possibly at the knee. If selecting the proper individual to meet Cyriax's criteria is essential for the use of this assessment method, then the benefit of the assessment model may be substantially reduced.

Cyriax's End-Feel Classification   The last aspect of Cyriax's selective tissue tension concept is the classification of the end-feel. One study questions the validity of reliability in identification of discrete **end-feel** categorization.[64] Cyriax and Cyriax[62] described an end-feel as "the extreme of each passive movement of the joint (that) transmits a specific sensation to the examiner's hands." He identified five specific end-feels, which are outlined in Table 2.4 ■. End-feel tends to suffer from poor interrater reliability but seems to exhibit better reliability when the presence of pain is assessed during detection of abnormal end-feel[68] or when an additional educational tool is used concurrently.[69]

Directional Coupling of the Cervical Spine Assessment of upper cervical **directional spine coupling** may suffer a lack of validity. Many disciplines still report the use of two-dimensional theories,[70] most notably the so-called *Laws of Physiologic Spinal Motion* outlined by Fryette.[71] In 1954, Fryette's findings were published and were largely based on the findings of Lovett.[72] Fryette's perception of coupling of the cervical region was that "sidebending is accompanied by rotation of the bodies of the vertebrae to the concavity of the lateral curve, as

■ TABLE 2.4 End-Feel Classification According to Cyriax and Cyriax (1993)

End-Feel Classification	Description
Bone to bone	The end-feel of the joint is hard as when a bone engages another bone.
Spring block	Per Cyriax, this may suggest internal derangement but may also represent a capsular or ligamentous end-feel.
Abrupt check	An unexpected restriction imposed by a muscular spasm.
Soft-tissue approximation	A normal end-feel where the joint can be pushed no further secondary to engagement to another body part.
Empty end-feel	No end-feel is felt since the movement is too painful and the examiner is unable to push the joint to its end range.

in the lumbar (spine)."[71] Recent three-dimensional analyses have confirmed that Fryette was correct on his assumption of cervical coupling direction from the cervical levels of C2-3 to C7-T1, but was incorrect at the levels of C0-1 through C1-2. Recent three-dimensional analyses of the cervical spine have demonstrated that variations in the upper cervical spine are present, thus exhibiting coupling patterns that are inconsistent.[73–77] Dogmatic use of Fryette's law during assessment of the upper cervical spine should be questioned.

Directional Coupling of the Lumbar Spine

Several authors have suggested that lumbar coupling biomechanics and Fryette's first and second *Laws of Physiological Spinal Motion* are poorly reliable and lack validity.[70,72,78] Cook[72] outlined the disparity between lumbar coupling directional movements specifically at lumbar segments L1-2, L4-5, and L5-S1. There seems to be little evidence to support that knowledge of lumbar spine coupling characteristics are important in understanding and treating patients with low back pain.[79] Many manual therapy techniques use coupling-based mobilizations and the validity of this approach is questionable. Several authors have suggested that the use of symptom reproduction to identify the level of pathology is the only accurate assessment method.[80–86] Because no pathological coupling pattern has shown to be consistent, an assessment method in absence of pain provocation or reduction methods may yield inaccurate results. Therefore, upper cervical and lumbar biomechanical coupling theory may only be useful if assessed with pain provocation or reduction within a clinical examination.[72,87]

Directional Coupling of the Thoracic Spine

Recently, Sizer et al.[88] found variability in thoracic coupling in eight studies that used three-dimensional assessment of movement patterns. The authors found no consistent coupling pattern was observed across the eight studies. In the cases examined, patients exhibited ipsilateral, contralateral, or mixed coupling behaviors. Higher quality, *in vivo* investigations are needed to evaluate thoracic coupling in symptomatic subjects in both a flexed and extended thoracic spinal position.

Postural Asymmetry and the Relationship to Impairment

A potential misjudgment is the emphasis placed on observational asymmetries found during assessment of spinal abnormalities. McKenzie[89] writes, "there is a mistaken belief among some physical therapists that articular asymmetry is a contributing factor to the onset of backache." In fact, there are no studies that have calculated any predictive observational relationship with any form of progression or predisposition to spinal impairment. Commonly identified maladies such as pelvic obliquity are as recognizable in patients with pain as those without pain[90] and in those with and without pelvis disorders. Postural asymmetry in the absence of a well-defined anatomical anomaly has no correlation with back pain and other forms of pelvic asymmetry are even less conclusive.[91] Additionally, it has been reported that asymmetries associated with the pelvis are too small to detect by manual examination, thus abnormalities have a high potential of being speculative assumption only.[92,93]

Assessment of Passive Accessory Spinal Movement

Passive spinal assessment methods such as **passive accessory intervertebral movements** (PAIVMs) are widely used in joint mobilization.[94–96] One particular method, the posterior–anterior (PA) mobilization applied specifically to the spinous process, is purported to be a fundamental technique in clinical judgment.[94,97–99] Use of the PA mobilization has been found to have a reasonable intertherapist reliability in the detection of the symptomatic lumbar segment level when accompanied with the verbal response of the subject.[100–102] Nonetheless, studies that have measured interrater reliability of forces without verbal response of the subject have reported a high degree of variability.[103–108] Additionally, studies that have focused on the presence of R1, defined as the point where stiffness is first perceived where the "feel" of the motion presents resistance to the therapist,[35,102,103,109–111] have demonstrated poor reliability.[35,112] There are many theories for the poor reliability, some of which include inconsistencies within the clinician education process,[109,113–118] differences in post-graduate training,[35,60,114,119] years of experience,[35,60,114] conflicting therapists' concept of stiffness,[102,118,120,121] the angle of mobilization force,[122] position of the patient during mobilization,[123,124] and teaching method.[96] Most notably, it appears that assessment of finite motions in the absence of patients' verbal feedback may lead to questionable findings.

The finite movement associated with a PAIVM involves displacements that are more complicated than a straight translation. In an *in vivo* analysis, Keller et al.[125] reported peak shear movements of 0.3 mm, axial movements of one millimeter, and sagittal rotation of one degree during manipulation forces. Although evidence does exist that movements of this magnitude are therapeutic, there is conflicting evidence to support that a clinician can "feel" such diminutive displacement, let alone discriminate between axial rotation and translation.

Biomechanic Theory of Disc Displacement with Repeated Movements Well-substantiated evidence to support the use of repeated end-range movements for patients with a suspected herniated disc exists.[126] In studies where patients have performed movements of this nature and have exhibited **centralization** of symptoms, outcomes have been favorable.[126] However, there is limited evidence to support that remodeling of the disc is the reason behind the benefit. Variations have been reported in studies that have examined the movement of intradiscal matter during repeated flexion and extension movements.[127,128] In some individuals and/or specimens, the discal matter moved anterior, posterior, or in both directions.

In place of remodeling of the disc there are other theories that may have merit. There is some evidence to support that the benefit of repeated movements may be associated with a change in the tension placed upon a nerve root during repeated loadings. In a cadaveric study, Schnebel et al.[129] reported that repeated extension decreased the tension and compression on the L5 nerve root. Repeated movements that reduce the tension and/or compression of a chemically sensitized disc would demonstrate the same patient-reported benefit as an alteration of a disc bulge.

An Overreliance on the Diagnostic Value of Special Testing There appears to be questionable validity associated with approaches that focus excessively on the use of "special" clinical tests to identify pathology or provide a diagnostic label prior to treatment. When examining reports on the diagnostic accuracy of a special test, a cohort of patients is subjected to at least two types of mutually exclusive testing: an index test (the special test) and the reference test, the latter usually being the best method available to detect the target condition. The accuracy of the index test is expressed in terms of sensitivity, specificity, or likelihood ratios.[130] Many commonly used special tests are subject to likelihood values that offer little conclusive diagnostic use to the clinician. The sacroiliac joint has a wealth of tests that have performed poorly in diagnostic studies,[131] as does other anatomical regions of the body such as the shoulder and knee. An overreliance on special tests may also reduce the pertinent information necessary during treatment selection.

Dogmatic Use of Clinical Prediction Rules on Patients Who Meet Criteria Clinical prediction rules (CPRs) are tools used to supplement clinical decision making. The clinical decision-making process is a complex and dedicated endeavor that involves ruling out sinister disorders outside a manual therapist's scope of practice and ruling in the possibility that a patient may benefit from dedicated care. Clinical decision making also requires the ability to sift through specific and concise information for patients that lack complexity and the ability to use treatment aids during cases of ambiguity. Clinical prediction rules are best used in well-defined cases (patient has been appropriately vetted from all other possibilities of pathologies) where the diagnosis or patient presentation is complex and vague.[132] Findings often lack precision, especially in small sample sizes. Clustering of clinical findings almost always leads to a specific set of findings, which should be used at the end of the decision-making cycle. When found after ruling out competing findings, the results are usually robust and useful. Decision making that is based only on whether patients meet clinical prediction rules is unwarranted and inappropriate, is beyond the intent of the tool, and should not be considered effective clinical decision making.

Summary

- There is strong evidence to support that the convex–concave rule does not apply to the glenohumeral joint. There is some evidence that the rule is effective for the ankle and knee.
- There is fair evidence that the Cyriax theory of selective tension is not applicable to all conditions.
- There is conflicting evidence that the Cyriax capsular pattern theory demonstrates validity and findings depend substantially on how patients are selected for assessment.
- There is some evidence that questions the reliability of Cyriax's end-feel classification.
- There is strong evidence to support that upper cervical spine coupling direction is unpredictable, thus Fryette's laws of physiological motions are invalid.
- There is substantial evidence to support that there is not a predictable coupling pattern for the lumbar or thoracic spine, thus Fryette's laws at the lumbar and thoracic spine are invalid.
- There is moderate evidence to support that postural asymmetry is not directly correlated to a specific impairment.
- There is moderate evidence that supports that the disc does not move in a specific direction or behave in a specific manner with repeated movements or specific postural positioning.
- There is strong evidence that suggests that manual therapy approaches that overutilize special tests will harbor inappropriate diagnoses and findings.

Assessment

The Patient Response-Based Model

Within this textbook, the "flavor" of the assessment most resembles a patient response-based model, which is an element of hypothetical-deductive decision making. Nonetheless, because the current best evidence does support a mixed model of decision making, probabilistic decision-making tools are also advocated, specifically if the tools were validated or captured in a high-quality study. Because of the weaknesses associated with clinical gestalt, guruism, and a sole focus on selected biomechanical principles that have not demonstrated decision-making value (or validity), a biomechanical approach is not routinely advocated.

Although not perfect, at present, the patient response approach (with unique, targeted, evidence-based examination findings) provides the greatest validity for evidence-based assessment in manual therapy. Additionally, this model, when performed in a sequential and specific manner, provides a rigorous system of what amounts to data collection and processing that is used to guide the clinician through a logical treatment format.[133] A patient response finding involves a positive or negative within-session (during the same session) or between-session (after the patient returns) response from a dedicated procedure. The clinician uses the within- and between-session findings to adjust their treatment dosage, intensity, and application for the optimal targeted result.

Primarily, the pioneers of this particular approach include G.D. Maitland, Robin McKenzie, numerous Australian-based researchers and physiotherapists, Brian Mulligan, and Gregory Grieve, and selected osteopathic approaches that have analyzed patient symptoms primarily with less emphasis on observation-based, visual abnormalities. To date, most research has addressed selected aspects of the patient response examination process but has only marginally examined the "model" of addressing within- and between-session changes.

Advantages of the Patient Response-Based Approach

There are several advantages to a patient response-based approach. These advantages are outlined below:

1. Adaptability to each patient and variability of symptoms.

2. Treatment is specific because it is driven by a positive response from the patient.
3. Treatment is derived from between-session changes.
4. The model is not based on biomechanical principles and since some biomechanical principles lack validity, have questioned validity, or are only valid in selected situations, the chance of error is substantially reduced.
5. The approach dictates an impairment-based approach that respects and selects a diagnosis, but bases much of the treatment decision making on impairment-based findings.
6. The model does not rely on the hypothetical presentation or protocol-based algorithm from a diagnostic label.
7. The treatment selection changes as the patient's symptoms change.
8. Several well-documented manual therapy models use a similar philosophy.
9. The model is intuitive and is relatively easy to learn.

Disadvantages of the Patient Response-Based Approach

Gregory Grieve[134] once wrote, "No test is perfect." Correspondingly, no clinical assessment method is perfect either. The patient response-based method does have notable flaws, which are listed below.

1. The patient response model is more time intensive because patient examination and treatment is not easily compartmentalized into common criteria.
2. The model assumes all findings are relevant and that each finding has the potential to influence decision making and prognosis.
3. In some cases, within-session treatments do not equate to a long-term improvement. In addition, there are many circumstances in which a within-session change can occur with a procedure (such as superficial heat, long-wave ultrasound, short-wave diathermy, and manual therapy)[135] and in many of these cases the finding is transient only.
4. The model requires dedicated communication between the clinician and the patient and will fail without concerted effort of both. In some situations when a patient does not commit to the approach, the result may yield poor outcomes.

5. Although no single model has been comparatively measured against another in a randomized clinical trial, the ability to indicate that the patient response model is better than another form of assessment model does not exist.

6. It does appear that the patient response model, which is mediated often by pain or impairment change, may not associate with long-term functional outcome.[29,135,136] This demands a function-specific program in combination with a patient response approach.

Summary

- This book has adopted a patient response-based approach.
- The patient response-based approach is similar to those pioneered by G.D. Maitland, Robin McKenzie, numerous Australian researchers and physiotherapists, Brian Mulligan, and selected Osteopaths who are not overly committed to purportedly visual biomechanical constructs.
- Both strengths and weaknesses of the patient response-based system are apparent. No assessment approach is perfect, yet the patient response-based system provides a fair amount of validity when both clinician and patient are committed to an effective outcome.

Chapter Questions

1. Compare and contrast the three decision-making models for manual therapists.

2. Describe the three manual therapy philosophical approaches (biomechanical, patient response, and mixed). Compare and contrast assessment methods.

3. Outline the weaknesses of the discussed manual therapy areas and how these weaknesses could alter assessment.

4. Outline the strengths of selected manual therapy areas and discuss how these lead to pertinent assessment.

References

1. Cahan A, Gilon D, Manor O, Paltiel O. Clinical experience did not reduce the variance in physicians' estimates of pretest probability in a cross-sectional survey. *J Clin Epidemiol.* 2005;58(11):1211–1216.

2. Kaul C, Bahrami B. Subjective experience of motion or attentional selection of a categorical decision. *J Neurosci.* 2008;28(16):4110–4112.

3. Szolovits P, Patil RS, Schwartz WB. Artificial intelligence in medical diagnosis. *Ann Intern Med.* 1988;108(1):80–87.

4. Sobri M, Lamont A, Alias N, Win M. Red flags in patients presenting with headache: Clinical indications for neuroimaging. *Br J Radiology.* 2003;76:532–535.

5. Boissonnault WG, Koopmeiners MB. Medical history profile: Orthopaedic physical therapy outpatients. *J Orthop Sports Phys Ther.* 1994;20(1):2–10.

6. Boissonnault WG. Prevalence of comorbid conditions, surgeries, and medication use in a physical therapy outpatient population: A multicentered study. *J Orthop Sports Phys Ther.* 1999;29(9):506–519; discussion 520–525.

7. Sizer P, Brismee JM, Cook C. Medical screening for red flags in the diagnosis and management of musculoskeletal spine pain. *Pain Pract.* 2007;7(1):53–71.

8. Swenson R. Differential diagnosis. *Neuro Clinics North Am.* 1999;17:43–63.

9. Bishop PB, Wing PC. Knowledge transfer in family physicians managing patients with acute low back pain: A prospective randomized control trial. *Spine J.* 2006; 6:282–288.

10. Leerar PJ, Boissonnault W, Domholdt E, Roddey T. Documentation of red flags by physical therapists for patients with low back pain. *J Man Manip Ther.* 2007;15(1):42–49.

11. Kabrhel C, Camargo CA, Goldhaber SZ. Clinical gestalt and the diagnosis of pulmonary embolism: Does experience matter? *Chest.* 2008;127:1627–1630.

12. Koontz NA, Gunderman RB. Gestalt theory: Implications and radiology education. *AJR.* 2008;190:1156–1160.

13. Davis SF, Palladino JJ. *Psychology: Media and research update.* 3rd ed. Upper Saddle River, NJ; Prentice Hall: 2002.

14. Croskerry P, Norman G. Overconfidence in clinical decision making. *Am J Med.* 2008;121:24–9.

15. Berner ED, Graber, ML. Overconfidence as a cause of diagnostic error in medicine. *Am J Med.* 2008;121:2–23.

16. Klein J. Five pitfalls in decisions about diagnosis and prescribing. *BMJ.* 2005;330:781–783.

17. Federspil G, Vettor R. Rational error in internal medicine. *Intern Emerg Med.* 2008;3:25–31.

18. Bauman A, Sallis JF, Dzewaltowski D, Owen N. Toward a better understanding of the influences on physical activity. The role of determinants, correlates, causal variables, mediators, moderators, and confounders. *Am J Prev Med.* 2002;23:5–14.

19. Kraemer H, Wilson T, Fairburn C, Agras S. Mediators and Moderators of Treatment Effects in Randomized Clinical Trials. *Arch Gen Psychiatry.* 2002; 59:877–883.

20. Koch G, Tangen C, Jung JW, Amara I. Issues for covariance analysis of dichotomous and ordered categorical data from randomized clinical trials and non-parametric strategies for addressing them. *Stat Med.* 1998;17:1863–1892.

21. Wong EC, Beutler L, Zane N. Using mediators and moderators to test assumptions underlying culturally sensitive therapies: An exploratory example. *Cult Diversity Ethnic Minority Psych.* 2007;13:169–177.

22. Swinkels-Meewisse EJ, Swinkels RA, Verbeek AL, Vlaeyen JW, Oostendorp RA. Psychometric properties of the Tampa Scale for kinesiophobia and the fear-avoidance beliefs questionnaire in acute low back pain. *Man Ther.* 2003;8:29–36.

23. George SZ, Zeppieri G. Physical therapy utilization of graded exposure for patients with low back pain. *J Orthop Sports Phys Ther.* 2009;39:496–505.

24. Cahan A, Gilon D, Manor O, Paltiel O. Probabilistic reasoning and clinical decision-making: Do doctors overestimate diagnostic probabilities? *QJM.* 2003; 96(10):763–769.

25. Soltani A, Moayyeri A. Deterministic versus evidence-based attitude towards clinical diagnosis. *J Eval Clin Pract.* 2007;13:533–537.

26. Cook C. Is clinical Gestalt good enough? *J Man Manip Ther.* 2009;17:1–2.

27. Beneciuk JM, Bishop MD, George SZ. Clinical prediction rules for physical therapy interventions: A systematic review. *Phys Ther.* 2009;89(2):114–124.

28. May S, Gardiner E, Young S, Klaber-Moffett. Predictor variables for a positive long-term functional outcome in patients with acute and chronic neck and back pain treated with a McKenzie approach: A secondary analysis. *J Man Manip Ther.* 2008;16L:155–160.

29. Tuttle N, Laasko L, Barrett R. Change in impairments in the first two treatments predicts outcome in impairments, but not in activity limitations, in subacute neck pain: An observational study. *Aust J Physiother.* 2006;52(4):281–285.

30. Tuttle N. Do changes within a manual therapy treatment session predict between-session changes for patients with cervical spine pain? *Aust J Physiother.* 2005;51(1):43–48.

31. Norman G, Young M, Brooks L. Non-analytical models of clinical reasoning: The role of experience. *Med Educ.* 2007;41(12):1140–1145.

32. Edwards I, Jones M, Carr J, Braunack-Mayer A, Jensen GM. Clinical reasoning strategies in physical therapy. *Phys Ther.* 2004;84(4):312–330; discussion 331–335.

33. Higgs J, Burn A, Jones M. Integrating clinical reasoning and evidence-based practice. *AACN Clin Issues.* 2001;12(4):482–490.

34. Olivero WC, Wang H, Hanigan WC, et al. Cauda eqina syndrome (CES) from lumbar disc herniations. *J Spinal Disord Tech.* 2009;22(3):202–206.

35. Farrell J, Jensen G. Manual therapy: A critical assessment of role in the professional of physical therapy. *Phys Ther.* 1992;72:843–852.

36. Bryan JM, McClune LD, Rominto S, Stetts DM, Finstuen K. Spinal mobilization curricula in professional physical therapy education programs. *J Physical Ther Education.* 1997;11:11–15.

37. Cook C, Showalter C. A survey on the importance of lumbar coupling biomechanics in physiotherapy practice. *Man Ther.* 2004;9:164–172.

38. Cook C. Subjective and objective identifiers of clinical lumbar spine instability: A Delphi study. *Man Ther.* 2006;11(1):11–21.

39. Gracey J, Suzanne M, Baxter D. Physiotherapy management of low back pain: A survey of current practice in Northern Ireland. *Spine.* 2002;27(4):406–411.

40. Foster N, Thompson K, Baxter D, Allen J. Management of nonspecific low back pain by physiotherapists in Britain and Ireland. *Spine.* 1999;24:1332–1342.

41. Hurley L, Yardley K, Gross A, Hendry L, McLaughlin L. A survey to examine attitudes and patterns of practice of physiotherapists who perform cervical spine manipulation. *Man Ther.* 2002;7(1):10–18.

42. Cookson J. Orthopedic manual therapy—an overview. Part II: The spine. *Phys Ther.* 1979;59:259–267.

43. Cookson J, Kent B. Orthopedic Manual Therapy—an overview. Part I: The extremities. *Phys Ther.* 1979; 59:136–146.

44. MacConail M. Joint Movement. *Physiotherapy.* 1964; 50:363–365.

45. Mennell J. *Back pain: Diagnosis and treatment using manipulative techniques.* Boston; Little, Brown: 1960.

46. Mitsch J, Casey J, McKinnis R, Kegerreis S, Stikeleather J. Investigation of a consistent pattern of motion restriction in patients with adhesive capsulitis. *J Manual Manipulative Ther.* 2004;12:153–159.

47. Wadsworth C. *Manual examination and treatment of the spine and extremities.* Baltimore; Williams and Wilkins: 1988.

48. McClure P, Flowers K. Treatment of limited should motion: A case study based on biomechanical considerations. *Phys Ther.* 1992;72:929–936.

49. Kaltenborn FM. *Manual mobilization of the extremity joints* (4th ed.). Minneapolis; OPTP: 1989.

50. MacConaill M, Basmajian J. *Muscles and movement: A basis for human kinesiology.* Baltimore; Williams & Wilkins: 1969.

51. Frankel V, Burstein A, Brooks D. Biomechanics of internal derangement of the knee: Pathomechanics as determined by analysis of the instant centers of motion. *J Bone Joint Surg (Am).* 1971;53:945–962.

52. Sammarco G, Burstein A, Frankel V. Biomechanics of the ankle: A kinematic study. *Orthop Clin North Am.* 1973;4:75–96.

53. Mercer S, Bogduk N. Intra-articular inclusions of the cervical synovial joints. *Brit J Rheumatol.* 1993;32: 705–710.

54. Baeyens J, Van Roy P, De Schepper A, Declercq G, Clarijs J. Glenohumeral joint kinematics related to minor anterior instability of the shoulder at the end of the later preparatory phase of throwing. *Clin Biomech.* 2001;16:752–757.

55. Baeyens J, Van Roy P, Clarjjs J. Intra-articular kinematics of the normal glenohumeral joint in the late preparatory phase of throwing: Kaltenborn's rule revisited. *Ergonomics.* 2000;10:1726–1737.

56. Hsu A, Ho L, Hedman T. Joint position during anterior–posterior glide mobilization: Its effect on glenohumeral abduction range of motion. *Arch Phys Med Rehabil.* 2000;81:210–214.

57. Harryman et al. Translation of the humeral head on the glenoid with passive glenohumeral motion. *J Bone Jnt Surg.* 1990;79A(9):1334–1343.

58. White A, Panjabi M. *Clinical biomechanics of the spine.* Philadelphia; J.B. Lippincott: 1990; 94.

59. Harryman D, Lazarus M. The stiff shoulder. In: Rockwood C, Matsen F, Wirth M, Lippitt S (eds). *The shoulder.* Vol. 2. 3rd ed. Philadelphia; W.B. Saunders: 2004.

60. Riddle D. Measurement of accessory motion: Critical issues and related concepts. *Phys Ther.* 1992;72:865–874.

61. Franklin M, Conner-Kerr T, Chamness M, Chenier T, Kelly R, Hodge T. Assessment of exercise-induced minor muscle lesions: The accuracy of Cyriax's diagnosis by selective tension paradigm. *J Ortho Sports Phys Ther.* 1996;24:122–129.

62. Cyriax J, Cyriax P. *Cyriax's illustrated manual of orthopaedic medicine.* Oxford; Boston; Butterworth-Heinemann: 1993.

63. Klassbo M, Larsson G. Examination of passive ROM and capsular patterns of the hip. *Physiotherapy Res International.* 2003;8:1–12.

64. Hayes K, Peterson C, Falconer J. An examination of Cyriax's passive motion tests with patients having osteoarthritis of the knee. *Phys Ther.* 1994;74:697–707.

65. Bijl D, Dekker J, van Baar M, Oostendorp R, Lemmens A, Bijlsma J, Voorn T. Validity of Cyriax's concept capsular pattern for the diagnosis of osteoarthritis of hip and/or knee. *Scand J Rheumatol.* 1998;27:347–351.

66. Kaltenborn F. *Manual mobilization of the joints. The Kaltenborn method of joint mobilization and treatment.* 5th ed. Oslo; Olaf Norlis Bokhandel: 1999.

67. Fritz J, Delitto A, Erhard R, Roman M. An examination of the selective tissue tension scheme, with evidence for the concept of a capsular pattern of the knee. *Phys Ther.* 1998;78:1046–1056.

68. Peterson C, Hayes K. Construct validity of Cyriax's selective tension examination: Association of end-feels with pain at the knee and shoulder. *J Orthop Sports Phys Ther.* 2000;30:512–521.

69. Chesworth B, MacDermid J, Roth J, Patterson S. Movement diagram and "end-feel" reliability when measuring passive lateral rotation of the shoulder in patients with shoulder pathology. *Phys Ther.* 1998;78:593–601.

70. Gibbons P, Tehan P. Patient positioning and spinal locking for lumbar spine rotation manipulation. *Man Ther.* 2001;6(3):130–138.

71. Fryette H. *The principles of osteopathic technique.* Carmel, CA; Academy of Applied Osteopathy: 1954.

72. Cook C. Lumbar coupling biomechanics: A literature review. *J Manual Manipulative Ther.* 2003;11(3):137–145.

73. Panjabi M, Oda T, Crisco J, Dvorak J, Grob D. Posture affects motion coupling patterns of the upper cervical spine. *J Orthop Research.* 1993;11:525–536.

74. Mimura M, Hideshige M, Watanbe T, Takahashi K, Yamagata M, Tamaki T. Three-dimensional motion analysis of the cervical spine with special reference to axial rotation. *Spine.* 1989;14:1135–1139.

75. Penning L. Normal movements of the cervical spine. *Am J Roentgenology.* 1978;130:317–326.

76. Iai H, Hideshige M, Goto S, Takahashi K, Yamagata M, Tamaki T. Three-dimensional motion analysis of the upper cervical spine during axial rotation. *Spine.* 1993;18:2388–2392.

77. Oda T, Panjabi M, Crisco J. Three-dimensional translation movements of the upper cervical spine. *J Spinal Disorders.* 1991;4:411–419.

78. Harrison D, Harrison D, Troyanovich S. Three-dimensional spinal coupling mechanics: Part one. *J Manipulative Physiol Ther* 1998;21(2):101–113.

79. Panjabi M, Oxland T, Yamamoto I, Crisco J. Mechanical behavior of the human lumbar and lumbosacral spine as shown by three-dimensional load-displacement curves. *Am J Bone Jnt Surg.* 1994;76:413–424.

80. Keating J, Bergman T, Jacobs G, Finer B, Larson K. The objectivity of a multi-dimensional index of lumbar segmental abnormality. *J Manipulative Physiol Ther.* 1990;13:463–471.

81. Hardy G, Napier J. Inter- and intra-therapist reliability of passive accessory movement technique. *New Zealand J Physio.* 1991;22–24.

82. Vilkari-Juntura E. Inter-examiner reliability of observations in physical examinations of the neck. *Phys Ther.* 1987;67(10):1526–1532.

83. Lee M, Latimer J, Maher C. Manipulation: Investigation of a proposed mechanism. *Clin Biomech.* 1993;8:302–306.

84. Maher C, Adams R. Reliability of pain and stiffness assessments in clinical manual lumbar spine examinations. *Phys Ther.* 1994;74(9):801–811.

85. Maher C, Latimer J. Pain or resistance: The manual therapists' dilemma. *Aust J Physiother.* 1992;38(4):257–260.

86. Boline P, Haas M, Meyer J, Kassak K, Nelson C, Keating J. Interexaminer reliability of eight evaluative dimensions of lumbar segmental abnormality: Part II. *J Manipulative Physiol Ther.* 1992;16(6):363–373.

87. Li Y, He X. Finite element analysis of spine biomechanics. *J Biomech Engineering.* 2001;18(2)288–289,319.

88. Sizer PS Jr, Brismée JM, Cook C. Coupling behavior of the thoracic spine: A systematic review of the literature. *J Manipulative Physiol Ther.* 2007;30(5):390–399.

89. McKenzie R. Mechanical diagnosis and therapy for disorders of the low back. In: Twomey L, Taylor J (eds). *Physical therapy of the low back.* 3rd ed. New York; Churchill Livingstone: 2000.

90. Fann A. The prevalence of postural asymmetry in people with and without chronic low back pain. *Arch Phys Med Rehabil.* 2002;83:1736–1738.

91. Levangie PK. The association between static pelvic asymmetry and low back pain. *Spine.* 1999;15;24(12):1234–1242.

92. Dreyfuss P, Michaelsen M, Pauza K, McLarty J, Bogduk N. The value of medical history and physical examination in diagnosing sacroiliac joint pain. *Spine.* 1996;21:2594–2602.

93. Freburger J, Riddle D. Using published evidence to guide the examination of the sacroiliac joint region. *Phys Ther.* 2001;81:1135–1143.

94. Sturesson B, Uden A, Vleeming A. A radiostereometric analysis of movements of the sacroiliac joints during the standing hip flexion test. *Spine.* 2000;25:354–368.

95. Battie M, Cherkin D, Dunn R, Ciol M, Wheeler K. Managing low back pain: Attitudes and treatment preferences of physical therapist. *Phys Ther.* 1994;4(3):219–226.

96. Fitzgerald G, McClure P, Beattie P, Riddle D. Issues in determining treatment effectiveness of manual therapy. *Phys Ther.* 1994;74(3):227–233.

97. Petty N, Bach T, Cheek L. Accuracy of feedback during training of passive accessory intervertebral movements. *J Man Manip Ther.* 2001;9(2):99–108.

98. Di Fabio R. Efficacy of manual therapy. *Phys Ther.* 1992;72(12):853–864.

99. Harms M, Milton A, Cusick G, Bader D. Instrumentation of a mobilization couch for dynamic load measurements. *J Med Engineering Tech.* 1995;9(4):119–122.

100. Goodsell M, Lee M, Latimer J. Short-term effects of lumbar posteroanterior mobilization in individuals with low-back pain *J Manipulative Physiol Ther.* 2000;23(5):332–342.

101. Jull G, Bogduk N, Marsland A. The accuracy of a manual diagnosis for cervical zygapophysial joint pain syndromes. *Med J Aust.* 1998;148:233–236.

102. Behrsin J, Andrews F. Lumbar segmental instability: Manual assessment findings supported by radiological measurement. *Aust J Physiother.* 1991;37:171–173.

103. Bjornsdottir S, Kumar S. Posteroanterior spinal mobilization: State of the art review and discussion. *Disabil Rehabil.* 1997;19(2):39–46.

104. Matyas T, Bach T. The reliability of selected techniques in clinical arthrometrics. *Aust J Physiother.* 1985;31:175–199.

105. Carty G. A comparison of the reliability of manual tests of compliance using accessory movements in peripheral and spinal joints. Abstract. *Aust J Physiother.* 1986;32:1,68.

106. Gibson H, Ross J, Alien J, Latimer J, Maher C. The effect of mobilization on forward bending range. *J Man Manip Ther.* 1993;1:142–147.

107. McCollam R, Benson C. Effects of poster–anterior mobilization on lumbar extension and flexion. *J Man Manip Ther.* 1993;1:134–141.

108. Simmonds M, Kumar S, Lechelt E. Use of spinal model to quantify the forces and motion that occur during therapists' tests of spinal motion. *Phys Ther.* 1995;75:212–222.

109. Binkley J, Stratford P, Gill C. *Intertherapist reliability of lumbar accessory motion mobility testing.* In: Proceedings of the International Federation of Orthopaedic Manipulative Therapists 5th International Conference, Vail, CO: 1992.

110. Lee M, Mosely A, Refshauge K. Effects of feedback on learning a vertebral joint mobilizations skill. *Phys Ther.* 1990;10:97–102.

111. Harms M, Cusick G, Bader D. Measurement of spinal mobilisation forces. *Physiother.* 1995;81(10):559–604.

112. Maitland GD. *Maitland's vertebral manipulation.* 6th ed. London; Butterworth-Heinemann: 2001.

113. Viner A, Lee M. Direction of manual force applied during assessment of stiffness in the lumbosacral spine. *J Manipulative Physiol Ther.* 1997;18(7):441–447.

114. Maitland G, Hickling J. Abnormalities in passive movement: Diagrammative representation. *Physiother.* 1970;56:105–114.

115. Latimer J, Lee M, Adams R. The effect of training with feedback on physiotherapy students' ability to judge lumbar stiffness. *Man Ther.* 1996;1(5):26–70.

116. Latimer J, Adams R, Lee R. Training with feedback improves judgments of non-biological linear stiffness. *Man Ther.* 1998;3(2):85–89.

117. Chiradenjnant A, Latimer J, Maher C. Forces applied during manual therapy to patients with low back pain. *J Manipulative Physiol Ther.* 2002;25:362–369.

118. Maher C, Simmonds M, Adams R. Therapists' conceptualization and characterization of the clinical concept of spinal stiffness. *Phys Ther.* 1998;78:289–300.

119. Cook C, Turney L, Ramirez L, Miles A, Haas S, Karakostas T. Predictive factors in poor inter-rater reliability among physical therapists. *J Man Manip Ther.* 2002;10:200–205.

120. Yahia L, Audet J, Drouin G. Rheological properties of the human lumbar spine ligaments. *J Biomed Eng.* 1991;13:399–406.

121. Shirley D, Ellis E, Lee M. The response of posteroanterior lumbar stiffness to repeated loading. *Man Ther.* 2002;7:19–25.

122. Caling B, Lee M. Effect of direction of applied mobilization force on the posteroanterior response in the lumbar spine. *J Manipulative Physiol Ther.* 2001;24:71–78.

123. Edmondston S, Allison G, Gregg S, Purden G, Svansson G, Watson A. Effect of position on the posteroanterior stiffness of the lumbar spine. *Man Ther.* 1998;3:21–26.

124. Lee R, Evans J. An *in-vivo* study of the intervertebral movements produced by posteroanterior mobilization. *Clin Biomech.* 1997;12:400–408.

125. Keller TS, Colloca CJ, Gunzburg R. Neuromechanical characterization of in vivo lumbar spinal manipulation. Part I. Vertebral motion. *J Manipulative Physiol Ther.* 2003;26(9):567–578.

126. Wetzel FT, Donelson R. The role of repeated end-range/pain response assessment in the management of symptomatic lumbar discs. *Spine J.* 2003;3(2):146–154.

127. Seroussi RE, Krag MH, Muller DL, Pope MH. Internal deformations of intact and denucleated human lumbar discs subjected to compression, flexion, and extension loads. *J Orthop Res.* 1989;7(1):122–131.

128. Edmondston SJ, Allison GT, Gregg CD, Purden SM, Svansson GR, Watson AE. Effect of position on the posteroanterior stiffness of the lumbar spine. *Man Ther.* 1998;3(1):21–26.

129. Schnebel BE, Watkins RG, Dillin W. The role of spinal flexion and extension in changing nerve root compression in disc herniations. *Spine.* 1989;14(8):835–837.

130. Mol BW, Lijmer JG, Evers JL, Bossuyt PM. Characteristics of good diagnostic studies. *Semin Reprod Med.* 2003;21(1):17–25.

131. Laslett M, Young S, Aprill C, McDonald B. Diagnosing painful sacroiliac joints: A validity study of a McKenzie evaluation and sacroiliac provocation tests. *Aust J Physiotherapy.* 2003;49:89–97.

132. Fritz JM. Clinical prediction rules in physical therapy: Coming of age? *J Orthop Sports Phys Ther.* 2009;39(3): 159–161.

133. Twomey L, Taylor J. *Physical therapy of the low back.* 3rd ed. New York; Churchill Livingstone: 2000.

134. Grieve G. *Common vertebral joint problems.* 2nd ed. Edinburgh; Churchill Livingstone: 1988.

135. Tuttle N. Is it reasonable to use an individual patient's progress after treatment as a guide to ongoing clinical reasoning? *J Manipulative Physiol Ther.* 2009;32:396–402.

136. Garrison JC, Shanley E, Thigpen C, McEnroe S, Hegedus E, Cook C. *Between session changes predict overall perception of improvement but not functional improvement in patients with shoulder impingement syndrome seen for physical therapy: An observational study.* American Academy of Orthopedic Manual Physical Therapist. Washington, DC: September 2009.

Orthopedic Manual Therapy Clinical Examination

Chad E. Cook

Chapter

3

Objectives

- Outline the absolute and relative contraindications to manual therapy.
- Define the purpose of the clinical examination.
- Outline the essential elements of the clinical examination.
- Review the two components of observation.
- Analyze the essential aspects of the subjective patient history.
- Analyze the essential aspects of the objective physical history.
- Associate the findings of the examination and the clinical reasoning hypotheses.

Determining Who Is and Is Not a Manual Therapy Candidate

Prior to determining who is and isn't a manual therapy candidate it is worth reviewing the exact nature of manual therapy benefits, discussed in Chapter 1. Manual therapy provides either a biomechanical benefit, a neurophysiological benefit, or a psychological benefit. Manual therapy is best viewed as a means to an end, or a stepwise method toward overall improvement of the patient. Prior to any instance of use it is worth weighing the known benefits of manual therapy toward the risks or costs of use.

Subsequently, step one of determining who is and isn't a manual therapy candidate involves ruling out the presence of conditions that are outside the scope of manual therapy intervention or are potentially hazardous. This step involves "recognition of" or "ruling out" the presence of red flags. Red flags are signs and symptoms that may tie a disorder to a serious pathology.[1,2] When combinations or singular representations of selected red flag features are encountered during an examination, a clinician may improve their ability to assess the risk of a serious underlying pathology.[3] Differential assessment for red flags in individual patients by a clinician involves the use of specific tests and measures that trigger a predetermined threshold effect for clinical decision making.

To improve the understanding and investigation of red flags, a categorization approach to findings is recommended. Moreover, organizing red flags into three distinct categories (Table 3.1 ■) can aid the clinician in making the appropriate management decisions.[4] The presence of potentially life-threatening red flags, such as pulsatile abdominal masses, unexplained neurological deficits, and recent bowel and bladder changes (Category I findings), suggests serious pathology outside the domain of musculoskeletal disorders and may require immediate intervention by an appropriate specialist.

Red flags such as a cancer history, long-term corticosteroid use, metabolic bone disorder history, age greater than 50, unexplained weight loss, and failure of conservative management (Category II findings) demand additional patient questioning and requires the clinician to adopt selected examination methods. Additionally, Category II findings are best evaluated in clusters with other examination findings. For example, when evaluated individually, an age greater than 50 and/or long-term corticosteroid use may not warrant immediate attention by a specialist. However, when both factors are present the likelihood of a spinal compression fracture is dramatically increased and may merit increased attention from a specialist.[5] Furthermore, isolated findings of failure of conservative management, unexplained weight loss, cancer history, or age greater than 50 represent only

■ TABLE 3.1 Categorical Classification of Red Flag Findings during Medical Screening

Category	Conditions
Category 1: Factors that require immediate medical attention	• Pathological changes in bowel and bladder • Patterns of symptoms not compatible with mechanical pain (after physical exam) • Blood in sputum • Numbness or paresthesia in the perianal region • Progressive neurological deficit • Pulsatile abdominal masses • Neurological deficit not explained by monoradiculopathy • Elevated sedimentation rate
Category 2: Factors that require subjective questioning or contraindications to selected manual therapy techniques	• Impairment precipitated by recent trauma • Writhing pain • Nonhealing sores or wounds • Fever • Clonus (could be related to past or present CNS disorder) • Gait defects • History of cancer • History of a disorder with predilection for infection or hemorrhage • Long-term corticosteroid use • History of a metabolic bone disorder • Recent history of unexplained weight loss • Age > than 50 • Litigation for the current impairment • Long-term worker's compensation • Poor relationship with the employment supervisor
Category 3: Factors that require further physical testing and differentiation analysis	• Bilateral or unilateral radiculopathy or paresthesia • Unexplained significant lower or upper limb weakness • Abnormal reflexes

minor concerns during a clinical screening[5] but should be considered as a whole during decision making as the cluster may be associated with the presence of cancer.

Selected red flag findings, such as referred or radiating pain (examples of Category III findings), are common, require further physical differentiation tests, and are likely to alter management. These symptoms have been described as "pain perceived as arising or occurring in a region of the body innervated by nerves or branches of nerves other than those that innervate the actual source of pain".[6,7] This form of pain may arise from a number of pain generators including (1) mechanically irritated dorsal root ganglia that are healthy, inflamed, or ischemically damaged; (2) mechanically stimulated nerve roots that have been damaged; (3) somatic structures such as muscle, intervertebral disc, zygapophyseal joint, or sacroiliac joint; or (4) visceral structures such as the kidneys and/or prostate.[8]

How clinicians respond to each of the three categories of red flags depends on the clinician's intent for management. Many red flag findings are either absolute or relative contraindications for selected treatment strategies. Other red flags should warrant immediate medical attention and, perhaps, surgery. Information obtained from present complaints may range from solicitation of appropriate medical consultation to the use of a multidisciplinary treatment plan. Any of the historical physical examination or laboratory findings may function as a trigger to perform further testing.

Contraindications to Orthopedic Manual Therapy

Absolute versus Relative Contraindications

Some red flags discovered during the subjective or objective examination will identify comorbidities that do not necessitate the referral to appropriate medical personnel but do require special consideration. In these cases, where risk may outweigh the benefit of a specific procedure, contraindications for selected manual therapy procedures exist. Two forms of contraindications are possible: absolute and relative.

An **absolute contraindication** involves any situation in which the movement, stress, or compression placed on a particular body part involves a high risk of a deleterious consequence. A **relative contraindication** involves a situation that requires special care.[9] The presence of a relative contraindication suggests there is risk of injury associated with a selected treatment and considerable reflection should occur prior to use. Because selected treatment types have dissimilar elements of risk, the contraindications are divided into treatment categories versus a single list of factors.

Active Movements   There are a variety of techniques utilized within physical medicine for the treatment of associated range-of-motion losses, most notably static stretching, mobilization (also known as nonthrust manipulation), and manipulation (also known as thrust manipulation). Active movements are those initiated and performed by the patient and do not involve effort from the manual therapy clinician. Typically, active movements are used as home programs to continue the benefit of a manual therapy technique applied during formal care. In some occasions active movement is contraindicated (Table 3.2 ■).

Passive Movements
Static Stretching, Mobilization, and Manually Assisted Movements   Static stretching, mobilization, and manually assisted movements have demonstrated comparable force magnitudes, directions, and principles of application and similar effect sizes. Because of this, the three methods have been consolidated (Table 3.3 ■). Few studies have reported dire complications associated with the application of these techniques; nonetheless, a prudent manual therapist must be well aware of the associative contraindications.

Manipulation   In general, the question of safety risks associated with thrust manipulation (and nonthrust mobilization) is relatively clear (Table 3.4 ■). Hurwitz et al.[10] performed a large-scale randomized trial that consisted of thrust- and nonthrust-based treatments. The authors reported that complications associated with thrust- and nonthrust-based treatments were minimal with respect to the total procedures performed. A majority of complications were associated with treatment of the cervical spine and occurred during treatment that negatively affected the vertebral basilar

---

■ TABLE 3.2 Absolute and Relative Contraindications of Active Movement

Absolute contraindications	a. Malignancy of the targeted physiological region
	b. Cauda equina lesions producing disturbance of bowel or bladder
	c. Red flags including signs of neoplasm, fracture, or systemic disturbance
	d. Rheumatoid collagen necrosis
	e. Coronary artery dysfunction (unless active movements involve stabilization procedures)
	• Drop attacks, blackouts, loss of consciousness
	• Nausea, vomiting, and general lack of wellness
	• Dizziness or vertigo
	• Disturbance of vision including diplopia
	• Unsteadiness of gait and general feelings of weakness (intermittent)
	• Tingling or numbness (especially dysaesthesia, hemianaesthesia, or facial sensation)
	• Dysarthria or difficulty swallowing
	• Hearing disturbances
	• Headaches
	f. Unstable upper cervical spine (unless active movements involve stabilization procedures)
Relative contraindications	a. Active, acute inflammatory conditions
	b. Significant segmental stiffness
	c. Systematic diseases
	d. Neurological deterioration
	e. Irritability
	f. Osteoporosis (depending on the intent and direction of movement)
	g. Condition is worsening with present treatment
	h. Hamstring and upper limb stretching on acute nerve root irritations

■ **TABLE 3.3** Absolute and Relative Contraindications to Passive Movements (i.e., Mobilization, Stretching, and Manually Assisted Movements)

Absolute contraindications	a. Malignancy of the targeted physiological region
	b. Cauda equina lesions producing disturbance of bowel or bladder
	c. Red flags including signs of neoplasm, fracture, or systemic disturbance
	d. Rheumatoid collagen necrosis
	e. Unstable upper cervical spine
	f. Coronary artery dysfunction
	• Drop attacks, blackouts, loss of consciousness
	• Nausea, vomiting, and general unwellness
	• Dizziness or vertigo
	• Disturbance of vision including diplopia
	• Unsteadiness of gait and general feelings of weakness (intermittent)
	• Dysarthria or difficulty swallowing
	• Hearing disturbances
	• Headaches (unless headache lessens with continued application)
	• Tingling or numbness (especially dysaesthesia, hemianaesthesia, or facial sensation)
Relative contraindications	a. Previously defined relative contraindications
	• Active, acute inflammatory conditions
	• Significant segmental stiffness
	• Systematic diseases
	• Neurological deterioration
	• Irritability
	• Osteoporosis (depending on the intent and direction of movement)
	• Condition is worsening with present treatment
	b. Acute nerve root irritation (radiculopathy)
	• When subjective and objective symptoms don't add up
	• Any patient condition (handled well) that is worsening
	• Use of oral contraceptives (if cervical spine)
	• Long-term oral corticosteroid use (if cervical spine)
	c. Immediately postpartum (if noncervical spine)
	d. Blood-clotting disorder

artery. Although some patients reported the occurrence of some symptoms associated with vertebral basilar artery testing, those individuals who recorded negative consequences had premeditating components associated with potential stroke such as smoking, hypertension, or arteriosclerosis. These considerations should be apparent during the patient history far prior to the application of thrust- and nonthrust-based manipulation.

In a comprehensive literature review, DiFabio[11] suggested that thrust- and nonthrust-based manipulation may be effective for the treatment of cervical conditions, but use does involve a risk of injury involving lesions of the brainstem, most specifically with disruption of the vertebral artery during cervical thrust manipulation. Physical therapists were less involved than other practitioners in injury totals, which accounted for less than 2%.[11] Physical therapists tend to be less involved in potential incidents, with less than one event for every 1,573 manipulations, while chiropractors were involved in one for every 476 cervical manipulations.

Summary

- Contraindications to manual therapy exist in two forms: relative and absolute.

- A relative contraindication involves a situation that requires special care, but does not negate the use of the technique.

- An absolute contraindication involves any situation in which the movement, stress, or compression placed on a particular body part involves a high risk of a deleterious consequence.

- Of the litany of manual therapy techniques, thrust manipulation displays the highest quantity of contraindications.

- Of the areas of the body that demonstrate the highest risk for manual therapy, the upper cervical spine has been linked to the most complications.

■ **TABLE 3.4** Absolute and Relative Contraindications to Manipulation

Absolute contraindications	a. Previously defined absolute contraindications
	• Malignancy of the targeted physiological region
	• Cauda equina lesions producing disturbance of bowel or bladder
	• Red flags including signs of neoplasm, fracture, or systemic disturbance
	• Rheumatoid collagen necrosis
	• Coronary artery dysfunction
	• Unstable upper cervical spine (unless active movements involve stabilization procedures)
	b. Practitioner lack of ability
	c. Spondylolisthesis
	d. Gross foraminal encroachment
	e. Children/teenagers
	f. Pregnancy
	g. Fusions
	h. Psychogenic disorders
	i. Immediately postpartum
Relative contraindications	a. Previously defined relative contraindications
	b. Active, acute inflammatory conditions
	c. Significant segmental stiffness
	d. Systematic diseases
	e. Neurological deterioration
	f. Irritability
	g. Osteoporosis (depending on the intent and direction of movement)
	h. Condition is worsening with present treatment
	i. Acute nerve root irritation (radiculopathy)
	j. When subjective and objective symptoms don't add up
	k. Any patient condition (handled well) that is worsening
	l. Use of oral contraceptives (if cervical spine)
	m. Long-term oral corticosteroid use (if cervical spine)
	n. Immediately postpartum (if noncervical spine)
	o. Blood-clotting disorder

Detailed Elements of the Clinical Examination Process

Once red flags or conditions that lie outside the scope of manual therapy are ruled out, a comprehensive clinical examination is warranted. There are a number of purposes to a clinical examination. First, an understanding of the patient's full condition, classification of impairments, and likelihood of recovery are essential in the long-term care of the patient. Some patients will benefit from a manual therapy treatment whereas others are more likely to benefit from a different form of intervention. The clinical examination helps determine this by examining the patient's response to the clinical examination sequence.

The purpose of a manual therapy clinical examination is to outline the movements, positions, or activities that produce, reduce, or selectively modify the patient's "familiar signs and symptoms," (**concordant signs**). Only during a systematic examination can a clinician outline the behavior of the patient's symptoms. This scheme is described as the *patient response method*, a method that relies less on theory and more on immediate and carryover patient responses. The patient response-based model is designed to determine selected impairments and does not focus on the isolation of a dedicated pathology.

Gregory Grieve[12] wrote:
the meaning of each sign and symptom in itself has much greater importance for treatment indications than for diagnosis. It is not especially difficult to decide "this is a degenerative joint condition." We have to note how, and in what kind of patient…(examples of multiple variables associated with patient type)…and has a bearing on how we proceed, as does coexistent disease and past history.

Three different examination domains—observation, patient history (subjective), and physical examination (objective)—impart essential information for treatment planning and endorse hypotheses of the type of physical impairment and related functional, physical, psychological, and social problems. These examination domains are outlined in detail in the following section of this chapter. Throughout the textbook, each region-specific section will follow the format outlined below.

1. Observation
2. Patient History
3. Physical Examination
   a. Structural Differentiation Tests
   b. Active Physiological Movements
   c. Passive Physiological Movements
   d. Passive Accessory Movements
   e. Special Clinical Tests

Structural differentiation tests are not always performed and may consist of highly sensitive special clinical tests or active movements with overpressure to "clear" a region. Although structural differentiation tests are generally performed earlier in the examination than special clinical tests, these tests are discussed (when pertinent) later in the special clinical tests section of each chapter. In many cases, special clinical tests are also used early to rule out the presence of red flags or conditions. The reader is recommended to closely scrutinize which special tests are actually useful at performing these methods by incorporating evidence-based summaries of special tests.

Observation

Observation is informally divided into two categories: general inspection and introspection. The process of "general inspection" includes the examination of outwardly apparent factors that may or may not associate to the patient's impairment. Introspection includes the aggregation of outwardly apparent information with selected psychological and social factors potentially related to the patient's condition.

General Inspection   The purpose of the **general inspection** is to examine visible static and movement-related defects for analysis during the subjective (history) and objective (physical) examination. Commonly, the static general inspection consists of skin (integument) inspection, posture, and body symmetry. Skin inspection may yield valuable information on past injuries (scars), inflammatory processes (redness, swelling), and sympathetic contributions to pain. Although posture and body symmetry alone do not dictate the presence of impairment, it is feasible to assume that these conditions may contribute to underlying pathologies. At present, there are no studies that have calculated any direct predictive observational relationship with any form of progression

or predisposition to spinal impairment.[13] Postural asymmetry has no correlation with back pain and other forms of pelvic asymmetry are even less conclusive.[14] Nonetheless, dramatic postural faults are worth further investigation and can be the basis for future exploration in many anatomical regions, especially when examined in conjunction with other assessment concepts.[15,16] Although the observations may not be exclusively predictive, these can provide clinically useful information that improves the expansion of the treatment hypothesis.

Introspection   **Introspection** allows the clinician to step back and analyze the relationship of nonphysical findings with physical findings. Examples include patient attitude, facial expressions during movement, expressions of pain, gender and the potential association to selected impairments, and believability. Patients may express a decreased willingness to move, a finding that has been related to poor treatment outcomes.[17,18] Avoidance of certain movements because of fear of reinjury or increased pain is common in patients with chronic low back impairment.[18] This reluctance to move may lead to a cascade of further problems associated with disuse.

Summary

- Observation involves the careful identification of potential contributors to the patient's impairments.
- The presence of a postural fault or body asymmetry does not dictate a pathology or impairment.
- Introspection involves the careful examination of both physical and nonphysical contributors to the impairment.

Patient History

Patient history is a useful guide in outlining the ease in which symptoms are aggravated, the activities that contribute to the concordant sign, and the relationship of the history findings to the physical measures assessed.[19] Generally, there are three major goals of a patient history: (1) to characterize the problem and to establish potential causes; (2) to determine the effect of the problem on patient lifestyle; and (3) to monitor the response to treatment for examination of effectiveness.[20]

Although history taking is often considered the most important aspect of a clinical evaluation, few studies have evaluated how subjective findings contribute to problem solving for treatment application.[20] Nonetheless, those that have investigated history taking are also stratified into diagnostic and impairment-based methods. For clinicians who use a diagnostic-based examination method, history taking appears to play a favorable part, providing a significant value in the diagnostic process.[21]

For clinicians who have adopted the impairment-based examination method, history and subjective findings have also demonstrated usefulness when combined with a purposeful physical examination. In studies that examined the history-taking strategies of clinical experts, engagement with the family and patient was more extensive, often prompting questions regarding the nature of the disorder versus questions that attempt to isolate a specific pathology.[19] Those who used the impairment-based model focused more on how the symptoms were related to movements and activities and less on how the symptoms were related to a diagnosis.[19]

The patient history involves both clinician and patient expectations. Patients aspire to fully characterize their current symptoms and the impact of the disorder in both physical and psychological terms. Often, clinicians are interested in clustering selected signs and symptoms for the appropriate selection of a treatment intervention[20,22] or interpreting the nature and severity of the condition at hand.[19] In many cases, the desires of the two are not the same or may address different purposes.

Some evidence exists that lends support to the idea that effective history taking is related to a desired outcome. Walker et al.[23] identified that subjective history, specifically report of activity requirements, was associated with future outcome and performance. By means of systematically obtaining information, the clinician can obtain information on the origin, contribution, and potential prognosis of a condition. Table 3.5 ■ outlines the appropriate components of an effective subjective history.

Mechanism and Description of Injury   The mechanism of the injury is the detailed recital of what the patient was doing when he or she injured themselves. In some circumstances, the mechanisms can provide useful information to the identification of the potential tissue. More importantly, the description of the injury provides a documentation of the "essence" of the problem. This involves two forms: (1) explanation and description of the injury-related pain and (2) the timing of when the event occurred. The identification of the pain from the injury is further expounded during the discussion of the concordant sign and nature of the problem, whereas the timing of the event is closely associated with the stage of the disorder. Both components enable the patient to meet their expectations of discussing the condition at hand.

Concordant Sign   The concordant pain response is an activity or movement that provokes the patient's "familiar sign".[24] Laslett et al.[24] define the concordant familiar sign as the pain or other symptoms identified on a pain drawing and verified by the patient as being the complaint that has prompted one to seek diagnosis and treatment. Maitland[25] described a similar focal point identified as the **comparable sign.** A comparable joint or neural sign refers to any combination of pain, stiffness, and spasm that the clinician finds during examination and considers comparable with the patient's symptoms. This text uses the two terms synonymously and recognizes that Maitland's contribution to this concept has been significant to orthopedic manual therapists.

Laslett et al.[24] suggests that one should focus on the patient's concordant (comparable) sign, and should distinguish this finding from other symptoms produced during physical assessment. They identify a finding that may be painful or abnormal, but not related to the concordant sign as the "discordant pain response." Essentially, a discordant pain response is the provocation of a pain that is unlike the pain for which the patient sought treatment. Maitland[25] identified a similar term called the "joint sign." Similar to

■ **TABLE 3.5** The Systematic Process of the Subjective History Examination

Category	Primary Purpose
Mechanism and description of problem	To determine the cause of the injury and to elicit a careful explanation of the symptoms.
Concordant sign	To determine the movement associated with the pain of the individual.
Nature of the condition	To determine the severity, irritability, kind, and stage of the impairment.
Behavior of the symptoms	To understand how the symptoms change with time, movement, and activities.
Pertinent past and present medical history	To determine if potential related medical components are associated with this disorder, or may lead to retardation of healing.
Patient goals	To understand the patient's goal behind organized care.
The baseline (function or pain)	To elicit a baseline measure to reevaluate over time.

a **discordant sign,** the joint sign may appear to implicate a guilty structure but may not be associated with the pathology whatsoever. Maitland[25] suggested avoidance of the tendency to focus on joint signs, which he defines as any aspect of a movement that is "abnormal." Because the term "joint sign" is somewhat confusing and infers that the pain or abnormality of the region is solely associated with a joint, the term "discordant sign" is used here.

Although the concordant sign is queried during the patient history, this phenomenon is also a physical response determined during the objective exam, requires inspection during the physical assessment, and requires further examination throughout the length of the intervention. The concordant sign is often used as a litmus test to determine both mechanical and pain-related changes over time.

The Nature of the Condition The nature of the condition is a reflection of the internalization of the patient's condition. The nature of the condition may alter how the examination and treatment is performed and may influence the aggressiveness of the clinician. Although many manual therapy models use variations of "nature," there are typically three representative aspects explored by each: (1) severity, (2) irritability, and (3) stage.

Severity of the Disorder Severity is the subjective identification of how significantly the problem has affected the patient. Typically, a severe problem will result in a reduction in activity of daily living functions, work-related problems, social disruption, and leisure activities. Severity may be associated with unwanted alterations or changes in lifestyle. The clinician should endeavor to determine where the patient's impairment lies on a continuum of nuisance or disability. Many functional outcomes scales are designed to measure the severity of the impairment and are effective in collecting aggregate data.

Irritability **Irritability** or "reactivity" is a term used to define the stability of a present condition. In essence, irritability denotes how quickly a stable condition degenerates in the presence of pain-causing inputs. Patients with irritability may often be leery of aggressive treatment because they will typically worsen with selected activities.[25–27] Patients who exhibit irritable symptoms may respond poorly to an aggressive examination and treatment approaches. Irritability is operationally defined using three criteria: (1) What does the patient have to do to set this condition off?; (2) Once set off, how long do the symptoms last and how severe are the symptoms?; and (3) What does the patient have to do to calm the symptoms down? The irritability of the patient will guide the comprehensiveness of the examination and will dictate the selection and aggressiveness of treatment procedures.

One common pitfall is the assumption that acute disorders are always irritable. Although irritability is seen more commonly in acute disorders, chronic disorders may also demonstrate irritability. Subjective clues to the likely presence of irritability are interrupted sleep, heavy doses of medications, limited levels of activity or activity avoidance, and/or a diagnosis suggesting serious pathology. Patients presenting with recent trauma, arachnoiditis, fractures, and acute arthritis are prone to being irritable. However, patients with chronic arthritis, especially osteoarthritis related to stiffness, are usually not irritable and may respond well to vigorous treatment.

Another pitfall is the supposition that irritability is synonymous with a patient who is in a significant amount of pain. This thinking ignores that patients without pain, or without significant pain, can be irritable. Patients with serious pathology may not always present with significant pain. Patients with noteworthy neurological changes are often irritable and may demonstrate little or no pain.

Stage Most impairments change over time. A skilled manual clinician is able to understand the path or progression of the disorder, a concept identified as the "stage".[25] The stage of an injury or impairment involves a snapshot of how the patient identifies their current level of dysfunction as compared to a given point in the past. This allows examination of whether the condition has stabilized, stagnated, or progressed. Consequently, there are only three potential reports for the stage of a disorder; worse, better, or the same, with variations in the level of "worse" or "better."

The stage of a disorder identifies the "snapshot" of that patient's condition in a cycle of natural progression. The cycle of an injury is very complicated and involves numerous steps. The onset of an injury often leads to an inflammatory process and a consequential cascade of comorbidities. First, muscle inhibition is common and can lead to decreased active stability at the site of injury. Decreased stability can lead to increased capsuloligamentous laxity and hypermobility.[28] As demand is placed upon the joint segment, reflexogenic spasm attempts to stabilize the region.[29,30] Unfortunately, this mechanism often contributes to muscular pain, ineffective stabilization, and supplementary weakness.[30,31] The joint no longer tracks or responds efficiently to required demands. Because the joint is unable to stabilize effectively against outside forces, continued trauma leads to degeneration of the segments. Throughout the process of degeneration, reflexive spasms continue in a subconscious attempt to stabilize the segment.[30] This degeneration culminates into boney, cartilage, and ligamentous changes that modify the arthrokinematics of the segment.[32] These changes are the hallmark components associated with losses in range of motion.[33]

Behavior of Symptoms   There are three aspects of the "behavior" of the pain: (1) time, (2) response to movements, and (3) area. First, it is critical to determine how the pain changes over a 24-hour period. Conditions associated with inflammation may worsen during rest or aggressive movements.[25] Noninflammatory conditions may worsen during very aggressive unguarded movements. Sinister problems (non-mechanical disorders that are potentially life threatening) often yield worsening symptoms at night. Second, the behavior of the symptoms is necessary to determine whether a specific movement pattern exists. Some conditions are worse in various postures or positions, whereas others demonstrate improvement or deterioration during repeated movements. Third, isolation of the area of the symptoms is necessary to determine potentially contributing structures. In some conditions, there may be more than one site of pain.[34] Regardless of the tissue diagnosis, the patient should be questioned regarding neighboring tissues. Failure to ascertain the total area of symptoms may lead to inappropriate or incomplete administration of treatment.

Pertinent Past and Present History   The pertinent past and present history assist in identifying contributing components that may affect the presence of the impairment. An investigation of similar past conditions, related disorders, and general health considerations yields valuable information. One may ask relevant medical questions as well within this domain, including information to distill potential red flags to recovery. Lastly, associative medications, surgeries, and comparable past and present treatment may generate ideas for effective care.

Patient Goals   The patient's goals will drive what the patient hopes to get out of the rehabilitation experience. The goals should also influence the treatment plan as these will be the milestones for the patient. Although there is little research in this area, there does appear to be a relationship between the selected goals and the patient and the likelihood of accomplishing the outcome. In a recent study that investigated return to work, the patient's return to work date (goal) was the single best predictor of return to work outcome. In contrast, the increased number of premorbid jobs, compensation status, patient's race, and gender were not predictive. This suggests that the

assessment of an individual's motivation (by using goal setting) may be a key factor in predicting a favorable outcome.[34]

Another benefit of obtaining a list of patients' goals is the ability to assess their perception or expectations of their outcomes. It is probable that a patient who does not expect an efficacious treatment outcome will recover as quickly as one who expects an efficacious outcome. Additionally, the patient goal is a reflection of his or her perceived assessment of the nature of the problem.

The Baseline   The **baseline** is the base functional performance or self-reported pain level prior to the treatment intervention. For a quick reference, one can use an iteration of a visual analog scale for pain (a 0–10 pain scale),[34,35] appropriate range-of-motion measurements, or some other easily repeatable value. Since the baseline is measured during each assessment position, each treatment, and during the beginning and end of each session, this simple comparative value should lack complexity but represent an overall picture of the condition at hand. Additionally, a baseline measure of function provides comparable and essential information for future measurement.

Putting the Subjective History Examination Findings Together

By the end of the subjective history, the clinician should have the following criteria:

1. A list (or no findings) that represents potential red flags or items that require further testing to "rule out" a condition.
2. Post-subjective set of competing hypotheses (an educated guess of the primary structures involved and the potential pain generators). The post-subjective hypotheses may allow the clinician to isolate certain components of the physical examination for more specific findings.
3. An understanding of the patient's appropriateness for manual therapy. Some clues within the patient history (such as report of stiffness) may drive the selection of manual therapy methods of examination and treatment.
4. The nature of the problem, characterized by the severity, irritability, and stage of the condition. These three areas provide information that can modify the vigor of the examination and treatment.
5. The patient's expectations and prediction of the outcome (through goals). Often, the patient's goals and expectations will drive their participation within the program. Additionally, this provides communication between the patient

and clinician for use later during the intent of the treatment.

6. The concordant sign of the patient and a hypothesis of what physical activities may be associated with it. The concordant sign will drive the examination and the treatment. The concordant sign, although also a manifestation of the physical examination, is the most important aspect of the manual therapist's examination.

Summary

- The history is a useful guide in outlining the ease in which symptoms are aggravated, the activities that contribute to the concordant sign, and the relationship to the physical measures assessed.
- The history is often considered the most important aspect of the examination.
- There are seven primary components of the subjective history: the mechanism and description of injury, the concordant sign, the nature of the problem, the behavior of the symptoms, the pertinent past and present medical history, the patient's goals, and the baseline. Each has a specific purpose.
- The purpose of the mechanism and description of the injury is to determine the cause of the injury and to elicit a careful explanation of the symptoms.
- The purpose of determining the concordant sign is to identify the movement or position associated with the pain of the individual.
- The purpose of determining the nature of the problem is to define the severity, irritability, kind, and stage of the impairment.
- The purpose of determining the behavior of the symptoms is to understand how the symptoms change with time, movement, and activities.
- The purpose of determining the pertinent past and present medical history is to determine if potential related medical components are associated to this disorder, or may lead to retardation of healing.
- The purpose in determining the patient's goals is to understand the patient's goal behind organized care.
- The purpose behind eliciting a baseline measure is to identify an easily obtainable value that allows reevaluation over time.

The Physical Examination

The physical examination's principal aim is to establish the influence of movement on the patient's concordant symptoms that were described during the patient history.[34] By assessing movement, the orthopedic manual therapist is more likely to determine the contributory muscles, joints, or ligaments involved in the patient's condition. Most importantly, the use of movement to alter symptoms enables determination of an appropriate treatment method and how that method would positively or negatively contribute to the patient's condition.

Orthopedic manual therapy treatment areas encompass innumerable methods of classification. In essence, most techniques will take the form of three particular categories, each based on the method of application and participation by the patient. For clarification, these skilled methods are outlined in the following three categories:

1. *Active movements* (includes active physiological techniques performed exclusively by the patient).
2. *Passive movements* (includes passive physiological, passive accessory, and occasionally combined passive movements performed exclusively by the clinician).
3. *Special clinical testing* (includes palpation, muscle provocation testing, upper and lower motor screening, differentiation tests, neurological testing, and any specific clinical tests designed to implicate a lesion).

Active Movements

Active movements are any form of physiological movement performed exclusively by the patient. In a clinical examination, the purpose of an active movement is to identify and examine the influence of selected active movements on the concordant sign. By determining the behavior of the concordant sign to selected movements, the clinician can identify potential active physiological treatment approaches.

It has been suggested that the pattern associated with active movements may be beneficial in identifying selected impairments. McKenzie has developed a classification scheme for the low back using this philosophy.[36] Using McKenzie's approach the patient's response to postural and repeated movements is recorded and classified for potential treatment application. Active movement patterns have also been suggested as helpful in implicating contractile versus noncontractile components; when scrutinized, this method of assessment is not precise and has not held up irrefutably.[37,38] Additionally, selected active movements are often assigned as home exercise programs and adjuncts to passive treatments.

The recommended procedure within this textbook for exploring the benefit of active movement assessment involves three stages of movements and an examination of the patient response during these stages. The initial movement involves a single active movement to the initiation of pain, if pain occurs prior to the limit or end range. The movement is held in this position and the patient's pain assessed for change. This procedure is followed by movement past the pain to the limit (if the patient is able to move to this point).

Again, the patient is asked to hold this position to determine the behavior of the pain. Lastly, the patient is asked to repeat the movement at end range to further assess the response of the patient.

1. The patient moves to the first point of pain (response is assessed).
2. The patient then moves beyond the pain and holds (response is assessed).
3. The patient then repeats the movement to determine if pain or range changes (response is assessed).

In the absence of pain, an **overpressure** is applied. The use of overpressure is designed to "rule out" potential movements and directions, which do not contribute to the patient's impairment and may be useful in isolating various impairments.[34] Overpressure is less effective when one attempts to dictate the presence of a specific pathology based on "feel" of the end range. An overpressure should be limited to differentiation between the concordant signs versus discordant signs and symptoms, or to identify if no symptoms are present.

There are several conjectures to examine when evaluating the influence of active movement on impairment. First, positive (or good) patient responses include an increase of range of motion, a reduction of pain, or both. The procedure (i.e., movement into flexion, abduction, internal rotation, etc.) that was responsible for the greatest abolition of pain or increase in range is considered the best potential selection for a treatment. Second, if symptoms were produced, how did the symptoms respond to single or repeated movements? Often, repeated movements will abolish symptoms, especially during mechanical dysfunction.[39] Third, where within the range did the symptoms worsen? End-range pain is typically associated with a mechanical impairment, whereas mid- or through-range pain may be indicative of an inflammatory impairment or instability.[25] Fourth, it is imperative to investigate how the patient yields to a particular movement. Since the intent to treat may require repeated movements into a movement that is initially painful, it is important to consider how faithfully the patient would commit to adoption of this potential strategy. Lastly, are there other factors that could potentially contribute to this problem? Is the movement sequential? Does there appear to be a range restriction or hypermobility? Is weakness a consideration?

Passive Movements

Passive movements are any planar or physiological motions that are performed exclusively by the clinician. The purpose of a passive movement is to identify and examine the influence of selected passive movements (repeated or static) on the concordant sign. Passive movements include (1) passive physiological motions, (2) passive accessory movements, and (3) combined passive movements.

Passive Physiological Movements Passive physiological movements are "movements which are actively used in the many functions of the musculoskeletal system."[34] Passive physiological movements are commonly defined in kinesiological literature as osteokinematic motions and generally are categorized using plane-based descriptors such as flexion, extension, adduction, abduction, and medial or lateral rotation. Passive physiological movements occur simultaneously with accessory motions; the degree of freedom and the availability of motion is a product of that accessory mobility.

Assessment of passive physiological movement is useful to differentiate total range of motion at a particular joint segment. Cyriax and Cyriax[38] claimed that passive physiological movements were necessary to assess the contribution of ligaments, capsules, and other inert structures to the cause of the impairment. On occasions where patients are unable or fearful to move the joint to end range, the apparent range may be mistakenly assessed as limited. To determine the true range of motion, a passive physiological movement is required.

The examination procedure for passive physiological movements is similar to the active physiological process. First, the patient is moved passively to the first point of pain identified by the patient. At that point, the amount and intensity of the pain is recorded by the clinician. Next, the patient is moved beyond the first point of pain and held in that position. Again, the patient is examined for response. Lastly, the patient is moved repeatedly near the limit of motion and changes in range or pain are recorded.

Procedure for Examination of Passive Physiological Range

1. The patient's selected body part is moved to the first point of reported pain (response is assessed).
2. The patient is then moved beyond the pain and held (response is assessed).
3. The clinician then repeats the movement to determine if pain or range changes (response is assessed).

This within-session process of examining symptoms has been shown to correctly identify patients who are most likely to demonstrate between-session changes.[45] Although laborious, this process provides the most specific marriage between the examination and potential treatment options.

Passive Accessory Movements Grieve[12] indicates that a passive accessory movement is "any movement mechanically or manually applied to a body with no voluntary muscular activity by the patient." Passive accessory mobilizations are best divided into two forms: regional and local mobilizations. Regional mobilizations involve directed passive movement to more than one given area, segment, or physiological component, whereas a local mobilization is specific and directed to one segment and/or joint region.[12] Within the spine, the majority of mobilization procedures advocated within this textbook involve regional mobilizations. Posterior–anterior (PA) mobilizations involve three-point movements of the primary targeted and neighboring segments[40,41] and move the adjacent segments as well as the targeted segment.[42]

Techniques that qualify as local or "targeted-specific" require a locking of the adjacent joint segments to foster greater movement at the targeted level. Generally, locking is facilitated through a procedure called apposition, which occurs when joint surfaces are most congruent and when ligamentous structures are maximally taut.[43] When treating the spine, targeting the appropriate level leads to better outcomes than when a randomly selected joint is treated in the lumbar spine[44] but not the cervical spine.[45,46] Locking a segment of the cervical spine is often not specific to the site of interest[47] and the overall specificity of treatment applications is indeed questionable. With regard to the periphery, a targeted-specific mobilization is less studied.

When addressing peripheral dysfunction, passive accessory movements are effective for engaging selected components of the capsule and ligament and for optimum assessment, passive assessment should occur at multiple ranges throughout the physiological availability to determine range–pain behavior. Additionally, passive movements throughout the range of motion will provide range–pain behavior.

Another consideration is whether or not to treat within open-packed or close-packed positions. Close-packed positions are those that theoretically tighten the ligaments and capsule maximally and create maximal congruency of a joint. Open-packed positions are those positions that do not place maximal tension on the capsule, and have been described by Cyriax and Cyriax[38] and Kaltenborn.[48] Treatment in open-packed positions may be useful if the patient is in significant pain. Mobilization at the close-packed position may be useful if gaining maximal range of motion is the primary interest. A particular close-packed position could vary from one individual to another or may be associated with the pathological condition of the individual. Despite the widespread use of paradigms such as capsular patterns and theoretical close-packed positions, this method of categorizing inert tissue has not stood up well to scrutiny and may be inappropriate for selected tissues.[49–51]

During the examination procedure for passive accessory movements, the articular movements are evaluated for reproduction of the concordant sign. Using either a translatory or rolling motion, the patient's segment is moved passively to the first point of pain identified by the patient; the intensity of the pain is then recorded by the clinician using some mechanism of scale. Next, the clinician applies a force that moves the segment beyond the first point of pain. The joint is held in that position and the response of the patient is re-elicited. Lastly, the clinician uses repeated movements near the limit of motion to determine if changes in range or pain have occurred.

1. The patient's selected body part is moved to the first point of reported pain (response is assessed).
2. The patient is then moved beyond the pain and held (response is assessed).
3. The clinician then repeats or sustains the movement to determine if pain or range changes (response is assessed).

Combined Movements Brian Edwards[19] purported that **combined movements** are habitual movements of the spine, and that "movements of the vertebral column occur in combination across planes rather than as pure movements in one plane." Movements of the periphery are also adopted in this definition. Therefore, a physical examination should be expanded to include combined movements because the standard movements of lateral flexion, extension, and flexion, and occasionally rotation are single-plane movements.

Combined movements are frequently used during manipulative procedures. Often, coupling movements are termed in osteopathic literature as a "locked" position.[43] Grieve[12] stated "the appreciation of the difference between the feel of a 'locked' joint and one that has not achieved a 'crisp or locked' end-feel is vital in determining the appropriate combined movement".[43] In reality, locking a joint has demonstrated less usefulness during outcomes and may not actually occur in the context originally considered.[47] Nonetheless, locking a joint is considered an essential skill for a manual therapist and is a requirement for targeted-specific techniques.

Cyriax and Cyriax[38] have proposed a measurement system to describe end-feels among various joints. Although the end-feel characterization is not specific to combined movements, the reliability of end-feel assessment based on Cyriax's theories is mixed.[52,53] Those studies that examined the presence of pain and abnormal end-feel concurrently[54] or provided further educational constructs associated with end-feel[55] demonstrated the best interrater reliability. The reliability of ligamentous detection methods that do not use a categorical system such as Cyriax and Cyriax's has fared much worse.[51,56]

In the periphery, combined movements are often necessary to place tension on selected ligamentous and capsular structures. For example, in the shoulder, maximal tension for the posteroinferior glenohumeral ligament occurs during internal rotation and elevation whereas maximal tension of the posterosuperior capsule occurs during internal rotation at lower shoulder elevations.[57,58] Subsequently, to engage the numerous capsular and ligamentous components, one would be required to move the shoulder into combined, multi-physiological positions.

The same process as active and passive movement examination is relevant for combined movements.

1. The patient's selected body part is moved to the first point of reported pain (response is assessed).
2. The patient is then moved beyond the pain and held (response is assessed).
3. The clinician then repeats the movement to determine if pain or range changes (response is assessed).

Combined movements may take many forms. For example, two active movements can be combined, as can two physiological or accessory motions. Additionally, the combination of an active physiological with a passive physiological, active physiological with a passive accessory, or a passive accessory with a passive physiological can increase the number of potential movements dramatically.

Fine-Tuning Mechanisms   During assessment of the influence of movement on a patient's condition, there are several conjectural considerations to examine. If the patient reports decreased pain, increased range, or both during the movement, the action that was responsible for the greatest abolition of pain or increase in range is considered the best potential selection for a treatment. Whether the best response occurred through single movements or repeated movements should be assessed. An investigation of best response during end range or mid range is also worth noting. Often, an assessment is made whether a patient is applicable for a manipulation during both passive physiological and passive accessory movements.[59]

Since assessment of passive accessory movement mandates an analysis of concordant pain behavior through various means, one should optimize the use of differentiation of targeted pain generators (i.e., one spine level vs. another; the origin of pain from the shoulder vs. the cervical spine). Many forms of impairment have associated aches and pains, yet the concordant sign is the passive movement that most appropriately isolates the true impairment.[24]

Lee and Svensson[60] outline variables that may alter both assessment findings and treatment outcome during application of accessory movements. Although the authors presented these variables with respect to application during spinal examination and treatment, there is overlay to peripheral tissues. Because each variable may be altered by the manual therapy clinician, we discuss these in the context of examination in this chapter, and in the context of treatment in Chapter 4.

Magnitude of Force   The magnitude of the force will clearly influence the amount of joint displacement.[61] In studies that have investigated the spine, a reasonable pattern has emerged. Increases in applied force will result in corresponding increases in linear displacement.[60] Most studies have suggested that a critical threshold exists before linear movement occurs. Prior to reaching the threshold, low load forces will most likely move soft tissues and will not result in linear movements. Lee et al.[61] claim that the range for linear assessment appears to exist in the order of 30–100 Newtons. Edwards[62] suggested that although the force for initial assessment is typically taken to the first point of pain, in some cases, it is necessary to push beyond to acquire reasonable joint behavioral characteristics. Often (i.e., inflammatory conditions), the first point of pain occurs early within the assessment and may not engage the 30–100 threshold. Failure to meet each joint's specific threshold most likely represents failure to comprehensively analyze the movement of that given segment.

Rate of Increase of Force   Fung[63] suggests that increases in the frequency of mobilization will result in an increase in resistance to deformation. Thus, it is expected that during a manual assessment, an increase in frequency during linear assessment of a given segment may appear stiffer. Consequently, frequency of the accessory motion during the assessment will alter the clinician's identification of stiffness, creating another intrinsic variable that alters interrater reliability.

Duration of Loading   There is some controversy regarding the influences of tissue mobility during the application of load over a given time. Lee et al.[61] reports that prolonged load results in an increase in deformation. Shirley et al.[64] reported an increase in stiffness and displacement over time. In other words, repeated loads over time will lead to greater stiffness assessment at end range, although linear movements prior to end range should increase.

Targeted Tissue to Which the Force is Applied   In the spine, the segment is a significant predictor of the detection of stiffness. Contributions from the pelvis, other segments, and from the respiratory system[64] can alter the assessment of stiffness per segment. Morphological characteristics may alter findings as well since soft tissue is both a supportive mechanism during application in force and is generally the first tissue displaced during assessment.

Location of Manual Force in Relation to the Center of the Targeted Structure   Maitland suggested that for optimum reliability across assessments, the starting point of assessment should be near the center of the targeted structures.[25] Lee[65] confirmed that a substantial effect does exist, depending on where the force is applied on the targeted segment.

Direction of Force   The direction of mobilization forces can alter the amount of stiffness measured by machines and perceived by therapists. Caling and Lee[66] determined that stiffness measured at plus or minus 10° from a perpendicular base direction (defined as the mean direction of force applied by experienced therapists), was 7–10% less than the stiffness measured in the perpendicular direction. Minor variations in joint assessment position can theoretically alter the response of the patient. However, Chiradejnant et al.[67] reported that the direction of the technique made little difference in the outcome of the patient. Randomly selected spine mobilization techniques performed at the targeted level demonstrated no difference when compared to therapist-selected techniques for patients with lumbar spine pain.

Contact Area over Which the Force is Applied   Lee et al.[61] state: "Although for many purposes, a manual force can be considered to be applied at one point, in reality there is a distribution of force over a finite area of skin surface." Consequently, differences of interpretation of joint mobility may occur based on the method used for skin contact. Several common assessment methods are currently used, including the thumbs, pisiform, and other contact points of the hand.

Special Clinical Testing

There are four purposes of a **special clinical test.** First, special clinical tests are used to determine the level of functional impairment or disability of

the patient (supportive information). For example, palpation and manual provocation tests lend support to the findings of certain impairments but yield little information in the absence of the movement examination. The second purpose is to provide diagnostic value to a set of findings using sensitivity and specificity values and the off-shoots of these (e.g., likelihood ratios, etc). Third, tests are used to determine prognosis of a patient. This is captured in one of two ways, either by directly tying a finding toward an outcome (less common) or by clustering findings that dictate the use of a decision rule. Fourth, special clinical tests may be useful in ruling out (structural differentiation) a particular region if the tests demonstrate a high degree of sensitivity. We initially discuss the first proposed set of benefits of a special clinical test.

The Use of Special Clinical Tests
As Supportive Information

Palpation   Cyriax and Cyriax write, "Palpation used by itself regularly deceives."[38] Palpation may be useful when performed near the end of treatment once the clinician has identified the series of concordant movements by the patient. Yet when used early or without clarification of a movement-based assessment, palpation may be of limited value. Palpation demonstrates poor reliability when tested during motion detection of the spine, but does yield useful information during analysis of the rotator cuff, temporomandibular joint, and tendonitis.[68,69] Additionally, palpation is useful to implicate a pain generator when referred pain of the patient's concordant sign occurs during palpation of a particular structure.[34]

Muscle Provocation Testing   The purpose of **muscle provocation testing** is to determine the "guilt" of contractile versus noncontractile tissue. A method described as "selective tension testing" was first acknowledged by Cyriax and Cyriax.[38] They proposed that contractile tissues (muscle, tendon, and bony insertion) are painful during an applied isometric contraction and inert structures (capsule, ligaments, bursae) are painful during passive movement. They furthered this definition by providing subdefinitions to the findings or the provocation tests. They suggested that a finding of *strong* and *painless* suggests that contractile tissue is not involved. *Strong* and *painful* indicates there is a minor lesion of the contractile tissue. *Weak* and *painless* may be a sign of complete rupture of the contractile tissue or it may be a disorder of the nervous system. *Weak* and *painful* indicates a major lesion. If all movements are painful, one should consider that an affective component or a sinister pathology may be the chief generator of pain. Lastly, if the tested muscle group is strong and painless but hurts after several repetitions, the examiner should suspect intermittent claudication.

As discussed in Chapter 2, the scientific evidence to support this elaborate set of findings is mixed. Pellecchia et al.[70] and Fritz et al.[71] found acceptable reliability and clinical usefulness with this tool. Others[72,73] have reported that the model lacks validity and reliability.

Finally, the traditional **manual muscle test** is also used as a special clinical test to implicate weakness at selected muscles. As a whole, the reliability of manual muscle testing, in absence of a mechanized tool is not strong.[74–78] A growing amount of evidence supports the use of this testing method when a hand-held device is used for more specific detection[79–82] and when the plus and minus categories are discarded.[74] Standardized criteria are outlined in Table 3.6 ■.

The Use of Special Clinical Tests for Diagnostic Value The second purpose of a special clinical test is to provide **diagnostic value.** Essentially, high-quality special clinical tests are designed to discriminate a subgroup of homogeneous characteristics from a heterogeneous pool of patients with dysfunction or to confirm a tentative diagnosis.[79] At best, special clinical tests add to hypotheses, but rarely have the clinical power to truly confirm a diagnosis. For further reading of clinical special tests and their ability to function as tools for diagnostic value, the reader is recommended to review the book *Orthopedic Clinical Special Tests: An Evidence-Based Approach.*[79]

The Use of Special Clinical Tests for Prognosis The third benefit of special clinical tests is to determine prognosis of a patient. This is captured in one of two ways, either by directly tying a finding toward an outcome (less common) or by clustering findings that dictate the use of a decision rule. For example, we know that a finding of centralization has demonstrated a positive outcome for patients with acute low back pain.[80] A finding such as this is useful for dictating prognosis and is considered a valuable finding. Recently, a decision rule for patients with mechanical neck pain was developed to predict who might benefit from thoracic manipulation.[81] The clinical findings of pain <30 days, no symptoms distal to the shoulder, no pain when looking up, a FABQPA score of <12, extension <30 degrees, and diminished upper thoracic kyphosis were included as the parsimonious variables for the model. Combinations of these "clinical findings" were predictive for a good outcome using thoracic manipulation.

The Use of Special Clinical Tests As Structural Differentiation Tests The fourth benefit of special clinical tests is for use during region and structure differentiation. Structural identification allows the clinician to target movement assessment at the appropriate bodily regions. Cues collected from the subjective examination outline on which area the clinician should focus the tests and measures. Generally, the clinician performs one to several structural differentiation tests to confirm the correct origin of the dysfunction. This is necessary when a patient is unable to provide a definitive region or when the symptoms suggest overlap or confusion between different bodily regions. When this occurs the clinician should differentiate each region using quick structural differentiation tests. Quality differentiation tests demonstrate a high degree of sensitivity and are easily provoked when impairment is present. Since the clinician is interested in differentiating structures, a negative test (for a test and measure with high sensitivity) is

■ TABLE 3.6 Six Categories of a Graded Traditional Manual Muscle Test

Grade	Description
V	Patient holds the position against maximum resistance throughout the complete range of motion.
IV	Patient holds the position against strong to moderate resistance and demonstrates full range of motion.
III	Patient tolerates no resistance but performs the movement through the full range of motion.
II	Patient demonstrates all or partial range of motion in the gravity-eliminated position.
I	The muscle(s) are palpable while the patient is performing the action in the gravity-eliminated position.
0	No contractile activity is felt in the gravity-eliminated position.

telling and suggests that symptoms are not present in that region. Selected special clinical tests with high sensitivity, such as the hip scour and cervical and lumbar quadrant, may be useful at ruling out regions. Otherwise, the use of overpressures after active movements help rule out a particular region as well.

Summary

- The purpose of the physical examination is to establish the effect of movement on the patient's symptoms that were described during the subjective history.
- There are three primary areas of the objective physical examination: (1) active movements, (2) passive movements, and (3) special clinical tests.
- Active movements include all motions performed exclusively by the patient.
- Passive movements include all motions performed by the clinician and may be physiological, accessory, or combined.
- Special clinical tests include palpation and manual muscle testing.

Putting the Objective Physical Examination Findings Together

By the end of the objective physical examination the clinician should have the following criteria:

1. A strong understanding of the causal pain-generating region.
2. An understanding of which active movements increase or decrease the pain associated with the concordant sign.
3. An understanding of which active movements increase, decrease, or normalize range of motion.
4. An understanding of which passive movements increase or decrease the pain associated with the concordant sign.
5. An understanding of which passive movements increase, decrease, or normalize range of motion.
6. An understanding of the potential pain generator based on movement, positional, and palpatory findings.
7. An understanding of a potential diagnosis based on the examination and clinical test findings.
8. A strong association between the subjective and objective findings (a marriage of the information).

Post-Examination Clinical Reasoning

Upon completion of the examination, the data presented by the patient should allow two primary theoretical conclusions. First, the clinician should have a strong understanding of the movements that negatively or positively influence the concordant sign of the patient. Second, the clinician should understand whether within- or between-session changes to the concordant sign were associated with the examination/intervention approach. Failure to identify a concordant sign during examination will yield three different consequences. First, since no mechanical pattern of symptoms was isolated, the patient could potentially receive a treatment approach that may or may not be associated with their underlying problem. Second, if the clinician is unable to isolate symptoms using appropriate clinical examination methods, it is possible that the patient exhibits a nonmechanical disorder and may be outside the scope of an orthopedic manual therapist's care. If manual therapy clinical examination methods that are mechanical in nature do not positively or negatively influence the patient's concordant sign, the patient may not benefit from manual therapy, and the patient may be best served by referring to a more appropriate medical provider. Third, some patients require preloading or cumulative loading of tissues to reproduce the concordant pain. This consequence occurs in many sport- or occupation-related injuries that require repetition before onset of symptoms.

Since the purpose of the physical examination was to analyze the response of the concordant sign to multiple movements, the clinician should have a strong understanding of which techniques improve or aggravate the patient's condition. Treatment selection should be selected based on these findings, and less on theoretical analysis or conjecture. Using probabilistic elements or decision rules improves one's ability to know the proper outcome with a selected intervention.

Summary

- Most methods that involve movement detection of finite quantities have demonstrated poor reliability and validity.
- Most methods that utilize patient report of symptoms during clinician-driven provocation procedures have demonstrated good reliability and validity.
- Clinical reasoning that focuses on pain provocation reduction and alteration of techniques to patient response is the focus of this book.

Chapter Questions

1. Describe the benefits and pitfalls of using observation-based methods during examination.

2. Define the concordant sign and discordant sign. How can an overemphasis on the discordant sign lead to false findings during an examination?

3. Define the irritability of a patient. Describe how irritability is a multidimensional concept.

4. Identify measures that are appropriate for a patient baseline. Please describe how these methods are used during treatment and reexamination.

5. Describe the appropriate procedural process of an active movement examination.

6. Describe the factors (methods) within a passive movement examination and describe the appropriate procedural process of a passive movement examination.

7. Describe how the patient response-based method provides usable information for a potential treatment program. Why is this method effective?

References

1. Sobri M, Lamont A, Alias N, Win M. Red flags in patients presenting with headache: Clinical indications for neuroimaging. *Br J Radiology.* 2003;76:532–535.
2. Sizer P, Brismee JM, Cook C. Medical screening for red flags in the diagnosis and management of musculoskeletal spine pain. *Pain Pract.* 2007;7(1):53–71.
3. Swenson R. Differential diagnosis. *Neuro Clin North Am.* 1999;17:43–63.
4. Kendall F, McCreary E. *Muscle testing and function.* 3rd ed. Baltimore; Williams and Wilkins: 1983.
5. Spurling R, Scoville W. Lateral rupture of the cervical intervertebral discs. *Surg Gyencol Obstet.* 1944;78:350–358.
6. McCombe PF, Fairbank JCT, Cockersole BC, et al. Reproducibility of physical signs in low-back pain. *Spine.* 1989;14:908–917.
7. Davidson R, Dunn E, Metzmaker J. The shoulder abduction test in the diagnosis of radicular pain in cervical extradural compression monomradiculopathies. *Spine.* 1981;6:441–446.
8. Partanen J, Partanen K, Oikarinen H, Niemitukia L, Hernesniemi J. Preoperative electroneuromyography and myelography in cervical root compression. *Electromyogr Clin Neurophysiol.* 1991;31:21–26.
9. Grieve G. *Common vertebral joint problems.* 2nd ed. Edinburgh; Churchill Livingstone. 1988.
10. Hurwitz EL, Morgenstern H, Harber P, et al. A randomized trial of medical care with and without physical therapy and chiropractic care with and without physical modalities for patients with low back pain: 6-month follow-up outcomes from the UCLA low back pain study. *Spine.* 2002;27(20):2193–2204.
11. Di Fabio RP. Manipulation of the cervical spine: Risks and benefits. *Phys Ther.* 1999;79(1):50–65.
12. Grieve G. *Common vertebral joint problems.* 2nd ed. Edinburgh; Churchill Livingstone: 1988.
13. Fann A. The prevalence of postural asymmetry in people with and without chronic low back pain. *Arch Phys Med Rehabil.* 2002;83:1736–1738.
14. Levangie PK. The association between static pelvic asymmetry and low back pain. *Spine.* 1999;15;24(12):1234–1242.
15. Astrom M, Arvidson T. Alignment and joint motion of the foot. *J Orthop Sports Phys Ther.* 1995;22:216–222.
16. Harris G, Wertsch J. Procedures for gait analysis. *Arch Phys Med Rehabil.* 1994;75:216–225.
17. Fritz J, George S. Identifying psychosocial variables in patients with acute work-related low back pain: The importance of fear-avoidance beliefs. *Phys Ther.* 2002;82:973–983.
18. Kilpikoski S, Airaksinen O, Kankaanpaa M, Leminen P, Videman T, Alen M. Interexaminer reliability of low back pain assessment using the McKenzie method. *Spine.* 2002;27(8):E207–214.
19. Edwards B. *Manual of combined movements.* Oxford; Butterworth-Heinemann: 1999.
20. Woolf AD. How to assess musculoskeletal conditions. History and physical examination. *Best Pract Res Clin Rheumatol.* 2003;17(3):381–402.
21. McGregor AH, Dore CJ, McCarthy ID, Hughes SP. Are subjective clinical findings and objective clinical tests related to the motion characteristics of low back pain subjects? *J Orthop Sports Phys Ther.* 1998;28(6):370–377.
22. Luime J, Verhagen A, Miedema H, et al. Does this patient have an instability of the shoulder or a labrum lesion? *JAMA.* 2004;292:1989–1999.
23. Walker W, Cifu D, Gardner M, Keyser-Marcus L. Functional assessment in patients with chronic pain: Can physicians predict performance? *Spine.* 2001;80:162–168.
24. Laslett M, Young S, April C, McDonald B. Diagnosing painful sacroiliac joints: A validity study of a McKenzie evaluation and sacroiliac provocation tests. *Aust J Physiother.* 2003;49:89–97.

25. Maitland GD. *Maitland's vertebral manipulation*. 6th ed. London; Butterworth-Heinemann: 2001.

26. Zusman M. Irritability. *Man Ther*. 1998;3(4):195–202.

27. Koury M, Scarpelli E. A manual therapy approach to evaluation and treatment of a patient with a chronic lumbar nerve root irritation. *Phys Ther*. 1994;74(6):548–559.

28. Tovin B. *Evaluation and treatment of the shoulder: An integration of the guide to physical therapist practice*. Philadelphia; F.A. Davis: 2001.

29. Fryer G, Morris T, Gibbons P. Paraspinal muscles and intervertebral dysfunction: Part one. *J Manipulative Physiol Ther*. 2004;27(4):267–274.

30. McQuillen MP, Tucker K, Pellegrino ED. Syndrome of subacute generalized muscular stiffness and spasm. *Arch Neurol*. 1967;16(2):165–174.

31. Kang YM, Choi WS, Pickar JG. Electrophysiologic evidence for an intersegmental reflex pathway between lumbar paraspinal tissues. *Spine*. 2002;27(3):E56–63.

32. Fitzgerald GK, Piva SR, Irrgang JJ. Reports of joint instability in knee osteoarthritis: Its prevalence and relationship to physical function. *Arthritis Rheum*. 2004;51(6):941–946.

33. Svanborg A. Practical and functional consequences of aging. *Gerontology*. 1988;34 Suppl 1:11–5.

34. Maitland GD. *Peripheral manipulation*. 3rd ed. London; Butterworth-Heinemann: 1986.

35. Tan V, Cheatle M, Mackin S, Moberg P, Esterhai J. Goal setting as a predictor of return to work in a population of chronic musculoskeletal pain patients. *Int J Neurosci*. 1997;92:161–170.

36. Donelson R. The McKenzie approach to evaluating and treating low back pain. *Orthopedic Review*. 1990;8:681–686.

37. Franklin M, Conner-Kerr T, Chamness M, Chenier T, Kelly R, Hodge T. Assessment of exercise-induced minor muscle lesions: The accuracy of Cyriax's diagnosis by selective tension paradigm. *J Ortho Sports Phys Ther*. 1996;24:122–129.

38. Cyriax J, Cyriax P. *Cyriax's illustrated manual of orthopaedic medicine*. Oxford; Butterworth-Heinemann: 1993.

39. Niere KR, Torney SK. Clinicians' perceptions of minor cervical instability. *Man Ther*. 2004;9(3):144–150.

40. Lee R, Evans J. An in vivo study of the intervertebral movements produced by posteroanterior mobilization. *Clin Biomech*. 1997;12:400–408.

41. Lee R, Tsung BY, Tong P, Evans J. Bending stiffness of the lumbar spine subjected to posteroanterior manipulative force. *J Rehabil Res Dev*. 2005;42(2):167–174.

42. Kulig K, Powers CM, Landel RF, et al. Segmental lumbar mobility in individuals with low back pain: In vivo assessment during manual and self-imposed motion using dynamic MRI. *BMC Musculoskel Disord*. 2007;8:8.

43. Hartman L. *Handbook of osteopathic technique*. 3rd ed. San Diego, CA; Singular Pub Group: 1997.

44. Chiradejnant A, Latimer J, Maher C, Stepkovitch N. Does the choice of spinal level treated during posteroanterior (PA) mobilization affect treatment outcome? *Physiother Theory Pract*. 2002;18:165–174.

45. Aquino RL, Caires PS, Furtado FC, Loureiro AV, Ferreira PH, Ferreira M. Applying joint mobilization at different cervical vertebral levels does not influence immediate pain reduction in patients with chronic neck pain: A randomized clinical trial. *J Man Manip Ther*. 2009;17:95–100.

46. Schomacher J. The effect of an analgesic mobilization technique when applied at symptomatic or asymptomatic levels of the cervical spine in subjects with neck pain: A randomized controlled trial. *J Man Manip Ther*. 2009;17:101–108.

47. Cattrysse E, Baeyens JP, Clarys JP, Van Roy P. Manual fixation versus locking during upper cervical segmental mobilization. Part 1: An in vitro three-dimensional arthrokinematic analysis of manual flexion–extension mobilization of the atlanto-occipital joint. *Man Ther*. 2007;12(4):342–352.

48. Kaltenborn F. Manual mobilization of the joints. *The Kaltenborn method of joint mobilization and treatment*. 5th ed. Oslo; Olaf Norlis Bokhandel: 1999.

49. Hayes K, Peterson C, Falconer J. An examination of Cyriax's passive motion tests with patients having osteoarthritis of the knee. *Phys Ther*. 1994;74:697–707.

50. Klassbo M, Larsson G. Examination of passive ROM and capsular patterns of the hip. *Physiother Res International*. 2003;8:1–12.

51. Mitsch J, Casey J, McKinnis R, Kegerreis S, Stikeleather J. Investigation of a consistent pattern of motion restriction in patients with adhesive capsulitis. *J Manual Manip Ther*. 2004;12:153–159.

52. Hayes K, Peterson C. Reliability of assessing end-feel and pain and resistance sequence in subjects with painful shoulders and knees. *J Orthop Sports Phys Ther*. 2001;31:432–445.

53. Peterson C, Hayes K. Construct validity of Cyriax's selective tension examination: Association of end-feels with pain at the knee and shoulder. *J Orthop Sports Phys Ther*. 2000;30:512–521.

54. Chesworth B, MacDermid J, Roth J, Patterson S. Movement diagram and "end-feel" reliability when measuring passive lateral rotation of the shoulder in patients with shoulder pathology. *Phys Ther*. 1998;78:593–601.

55. Anson E, Cook C, Comacho C, et al. The use of education in the improvement in finding R1 in the lumbar spine. *J Man Manip Ther*. 2003;11:204–212.

56. Bijl D, Dekker J, van Baar M, et al. Validity of Cyriax's concept capsular pattern for the diagnosis of osteoarthritis of hip and/or knee. *Scand J Rheumatol*. 1998;27:347–351.

57. McClure P, Flowers K. Treatment of limited should motion: A case study based on biomechanical considerations. *Phys Ther*. 1992;72:929–936.

58. Harryman D, Lazarus M. The stiff shoulder. In: Rockwood C, Matsen F, Wirth M, Lippitt S (eds). *The shoulder.* Vol 2. 3rd ed. Philadelphia; W.B. Saunders: 2004.

59. Haldeman S. Spinal manipulative therapy. A status report. *Clin Orthop.* 1983;(179):62–70.

60. Lee M, Svensson NL. Effect of loading frequency on response of the spine to lumbar posteroanterior forces. *J Manipulative Physiol Ther.* 1993;16(7):439–446.

61. Lee M, Steven J, Crosbie R, Higgs J. Towards a theory of lumbar mobilization: The relationship between applied manual force and movements of the spine. *Man Ther.* 1996;2:67–75.

62. Edwards B. Examination. In: Maitland GD. *Maitland's vertebral manipulation.* 6th ed. London; Butterworth-Heinemann: 2001.

63. Fung Y. Biomechanics. *Mechanical properties of living tissues.* 2nd ed. New York; Springer-Verlag: 1993.

64. Shirley D, Ellis E, Lee M. The response of posteroanterior lumbar stiffness to repeated loading. *Man Ther.* 2002;7:19–25.

65. Lee M. Mechanics of spinal joint manipulation in the thoracic and lumbar spine: A theoretical study of posteroanterior force techniques. *Clin Biomech.* 1989;4:249–251.

66. Caling B, Lee M. Effect of direction of applied mobilization force on the posteroanterior response in the lumbar spine. *J Manipulative Physiol Ther.* 2001;24:71–78.

67. Chiradejnant A, Maher C, Latimer J, Stepkovitch N. Efficacy of therapist selected versus randomly selected mobilization techniques for the treatment of low back pain: A randomized controlled trial. *Aust J Physiotherapy.* 2003;49:233–241.

68. Manfredini D, Tognini F, Zampa V, Bosco M. Predictive value of clinical findings for temporomandibular joint effusion. *Oral Surg Oral Med Oral Pathol Oral Radiol Endod.* 2003;96(5):521–526.

69. Cook JL, Khan KM, Kiss ZS, Purdam CR, Griffiths L. Reproducibility and clinical utility of tendon palpation to detect patellar tendinopathy in young basketball players. Victorian Institute of Sport tendon study group. *Br J Sports Med.* 2001;35(1):65–69.

70. Pellecchia GL, Paolino J, Connell J. Intertester reliability of the Cyriax evaluation in the assessing patients with shoulder pain. *J Orthop Sports Phys Ther.* 1996;23:34–38.

71. Fritz J, Delitto A, Erhard R, Roman M. An examination of the selective tissue tension scheme, with evidence for the concept of a capsular pattern of the knee. *Phys Ther.* 1998;78:1046–1056.

72. Jepsen J, Laursen L, Larsen A, Hagert C. Manual strength testing in 14 upper limb muscles: A study of inter-rater reliability. *Acta Orthop Scand.* 2004;75:442–448.

73. Wadsworth C, Krishnan R, Sear M, Harrold J, Nielson D. Intrarater reliability of manual muscle testing and hand held dynametric muscle testing. *Phys Ther.* 1987;67:1342–1347.

74. Ottenbacher K, Branch L, Ray L, Gonzales V, Peek M, Hinman M. The reliability of upper- and lower-extremity strength testing in a community survey of older adults. *Arch Phys Med Rehabil.* 2002;83:1423–1427.

75. Perry J, Weiss W, Burnfield J, Gronley J. The supine hip extensor manual muscle test: A reliability and validity study. *Arch Phys Med Rehabil.* 2004;85:1345–1350.

76. Frese E, Brown M, Norton B. Clinical reliability of manual muscle testing. Middle trapezius and gluteus maximus muscles. *Phys Ther.* 1987;67:1072–1076.

77. Kelly B, Kadrmas W, Speer K. The manual muscle examination for rotator cuff strength. An electromyographic investigation. *Am J Sports Med.* 1996;24:581–588.

78. Hsieh C, Phillips R. Reliability of manual muscle testing with a computerized dynamometer. *J Manipulative Physiol Ther.* 1990;13:72–82.

79. Cook C, Hegedus E. *Orthopedic physical examination tests: An evidence-based approach.* Upper Saddle River, NJ; Prentice Hall: 2008.

80. Werneke M, Hart DL. Centralization phenomenon as a prognostic factor for chronic low back pain and disability. *Spine.* 2001;26(7):758–764; discussion 765.

81. Cleland JA, Childs JD, Fritz JM, Whitman JM, Eberhart SL. Development of a clinical prediction rule for guiding treatment of a subgroup of patients with neck pain: Use of thoracic spine manipulation, exercise, and patient education. *Phys Ther.* 2007;87(1):9–23.

Treatment and Re-Examination

Chad E. Cook

Objectives

- Define the patient response treatment philosophy.
- Define how the different determinants of treatment alter the outcome of the treatment.
- Describe the various treatment techniques used by orthopedic manual clinicians.
- Describe the patient's role in "intention to treat" and how this role may alter the outcome of the treatment.

Treatment

Treatment Philosophy

The purpose of a manual therapy-directed treatment is to apply purposeful techniques that reduce, centralize, or abolish the patient's signs and symptoms. Techniques are selected based on within-session changes during the patient encounter. The selection of a *set* of treatment techniques follows the same philosophy as the examination,[1] a procedure defined as the patient response-based method. The patient response-based method requires a diligent effort of the patient and the clinician to determine the behavior of the patient's pain and/or impairment by analyzing concordant movements and the response of the patient's pain to repeated or applied movements. The repeated or sustained movements that positively or negatively alter the signs and symptoms of the patient deserve the highest priority for treatment selection[2,3] and should be similar in construct to the concordant examination movements. Examination methods that fail to elicit the desired patient response (within-session change) may offer nominal or imprecise value.[4]

A patient response method requires careful and dedicated participation by the patient and the manual therapy clinician. Christensen et al.[5] state: "A patient's full understanding of and participation in the management of his or her problem, resulting in an increase in understanding and, in turn, self-efficacy, is thought to have a significant positive impact on treatment outcomes." The idea of involving the patient in his or her own care is not new and is purported to lead to beneficial outcomes.[6] By empowering the patient to participate in the treatment the patient improves their ability to adjust to symptomatic changes.

To accomplish this concept, the patient must be made aware of the intention of treatment. The intention of treatment is the cooperative understanding of the goals of the treatment, developed in a format in which the patient can understand. Although there are several goals to a manual therapist's intervention, there are essentially three potential treatment objectives: (1) pain reduction, (2) normalizing or improving movement, and (3) education of the patient to allow self-treatment.

Normalizing range of motion may occur through the physiological benefits obtained through neurophysiological improvements.[7] Passive manual therapy techniques are designed to increase range of motion of a targeted, specific region and normalize **arthrokinematic** gliding and rolling movement. It is suggested that the improvement in arthrokinematic gliding and rolling will normalize osteokinematic rotation and enable the normalization of active movements.[8] Assessment of range or normality of movement is a within-session procedure associated with biomechanical change.

Targeted procedures may be oriented toward the concordant sign of the patient. Normalizing movement may be a better choice than "detection of stiffness" or "biomechanical theories" since stiffness may encompass differences in theoretical constructs among physical therapists[9] and biomechanical theories may lack validity or prognostic influence. Maher and Adams[10] suggested that the treatment focus should remain on the concordant sign and modifications based on the response of the patient should dictate the progression of the treatment plan. Treatment of the source of the problem may increase the likelihood of a neurophysiological and/or biomechanical response, and may provide a greater chance of a within-session change. Because the objective of the technique is to reproduce or reduce the patient's pain or improve range during the treatment process, the patient must be made well aware of the intent and the prospective outcome.

This also emphasizes the suggestion that individual techniques alone offer little in isolation and should always represent a means to an end, or need to be specific for that patient.[2] The selection of a technique is based on the presentation of the particular patient, indicating that the technique selection will most likely be different from patient to patient and will often change throughout the course of the patient's progression. The determination of method, dosage, and progression is dependent on the direct response of the patient and will differ over time.

Gregory Grieve[11] outlined common treatment-related goals in his 1988 textbook, goals that are salient to this date. If analyzed, Grieve's eight goals reflect the three principle objectives of treatment that include reduction of pain, restoration of normalized range of movement, and patient education for self-treatment. Changes in these areas should result in alterations of function, pain, and reductions of perceived disability. Table 4.1 ■ outlines the eight goals, broken down into the three objectives with some degree of overlap.

Summary

- Treatment is based on patient response and should accurately reflect the findings during the examination.
- Examination methods that fail to elicit the patient response may offer nominal or imprecise value.
- An understanding and participation from the patient in the management of his or her problem should have a significant positive impact on treatment outcome.
- Manual therapy should lead to within- and between-session changes.
- Inflammatory conditions are generally described using pain-related verbiage, and frequently patients with this primary disorder are considered "pain dominant."
- Certain clues regarding treatment of a patient with predominant range loss may help improve the understanding of a mechanically based dysfunction that responds well to aggressive movements.

Manual Therapy Techniques

It has been stated that most manual therapy techniques are highly specified and require a formal education and skill levels beyond an entry-level practitioner.[12] In reality, even unspecified manual therapy is likely beneficial when applied to the correct candidate. Failure to apply manual therapy to an appropriate candidate should be considered therapeutic nihilism. Within this textbook, the preponderance of orthopedic manual therapy techniques encompasses three major categories, discussed in Chapter 1: (1) stretching, (2) mobilization (also known as nonthrust manipulation), and (3) manipulation (also known as thrust manipulation). In addition, combined techniques involve the use of two or more of one technique or disparate techniques. As discussed in Chapter 1, each of the techniques provides evidence of biomechanical or neurophysiological changes.

Manual therapy techniques are applied to the joint, soft tissue, or nerve tissue.[13] The majority of this book

■ TABLE 4.1 Goals of Manual Therapy Treatment

Objectives	Description
Objective One: Reduction of Pain	1. Relief of pain and reduction of muscle spasm 2. Relief from chronic postural or occupational stress
Objective Two: Alteration of Stiffness	1. Restoration of normal tissue pliability and extensibility 2. Correction of muscle weakness or imbalance 3. The stabilization of unstable segments 4. Restoration of adequate control of movement
Objective Three: Patient Education	1. Prevention of reoccurrence 2. Restoration of psychological well-being and confidence

■ TABLE 4.2 Manual Therapy Technique Types

Region	Type	Nature
	Manipulation	Passive technique beyond normal range of movement
Joint	Mobilization	Passive or combined passive/active technique within normal range of movement
	Muscle Energy	Active assist technique within or beyond normal range of movement
	Myofascial	Deep techniques designed to lengthen tissue or increase range of movement
Soft Tissue	Muscular	Deep techniques designed to improve actual performance
	Lymphatic	Light, superficial techniques designed to improve circulation
Nerve	Neurodynamic	Passive or active movements designed to elongate or glide targeted nerve roots using movements and body postures

(and the techniques associated with manual therapy) are joint related. Nonetheless, soft-tissue techniques (demonstrated in Chapter 16) and nerve techniques (demonstrated in Chapter 15) can be useful as well when applied to the appropriate population. See (Table 4.2 ■).

Static Stretching Techniques

Stretching techniques allow lengthening of targeted tissue. Stretching techniques can be active assisted, applied by the patient, or passive movements applied by a clinician. **Static stretching** has received a fair amount of experiential investigation and an overwhelming majority identify that static stretching does lead to mechanical changes in range of motion. It has been suggested that passive static stretching does lengthen muscle fibers[14] and can assist in prevention of muscular atrophy secondary to immobilization.[15] However, less is known about the long-term benefit of static stretching on range of motion. The majority of these studies used measurements that were limited to pre- and post-analysis, which hampers the ability to determine the lasting influences of static stretching.

A number of studies, mostly pseudorandomized controlled trials, have independently examined the benefit of static stretching with a focus on a biomechanical outcome (e.g., range of motion).[16–30] Within these studies, variations in static hold associated with the length of time required to obtain optimal results has been presented. Although there is no consensus on a single specific time, it is apparent that a static hold of 15–30 seconds provides equitable gains in range of motion when compared to longer time periods and better outcomes when compared to shorter durations.

The role of static stretching for preventing sports-related injuries is less precise,[31] although there is some evidence that stretching may reduce work-related injuries.[32] Evidence to support stretching for spasticity is mixed.[33] For tendon-related injuries, ballistic stretching may have more benefit than static holds, although further research is needed for clarification and dosage.[34]

Collectively, there are methodological weaknesses in most studies. Although a preponderance of investigations have shown that static stretching does lead to increases in range of motion, an overwhelming majority used asymptomatic subjects and most limited the investigation to outcomes associated with hamstring stretching. Another consideration was the small sample sizes and younger populations. This aspect and the failure to use comparable controls prevented most studies from demonstrating high quality.

Summary

- Joint displacement may be associated with passive movement to mechanoreceptors and may be a reason behind neurophysiological change. Static stretching does improve range of motion in asymptomatic subjects.
- Static stretching does lead to temporary improvements in tissue mobility.
- Whether static stretching leads to long-term or permanent changes beyond the application data is unknown.
- Static stretching may be beneficial to prevent work-related injuries.

Mobilization (Nonthrust Manipulation)

Mobilizations typically fall within the treatment domain of passive movements.[12] **Mobilization** techniques are designed to restore a full painless joint function by rhythmic, repetitive, passive movements, generally to the patients' tolerance, in voluntary and/or accessory ranges.[35] Several studies have analyzed range-of-motion changes concurrently during outcome analyses and have supported the benefit of mobilization for mechanical range-of-motion improvement.[36–44] There does appear to be four specific trends. First, the most significant effects are confined to those who are symptomatic. Second, most studies are limited to immediate effects only. This finding diminishes the value of the findings and does not indicate whether the outcome is long term in nature. Third, in most studies, mobilization was used in conjunction with other forms of treatment. Lastly, it does appear that the disorder may contribute to the likelihood of success.

Mobilization methods may involve segmental/joint or soft-tissue mobilization. There are two forms of segmental/joint mobilizations: regional and local. **Regional mobilization** involves directed passive movement to more than one given area, segment, or physiological component, whereas **local mobilization** is specific and directed to one segmental and/or joint region.[9]

Segmental/Joint Mobilization   Segmental/joint mobilization techniques are designed to restore a full painless joint function by rhythmic, repetitive, passive movements, generally to the patients' tolerance, in voluntary and/or accessory range and graded according to examination findings.[9] Generally, segmental/joint techniques involve static and/or oscillatory movements. Static techniques (prolonged stretch into restricted tissue) are sustained forces applied manually or mechanically to one aspect of a body part to distract the attachments or shortened soft tissue. Oscillatory techniques (small or large passive movements) are applied movements to a segment/joint anywhere in a range, whereas the joints are held or compressed.[2] Both techniques appear to exhibit similar mechanical characteristics.

Motion at a joint is the result of movement of one joint surface in relation to the other.[45] Mobilization movements of a segmental region may include any biomechanical form of accessory motion including distraction, compression, sliding, spinning, and rolling. Techniques that encourage distraction (joint surface separation without injury or dislocation of the parts) are sustained or rhythmic in nature, manual or mechanical, and are applied in a longitudinal manner that results in the distancing of two joint surfaces. Mennell[46] and Cyriax and Cyriax[47] frequently described distraction mobilization as useful treatment methods.

Techniques that encourage compression result in joint surfaces that are compressed together, allowing shorter distances between articular structures. Several authors have advocated the benefit of compression mobilization, although in most cases, the compressions were actually combined with other accessory movements such as gliding or rolling. Techniques that encourage sliding refer to the gliding of one articular component over another. The majority of simple planer mobilizations are sliding techniques. The convex–concave rule particularly emphasizes the proposed benefit to following appropriate sliding rules during mobilization application.[48]

Techniques that encourage rolling refer to the rolling of one body surface over another. For example, when a convex surface moves osteokinematically on a fixed concave surface, the majority of the hypothetical movement should include rolling. Whether or not rolling and the convex–concave rule are transferable to all synovial joints is questionable.

Nerve Mobilization   Nerve mobilization techniques involve tension or gliding maneuvers that are designed to reduce or reproduce neuropathic pain at the site of an entrapment or may be targeted at the nerve root itself. Nerve mobilization techniques are used as test measures and treatments and are discussed in Chapter 15.

Soft-Tissue Mobilization   Soft-tissue mobilization techniques are typically defined as massage or myofascial release. Soft-tissue mobilization is the intentional and systematic manipulation of the soft tissues of the body to enhance health and healing.[49] Multiple forms of soft-tissue techniques exist, and may include gliding, sliding, percussion, compression, kneading, friction, vibrating, and stretching.[49] The variant forms of soft-tissue mobilization are discussed in Chapter 16.

Summary

- Most studies that have analyzed mechanical changes using mobilization demonstrated fair design.
- Mobilization appears to lead to mechanical range-of-motion (ROM) changes during single and repeated applications.
- Mobilization is as effective as other pragmatic methods during mechanical range-of-motion intervention.
- Nerve mobilization techniques involve tension or gliding maneuvers that are designed to reduce or reproduce neuropathic pain at the site of an entrapment or may be targeted at the nerve root itself.
- Soft-tissue techniques are typically defined as massage or myofascial release.

Manipulation (Thrust Manipulation)

Manipulations are used in both passive and assisted movements. **Manipulation** is an accurately localized or globally applied, single, quick, and decisive movement (thrust) of small amplitude, following a careful positioning of the patient.[50] There are four primary lesions that may respond to manipulative treatment:[51] (1) entrapped synovial folds or plica, (2) hypertonic muscle, (3) articular or periarticular adhesions, and (4) segmental displacement. Although a majority of studies have demonstrated mechanical range-of-motion changes directly after a manipulative treatment, or a large effect size associated with the manipulation, most were poorly designed.

Cramer et al.[52] demonstrated an increase in facet joint space after high-velocity manipulation to the lumbar spine. However, the subjects in the study had no history of low back pain, thus extrapolation to pathological conditions is questionable. Others have investigated range-of-motion gains after manipulative treatment. A number of studies examined improvement of cervical spine movements with manipulation in patients with pathology, some in which the manipulation was targeted to the neck, others to the thoracic spine. In nearly every study, manipulation does provide immediate effects (short-term changes) in pain and range of motion.[53–62] In the studies that compared against pragmatic controls (such as muscle energy techniques), the effects of manipulation proved similar in between-groups treatment, but substantially better than the baseline measure (within-groups changes). Additionally, although manipulation appears to significantly improve range of motion, these studies fail to measure the long-term effects. Typically manipulation techniques are classified as localized or general.

Targeted Specific Manipulation **Localized manipulative** or targeted specific techniques involve the intent of applying a passive or assisted movement toward one specific functional region (i.e., spinal unit or single joint).[63] These techniques are occasionally termed short-lever manipulative procedures. During a localized manipulative technique the application of a high-velocity, low-amplitude thrust occurs at the end of range of movement for the joint. Generally, the joint is appropriately prepositioned in such a manner that allows an end-range feel to be produced in a combination of mid-range positions.[64] Thus the high-velocity, low-amplitude thrust is applied in a position where the joint was placed in a clinician-determined, end-range movement, in a particular combination of plane movements to allow application isolated to that segment.[65] Manipulation is distinguished from mobilization by the prepositioning, the administration of the high-velocity, low-amplitude thrust, and that the clinician manages the direction force and application beyond the patient's control.[66]

Generalized Manipulation **Generalized manipulative** techniques involve less defined prepositioning methods and are designed in such a manner as to isolate the thrust to a dedicated region. These techniques are frequently described as long-lever manipulative techniques. Force is directed through a long-lever arm, which is distant from the specific contact.[67] Generalized manipulative techniques allow the thrust to transcend throughout the regional anatomical site dispensing the force through multiple segmental levels or peripheral joints. Muscle energy techniques used for manipulation purposes are examples of a generalized manipulation technique.

Summary

- The majority of manipulation studies measuring mechanical range-of-motion (ROM) changes demonstrate only fair design.
- The majority of manipulation studies measuring mechanical ROM changes did demonstrate direct ROM improvements after application.
- Most studies that measure mechanical ROM changes during manipulation demonstrated significant improvement over baseline and had similar improvements when compared to pragmatic controls.
- Manipulation appears to provide short-term mechanical ROM changes in both symptomatic and asymptomatic patients.
- Manipulation may provide short-term benefit even when applied at regions away from the targeted pathology.
- Manipulation involves a clinician-driven method that is accurately localized, singularly performed, and involves a quick and decisive small amplitude movement.
- Localized manipulative techniques involve the intent of applying a passive or assisted movement toward one specific functional region.
- Generalized manipulative techniques involve less defined prepositioning methods and are designed in such a manner as to isolate the thrust to a dedicated region.

Combined Techniques

Any procedure that combines any of the previously described techniques is considered a combined method. The most common form of combined technique is the manually assisted technique. This method requires variations in active contraction by the subject against passive application of a stress by the clinician. Often, these methods are described as **proprioceptive neuromuscular facilitation** (PNF). PNF exercises are designed to "hasten the response of the neuromuscular mechanism through stimulation of the proprioceptors."[68] Although PNF techniques were theoretical when created, the basis of the theory is fairly well substantiated.[69]

A **muscle energy technique** (MET) is another manually assisted method of stretching/mobilization. METs are performed when the patient actively uses their muscles, on request, while maintaining a targeted preposition, against a distinctly executed counterforce.[70] METs may be classified as isotonic or isometric contractions, each with opposite desired outcomes. In an isometric contraction, the overall muscle belly length (of the activated muscle) shortens (the tendon lengthens), whereas during an isotonic contraction the muscle may lengthen or shorten. Goodridge[71] suggests that localization of force by appropriate patient positioning is essential to the benefit of MET, and is more important than force intensity.

A number of studies[69,70,72–75] have enlisted a mixed set of subjects, some symptomatic, others not. Additionally, a minority did not perform mutually exclusive stretching nor did the studies compare the methods to a control group. Nonetheless, manually assisted movements, specifically PNF techniques, appear to provide similar outcomes as static stretching. In addition, it is projected that PNF techniques may have a pain-modulating mechanism that contributes to overall mobility.[76]

One popular form of manually assisted movement is "**mobilization with movement**," a term coined by Brian Mulligan. Mobilization with movement is defined as the application of an accessory glide during the patient-driven active physiological movement.[77–79] The underlying principle recommends accessory application along biomechanical joint orientations.[8] This concept may involve the application of sustained, through-range, manually derived forces that guide the joint in such a manner that superimposed active movement, which previously produced pain, can then occur painlessly. Essentially, the nature of these techniques involves the simultaneous combination of passive accessory mobilization and active patient originated movement.[80] Mobilization with movement has its foundation based on Kaltenborn's principles of restoring the accessory component of active and passive physiological joint movement.[8]

Summary

- PNF stretching methods have been demonstrated to be as effective as other pragmatic models and significantly effective when compared to placebo.
- METs have demonstrated effectiveness when compared to controls and can lead to increases in spine mobility.
- There is fair evidence that manually assisted techniques lead to ROM increases in both symptomatic and asymptomatic subjects.
- Any method that combines active and/or passive movements is considered a combined method.
- The most common methods of combined movements involve mobilization with movement, muscle energy techniques, and proprioceptive neuromuscular facilitation.

General versus Targeted Specific Techniques

So far, all techniques described have been variations of general techniques and all literature that has investigated the benefits of manual therapy has involved general procedures. Nonetheless, experienced clinicians often attempt to localize a procedure to a specific joint, a mechanism that is called a **targeted specific technique**. The targeted specific technique is a technique that is designed to facilitate the range-of-motion restriction (or limitation) of the patient by (1) targeting force in the direction of the restriction, or (2) prepositioning the patient in the position of the restriction. Although there is no evidence that this form of procedure is more useful than a general technique, clinical findings do seem to support the use of this method on troublesome patients or patients that have reached a plateau in their progression.

An example of a targeted specific technique is as follows. Suppose a patient exhibits pain during cervical side flexion to the right, or during closing of the intervertebral foramen on the right. The clinician may decide to preposition the patient in right-side bending (the position of restriction) and follow with a manipulation that emphasizes a downward glide to the right upper facet (which further closes the intervertebral foramen on the right). This targeted specific technique encourages closing of the right side (the restriction) in a fashion that is much greater than a general manipulative technique.

Within this book, general techniques and targeted specific techniques using restrictions associated with movements are both taught. It is important to note there is no evidence that supports one method over another.

Fine-Tuning the Techniques

There is little evidence that suggests that there is one "right" way to do a specific technique. In fact, there is more evidence toward the opposite: the nonspecific nature of selected applications (various techniques) yield similar consequences.[18,19] Fundamentally, there are many different ways to apply techniques and many methods to alter the selected technique once chosen. The fine-tuning mechanisms suggested by Lee et al.[20] outline variations for the treatment application that could yield different outcomes for the concordant sign.

Magnitude of Force

There is no "gold standard" for determining the ideal magnitude of force applied during segmental movements.[21–26] In theory, the "ideal" force should vary from subject to subject and will directly rely on the type and location of the signs and symptoms of the patient. For example, if a patient exhibits inflammatory-based pain, light movements designed to alter the affected substance composition may encourage normalization of the tissue chemical environment.[27] Symptoms associated with segmental restrictions may require treatment techniques that lengthen the tissue and provide a mechanical change. Mechanical symptoms associated with muscle reflexive spasm may require forces that result in a reduction in protective spasm, thus allowing osteokinematic movements.

Although there is a theoretical concept associated with the ideal force during treatment, there are few examples within the literature of measured forces during mobilization and manipulation among various professions. While the reliability and consistency of force during application is somewhat suspect, the forces can be generalized based on several studies. Measurement devices have ranged from subjective scales, force platforms, pinch grips, and mechanical spinal mobilization devices. The difficulty in standardizing a measurement point may be one of the reasons for the sparseness within the literature. Many studies have utilized a posterior–anterior (PA) force to the spine as their measurement point within studies.

In a study performed to measure the educational effects of using the force plate, Lee, Moseley, and Refshauge[81] found that most physical therapy students applied consistent mobilization forces that ranged from 20 to 45 Newtons. Latimer, Lee, and Adams[82] determined the range of applied force of manual therapists varied from 30 to 200 Newtons. The authors suggested that most clinicians routinely applied forces of 30 to 429 Newtons during mobilization. Others have reported[83] average mobilization forces ranging from 50.1 Newtons to 194.8 Newtons during actual patient care intervention of the lumbar spine. The lower numbers reflected lower grades and, correspondingly, the upper numbers reflected upper grades.

Herzog et al.,[84] reported consistent use of 500–600 Newtons of force during the fourth thoracic vertebral (T4) manipulation techniques from chiropractors. Additionally, most chiropractic techniques require a preload of forces that are often higher than a mobilization-based force, used by many physical therapists. Cervical and sacroiliac techniques were observed with smaller torque values, 100 Newtons and 300-plus Newtons, respectively. These forces occurred with a population of symptomatic patients without incident or plastic failure of the tissues.

Based on the literature it is reasonable to assume normal treatment ranges for both mobilization and manipulation from 30 to 500 Newtons of force. This force application must be selective toward the proper targeted tissue. For instance, the connective tissue of the low back, including the shear forces absorbed by the disc and surrounding tissues, may tolerate more force than the connective tissue of the anterior talofibular ligament.

Rate of Increase of Force

It has been suggested that the rate of increase in force application can alter the perception of stiffness.[20] A similar suggestion from Maitland[2] hypothesized that differences in frequency are necessary depending on the response of the patient to various mobilization movements. Variations include faster frequencies during the application "on" and slower frequency for load "off" or a steady pace when patients exhibit fair to strong symptoms.

Duration of Loading

Maitland[85] also suggested that a sustained load in the presence of a muscle spasm may yield positive responses and a reduction in muscle spasm. Nonetheless, there is little information to support the suggestion that duration significantly alters the treatment outcome. Essentially, modification of the duration of the load is purely patient response based and may yield different results with each patient.

Targeted Tissue to Which the Force is Applied

Information has suggested that a technique applied in any direction within the region of the spine is as beneficial as a therapist-selected force to the pathological segment. This concept is a paradigm shift from most philosophies and further studies are suggested. Furthermore, evidence exists that manual therapy to the thoracic spine is helpful for patients complaining of a cervical spine disorder.[19] This suggests a link between various aspects of the cervical and thoracic spine pain generators.

Location of Manual Force in Relation to the Center of the Targeted Structure

Maitland[85] recognized that mobilization methods performed at various locations on the targeted structure (i.e., interspinous space, laminar trough, transverse process, and zygopophyseal joint) will yield different results. Since the application of a technique that identifies the patient's most concordant reproduction is the goal of the treatment, movements outside the "center" of the targeted structure are warranted. The manner in which the symptoms are reproduced demonstrate equal importance to the diagnosis of the patient.[85]

Direction of Force

Selected authors have suggested that patient position and direction (angle) of force may lead to differences in stiffness detection.[33,85] Increased stiffness, or resistance, begins as soon as force is applied to a spinous process during a posterior–anterior mobilization and is increased or decreased by changing the position of the spine.[33] Edmondston and colleagues[33] found that prepositions of flexion or extension by the patient during prone lying significantly increased the stiffness coefficient of the lumbar spine. To maintain continuity between raters, the patient is required to assume the exact position he or she assumed from the previous rater. This difficulty in maintaining a standard position for assessment combined with the small overall joint movement expected during a movement assessment will reduce the possibility of obtaining reliable results.[86,87]

The direction of mobilization forces can alter the amount of stiffness measured by machines and perceived by therapists. Caling and Lee[85] determined that stiffness measured at plus or minus 10° from a perpendicular base direction (defined as the mean direction of force applied by experienced therapists) was from 7 to 10% less than the stiffness measured in the perpendicular direction.

Contact Area over Which the Force is Applied

Several common treatment methods currently use different contact aspects of a clinician's hands. For example, the use of the thumbs, pisiform, and/or other contact points of the hand could alter the pain reproduction associated with the treatment approach. It is common to produce "false pain" during a treatment that is purely associated with a painful contact versus the movement reproduction of the pain.

Summary

- Fundamentally, there are many different ways to apply techniques and many methods to alter the selected technique once chosen.
- Methods to alter the treatment include changes in force magnitude and direction, contact area, duration of loading, rate of increased force, and alterations in the tissue in which the force is applied.

Re-Examination

The careful marriage of the examination and treatment often results in reduction of pain or normalization of range of motion. These impairment-based changes should result in an improvement in dysfunction or reduction in disability. In reality, a patient's condition is capricious and requires an ever-changing clinician's response. Analysis of the patient's change is the purpose behind careful re-examination. Additionally, the re-examination determines when and how the treatment would benefit from modification based on new findings.

Sizer et al.[88] reported that adaptation to patient response was one of the most imperative aspects of orthopedic manual therapy treatment. Included within these skill descriptors were force management, technique modifications, and velocity management methods. Ladyshewsky and Gotjamanos[35] suggested that adaptation is only possible during effective verbal and nonverbal communication between the patient and the clinician. Others have identified this form of communication as an essential trait of orthopedic clinical experts.[89]

A positive outcome will represent as a within-session (during the same session) or between-session (after the patient returns) change of the patient. Within- and between-session changes are used to adjust treatment dosage, intensity, and application for the optimal targeted result, advocating primarily the use of within-session (immediate response) changes toward a positive long-term outcome. If manual therapy is applied, and there are no within- or between-session changes, then one of three possible outcomes is probable:

1. The patient does not benefit from manual therapy.
2. The patient is doing something to "undo" the positive within-session findings of manual therapy and this needs to be further vetted out.
3. The clinician is using a technique that is inappropriate in dosage, intensity, or application.

By understanding these possible consequences, one can target the appropriate choices involved in selection of treatment techniques, dosage, and progression.[5] It emphasizes the suggestion that techniques by themselves offer little in isolation and should always represent a means to an end or need to be specific for that patient.[2] The selection of a technique is based on the presentation of the particular patient, indicating that the technique selection will most likely be different from patient to patient and will often change throughout the course of the patient's progression. The determination of method, dosage, and progression is dependent on the direct response of the patient and will differ over time.

By using both methods during assessment, the accurate ability to quantify changes in a patient's condition significantly improves. Bias associated with discordant measures or by analyzing methods that are steeped in clinician perception is reduced dramatically. Perhaps most importantly, since the model is patient response based, alterations in the treatment are applied automatically, and are based on the results of a patient's concordant and functional changes.

Summary

- Re-examination involves the analysis of the change associated with the targeted intervention.
- There are two primary considerations during re-examination of a patient: changes in the patient's concordant sign and alterations in the baseline function of the patient.

Chapter Questions

1. Why is a careful analysis of the patient's response a necessity in determining the appropriate treatment technique selection?

2. Outline the various passive treatment techniques. Compare and contrast the methods.

3. What findings are most important during re-examination, which dictate whether the treatment approach selected is correct?

4. What impact does the patient have on his or her outcome?

References

1. Edwards B. *Manual of combined movements*. Oxford; Butterworth-Heinemann: 1999.
2. Maitland GD. *Peripheral manipulation*. 3rd ed. London; Butterworth-Heinemann: 1986.
3. Edmondston SJ, Allison GT, Gregg CD, Purden SM, Svansson GR, Watson AE. Effect of position on the posteroanterior stiffness of the lumbar spine. *Man Ther*. 1998;3(1):21–26.
4. Trott P. Management of selected cervical syndromes. In: Grant R (ed). *Physical therapy of the cervical and thoracic spine*. 3rd ed. New York; Churchill Livingstone: 2002.
5. Christensen N, Jones M, Carr J. Clinical reasoning in orthopedic manual therapy. In: Grant R (ed). *Physical therapy of the cervical and thoracic spine*. 3rd ed. New York; Churchill Livingstone: 2002.
6. Gifford L. Pain, the tissues and the nervous system: A conceptual model. *Physiotherapy*. 1998;84:27.
7. Vicenzino B, Collins D, Wright A. Sudomotor changes induced by neural mobilization techniques in asymptomatic subjects. *J Man Manip Ther*. 1994; 2:66–74.
8. Exelby L. The Mulligan concept: Its application in the management of spinal conditions. *Man Ther*. 2002; 7(2):64–70.
9. Maher C, Latimer J. Pain or resistance: The therapists' dilemma. *Aust J Physiother*. 1993;38:257–260.
10. Maher C, Adams R. Reliability of pain and stiffness assessments in clinical manual lumbar spine examination. *Phys Ther*. 1994;74:10–18.
11. Grieve G. *Common vertebral joint problems*. 2nd ed. Edinburgh; Churchill Livingstone: 1988.
12. Guide to Physical Therapist Practice. 2nd ed. *Phys Ther*. 2001;81:9–744.
13. Bialosky JE, Bishop MD, Price DD, Robinson ME, George SZ. The mechanisms of manual therapy in the treatment of musculoskeletal pain: A comprehensive model. *Man Ther*. 2009;14(5):531–538.
14. Hubbard A. Homokinetics. Muscular function in human movement. In: Johnson W, Buskirk R. *Science and medicine of exercise and sport*. New York; Harper and Row: 1974.
15. Ferber R, Osternig L, Gravelle D. Effect of PNF stretch techniques on knee flexor muscle EMG activity in older adults. *J Electomyography Kinesiology*. 2002;12: 391–397.
16. Wilson E. Central facilitation and remote effects: Treating both ends of the system. *Man Ther*. 1997;2(3):165–168.
17. Prentice W. A comparison of static stretching and PNF stretching for improving hip joint flexibility. *Athletic Training*. 1983;18:56–59.
18. Childs J. Risk associated with the failure to offer manipulation for patients with low back pain. Platform Presentation. *American Academy of Orthopaedic Manual Physical Therapists Conference*. Louisville, KY. 2004.
19. Cleland J, Childs J, McRae M, Palmer J. Immediate effects of thoracic spine manipulation in patients with neck pain: A randomized clinical trial. Platform Presentation. *American Academy of Orthopaedic Manual Physical Therapists Conference*. Louisville, KY. 2004.
20. Lee M, Steven J, Crosbie R, Higgs J. Towards a theory of lumbar mobilization: The relationship between applied manual force and movements of the spine. *Man Ther*. 1996;2:67–75.
21. Anson E, Cook C, Comacho C, Gwillian B, Karakostas K. The use of education in the improvement in finding R1 in the lumbar spine. *J Man Manip Ther*. 2003;11(4): 204–212.

22. Bjornsdottir SV, Kumar S. Posteroanterior spinal mobilization: State of the art review and discussion. *Disabil Rehabil.* 1997;19:39–46.

23. Yahia L, Audet J, Drouin G. Rheological properties of the human lumbar spine ligaments. *J Biomed Eng.* 1991;13:399–406.

24. DiFabio R. Efficacy of manual therapy. *Phys Ther.* 1992;72(12):853–864.

25. Petty N, Messenger N. Can the force platform be used to measure the forces applied during a PA mobilization of the lumbar spine? *J Man Manip Ther.* 1996;4(2): 70–76.

26. Chesworth B, MacDermid J, Roth J, Patterson S. Movement diagram and "end-feel" reliability when measuring passive lateral rotation of the shoulder in patients with shoulder pathology. *Phys Ther.* 1998;78: 593–601.

27. Holm S, Nachemson A. Variations in the nutrition of the canine intervertebral disc induced by motion. *Spine.* 1983;8:866–873.

28. Maitland G, Hickling J. Abnormalities in passive movement: Diagrammative representation. *Physiother.* 1970;56:105–114.

29. Carroll W, Bandura A. The role of visual monitoring in observational learning of action patterns: Making the unobservable observable. *J Motor Behavior.* 1982;14: 153–167.

30. Carroll W, Bandura A. Representational guidance of action production in observational learning: A causal analysis. *J Motor Behavior.* 1990;22:85–97.

31. Yahia L, Audet J, Drouin G. Rheological properties of the human lumbar spine ligaments. *J Biomed Eng.* 1991;13:399–406.

32. Lee R, Latimer J, Maher C. Manipulation: Investigation of a proposed mechanism. *Clin Biomech.* 1994;8:302–306.

33. Edmondston S, Allison G, Gregg S, Purden G, Svansson G, Watson A. Effect of position on the posteroanterior stiffness of the lumbar spine. *Man Ther.* 1998;3(1):21–26.

34. Hardy GL, Napier JK. Inter and intra-therapist reliability of passive accessory movement technique. *NZ J Physiother.* 1991;22–24.

35. Ladyshewsky R, Gotjamanos E. Communication skill development in health professional education: The use of standardised patients in combination with a peer assessment strategy. *J Allied Health.* 1997;26(4):177–186.

36. Haldeman S. The clinical basis for discussion of mechanisms of manipulative therapy. In: Korr I (ed). *The neurobiologic mechanisms in manipulative therapy.* New York; Plenum Press: 1978.

37. Raftis K, Warfield C. Spinal manipulation for back pain. *Hosp Pract.* 1989;15:89–90.

38. Glover J, Morris J, Khosla T. Back pain: A randomized clinical trial of rotational manipulation of the trunk. *Br J Physiol.* 1947;150:18–22.

39. Denslow JS. Analyzing the osteopathic lesion. *J Am Osteopath Assoc.* 2001;101(2):99–100.

40. Farfan H, The scientific basis of manipulation procedures. In: Buchanan W, Kahn M, Rodnan G, Scott J, Zvailfler N, Grahame R (eds). *Clinics in rheumatic diseases.* London; WB Saunders: 1980.

41. Giles L. *Anatomical basis of low back pain.* Baltimore; Williams and Wilkins: 1989.

42. Terrett AC, Vernon H. Manipulation and pain tolerance. A controlled study of the effect of spinal manipulation on paraspinal cutaneous pain tolerance levels. *Am J Phys Med.*1984;63(5):217–225.

43. Vernon H, Dhami M, Howley T, Annett R. Spinal manipulation and beta-endorphin: A controlled study of the effect of a spinal manipulation on plasma beta-endorphin levels in normal males. *J Manipulative Physiol Ther.* 1986;9:115–123.

44. Petersen N, Vicenzino B, Wright A. The effects of a cervical mobilization technique on sympathetic outflow to the upper limb in normal subjects. *Physiother Theory Pract.* 1993;9:149–156.

45. Norkin C, Levangie P. Joint structure and function: *A comprehensive analysis.* 2nd ed. Philadelphia, PA; F. A. Davis: 1992.

46. Mennell J. *Back pain: Diagnosis and treatment using manipulative techniques.* Boston; Little, Brown: 1960.

47. Cyriax J, Cyriax P. *Cyriax's illustrated manual of orthopaedic medicine.* Oxford; Butterworth-Heineman: 1993.

48. Kaltenborn F. Manual mobilization of the joints. *The Kaltenborn method of joint mobilization and treatment.* 5th ed. Oslo; Olaf Norlis Bokhandel: 1999.

49. Benjamin P, Tappan F. *Tappan's handbook of healing massage techniques.* 4th ed. Upper Saddle River, NJ; Prentice Hall: 2004.

50. Sizer P. Manual therapy skills: Results of the Delphi study. Breakout Presentation. *American Academy of Orthopaedic Manual Physical Therapists Conference.* Reno, NV. 2003.

51. Wood T, Collaca C, Matthews R. A pilot randomized clinical trial on the relative effect of instrumental (MFMA) versus manual (HVLA) manipulation in the treatment of cervical spine dysfunction. *J Manipulative Physiol Ther.* 2001;24:260–271.

52. Cramer G, Tuck N, Knudsen J. et al. Effects of side-posture positioning and side-posture adjusting on the lumbar zygopophyseal joints as evaluated by magnetic resonance imaging: A before and after study with randomization. *J Manipulative Physiol Ther.* 2000;23: 380–394.

53. Angstrom L, Lindstrom B. (abstract). Treatment effects of traction and mobilization of the hip joint in patients with inflammatory rheumatological diseases and hip osteoarthritis. *Nordisk Fysoterapi.* 2003;7:17–27.

54. Collins N, Teys P, Vicenzino B. The initial effects of a Mulligan's mobilization with movement technique on dorsiflexion and pain in subacute ankle sprains. *Man Ther.* 2004;9:77–82.

55. Conroy D, Hayes K. The effect of joint mobilization as a component of comprehensive treatment for primary shoulder impingement syndrome. *J Orthop Phys Ther.* 1998;28:3–14.

56. Gibson H, Ross J, Allen J, Latimer J, Maher C. The effect of mobilization on forward bending range. *J Man Manip Ther.* 1993;1:142–147.

57. Ginn K, Cohen M. Conservative treatment for shoulder pain: Prognostic indicators of outcome. *Arch Phys Med Rehabil.* 2004;85:1231–1235.

58. Green T, Refshauge K, Crosbie J, Adams R. A randomized controlled trial of a passive accessory joint mobilization on acute ankle inversion sprains. *Phys Ther.* 2001;81:984–994.

59. Hjelm R, Draper C, Spencer S. Anterior–inferior capsular length insufficiency in the painful shoulder. *J Orthop Sports Phys Ther.* 1996;23:216–222.

60. Hoeksma H, Dekker J, Ronday K, Heering A, van der Lubbe N, Vel C, Breedveld F, van den Ende C. Comparison of manual therapy and exercise therapy in osteoarthritis of the hip: A randomized clinical trial. *Arthritis Rheum.* 2004;51:722–729.

61. Randall T, Portney L, Harris B. Effects of joint mobilization on joint stiffness and active motion of the metacarpal–phalangeal joint. *J Orthop Sports Phys Ther.* 1992;16:30–36.

62. Shamus J, Shamus E, Gugel R, Brucker B, Skaruppa C. The effect of sesamoid mobilization, flexor hallucis strengthening, and gait training on reducing pain and restoring function in individuals with hallux limitus: A clinical trial. *J Orthop Sports Phys Ther.* 2004;34: 368–376.

63. Herzog W. *Clinical biomechanics of spinal manipulation.* London; Churchill Livingstone: 2000.

64. McCarthy CJ. Spinal manipulative thrust technique using combined movement theory. *Man Ther.* 2001;6: 197–204.

65. Nyberg R. Manipulation: Definition, types, application. In: Basmajian J, Nyberg R (eds). *Rational manual therapies.* Baltimore; Williams and Wilkins: 1993.

66. Sprague R, Cook C. Differential assessment and mobilization of the cervical and upper thoracic spine. In: Donatelli R, Wooden M (eds). *Orthopedic physical therapy.* Philadelphia; Churchill Livingston: 2010.

67. Grice A, Vernon H. Basic principles in the performance of chiropractic adjusting: Historical review, classification and objectives. In: Haldeman S. (ed) *Principles and practice of chiropractic.* 2nd ed. Norwalk; Appleton & Lange: 1992;443–458.

68. Lenehan K, Fryer G, McLaughlin P. The effect of muscle energy technique on gross trunk range of motion. *J Osteopathy Med.* 2003;6:13–18.

69. Schenk R, MacDiarmid A, Rousselle J. The effects of muscle energy technique on lumbar range of motion. *J Man Manip Ther.* 1997;5:179–183.

70. Schenk R, Adelman K, Rousselle J. The effects of muscle energy technique on cervical range of motion. *J Man Manip Ther.* 1994;2:149–155.

71. Goodridge JP. Muscle energy technique: Definition, explanation, methods of procedure. *J Am Osteopath Assoc.* 1981;81(4):249–254.

72. Winters M, Blake C, Trost S, Marcello-Brinker T, Lowe L, Garber M, Wainner R. Passive versus active stretching of hip flexor muscles in subjects with limited hip extension: A randomized trial. *Phys Ther.* 2004;84:800–807.

73. Grieve G. *Common vertebral joint problems.* 2nd ed. Edinburgh; Churchill Livingstone: 1988.

74. Shekelle PG. Spinal manipulation. *Spine.* 1994;19: 858–861.

75. Whittingham W, Nilsson N. Active range of motion in the cervical spine increases after spinal manipulation. *J Manipulative Physiol Ther.* 2001;24:552–555.

76. Andersen S, Fryer G, McLaughlin P. The effect of talocrural joint manipulation on range of motion at the ankle joint in subjects with a history of ankle injury. *Australas Chiropract Osteopathy.* 2003;11:57–62.

77. Mulligan B. Mobilisations with movement (MVM's). *J Man Manip Ther.* 1993;1:154–156.

78. Mulligan B. *Manual therapy "NAGS", "SNAGS", "MWM's" etc.* 4th ed. Wellington; Plane View Services Ltd: 1999.

79. Mulligan BR. Spinal mobilisation with leg movement (further mobilisation with movement). *J Man Manip Ther.* 1995;3(1):25–27.

80. Konstantinou K, Foster N, Rushton A, Baxter D. The use and reported effects of mobilization with movement techniques in low back pain management; a cross-sectional descriptive survey of physiotherapists in Britain. *Man Ther.* 2002;7(4):206–214.

81. Lee M, Mosely A, Refshauge K. Effects of feedback on learning a vertebral joint mobilizations skill. *Phys Ther.* 1990;10:97–102.

82. Latimer J, Lee M, Adams RD. The effects of high and low loading forces on measured values of lumbar stiffness. *J Manipulative Physiol Ther.* 1998;21: 157–163.

83. Chiradejnant A, Latimer J, Maher CG. Forces applied during manual therapy to patients with low back pain. *J Manipulative Physiol Ther.* 2002;25(6):362–369.

84. Herzog W, Conway PJ, Kawchuk GN, Zhang Y, Hasler EM. Forces exerted during spinal manipulative therapy. *Spine.* 1993;18(9):1206–1212.

85. Caling B, Lee M. Effect of direction of applied mobilization force on the posteroanterior response in the lumbar spine. *J Manipulative Physiol Ther.* 2001;24: 71–78.

86. Lee R, Evans J. An *in-vivo* study of the intervertebral movements produced by posteroanterior mobilization. *Clin Biomech.* 1997;12:400–408.

87. Frank C, Akeson WH, Woo SLY, Amiel D, Coutts RD. Physiology and therapeutic value of passive joint of motion. *Clin Ortho.* 1984;185:113–124.

88. Sizer PS, Matthijs O, Phelps V. Influence of age on the development of pathology. *Curr Rev Pain* 2000;4:362–373.

89. Jensen G, Shepard K, Hack L. The novice versus the experienced clinician: Insights into the work of the physical therapist. *Phys Ther.* 1990;70:314–323.

Manual Therapy of the Cervical Spine

Chad E. Cook and Rogelio Coronado

Objectives

- Outline the pertinent clinically relevant anatomy of the cervical spine.
- Outline the three-dimensional coupling patterns of the cervical spine.
- Outline and describe the anatomical considerations of the coronary artery system.
- Perform the clinical examination of the cervical spine.
- Outline an effective treatment program for various cervical spine impairments.
- Identify the outcomes associated with manual therapy to the cervical spine.

Clinical Examination

Pretesting

The cervical spine is unique to other musculoskeletal regions because manual therapy techniques are associated with more risk in this region than any other area of the body. Consequently, pretesting for ligamentous integrity and the potential for vascular compromise may be useful. Life-threatening consequences have been associated with a condition called **cervical arterial dysfunction (CAD)**. CAD may be associated with hypermobility, a lack of ligamentous stability, or predisposing factors such as atherosclerosis or spondylosis. Ligamentous testing and CAD testing are discussed in detail below.

Ligamentous Testing Ligamentous testing is useful after trauma or in special populations such as rheumatoid arthritis, in which degradation of ligamentous tissues is suspected. Testing may include the Modified Sharp Purser test (Figure 5.1), the Alar Ligament Stress Test (Figure 5.2), and the Transverse Ligament of Atlas test (Figure 5.3).

Cervical-Arterial Dysfunction (CAD) Testing For manual therapy of the cervical spine, the most significant cause for concern is associated with the stresses to the arterial vessels around the neck.[3]

Complications may occur with the vertebrobasilar artery and the internal carotid artery of the neck. Damage to the vertebrobasilar artery may lead to the following signs and symptoms associated with CAD: diplopia, dizziness, drop attacks, dysarthria, dysphagia, nystagmus, nausea, and numbness.[4] Other findings may include ataxia, clumsiness and agitation, facial numbness, hearing disturbances, hoarseness, loss of short-term memory, malaise, papillary changes, photophobia, or vomiting.[3]

Damage to the internal carotid artery (ICA) may lead to the ischemic complications of transient ischemic attack, ischemic stroke, and retinal infarction.[3] Nonischemic signs and symptoms of ICA dissection may include Horner's syndrome, pulsatile tinnitus, cranial nerve palsy, scalp tenderness, neck swelling, cranial nerve VI palsy, and orbital pain.[3]

Although manual therapists have "screened" for CAD for years, the effectiveness of these methods is questionable. For starters, the predictive value of current pretreatment screening guidelines/guidance is poor, and blood flow reduction as tested in asymptomatic subjects is not necessarily transferable to symptomatic subjects. In addition, the absence of cardinal signs during testing does not decrease the incidence of CAD. Recent recommendations suggest extension may decrease blood flow as well as rotation. Lastly, a number of comorbidities are associated with an

Modified Sharp-Purser Test

The Modified Sharp-Purser Test is designed to assess upper cervical instability, specifically instability associated with disruption of the transverse ligament of the dens. Cattryesse et al.[1] found that the Modified Sharp-Purser Test was not reliable for "feel" or valid for provocation of symptoms when testing hypermobility. In their study, the clinicians were unable to identify patients with congenital hypermobility in the upper cervical spine. It is important to note that if the clinician suspects a fracture, this test should not be performed until appropriate imaging is used to screen the patient, since the test does involve some risk of injury. In addition, if disruption of the transverse ligament is present, the passive migration of the axis anteriorly could place considerable pressure upon the spinal cord.

The test has been taught using two ways and has two potential "positive findings." The first is associated with any movement felt during a passive translation of the head posteriorly during the blocking of C2. The other "positive" occurs when symptoms that were present during forward flexion of the head are relieved during posterior translation of the head. The original study by Sharp-Purser failed to define the procedure and manual therapists have since altered the test to meet their needs. Most commonly, the test is performed in a sitting position.

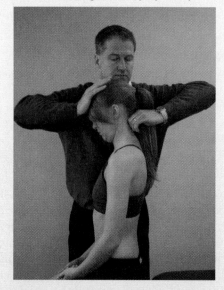

■ **Figure 5.1**   The Sharp-Purser Test

1. The patient's head should be slightly flexed.

2. The clinician should query the patient for symptoms while in the flexed position.

3. The clinician stands to the side of the patient and stabilizes (blocks) the C2 spinous process posteriorly using a pincer grasp.

4. Gently at first, the clinician applies a posterior translation force from the palm of the hand on the patient's forehead toward a posterior direction. Symptoms are assessed for both degree of linear displacement and symptom elimination during posterior translation (Figure 5.1 ■).

Alar Ligament Stress Test

The Alar Ligament Stress Test has long been advocated as a maneuver to assess the integrity of the Alar ligament. There are many iterations of the test but all have the same underlying philosophy. Because the Alar ligament controls axial rotation between the atlas and axis (i.e., right axial rotation is limited by the left Alar ligaments and vice versa), and because the ligament also controls excessive side flexion, both movements are often examined during testing. During the test, if no rotation or side flexion is felt on the axis spinous process (C2), then it is assumed that damage has occurred to the

Alar ligament. In normal situations, C2 attempts to move during side flexion and rotation. Both reproduction of symptoms and abnormal feel are considered positive.

1. The patient assumes a sitting or supine position.

2. The head is slightly flexed to further engage the Alar ligament.

3. The clinician stabilizes the C2 spinous process using a pincer grasp (Figure 5.2 ■). A firm grip ensures appropriate assessment of movement.

4. Either side flexion or rotation is passively initiated. During these passive movements, the clinician attempts to feel movement of C2. A positive test is the failure to "feel" movement of the C2 process during side flexion and/or rotation.[2]

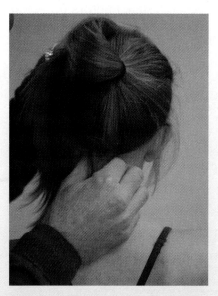

■ **Figure 5.2**   Alar Ligament Stress Test

The Transverse Ligament of Atlas Test

The Transverse Ligament of Atlas Test also assesses the integrity of the transverse ligament. Essentially, this test is redundant to the Modified Sharp-Purser Test. As with the Modified Sharp-Purser, both movement and symptom provocation assessment is the objective of this test. Because the anterior translation is focused on the C1 transverse processes, the test theoretically assesses excessive movement of C1 into the spinal canal. Additionally, since the transverse ligament functions to resist anterior shear and since failure to this ligament may result in symptoms such as dizziness, nausea, lip, face, or limb paresthesia, nystagmus, or any form of myelopathic symptoms, this test is extremely beneficial following a trauma to the cervical spine[2].

1. The patient assumes a supine position.

2. The clinician assesses resting symptoms prior to contacting the posterior aspect of the bilateral C1 transverse processes with their fingers.

3. The palms of the clinician are placed under the occiput of the patient.

4. The clinician applies an anterior force to the C1 transverse processes (using their fingers), lifting the head as the force is applied (Figure 5.3 ■). This position is held for 15–20 seconds, and if no symptoms occur the clinician can apply a downward force on the patient's forehead using the anterior aspect of the shoulder.

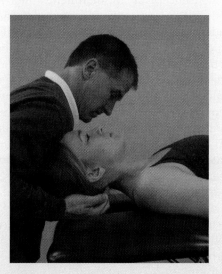

■ **Figure 5.3**   The Transverse Ligament of Atlas Test

■ TABLE 5.1 Risk Factors for Arterial Intimal Damage (Stroke Risk)

Major Risk Factors	Minor Risk Factors
Hypertension (BP >140/90)	Estrogen-based contraceptive
Hypercholesterolemia	Hormone replacement therapy
Hyperlipidemia	Infection (systemic)
Diabetes	Poor diet
Family history of myocardial infarction, angina, transient ischemic attacks, stroke, or peripheral vascular disorder	RA or other connective tissue syndrome
Smoking	Blood-clotting disorder
BMI >30	Fibromuscular dysplasia
Repeated or recent injury (including repeated manipulations)	Hypermobility
Upper cervical instability	Erectile dysfunction
	BMI 25–29

BP, blood pressure; BMI, body mass index.

increased risk of CAD and are worth examining during clinical practice[4,5] (Table 5.1 ■). To assess these comorbidities, Kerry and Taylor[5] have suggested mandatory assessment of resting blood pressure, upper cervical spine instability testing, and body mass index.

Barker et al.[6] outline several important premanipulative testing procedures prior to selection of a manipulative maneuver. The cornerstones of their suggestions outline the risk factors associated with CAD assessment using both subjective and objective criteria. They suggest that premanipulative tests such as CAD testing maneuvers should be performed upon patient consent prior to treatment intervention. Nonetheless, this suggestion is controversial as there is no evidence to support that screening for CAD leads to a reduction of consequences after manual therapy.

Vertebral basilar insufficiency (VBI), which is a component of CAD, is a localized or diffuse reduction in blood flow through the vertebrobasilar arterial system. This system supplies the posterior aspects of the brain and includes the brainstem, cerebellum, occipital lobe, medial temporal lobe, and thalamus. VBI-related problems associated with manipulation have been reported to range from one occurrence in 20,000 to five in 10,000,000 during cervical spine manipulations[7]. The most frequently reported form of injury is arterial dissection, which can result in a variety of outcomes including death in 18% of cases [8]. Although the causes of arterial dissection associated with manipulation are not completely known, it is apparent that the most frequently injured site for the artery is at C1–C2,[9] most likely because the artery experiences elongation and kinking during cervical rotation, mostly at this region. For example, during right rotation the left vertebral artery experiences elongation.

CAD tests are used with some degree of controversy and as previously stated do not likely result in a known outcome after testing. Johnson et al.[10] found unreliable evidence that upper cervical manipulation influences upper vertebral artery flow. However, participants for the study were a mean age of 33 and were asymptomatic with no CAD-related symptoms. In other experimental studies, tests have shown mixed overall results regarding the occlusion of blood flow to the brain with cervical motion. Some studies confirm that collateral circulation is present during the provocative movements, whereas others have been inconclusive.[11–14] As stated previously, the relationship between reduced blood flow during a physical test and a negative consequence during a manipulative procedure is speculative at best.

Nonetheless, several physical testing methods have been defined within the literature. Maitland[15] suggested placing an individual in the premanipulative position (Figure 5.5) prior to performing the procedure in order to assess their tolerance to the position. Of all the tests identified, sustained end-range rotation of the cervical spine has long been suggested as the most effective method of CAD assessment of the upper cervical spine (Figure 5.4). This test was first described by Maitland in 1968,[16,17] and is currently recommended in the premanipulation guidelines for the cervical spine[6,18,19] that are used by physiotherapists and other manual therapists. The purpose of the test is to reproduce potential signs or symptoms of CAD in a safe, gradual progression of neck rotation. If central neurological signs or symptoms are reproduced, immediate referral to a physician for further testing is warranted.

It is the discretion of the clinician to perform a CAD test prior to treatment; however, screening for CAD should occur prior to every manipulative session.[6] Barker et al.[6] report that despite thorough screening, there is still an element of risk associated with spontaneous accident. Additionally, the subjective examination will often dictate who may have a positive CAD response prior to testing. Since there is some risk of causing a positive CAD using the testing method, it may be advisable to avoid the performance of the test or treatment in cases where subjective symptoms are already reported or past tests have demonstrated positive findings. In the event of a positive CAD during testing, the treatment should be stopped immediately and appropriate medical assistance should be consulted.[6]

Cervical Arterial Dysfunction (CAD) Testing

The first component of the examination requires a patient interview to extract signs and symptoms of CAD. If findings are remarkable, the patient is referred out for appropriate medical consult.

1. Prior to a comprehensive clinical examination, the clinician performs end-range cervical rotation tests or rotation and extension on the patient in a sitting or supine position (Figures 5.4 ■ and 5.5 ■).

2. The position is held for 10 seconds with observation for signs and symptoms of CAD.

3. The head is returned to a neutral position and held for a minimum of 10 seconds.

4. Rotation is repeated to the opposite side and held for 10 seconds. Rotation and extension is suggested with the same holds and visual assessments. This assessment method can also be examined in supine. If minor dizziness is present the clinician may choose to perform vestibular testing, which is beyond the scope of this book.

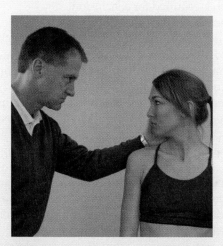

■ Figure 5.4   Cervical Rotation Test in Sitting

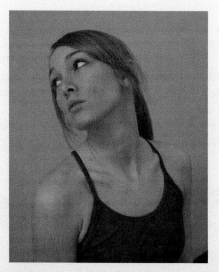

■ Figure 5.5   Cervical Rotation and Extension Test in Sitting

Premanipulative Position Test

The last procedure performed is the premanipulative position test (Figure 5.6 ■) to determine the patient's tolerance to combined movements of the mid and lower cervical spine. The procedure is performed in a supine position. The patient's symptoms require a preassessment prior to the examination.

1. The patient's neck is side-glided toward an end point.

2. Using the lateral aspect of the first metacarpalphalangeal joint, the clinician provides a fulcrum force to the neck. The contact point should consist of the articular pillars or the transverse processes. The patient's neck is side-flexed (Figure 5.6, left) to the level of the contact point. Since combined movements are often used when single-plane movements are less sensitive, pain should not be as critical a consideration.

3. The patient neck is rotated in the opposite direction as the side flexion (to the right in the photo), but not beyond. The clinician should feel the neck "lock."

4. The patient's condition should be reassessed, specifically for signs of CAD. The position is held for 10 seconds and if symptoms are remarkable (during or after assessment), the patient is referred to appropriate medical personnel.

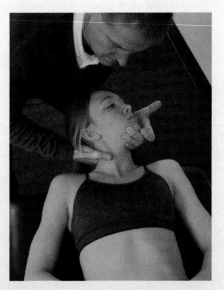

■ **Figure 5.6**   The Premanipulative Position

Summary

- The cervical spine is unique to other musculoskeletal regions because of the consequences associated with CAD. Consequently, premanipulative testing is required for safety considerations.

- Sustained end-of-range rotation of the cervical spine has long been suggested as the most effective method of CAD assessment of the upper cervical spine.

- Despite thorough CAD screening prior to the initiation of treatment, there is still an element of risk associated with spontaneous accident.

Observation

Visual assessment of cervical posture is frequently used during clinical examination.[20, 21] It has long been postulated that posture directly influences temporomandibular disorder (TMD). Studies that have investigated this hypothesis have found mixed results. Selected authors have reported no such relationship exists,[22–24] whereas others have identified a relationship, most notably muscle imbalances.[25] Wright et al.[26] report that postural training with TMD self-management methods was more effective than self-management methods alone. Further research is required for conclusion.

Selected authors[27,28] have reported a notable association between forward head posture and headaches. Watson and Trott[27] found that a preponderance of subjects examined with chronic headaches demonstrated abnormal posture, specifically forward head posture (Figure 5.7 ■), while the control subjects did not.

A decreased willingness to move may be associated with spine instability or an upper cervical fracture. Because cervical spine instability may only demonstrate subtle clinical examination features,[29,30] it is important to recognize certain attributes associated with this potentially serious complication. These attributes have been described as aberrant cervical movements,[31] referred shoulder pain,[31,32] radiculopathy and/or myelopathy,[33] paraspinal muscle spasms, decreased cervical lordosis,[31] tinnitus,[34] pain during sustained postures[31], and altered range of motion.[29,35–37] Because these symptoms are similar to other, less complicated disorders, it is essential to determine if a history of major

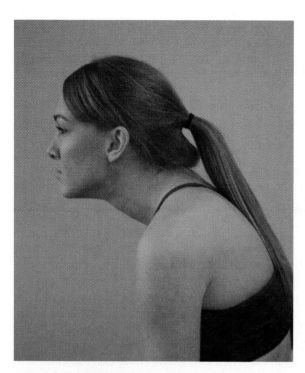

■ **Figure 5.7** Forward Head Posture

trauma or repetitive microtrauma has predated the report of symptoms.[29]

In patients with cervical instability from a dens fracture, neurological symptoms associated with myelopathy may be present. Occasionally, these neurological symptoms are limited to one transitory episode of diffuse paresis following trauma, whereas in other patients, cervical myelopathy is notable and profuse. Progressive myelopathy causes weakness and ataxia, which predominates over sensory changes.[38] In severe cases a dens fracture may lead to neurovascular symptoms and vertebral artery compression. Subsequently, this compression may cause cervical and brainstem ischemia with signs and symptoms such as gait ataxia, syncope, vertigo, and visual disturbances. This serious phenomenon is beyond the scope of a manual therapist's treatment and should be discovered during pretesting.

Since less than 3% of trauma radiographic series have positive findings[39] and provide very low yield, many authors consider universal C-spine radiography inefficient and costly.[40,41] Occasionally, to effectively clear the C-spine, repeated imaging attempts are required, a mechanism that adds to the total costs.[42] Subsequently, the **Canadian C-Spine rules** were devised to rule out those who may not need a radiograph after acute trauma. Bandiera et al.[43] have reported that the sensitivity of this instrument was higher than the clinical judgment of emergency room physicians, demonstrating 100% sensitivity in a large population of patients with cervical spine trauma. Patients who are (1) cognitively intact and have no neurological symptoms; (2) are under the age of 65; (3) are not fearful of moving the head upon command; (4) who were not involved in a distraction-based injury; and (5) who demonstrate no midline pain are spared a radiograph.[43]

Summary

- Selected postures such as forward head are commonly associated with cervical pain.
- There is mixed information regarding the postural contribution of the cervical spine to TMD.
- After a traumatic incident, a decreased willingness to move could be a red flag associated with upper C-spine instability.
- The use of the Canadian C-Spine Rules is beneficial in determining whether a medical referral for a radiograph is warranted.

Patient History

Gregory Grieve[44] outlined three mandatory questions for the cervical spine:

1. Any dizziness (vertigo), blackouts, or "drop" attacks?
2. Any history of rheumatoid arthritis or other inflammatory arthritis, or treatment by systemic steroid?
3. Any neurological symptoms in the arms and legs?

Often, dizziness, blackouts, and drop attacks are associated with a CAD disorder, characterized by restriction of blood flow through the cervical arteries, thus restricting the flow of blood to the rear portions of the brain; including the occipital lobe, cerebellum, and brainstem.[8] Further discussion of detection of CAD is provided in the pretesting section.

Neurological symptoms are frequent in patients with instability-based disorders. Rheumatoid arthritis (RA) is the most common inflammatory disorder that may influence the integrity of the cervical spine, with a predilection for the atlantoaxial joint complex.[45] RA is associated with instability and should always be determined prior to assessment.[46]

Neurological symptoms in the legs associated with cervical disorders or movements may be indicative of myelopathy. Myelopathy is characterized by the clinical finding that the lower extremities are affected first, with subsequent spasticity and paresis. The patient often complains of a gait disturbance due to abnormalities in the corticospinal tracts and spinocerebellar tracts. Later, the upper extremities become involved with loss of strength and difficulty in fine finger movements.[47,48] Significant complaints associated with myelopathy are best served by referral to a medical physician trained in neurological assessment. Nonetheless, it is important to note that the diagnosis is extremely difficult to make without imaging support and that most tests and measures lack sensitivity, resulting in a number of false-positive findings.[47]

Summary

- Dizziness, blackouts, and drop attacks are associated with CAD.
- CAD is a disorder characterized by restriction of blood flow through the cervical arteries, thus restricting the flow of blood to the rear portions of the brain, including the occipital lobe, cerebellum, and brainstem.
- RA is the most common form of inflammatory disorder, which influences the integrity of the cervical spine.
- Myelopathy is a difficult diagnosis to make but does involve initial problems in the lower extremities, with subsequent spasticity and paresis.

Physical Examination

Active Physiological Movements

Active movements are any form of physiological movements performed exclusively by the patient. In a clinical examination, the purpose of an active movement is to identify and examine the effect of selected active movements on the concordant sign. By determining the behavior of the concordant sign during selected movements, the clinician can effectively identify potential active physiological treatment approaches. Active physiological assessment of the cervical spine purportedly examines the contractile elements of the cervical spine.[49] Range-of-motion testing is an efficient screening technique and is effective for assessment of age-related changes and degeneration. In many cases, degenerative changes of the cervical spine result in losses of range of motion in all movements except rotation.[49]

Sandmark and Nisell[50] deemed active assessment that consisted of visual observation of movement patterns insufficiently sensitive in detecting concordant patients' complaints. The authors used reproduction of pain as their sensitivity instrument during detection. Lee et al.[51] reported active range-of-motion differences between symptomatic and asymptomatic patients in a controlled comparison. Their findings indicate that when compared to normal subjects, symptomatic patients exhibited decreased lower cervical extension and left rotation but exhibit greater chin retraction. The work of Sterling et al.[52] indicates that the active range-of-motion values are consistent over time and do not

Upper Cervical Flexion

A systematic process is helpful in detecting the concordant sign of the patient and since multiple movements in several degrees of freedom are capable in the cervical spine, there are many movements to assess. The first motion of assessment is upper cervical spine flexion.

1 The clinician positions the patient's head in a designated neutral position.

2 The clinician instructs the patient to retract his or her chin, or to "make a double chin" (Figure 5.8 ▪). The patient should be instructed to retract up to the first point of pain.

3 The clinician instructs the patient to retract beyond his or her first point of pain, or if no pain is present, go toward the end range.

4 The clinician then instructs the patient to gently nod his or her chin to further provoke the region with repeated movements.

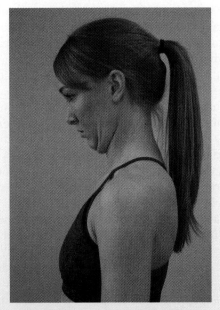

▪ Figure 5.8   Upper C-Spine Flexion

Upper Cervical Extension

Upper cervical spine extension is a movement that is commonly associated with forward head postures.

1. The clinician positions the patient's head in a designated neutral position.

2. The clinician then instructs the patient to protract his or her chin, or to "stick your chin out" (Figure 5.9 ■). The patient should be instructed to protract up to the first point of pain.

3. Then the clinician instructs the patient to protract beyond his or her first point of pain, or if no pain is present, the patient is instructed to move toward the end range.

4. The clinician instructs the patient to gently nod his or her chin to further provoke the test through repeated movements. The patient's signs and symptoms are readdressed.

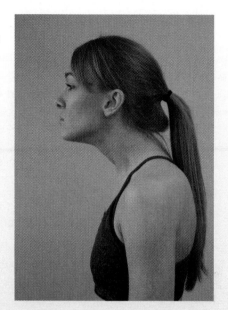

■ **Figure 5.9**   Upper C-Spine Extension

reflect artifact or changes associated with the presence of pain during the time of assessment. Subsequently, it appears that range-of-motion abnormalities that also reproduce the patient's current complaint of pain are helpful in identifying the impaired movement as compared to painful movements alone.

Active Physiological Motion of the Upper Cervical Spine   As previously stated, in a clinical examination, the purpose of an active movement is to identify and examine the effect of selected active movements on the concordant sign.

The use of overpressure may be useful in isolating various impairments, and is designed to "rule out" potential joints that do not contribute to the patient's impairment.[29,53] Overpressure is less effective when one attempts to dictate the presence of the impairment based on "feel" of the end range. Assessment of end-feel appears to be a valuable skill for manual therapists, although investigators have reported mixed outcomes regarding the reliability and clinical utility in several different joint systems.[54,55] Test effectiveness may vary according to other factors including the joint position, the tester's educational background,[56] and the presence of pain.[57]

Active Physiological Motion of the Lower Cervical Spine   As previously stated, in a clinical examination, the purpose of an active movement is to identify and examine the effect of selected active movements on the concordant sign.

Lower Cervical Flexion

The lower cervical spine harbors different movements and responsibilities when compared to the upper cervical spine. Subsequently, it is beneficial to disassociate the movement of the upper cervical spine. Because it is impossible to eliminate movement, the following provides a guideline that emphasizes the flexion-based motion to the lower cervical spine.

1. The clinician positions the patient's head in a designated neutral position.

2. The clinician then instructs the patient to retract his or her chin, or to "make a double chin." The clinician instructs the patient to bend the neck forward, up to the first point of pain, while keeping the chin tucked.

3. As with the upper cervical spine, the clinician instructs the patient to move beyond the first point of pain.

4. (If no pain) The clinician applies a gentle overpressure into physiological flexion (pictured), while concurrently stabilizing the lower posterior neck (Figure 5.10 ■). The clinician applies traction with the flexion-based overpressure and the patient's signs and symptoms are reassessed.

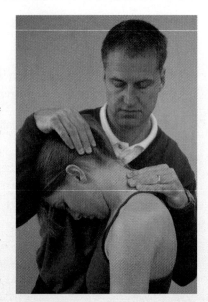

■ **Figure 5.10** Lower Cervical Flexion and Flexion with Overpressure

Lower Cervical Extension

A forward head posture places the lower cervical spine into a position of flexion. Assessing extension is beneficial to determine if the postural problem is structural or positional.

1. The clinician positions the patient's head in a designated neutral position.

2. The clinician then instructs the patient to retract his or her chin, or to "make a double chin."

3. The clinician instructs the patient to bend the neck backward up to the first point of pain, or to "keep your chin tucked in while bending your neck backward."

4. The clinician instructs the patient to move beyond the first point of pain to his or her end range. (If no pain)

5. The clinician applies a gentle overpressure into physiological extension while supporting the thoracic spine with his or her elbow and forearm and cupping the posterior aspect of the head of the patient (Figure 5.11 ■). Upon completion, the patient's signs and symptoms are reassessed.

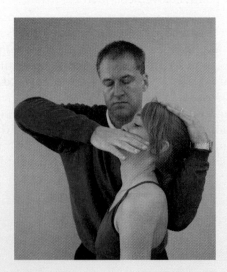

■ **Figure 5.11** Lower Cervical Extension and Extension with Overpressure

Physiological Side Flexion

Physiological side flexion is a movement that requires six degrees of accessory motion.[58]

1. The clinician positions the patient's head in a designated neutral position.

2. The clinician instructs the patient to side-flex the neck up to the first point of pain, or to "touch your ear to your shoulder."

3. The clinician instructs the patient to move beyond the first point of pain to his or her end range.

4. (If no pain) The clinician gently applies overpressure into physiological side flexion. Typically, this is performed using the ulnar aspect of the hand as a "fulcrum" to the neck. The clinician should place his or her palm on the zygomatic arch of the patient and stabilize the head with the fingers for maximum patient comfort (Figure 5.12 ■). The patient's signs and symptoms should be reassessed and the technique repeated on the opposite side.

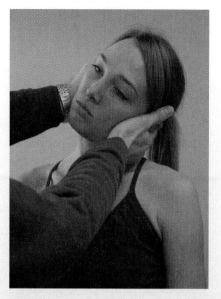

■ **Figure 5.12**   Side Flexion and Side Flexion with Overpressure

Physiological Rotation

Physiological rotation is guided primarily by zygopophyseal joint translation.[59]

1. During rotation, the clinician positions the patient's head in a designated neutral position. The clinician then instructs the patient to rotate the neck up to the first point of pain, or to "turn to your right (or left) while keeping your eyes level."

2. The clinician instructs the patient to move beyond the first point of pain to his or her end range.

3. (If no pain) The clinician gently applies overpressure into physiological rotation. If right rotation (pictured), the right shoulder is stabilized with the clinician's left forearm (the opposite for left rotation). The clinician places his or her palms on both zygomatic arches while stabilizing the head (as in side flexion) (Figure 5.13 ■). The forearm is used as a counterforce to prevent the body from turning.

4. The patient's signs and symptoms are then assessed and the process is repeated on the opposite side.

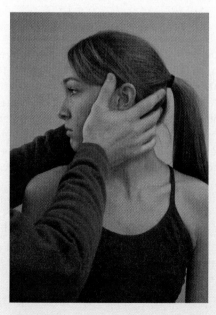

■ **Figure 5.13**   Rotations with Overpressure

Active Cervical Flexion and Rotation

A well-described combined movement designed to narrow the anatomical space in the intervertebral foramen is the lower quadrant maneuver described by Maitland.[15] This movement is somewhat similar to the Spurling's test and is sometimes used during detection of cervical radiculopathy.[60] Maitland[15] reported that the quadrant test is effective in ruling out pain of cervical origin. A positive test could reflect nerve root compression of spondylogenic-based dysfunction on the side tested.

1. The patient assumes a sitting position.
2. The head is positioned in a designated neutral position.
3. The clinician stands to the side of the patient on the tested side.
4. The clinician then places his or her hand on the top of the patient's scapula while the clinician stabilizes the patient's thorax with his or her forearm.
5. The clinician instructs the patient to look back to the clinician's hand, which involves side flexion and rotation to the same side with extension. The patient should be instructed to stop at the first point of pain. (If no pain)
6. The clinician applies a gentle overpressure into the combined range of side flexion, rotation, and extension by placing the palm of his or her hand on the zygomatic arch and applying a very brief and quick force (Figure 5.14 ■). The process can be repeated on the opposite side if needed.

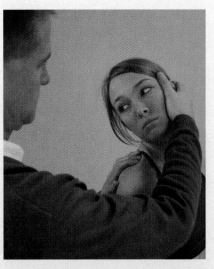

■ **Figure 5.14** Lower Cervical Quadrant with Overpressure

Combined Movements Combined movements are useful to identify concordant movements that are not identified during single plane movements and may further flesh out the behavior of movement and its contribution to the patient's cervical problem.

An upper quadrant test involves concurrent upper cervical extension with side flexion and rotation to the same side. Full upper cervical extension is necessary; however, the movements of side flexion and rotation should be minimal in magnitude. It is useful to load (press downward) through the upper aspect of the skull to move the patient toward end range. The technique is difficult to do and should be learned during an educational course or from a clinician that is competent with the technique.

Summary

- Active physiological assessment of the cervical spine purportedly examines the contractile elements of the cervical spine, but also assesses the patient's tolerance to a given position.

- The use of overpressures may be useful in isolating various impairments and are designed to 'rule out' joints that do not contribute to the patient's impairment.

- Selected combined movements may be beneficial to isolate the origin of the pain by increasing the tension or compression placed on articular and surrounding structures.

- Range-of-motion abnormalities that reproduce the patient's current complaint of pain are helpful in identifying the impaired movement.

Passive Movements

Passive Physiological Movements   The movement planes applied during passive physiological examination are similar to those tested during active physiological movements, and are used to further confirm the concordant sign of the patient. In some cases, these movements are used only to determine abnormal mobility. Fjellner et al.[61] reported that passive physiological movements demonstrated acceptable interclinician reliability in six of the eight plane-based testing movements.

Passive physiological movements are commonly used to dictate the appropriate level for manipulation or mobilization of the cervical spine. In a study performed by Haas et al.,[62] manipulation based on clinical physiological end-feel assessment was compared against a randomized selection of a targeted level. These findings were based on one day's worth of treatment and displayed no differences in pain or stiffness outcomes. This finding is analogous to the thoracic and lumbar spine that there is little information to support the need to identify a specific level for manipulative intervention.[63,64] Nonetheless, passive physiological movements have long been considered important for manual therapy assessment, thus it is intuitive to consider isolating the appropriate segment as crucial for appropriate care.

Passive Physiological Flexion

The first passive physiological assessment method during examination is flexion. This procedure is not discriminatory in detecting concordant pain, but is helpful in detecting asymmetries in cervical flexion.

1. The patient should assume a supine position.

2. The head should extend beyond the end of the plinth up to the T2 spinous process.

3. The head is stabilized using digits 1 and 2 to support the posterior articular pillars and the thumb anteriorly. The clinician applies a gentle cephalic to caudal movement, allowing passive flexion to occur in the spine, stopping at the first point of pain (Figure 5.15 ■). The clinician should feel for symmetry of motion and assess reproduction of pain while moving beyond the first point of pain and progressing to end range. If no pain is present the clinician may increase the sensitivity of the test by applying force through the top of the skull (using the abdomen to increase compression).

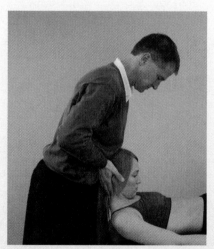

■ **Figure 5.15**   Passive Physiological Flexion

Passive Physiological Extension

The second passive physiological assessment method during examination is extension. Because of the angle of the facets, this procedure provides fair discriminatory capabilities in detecting concordant pain, and is very helpful in detecting asymmetries in cervical extension.

1. The patient assumes a supine position and the head should extend beyond the end of the plinth up to the T2 spinous process.

2. The head is stabilized using digits 1 and 2 to support the posterior articular pillars and the thumb anteriorly.

3. The clinician applies a gentle cephalic to caudal movement, allowing passive extension to occur in the spine (Figure 5.16 ■). The head is extended to the T2 process but is stopped at the first reported presence of pain. The clinician moves the patient's cervical spine into further extension beyond the first point of pain, while feeling for symmetry of motion and assessing reproduction of concordant pain.

4. If no pain is present the clinician may increase the sensitivity of the test by applying force through the top and front of the skull using the abdomen to increase compression.

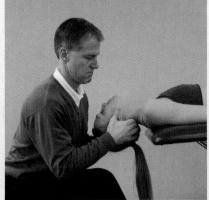

■ **Figure 5.16** Passive Physiological Extension

Chin-Cradle Grip

The "**chin-cradle grip**" is a useful handling mechanism for assessment and treatment of the cervical spine.[15] The chin-cradle grip permits one arm to perform the physiological movement activities while the other is free to apply force, palpate a segment, or stabilize a particular region.

1. The patient should assume a supine position.

2. The patient's head should extend beyond the end of the plinth up to the T2 spinous process.

3. Using the ulnar-most digits, the clinician "hooks" the chin of the patient and curls the forearm around and posterior to the ear in order to provide a stable "base" upon which the head can sit. For rotations to the right, the right arm supplies the stabilization. For rotations to the left (pictured), the left arm supplies stabilization.

4. The clinician then places his or her shoulder gently on the patient's forehead and applies a gentle force to "lock" the head in the arm cradle (Figure 5.17 ■).

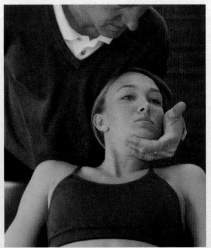

■ **Figure 5.17** The Chin-Cradle Grip

Passive Physiological Side Flexion

The third passive physiological assessment method during examination is side flexion. This procedure assesses the collective mobility of all structures and may be helpful in assessing the uncovertebral joint.

1. The procedure is performed in a supine position, and the head should extend beyond the end of the plinth up to the T2 spinous process.

2. The clinician uses the chin-cradle grip to support the patient's cervical spine.

3. The clinician places his or her radial border of the first metatarsal joint against the posterior articular pillars of the desired cervical level and applies a fulcrum-like force with the metatarsal joint (Figure 5.18 ■).

4. The clinician then gently provides physiological side flexion toward the fulcrum force. The movement should "break" at the level of the radial border and should stop at the first reported pain response of the patient.

5. The patient is then moved beyond the first reported pain toward end range and the patient's response is again reassessed. To target different levels, the clinician may move the radial border up and down the posterior articular pillars to identify the "guilty" level.

6. The process is repeated on the opposite side.

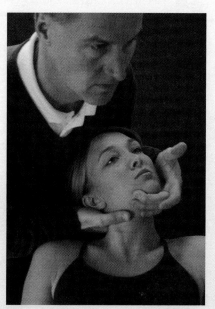

■ **Figure 5.18** Side Flexion using Chin Cradle

Passive Physiological Rotations

The fourth passive physiological assessment method during examination is rotation. This procedure is performed in a supine position and assesses the collective mobility of all structures and may be helpful in assessing the zygopophyseal joints.

1. The patient should assume the supine position.

2. The head should extend beyond the end of the plinth up to the T2 spinous process.

3. The clinician uses the chin cradle grip to support the patient's cervical spine.

4. The clinician then "grabs" the posterior tissue of the neck (Figure 5.19 ■), the "scruff of the neck," to emphasize the rotation at that particular level, moving into rotation to the first point of the patient's pain.

5. The patient is then moved beyond the first reported pain toward end range and the patient's response is assessed (Figure 5.20 ■). The clinician may move the posterior grip up and down the cervical spine to isolate different cervical segments to identify the "guilty" level.

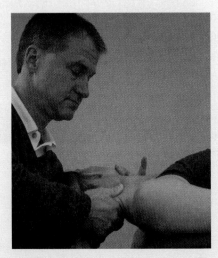

■ **Figure 5.19**   Posterior Hand Position for Rotation

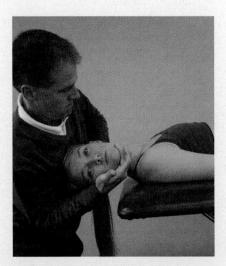

■ **Figure 5.20**   Passive Physiological Rotation

Combined Physiological Movements

Combined passive physiological movements are useful in detection of articular or capsular structures. Since there are several potential movements, it is helpful to divide the groups into supine and sitting assessment methods. The following four procedures are supine techniques.

Summary

- Passive physiological examination techniques help identify cervical movements that contribute to concordant patient complaints.

- Passive physiological movements have demonstrated acceptable interclinician reliability.

- Passive physiological movements may be single plane or combined to engage the articular or surrounding structures.

Extension and Rotation

The combined movement of extension and rotation can target different aspects of the articular regions beyond the assessment of a neutral position. The procedure is performed in a supine position, and the head should extend beyond the table to approximately T2. The patient's symptoms require a preassessment prior to the examination.

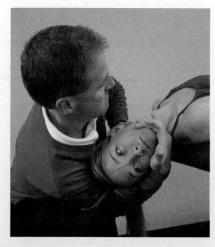

■ **Figure 5.21**   Combined Extension with Rotation

1. Using the chin-cradle grip, the clinician extends the cervical spine, carefully controlling the amount of upper cervical extension.

2. Upon completion of passive extension, the clinician then provides a rotational force toward the direction of the cradle arm (right hold, rotation right) (Figure 5.21 ■). The clinician should feel the neck's range tighten up.

3. The patient's condition should be reassessed for concordant pain but also for the possibility of CAD-related symptoms.

Combined Flexion and Rotation

Following the combined movement of extension and rotation is the combined movement of flexion and rotation. This procedure primarily solicits movement from the upper cervical spine and may be useful in detecting cervicogenic headache complaints. The procedure is performed in a supine position and the patient's symptoms require a preassessment prior to the examination.

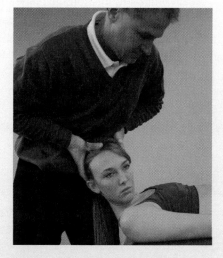

■ **Figure 5.22**   Combined Flexion with Rotation

1. Placing both hands behind the occiput, the clinician flexes the cervical spine, carefully controlling the amount of upper cervical extension.

2. Upon completion of passive flexion, the clinician then provides a rotational force until palpable end range (Figure 5.22 ■). The clinician should feel the neck's range tighten up.

3. The patient's condition should be reassessed for concordant pain but also for the possibility of CAD-related symptoms.

Cervical Distraction

Cervical distraction qualifies as a combined technique because it provides a general distraction to all segments. Cervical distraction is an assessment method that may also be useful as a treatment approach. Typically, the movement is beneficial for pain relief.

1. The patient assumes a supine position. The patient's symptoms require a preassessment prior to the examination.

2. Using the chin-cradle grip (with one hand pulling posteriorly on the occiput), the clinician provides a traction force while simultaneously querying symptoms (Figure 5.23 ■).

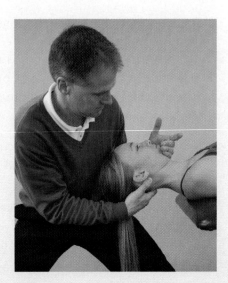

■ **Figure 5.23**   Cervical Distraction

Physiological Side Glide

A physiological side glide is a combined movement that involves both a translatory force and a blocking method. Although the movement is typically limited to the coronal plane, the procedure is highly stimulatory[65] and has been shown to elicit central nervous system responses.[66]

1. The procedure is performed by side-gliding the head to one direction (to the left in Figure 5.24 ■).

2. The procedure can be exaggerated by blocking the segment below the targeted region with the radial aspect of the hand (not pictured).

3. Reproduction of the concordant sign is considered beneficial and the response to repeated movements dictates the usefulness of the technique.

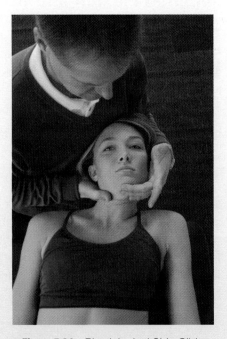

■ **Figure 5.24**   Physiological Side Glide

Passive Accessory Movements Jull et al.[67] demonstrated 100% accuracy in isolating the appropriate level of pathology using passive accessory movements. They found that when used as a method to isolate the concordant sign the posterior–anterior passive accessory movement was very useful. The use of pain provocation during the examination is a concept supported by many authors[67–69] and a number of studies have shown the **intertester reliability** of examination methods that fail to concurrently elicit the joint movement and verbal pain reproduction is abysmal.[61,68]

There may be several reasons for the poor reliability in these studies.[70,71] First, the majority of studies tested students versus experienced clinicians. Second, a preponderance of studies tested asymptomatic subjects. Third, the majority of the tests included stiffness detection in the absence of pain provocation. There is substantial evidence to support that this method of examination is unreliable secondary to the very small movements associated with passive neck glides.[71]

Nonetheless, some argue that a detection of stiffness is imperative to guide the clinician to appropriate treatment decision making. Jull and colleagues[67] wrote, "selection of a treatment technique . . . will differ if the tissue stiffness limiting movement is muscle spasm rather than capsular tightness." Subsequently, this book recognizes the importance of a stiffness assessment but also recognizes the limitations associated with stiffness assessment in absence of pain provocation. As discussed in Chapter 3, the passive accessory examination should be focused on the concordant movement or segment, allowing the clinician to further their analysis of the patient's responses.

Central Posterior Anterior (CPA)

A central posterior anterior is often called a CPA. CPAs are used to detect concordant pain during a posterior to anterior glide. Maitland suggested that the CPA is beneficial for patients who demonstrate bilateral or midline pain.[15] The tests are commonly used in examination and are often used as treatment methods as well[15].

1 For this assessment, the patient may lie in prone or sidelying. The neck is positioned in neutral and resting symptoms are assessed.

2 The clinician palpates the C2 spinous process using the tips of the thumb.

3 Using a thumb-to-thumb application the clinician applies a gentle downward force up to the first point of the patient's complaint of pain and the pain response is assessed (Figure 5.25 ■).

4 The clinician then pushes beyond the first point of pain, toward end range, and reassesses pain and quality of movement. Additionally, one should assess splinting or muscle spasm and assess if pain is concordant.

5 The clinician repeats the movements toward end range while assessing pain. One should use caution if patient reports significant pain that is unrelenting.

6 The process is repeated on each spinous process to T4 to identify the concordant segment.

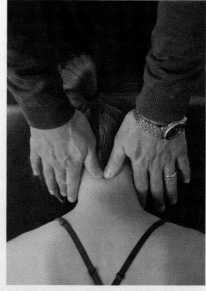

■ **Figure 5.25** CPA of the Cervical Spine

Unilateral Posterior–Anterior (UPA)

A unilateral posterior–anterior is frequently called a UPA. The unilateral posterior–anterior provides a combined extension-based movement with rotation to the same side the examination is applied. Maitland suggested that UPAs are useful in patients who demonstrate unilateral pain. UPAs are also commonly used as examination and treatment techniques and are useful in identifying the concordant sign of the patient[67].

1. The patient is positioned in prone or sidelying, and the neck is placed in neutral.
2. The clinician then pulls the paraspinals that lie just to the side of the spinous process medially to expose the articular pillars (facets).
3. To isolate the articular pillar, the clinician finds the spinous process of C2, slides approximately a thumb-width lateral, and moves his or her thumb in a caudal and cephalic direction (Figure 5.26 ■). The raised area felt under the thumb is the articular pillar, which is the targeted region for the mobilization.

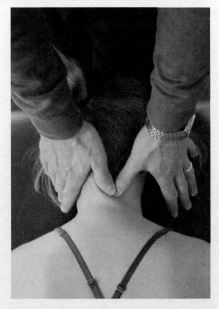

4. Using a thumb-to-thumb application, the clinician applies a gentle downward force up to the first point of the patient's complaint of pain.
5. The clinician then pushes beyond the first point of pain toward end range, reassesses pain and quality of movement, and checks for splinting or muscle spasm.
6. The clinician then repeats the movements at end range while assessing pain, using caution if patient reports significant pain that is unrelenting.
7. The clinician repeats the process on each articular pillar to T4 attempting to identify the concordant segment.
8. The process is repeated on the opposite side.

■ **Figure 5.26**   UPA of the Cervical Spine

Transverse Glides

A transverse glide is a technique that applies a lateral glide to the lateral aspects of the spinous processes of the spine.

1. The patient is positioned in prone or sidelying, and the neck is placed in neutral.
2. The clinician palpates the C2 spinous process using the tips of the thumb. Using one thumb pad, the clinician applies a very broad and deep contact to the side of the spinous process, applying more force on the base of the spinous process than the posterior tip.
3. The clinician then aligns the forearm so that it is parallel to the force to the spinous process and pushes to the first point of reported pain.

4 The clinician then pushes beyond the first point of pain toward end range, reassesses pain and quality of movement, and checks for splinting or muscle spasm (Figure 5.27 ■).

5 Passive repeated movements are performed at end range and changes in pain level are determined as is the assessment if whether the pain is concordant.

6 The process is repeated on each spinous process to T4 to identify the concordant segment.

7 The process is repeated on the opposite side.

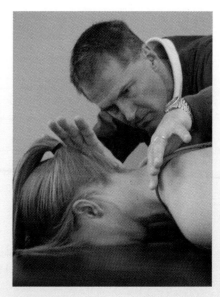

■ **Figure 5.27**   Transverse Glide of the Cervical Spine

Unilateral Anterior–Posterior (UAP)

Unilateral anterior–posteriors are often identified as UAPs. UAPs are also well studied[72] and are considered to have a very strong neurophysiological affect on the spine and upper extremities. UAPs are often considered useful when referred pain to the upper extremity is reported during the patient history and examination.

1 The patient is positioned in supine or sidelying, and the neck is placed in neutral.

2 The patient is informed of the specifics of the technique, including that the clinician's hands will be around the front of his or her throat.

3 Using a thumb, the clinician hooks the anterior cervical musculature (SCM specifically) and pulls the tissue medially. This will expose the anterior aspect of the transverse process.

4 The clinician then applies a broad and thick thumb contact (dummy thumb) to the anterior transverse processes while using the other thumb to apply a force downward on the "dummy" thumb (Figure 5.28 ■).

5 The clinician pushes to the first point of reported pain by the patient.

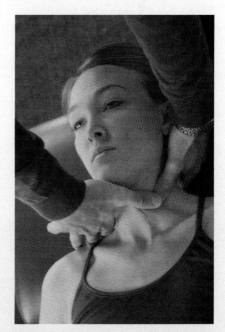

■ **Figure 5.28**   UAP of the Cervical Spine

(Continued)

6. The clinician then pushes beyond the first point of pain, reassesses symptoms, and assesses if the pain is concordant.

7. The clinician then performs repeated movements toward end range while reassessing the patient's pain.

8. The process may be repeated on the opposite side. It is not uncommon to elicit discordant referred symptoms into the shoulder of the patient during the assessment.

Summary

- Passive accessory movements, when combined with elicitation of the concordant sign of the patient, are reliable and useful assessment tools.
- Passive accessory movement in absence of elicitation of the concordant sign demonstrates little usefulness.
- Transverse glides and UAPs are more likely to elicit profound neurophysiological responses than UPAs and CPAs.

Special Clinical Tests

Palpation   Trigger points have been defined as hyperirritable foci that lie within taut bands of muscle that are painful upon compression and that often refer pain to a distal site or a site away from the point of origin.[73] Trigger points may also manifest as tension headache, tinnitus, or temporomandibular joint pain.[74] Trigger points are often (but not always) at neuromuscular junction sites and the muscles associated with the trigger points are often painful when contracted. Active trigger points can cause peripheral sensitization of muscle nociceptors, which can enhance pain mechanisms experienced by the patient. Lastly, trigger points have been associated with neighboring joint dysfunction, although the relationship is mostly theoretical at this point.[75]

Trigger points are identified through palpation. Palpation consists of a firm pressure applied directly over the trigger point, often perpendicular to the muscle (Figures 5.29 ■ and 5.30 ■). In some cases, there is a transient visible or palpable contraction or dimpling of the muscle and skin as the tense muscle fibers (taut band) of the trigger point contract when pressure is applied.[74] Often maintenance of pressures results in a reduction of the spasm and a decrease in report of pain.

Manual Muscle Testing   Manual muscle testing may implicate strength or endurance as a contributor to the patient's symptoms. Specific manual muscle testing such as anterior neck flexor endurance testing and posterior neck extensor testing are particularly valuable.

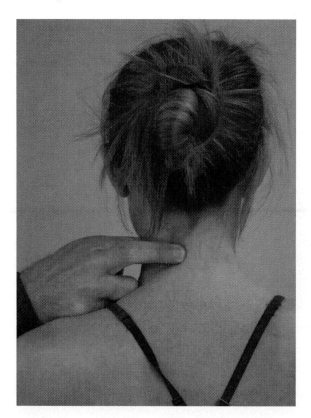

■ Figure 5.29   Trigger Point Palpation of the Levator
Scapulae

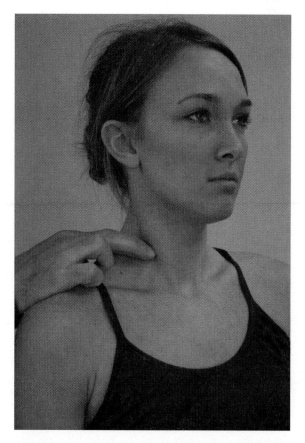

■ Figure 5.30   Trigger Point Palpation of the Scalenes

Anterior Neck Flexor Endurance Test

The anterior neck flexor endurance test is a commonly used test to identify patients with weak anterior neck flexors. Weakness and endurance losses in the anterior neck are common in patients with cervical headache[76] and in other conditions such as postural abnormalities.

1 The technique is performed in supine and involves patient chin retraction to create a skin fold below the mandible while the clinician cradles the head with his or her fingers.

2 The patient is told to hold this position while the clinician removes his or her hand support under the head (Figure 5.31 ■).

3 The patient is instructed to hold the position while maintaining the skin fold under the mandible. The mean holding time for patients in a recent study is approximately 46.9 seconds (standard deviation [SD] = 22.7).[77]

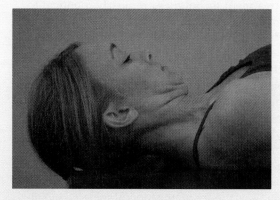

■ Figure 5.31   Neck Flexor Endurance Test

Posterior Neck Extensor Endurance Test

The posterior neck extensor endurance test (a variant of the Biering-Sorensen test for muscle endurance) is performed in prone and involves a similar concept to the anterior neck flexor test.

1. The patient is stabilized at T2–T4 with a belt.

2. The patient is instructed to perform a chin tuck and to hold his or her neck in a neutral posture (Figure 5.32 ■). The mean holding time for subjects in a recent trial was 151 seconds (SD = 71.4)[78] and the test is designed to target endurance assessment of the extensor muscles.

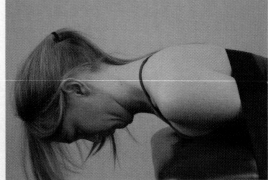

■ **Figure 5.32**   Neck Extensor Endurance Testing

Treatment Techniques

The patient response-based method endeavors to determine the behavior of the patient's pain and/or impairment by analyzing concordant movements and the response of the patient's pain to applied or repeated movements. The applied or repeated movements that positively or negatively alter the signs and symptoms of the patient deserve the highest priority for treatment selection[79,80] and should be similar in construct to the concordant examination movements. Examination methods that fail to elicit the patient response may offer nominal or imprecise value as do methods that focus solely on treatment decision making based on a single diagnostic label.[81]

With the exception of manipulation, which is not an examination procedure, the majority of active and passive treatment techniques are nearly identical to the examination procedures. In all cases of manual therapy treatment, there should be a direct mechanical relationship between the examination and treatment techniques selected.

In situations where the examination has failed to outline the appropriate treatment selection, a classification system may be useful. Classification allows large amounts of data to be broken down into common components and may improve the treatment outcome by homogeneity. This book advocates a Treatment Based Classification (TBC)-based cervical classification tool, which outlines five classification groups for the cervical spine: (1) mobility, (2) centralization, (3) conditioning and increased exercise tolerance, (4) pain control, and (5) reduction of headache.[82] Mobility techniques may include thrust and nonthrust procedures, muscle energy techniques, and stretching. Active physiological movements and traction are useful for centralization. General strengthening exercises (outside the scope of this book) are useful for conditioning whereas pain control may include palliative techniques such as modalities, nonaggressive manual therapy, and massage. Headache-based techniques include a number of manual therapy procedures.

Active Physiological Movements

Active physiological movements that consist of postural exercises or strengthening are plausible additions for treatment and may be appropriate for adjunctive care as a home program. Studies have shown some degree of success with implementation of an active exercise program,[83] specifically those that focus on postural exercises[84,85] or strengthening.[86] Repeated neck retraction in sitting (Figure 5.33 ■), a common intervention, has been shown to recover the Hoffmann (H) reflex amplitude, decompress cervical neural elements, and reduce cervical pain when compared against normal controls.[87]

Supine chin retraction (Figure 5.34 ■) allows gravity to assist during the active movements and may be useful to initiate. Another common postural exercise is the prone cervical retraction technique (not pictured), which is designed to incorporate a passive stretch during an active strengthening movement.

Passive Physiological Movements

Passive physiological stretching techniques have demonstrated strong association to range-of-motion

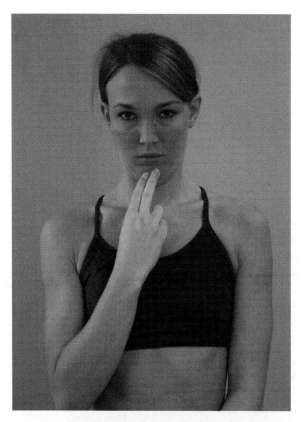

■ **Figure 5.33**   Sitting Chin Retractions

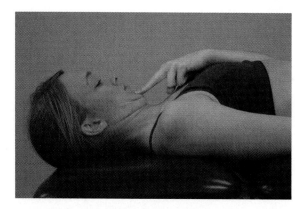

■ **Figure 5.34**   Supine Chin Retraction

gains in patients with neck dysfunction.[84,88] However, over time, when compared in isolation with active approaches, a passive physiological stretching program is less effective. Subsequently, passive physiological exercises should be adjuncts to concurrent active strengthening programs that include active postural exercises.

All of the examination methods used previously qualify as potential treatment techniques. For example, if a patient demonstrated concordant pain with restriction to the left during lateral side-flexion, which benefited from repeated movements during the examination, a passive physiological treatment into side-flexion is the treatment of choice. This concept is consistent throughout all planar movements.

Suboccipital Distraction

Easing techniques are often used during occasions where the patient complains of pain or an irritable headache. Easing techniques may be helpful in reducing treatment soreness or reducing pain in a pain-dominant individual. One easing technique is the suboccipital distraction technique.

1 The technique is performed in a supine position with the head on the plinth. The resting symptoms of the patient are assessed.

2 Using all the fingertips in both hands from digits 2 through 5, the clinician cups the suboccipital region of the patient and supports the posterior skull.

3 The clinician provides a light cephalic distraction to the posterior skull (Figure 5.35 ■).

4 The patient may perform extension-based isometric exercises for a hold relax stretch or allow a passive-specific treatment.

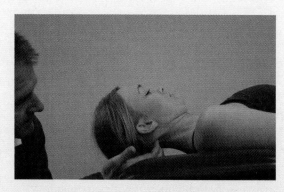

■ **Figure 5.35**   Suboccipital Distraction

Passive Chin Retraction

A compliment to the active chin retraction technique is a passive technique. Since a passive physiological technique is designed to stretch beyond the ranges of an active method, this technique may provide a more vigorous stretch to the patient.

1. The patient assumes a supine position.

2. Using the chin-cradle grip, the clinician provides a retraction force to the patient's head (Figure 5.36 ■). The clinician can also incorporate extension with the retraction to embellish the procedure.

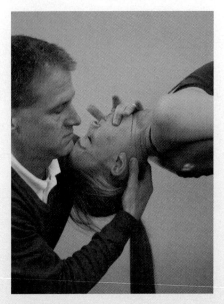

■ **Figure 5.36** Chin Retraction with Overpressure

Physiological Side Glide

1. A physiological side glide involves placing the patient in a supine position and a stabilized chin-cradle grip.

2. The patient's head is side-glided toward a specific direction through facilitation of the clinician's lateral aspect of his or her index finger (Figure 5.37 ■). The technique may be useful if side flexion is painful and concordant during the examination.

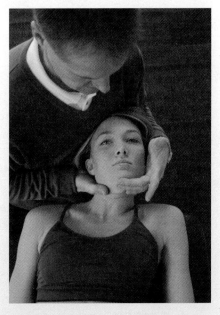

■ **Figure 5.37** Physiological Side Glide

General Techniques

Passive Accessory Movements (PAIVMS)

There is a moderate amount of evidence to support that passive accessory techniques provide an excitatory effect on the sympathetic nervous system.[89–91] Mobilizations have produced skin temperature changes and an increase in skin conductivity.[92] Stimulation of the cervical spine has demonstrated upper extremity changes in pain response (pressure pain) and a measurable sympathoexcitatory effect.[91,93] An excitatory effect on the sympathetic nervous system occurs concurrently with a reduction of hypoalgesia and may parallel the effects of stimulation of the dorsal periaqueductal gray area of the midbrain, a process that has occurred in animal research.[94] Since mobilization does lead to a reduction of pain using the same procedures as those performed during examination, it makes sense to use the very mechanism that has been shown to be specific.

There is also evidence that cervical posterior–anterior (PA) mobilizations are effective in reducing pain.[92] PAs helped to increase pain thresholds and led to significant reductions against controlled comparisons on a visual analog scale.[92] Treatment benefits were present during the treatment and over a 2-week period.[92]

The most commonly used treatment technique from a past survey of manipulative physical therapists was the passive accessory intervertebral glide[95]. While detecting spinal accessory stiffness alone has not been shown to be consistently reliable, several authors have suggested that palpating for pain accompanying stiffness is both reliable and valid.[50,67,91] Jull et al.[96] demonstrated a very high degree of agreement among clinicians in isolating the painful cervical segment in patients with chronic cervicogenic headaches. The use of subjective responses while identifying stiffness through PA mobilization is consistently used in clinical situations, and reigns supreme over stiffness detection alone.

Lee et al.[51] reported that the movement of a PA causes three-point axial movements. Although these movements have been purported to produce isolated linear glides, significant axial or sagittal rotation is common during the movement application. This results in significant spinal bending under the application of PA loads, and variability in direction of the bend. Mobilization forces on the C5 processes resulted in extension at the C2–3 and C3–4 segments and flexion at the C7–T1 segments. Variability was found in the mid-cervical segments, which demonstrated both flexion and extension behavior.

Although the magnitude of intervertebral movements produced by mobilization was generally small, the forces applied at one spinous process produced not only movements at the target vertebra but also movements of the entire cervical spine. These findings are consistent with the findings of low back research.[97,98] Based on these findings, it is imperative to recognize that PAs are recognized as a *global mobilization*, not just a simple gliding of one vertebra upon another.

C0–C1 Passive Mobilization for Headaches

A commonly used mobilization method for headaches targets the upper cervical structures of C0–1, C1–2, and C2–3. This method, first described by Maitland[15], has been successful in a randomized trial that focused treatment on cervicogenic headaches[86].

C0–1 Cervicogenic Treatment

1. The patient is placed in a prone position. The patient's resting symptoms are assessed.

2. The clinician palpates the suboccipital region of the posterior skull. The ring finger should fall within a depression in this region, which is the area that lies over the C0–1 joint. A light pressure is applied using one thumb over the other (Figure 5.38 ■). Initially, the clinician should press only to the first point of pain since the technique is quite powerful.

3. Then, the clinician pushes beyond pain and the patient's symptoms are reassessed.

4. If tolerated well, the clinician repeats the movements and routinely reassesses the patient's condition.

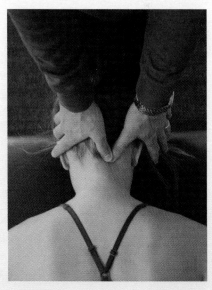

■ **Figure 5.38** C0–1 Passive Accessory Treatment

(Continued)

C2–3 Cervicogenic Treatment

1. The patient assumes a prone position. The patient's resting symptoms are assessed.

2. Using his or her thumb, the clinician palpates the C2 spinous processes, moves the thumb just lateral to the spinous process, and pulls the muscles and soft tissue medial to expose the articular pillars (Figure 5.39 ▪). The C2–3 segment lies just laterally to the C2 spinous process. The clinician provides a light pressure using one thumb over the other. Initially, the clinician should press only to the first point of pain.

3. The clinician then pushes beyond pain and the patient's symptoms are reassessed.

4. If tolerable, repeat the movements.

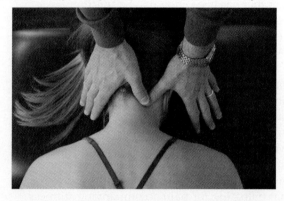

■ **Figure 5.39** C2–3 Passive Accessory Treatment

C1–2 Cervicogenic Treatment

C1–2 mobilization involves a very similar process to C2–3.

1. The patient assumes a prone position and their resting symptoms are assessed.

2. Using his or her thumb, the clinician palpates the C2 spinous processes, moves the thumb just laterally to the spinous process, and pulls the muscles and soft tissue medially to expose the articular pillars.

3. While keeping the fingers on the C2–3 facet, the head is rotated to the same side of the facet (approximately 30 degrees). The rotation enhances the amount of movement that is applied through C1–2, but most likely does not eliminate all of the movement through C2–3. A light pressure is applied using one thumb over the other to the first point of pain with a direction of force toward the patient's mouth (Figure 5.40 ▪).

4. Then, the clinician pushes beyond pain and the patient's symptoms are reassessed. If tolerated, the clinician should repeat the movements.

If pain is concordant in any of the levels assessed, the treatment is isolated to those levels. Solid evidence exists that strengthening exercises in conjunction with mobilization is effective for reduction of pain in some headache patients[7].

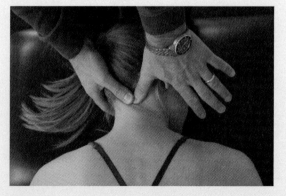

■ **Figure 5.40** C1–2 Passive Accessory Treatment

Mobilizations with Movement

Mobilizations with movement are techniques that incorporate active movements of the patient with passive movements by the clinician. The techniques may take many different forms.

Sitting Accessory Glide into Upper Cervical Flexion or Lower Cervical Extension

A mobilization with movement technique designed to encourage upper cervical flexion and/or lower cervical extension can be used for treatment of cervicogenic headache and cervical dizziness.[99]

1. The technique is performed in sitting, and the clinician glides the head posteriorly during concurrent active movement of chin retraction by the patient (or passive movement by the clinician).

2. The clinician typically blocks the level below the targeted site to enhance the movement of the desired region. Although taught as a "pain-free" mobilization, the technique can be worked into the concordant sign and is useful as a bridge to an active program (Figure 5.41 ■).

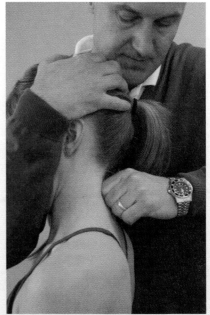

■ **Figure 5.41**   Sitting Accessory Glide into Upper Cervical Flexion or Lower Cervical Extension

Sitting Accessory Glide into Upper Cervical Extension and Lower Cervical Flexion

A mobilization with movement technique designed to encourage upper cervical extension and/or lower cervical flexion is another option for treatment.

1. The technique is performed in sitting, and the clinician glides the head anteriorly during concurrent active movement of chin protraction (Figure 5.42 ■) by the patient (or passive movement by the clinician).

2. The clinician typically glides the level at the targeted site to enhance the movement of the desired region. Although taught as a "pain-free" mobilization, the technique can be worked into the concordant sign and is useful as a bridge to an active program.

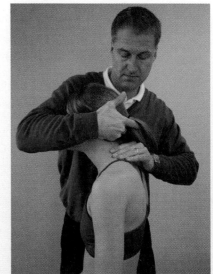

■ **Figure 5.42**   Sitting Accessory Glide into Upper Cervical Extension or Lower Cervical Flexion

Sitting Accessory Glide for Upper Cervical (C1–C2) Rotation

A mobilization with movement technique designed to encourage upper cervical rotation at C1–C2 can be used as a home program and follow-up to mobilization, especially in the treatment of cervicogenic dizziness.[99,100]

1. A belt (or towel) is placed around the C1 arch on the left and wrapped across the mandible.

2. Gentle pressure is applied along the belt by the patient as the patient actively rotates his or her head to the right (Figure 5.43 ■).

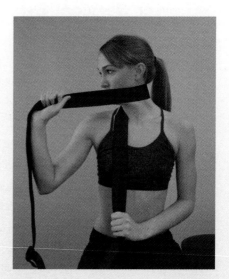

■ **Figure 5.43**   Sitting Accessory Glide for Upper Cervical (C1–C2) Rotation

Sitting Extension with a Belt

A mobilization with movement technique that is useful as a home program for improving neck extension is the extension with belt technique.

1. A belt (or a towel if a belt is not available) is placed at the region where the desired extension is targeted.

2. The patient is instructed to perform a chin tuck, then extension of his or her lower cervical region while concurrently applying an anterior force (and if warranted, an upward force) onto the posterior neck with a towel or belt (Figure 5.44 ■).

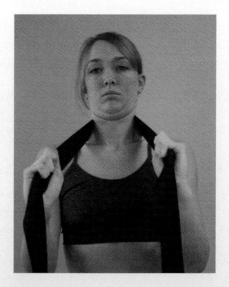

■ **Figure 5.44**   Sitting Extension with a Belt

Sitting Rotation for Opening with Enhancement

A mobilization with movement technique used as a home program for enhancing movement created during a passive procedure is useful to provide carryover effects. For patients who struggle with pain on the opposite side of rotation, a limitation in opening may be the culprit.

1 The technique is typically performed in sitting.

2 By enhancing rotation with one's hand while pulling over the restricted area, the movements into opening are improved.

3 The fingers used in pulling the neck into rotation should be applied at the restricted area of the neck and movement should be performed at the same time of the pulling (Figure 5.45 ■).

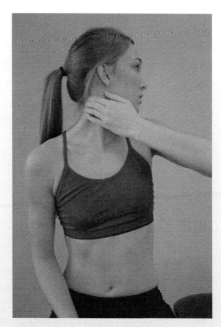

■ **Figure 5.45**   Sitting Rotation for Opening with Enhancement

Sitting Rotation for Closing with Enhancement

This mobilization with movement technique can be used as a home program for enhancing closure of intervertebral foreman on a target side. For patients who struggle with pain on the same side of rotation, a limitation in closing may be the culprit.

1 The technique is typically performed in sitting.

2 By pulling over the restricted area during concurrent rotation toward that area (pictured as a limitation to the right), the movements into closing are improved.

3 The fingers used in pulling the neck into rotation should be applied at the restricted area of the neck (Figure 5.46 ■).

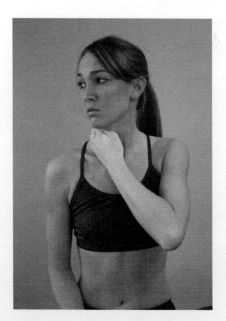

■ **Figure 5.46**   Sitting Rotation for Closing with Enhancement

Cervical

Traction

Traction is applicable for use in patients who exhibit a centralization or peripheralization of symptoms during selected examination movements. Traction is usually provided in a supine position. One method involves the use of a chin-cradle grip with equal force anterior and posterior (Figure 5.47 ■). If the patient demonstrates a temporomandibular disorder or has dental work not conducive to compression, the posterior force using a towel may be beneficial.

1. The clinician supplies a light traction force of approximately 5–10 pounds and the patient's symptoms are assessed for change.

2. The force is held for approximately 1 minute and the patient is reevaluated. Force and time is modulated based on patient response. In most cases, it is not necessary to provide very high forces for traction as lighter forces generally provide successful treatment outcomes.

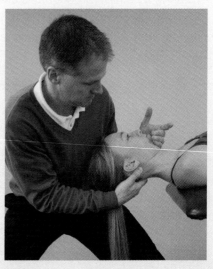

■ **Figure 5.47** Cervical Distraction Using the Chin and Occipital Grip

Manually Assisted Movements

Manually assisted movements consist of muscle energy methods of patient-assisted stretching. Muscle energy techniques (METs) are a technique in manual therapy where the patient actively uses his or her muscles, on request, while maintaining a targeted preposition against a distinctly executed counterforce.[101] METs make use of proprioceptive stimulus for strengthening of selected and targeted muscle groups. Both are manually assisted methods and both have established benefit during manual therapy treatment. There are numerous different treatment techniques and this book only demonstrates a few.

Upper Trapezius Stretching

Chronic forward head posture may lead to alterations of the anterior and selective posterior muscles such as the trapezius. One method designed to reduce pain and stiffness of the soft-tissue regions of the spine is a lateral stretch.

1. The patient assumes a supine position.

2. After assessment of resting symptoms, the clinician stabilizes the lower fibers of the trapezius by applying a downward pressure posterior to the distal clavicle (Figure 5.48 ■).

3. The cervical spine is side-flexed away and forward-flexed to engage the trapezius fibers.

4. The patient may provide an isometric side flexion and extension contraction against the stretching force of the clinician.

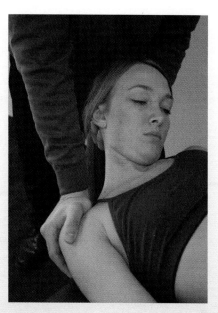

■ **Figure 5.48**   Upper Trapezius Stretching

Side Flexion Physiological Glide

A lateral physiological glide is used to target structures other than the trapezius. A side flexion stretch may be helpful if the pain during the passive physiological examination was felt on the opposite side of the side flexion. One may also mobilize the lateral joint structures as well.

1. With this technique, the patient assumes a supine position and the resting symptoms of the patient are assessed.

2. The clinician stabilizes the lower fibers of the trapezius and the origin of the scalenes and lateral musculature by applying a downward pressure to the posterior-medial aspect of the neck (Figure 5.49 ■).

3. The clinician provides a light static stretch in the direction of side flexion away from the stabilization.

4. The patient may provide an isometric contraction against the clinician's stretch.

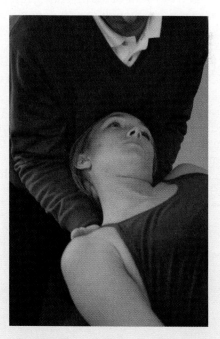

■ **Figure 5.49**   Lateral Flexion Stretching

Chin Retraction with Overpressure

Chin retraction with compression of forehead is a technique used to reduce forward head.

1 The patient assumes a supine position and the patient's resting symptoms are assessed.

2 Using the chin-cradle grip, the clinician provides a retraction force to the patient's head.

3 The clinician may now add a downward stretch into extension using one of two possible contact points: a downward glide by providing a force downward through the forehead using the anterior aspect of his or her shoulder, or a downward force manually through the maxilla using the web space of the free hand (Figure 5.50 ■).

4 The patient may apply a further downward force or a light upward force against the clinician's resistance.

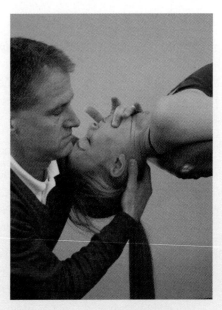

■ **Figure 5.50** Chin Retraction with Compression of the Forehead

Manipulation Techniques

Manipulation is a commonly performed treatment technique used by 84.5% of the practicing respondents in a past survey.[95] Although manipulation was used less frequently in the upper cervical spine when compared to the middle and lower regions (83.4%, 84.7%, and 98.3%, respectively), the technique still demonstrated a high frequency of use in all regions of the cervical spine.[102]

Several different forms of manipulative treatments are used. Specific high-velocity thrust techniques commonly include lateral flexion, longitudinal, posterior–anterior (PA) thrust, and transverse and rotary techniques.[95] Thrust manipulation techniques involve highly skilled psychomotor skills that require supervised practice.[102] Although the use of a textbook and didactic knowledge is helpful in understanding the components of manipulation, there is no substitute for safe practice and psychomotor learning in a well-organized environment.[102] This book is not designed to be a substitute for traditional laboratory-based learning.

Prior to upper spine manipulation, assessment of CAD and instability are warranted. In addition, one should feel quite comfortable that they know the outcome of the intervention will be successful, as the techniques do involve risk. Nonthrust mobilization methods are safer applications that involve less risk for potentially similar benefit.

Longitudinal Distraction

For manipulation of the upper C-spine, this text advocates the use of the C0–1 distraction maneuver. This technique may be useful in patients with upper cervicogenic headaches or unilateral pain and stiffness of origin in the upper C-spine. The following describes the technique procedure.

1. The patient is positioned in supine with the head and neck placed beyond the table to T2.

2. The head of the patient is prepositioned toward rotation (pictured in Figure 5.51 ■ as a right rotation in which the left side is treated) and the lateral border of the first metacarpal bone is placed against the mastoid process of the patient.

3. The clinician applies a light distraction to the patient's mastoid process using a chin-cradle grip and the patient's head is rotated back toward midline to approximately 15–20 degrees. The head is held firmly within the chin-cradle grip and against the body of the clinician.

4. After several small oscillations, a longitudinal force is provided (traction) using a light thrust (Figure 5.52 ■).

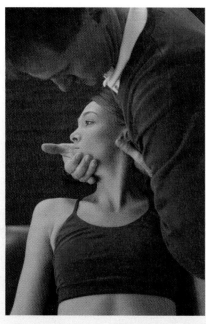

■ **Figure 5.51** Upper C-Spine C0–C1 Distraction; Preposition in Right Rotation

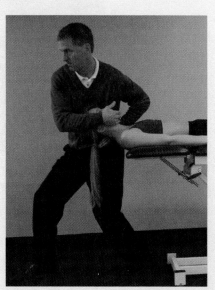

■ **Figure 5.52** Upper C-Spine Manipulation Targeting the Left C0–C1 Region

Manipulation of the Mid and Lower Cervical Spine

The ability to lock the joint using apposition is more difficult to perform on the cephalic segments of the cervical spine. Most likely, this is associated with the angulations of the facet joints. In some cases, there is a need to place the neck in slight extension to fully engage the joints and "lock" out the neck for the upper mid-cervical segments. As with the upper cervical spine, a comprehensive CAD assessment is essential prior to treatment. The determination of the appropriate side to manipulate is best selected using patient report of symptoms and is usually identified during passive physiological and passive accessory testing.

1. The patient is positioned in supine and the baseline symptoms are assessed.

2. The patient's head is held in a chin-cradle grip.

3. To manipulate the right mid or lower cervical segments, the head should be cradled using the left hand (Figure 5.53 ■). The opposite hold is used to manipulate the left segments. A translatory force (Figure 5.53, left) is applied to the lower cervical spine (contact point is the isolated lower cervical transverse process or articular pillar). Simultaneously, a side flexion force (to the opposite direction as the translation; Figure 5.53, right) is applied.

4. The clinician provides a rotational force of approximately 10–20 degrees to the opposite side of side flexion (Figure 5.53, left) to lock the segments. The rotation should not go beyond the contact point of the side glide (thrusting knuckle).

5. The patient's sagittal flexion and extension is modified to further "tighten" the position. Extension tends to target the anterior capsule whereas flexion targets the posterior aspect of the capsule and is usually the best selection for the mid-cervical region. The technique does provide a general force to the complete region. A light thrust is applied in the same translatory preposition described earlier.

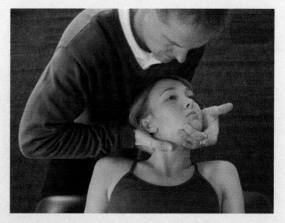

■ **Figure 5.53** Chin-Cradle Manipulation of the Mid or Lower Cervical Spine

Cervical–Thoracic Junction Manipulation

The transition zone between the cervical and thoracic spine is difficult to access, secondary to a large amount of soft-tissue structures that cover the area. Consequently, innovative methods are necessary to mobilize this particular region. The following describes a lower C-spine manipulative procedure performed in sitting.

1. The patient is seated with their back facing the clinician.

2. The clinician stands or kneels directly behind the patient and the patient is positioned so that he or she leans back against the clinician.

3. The opposite arm of the patient from the side being treated is placed over the knee of the clinician. In Figure 5.54 ■, the left arm of the patient is placed over the knee of the clinician and the clinician is treating the right cervical–thoracic junction site.

4. The clinician controls the head of the patient with the nonthrusting arm and leans his or her arm on the shoulder of the patient on the opposite side that is treated (Figure 5.54, left).

5. A lateral force is applied to the spinous process (on the right in the photo) using the thumb of the clinician. The patient simultaneously side-flexed to the right and, using the body of the clinician, leaned to the left (the body of the patient; Figure 5.54) to increase the movement at the cervical–thoracic junction.

6. A small thrust is performed at the end range of side flexion.

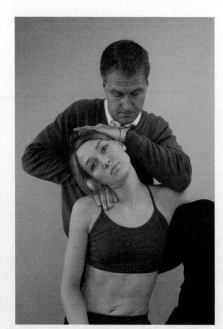

■ **Figure 5.54** Lower C-Spine, Upper T-Spine Thrust

Cervical–Thoracic Junction Manipulation in Prone

A technically similar method to the sitting cervical–thoracic junction manipulation that involves less psychomotor skill can be performed in prone. The following procedure outlines the prone manipulative technique.

1. The patient is positioned in prone.

2. The head is rotated away from the direction the clinician desires to manipulate (the left side is being manipulated in Figure 5.55 ■).

3. A towel is placed under the patient's face to allow gliding on the plinth, and the patient's

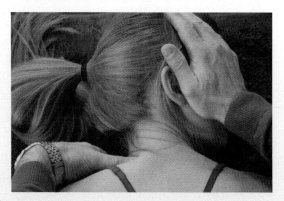

■ **Figure 5.55** Prone Lower C-Spine, Upper Thoracic Thrust

(Continued)

baseline symptoms are assessed. A lateral block at the spinous process (on the left side) is used for stabilization of the desired segment.

4 The clinician's thumb should engage the deepest aspect of the spinous process, targeting the lamina's connection to the spinous process.

5 Using the palm of the hand, the patient's head is prepositioned into extension, side flexion, and rotation to the opposite side. In many cases, just moving the patient into the preposition (extension, left side flexion, and right rotation in Figure 5.55) will result in a lock or an audible.

6 At the "end point" of preposition, a light thrust toward left side flexion is provided by the clinician.

Thoracic Manipulation

Thoracic manipulation may be useful for improvements of selected forms of mechanical cervical pain. Thoracic manipulation involves less risk than cervical spine manipulation and is a manipulative method that is less challenging to perform. There are two potential techniques: one performed in a sitting position, the other performed in a supine position.

Sitting

1 The subject is seated, and the therapist places his or her upper chest at the level of the subject's middle thoracic spine. In some cases, the use of a rolled-up towel placed between the clinician's chest and the patient's thoracic spine will further emphasize the force to the targeted region.

2 The clinician reaches around the patient and grasps the opposite elbows (e.g., the right hand of the clinician grasps the left elbow and the left hand of the clinician grasps the right elbow).

3 The patient is prepositioned into flexion of the thoracic spine and the clinician pulls firmly on the arms to take up the slack in the spine of the patient.

4 A high-velocity distraction thrust is performed in an upward direction using a "scooping method" at the arms. During the thrust, the therapist uses his or her sternum as a fulcrum on the subject's middle thoracic spine (Figure 5.56 ■).

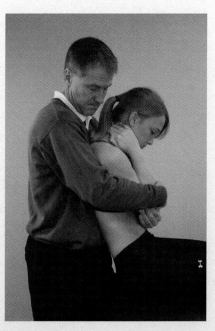

■ **Figure 5.56** Sitting Thoracic Distraction Technique

Supine

The supine technique is often termed the "pistol."

1. The pistol requires that the patient place their arms in an over- and undercrossing technique (not crossing the arms) while firmly gripping their own thoracic region with their hands.

2. The clinician stands to the opposite side of the targeted segment (right side to treat the left side; Figure 5.57 ■).

3. Using the arm furthest from the targeted side, the clinician gently pulls the patient into sidelying.

4. The clinician then leans over the patient and places the hand behind the patient's back just caudal to the targeted segment. The pistol grip allows the transverse processes to articulate with the thenar eminence and the folded digits of the clinician's hand.

5. The patient is "scooped" into flexion (using his or her arms as a lever) and is gently placed over the pistol hand of the clinician (careful effort is made to keep the patient in thoracic flexion) (Figure 5.57). The clinician may further enhance the contact point on the patient's transverse process by pronating the wrist or through ulnar deviation of the forearm. The clinician's thrust should be through the shaft of the humeri with careful attention toward keeping the flexed thoracic position of the patient. The force of the thrust should go through the chest of the clinician to ensure enough vigor is applied.

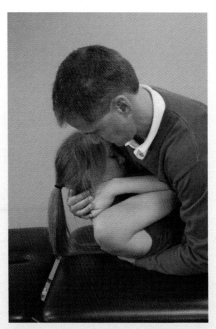

■ **Figure 5.57** Pistol Manipulation

Summary

- Strong association between examination and treatment should improve the outcome of a dedicated treatment program.
- Active physiological movements are beneficial in creating home exercise programs, working on abnormal posture, or strengthening the selected cervical musculature.
- Although slightly less effective than active physiological methods, passive physiological stretching techniques have demonstrated strong association to range-of-motion gains in patients with neck dysfunction.

Targeted Specific Techniques

Passive Accessory Movements (PAIVMS)

Passive accessory movements are typically targeted if the same assessment procedures were concordant during the examination.

Central Posterior–Anterior (CPA) in Physiological Extension

A CPA in physiological extension is a combined movement that is also a targeted specific technique. The technique may be useful in patients with mechanical neck pain who demonstrate difficulty with extension.

① The patient is positioned in prone and the neck is placed in extension.

② The clinician palpates the desired spinous process using the tips of his or her thumbs.

③ Using a thumb-to-thumb application the clinician applies a gentle downward force up to the first point of patient complaint of pain, assessing if the pain is concordant (Figure 5.58 ■).

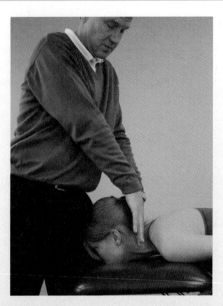

■ **Figure 5.58**   CPA in Extension

④ The clinician then pushes beyond the first point of pain toward end range, reassesses pain and quality of movement, and checks for splinting or muscle spasm.

⑤ The clinician performs repeated movements toward end range and reassesses pain.

Unilateral Posterior Anterior (UPA) during Physiological Rotation

The UPA during physiological rotation enhances the movement that the UPA produces in small, isolated quantities. Specifically, the procedure may increase the tension placed on the posterior capsule of the facet, an area thickened and altered during degenerative processes. Rotation increases the tension placed on this capsule.[58]

① The patient is positioned in prone and the neck is placed in rotation (Figure 5.59 ■, left).

② The clinician pulls the paraspinals that lie just to the side of the spinous process medially, which exposes the articular pillars.

③ The clinician then finds the spinous process of C2, slides approximately a thumb-width lateral, then moves his or her thumb in a caudal and cephalic direction to "feel" the articular pillar. The raised area felt under the thumb is the articular pillar.

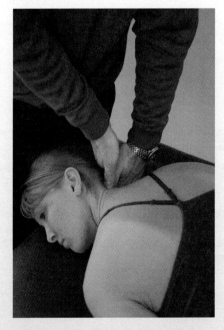

■ **Figure 5.59**   UPA in Physiological Rotation

④ Using a thumb-to-thumb application, the clinician applies a gentle downward force up to the first point of patient complaint of pain, assessing if the pain is concordant. In the photo the clinician is treating the left side.

⑤ The clinician then pushes beyond the first point of pain toward end range, reassessing pain, quality of movement, and checking for splinting or muscle spasm.

⑥ The clinician then repeats the movements toward end range, reassessing pain and determining if the pain is concordant.

UPA during Physiological Side Flexion

The UPA during physiological side flexion may increase the tension placed on the anterior and posterior capsule of the facet and theoretically may be beneficial in individuals that have demonstrated degeneration associated with the uncovertebral joint.

① The patient is positioned in prone and the neck is positioned in side flexion toward the directed joint of interest (Figure 5.60 ■, left).

② The clinician pulls the paraspinals that lie just to the side of the spinous process medially, thus exposing the articular pillars.

③ The clinician palpates the spinous process of C2 and slides approximately a thumb-width lateral, then moves his or her thumb in a caudal and cephalic direction. The raised area felt under the thumb is the articular pillar.

④ Using a thumb-to-thumb application, the clinician applies a gentle downward force up to the first point of patient complaint of pain (treating the left side in Figure 5.60), assessing if the pain is concordant.

⑤ The clinician then pushes beyond the first point of pain toward end range, reassessing the pain, quality of movement, and checking for splinting or muscle spasm.

⑥ The process is repeated toward end range, further assessing the pain.

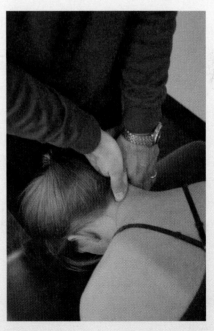

■ **Figure 5.60** UPA in Physiological Side Flexion

Combined Unilateral Posterior–Anterior (UPA), Unilateral Anterior–Posterior (UAP) with Rotations

Perhaps the most difficult combined method to perform involves the combined movements of physiological rotation, a UAP, and a UPA. This procedure enhances the vigor of physiological rotation and concentrates the force of the examination to both sides of the joint segment.

1. The patient is positioned in supine and the neck is placed in neutral.

2. The clinician holds the patient's head in a chin-cradle grip (a left chin-cradle grip is pictured in Figure 5.61 ■).

3. Using the tips of digits 2 and 3, the clinician hooks the anterior aspect of the transverse processes on the same side of the neck in which rotation is initiated (Figure 5.61, left).

4. Using the thumb of the same hand (the right hand in Figure 5.61), the clinician applies a direct UPA force on the articular pillar (right articular pillar in Figure 5.61) at the same level that digits 2 and 3 pull posteriorly using a UAP force (on the left side of the patient's neck).

5. In a combined sequence, the clinician provides a physiological rotation concurrently with the UAP and UPA motion.

6. The process is performed up to the first point of pain, while assessing and targeting the pain that is concordant. The clinician then takes the combined movement beyond the first reported point of pain and reassesses the patient, specifically the concordant sign.

7. The clinician takes the combined movements to the end range, repeating the rotations while reassessing the patient.

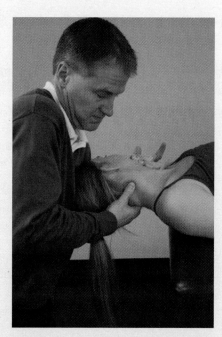

■ **Figure 5.61** UPA and UAP during Physiological Rotation

Opening Technique for the Cervical Spine

An opening dysfunction occurs when the patient's complaint of pain is on the opposite side of the direction that he or she side-bends or rotates (e.g., pain on the left during side flexion to the right or rotation to the right). In these cases, it is sometimes beneficial to treat into the opening restriction.

1. To target opening of the cervical spine, the clinician should contact the level below the desired facet with his or her hand that will apply the thrust technique.

2. Next, the clinician lifts the neck into flexion of the lower cervical spine.

3. The clinician then provides a transverse glide (Figure 5.62 ■, left) to take up slack (similar to what was used during the general manipulation technique).

4. Side flexion (slight) to the affected side (Figure 5.62, right) is then used to oppose the joint followed by slight rotation away (Figure 5.62, left) from the affected side (side flexion is opposite of rotation). The

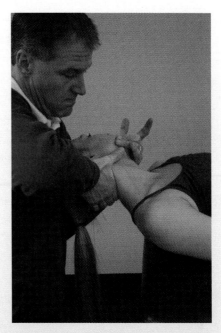

■ Figure 5.62 Opening Technique for the Cervical Spine: Right-Sided Opening

thrust involves a rotation (to the left) and cephalic movement to open the facet on the right side. In Figure 5.62, the clinician is treating an opening restriction on the right side.

Closing Technique for the Cervical Spine

Patients will sometimes complain of pain on the same side that they side flex or rotate toward. This type of distribution is often considered a closing dysfunction.

1. To target closing of the cervical spine, the clinician should target the level above the desired facet (the clinician is treating a closing restriction on the right in Figure 5.63 ■). The neck is kept in neutral or slight extension to enhance closing.

2. The clinician then provides a transverse glide (Figure 5.63, left) to take up slack. Side flexion (slight) to the affected side (Figure 5.63, right) is then used to oppose the joint, followed by slight rotation away from the affected side (side flexion is opposite of rotation).

3. The thrust involves a side flexion and downward glide movement to close the facet on the right side.

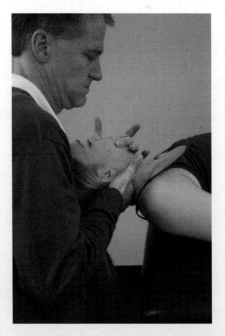

■ Figure 5.63 Targeted Specific Closing Technique for the Right Side

Manually Assisted Opening Technique of the Cervical Spine

1. The clinician should target the level below the desired facet. Next, the clinician lifts the neck into flexion of the lower cervical spine.

2. The clinician then provides a transverse glide to take up slack.

3. Side flexion (slight) to the affected side is then used to oppose the joint, followed by slight rotation away from the affected side (side flexion is opposite of rotation) (Figure 5.64 ■).

4. The clinician then asks the patient to actively rotate into his or her thumb while holding the head stable.

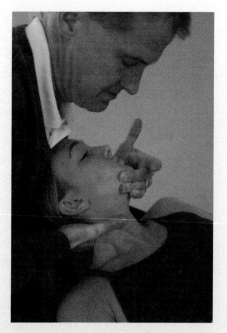

■ **Figure 5.64** Manually Assisted Opening Technique of the Cervical Spine

Manually Assisted Closing Technique of the Cervical Spine

1. The clinician should target the level above the desired facet. The neck is kept in neutral or slight extension to enhance closing.

2. The clinician then provides a transverse glide to take up slack.

3. Side flexion (slight) to the affected side is then used to oppose the joint, followed by slight rotation away from the affected side (side flexion is opposite of rotation) (Figure 5.65 ■).

4. The clinician then asks the patient to actively side-flex away from the current side flexion while holding the head stable.

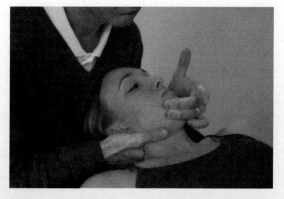

■ **Figure 5.65** Manually Assisted Closing Technique of the Cervical Spine

Treatment Outcomes

The Evidence

Overall, there is Level A evidence that a treatment approach that consists of some element of orthopedic manual therapy is associated with a positive outcome.[103,104] Treatment elements such as nonthrust and thrust manipulation have functioned similarly when performed in isolation[105] but exhibit stronger outcomes when combined with exercise[105] or some other form of intervention.[106,107]

Evidence for Cervical Manipulation and Mobilization

There is Level A evidence that treatment with cervical thrust manipulation and nonthrust mobilization is beneficial for patients with subacute or chronic mechanical neck pain.[104,108,109] Several authors have reported that outcomes of thrust manipulation compared with nonthrust mobilization show similar benefit.[104,105] In a 2004 Cochrane review of manipulation and mobilization for mechanical neck disorders, Gross et al.[104] suggested that mobilization and manipulation displayed similar outcomes but were not beneficial when performed alone on a heterogeneous group of patients. In 1996, Hurwitz et al.[110] concluded in a systematic literature review that (1) mobilization provided short-term benefit for patients with acute neck pain, (2) manipulation was probably more effective than mobilization for patients with subacute or chronic neck problems, (3) both were more effective than conventional medical care, and (4) manipulation and mobilization were beneficial for cervicogenic headaches.

When combined with exercise, both methods of treatment also demonstrate Level A evidence for pain reduction and functional improvements in patients with or without cervicogenic headaches. Although Gross et al.[104] reported there was insufficient evidence available to draw conclusions regarding patients with radiculopathy, two recent articles have demonstrated benefit using either indirect cervical mobilization methods[106] or selective mobilization of the nerve tissue.[111]

There is also Level A evidence to support the use of mobilization and manipulation combined with a targeted local musculature strengthening program for the neck.[29] One substantiated program is the cervical strengthening program suggested by Jull et al.[86] This program targets the anterior cervical deep flexors in a sequence of targeted progressive steps. Harris and colleagues[112] recently demonstrated differences in neck flexor endurance between subjects with and without neck pain, using the neck flexor endurance test. The test purportedly isolates the ability of the deep neck flexors for stability and endurance.

Evidence for Cervical Mobilization with Movement

There is Level B evidence specifically supporting the use of mobilization with movement techniques in patients with cervical dysfunction. Two studies have investigated the effects of upper cervical mobilizations with movement on patients with cervicogenic headache and dizziness.[99,100] Four to six treatments of upper cervical mobilizations with movement were shown to improve neck pain, dizziness, and disability, immediately post-treatment and at 6- and 12-week follow-up.[99] Similarly, Hall et al.[100] reported significant improvements in range of motion and headache in favor of a group performing self-C1–2 mobilizations with movement (also called SNAGs).

Evidence for Thoracic Manipulation and Mobilization

Several recent studies have investigated the benefits of performing thoracic thrust manipulation and nonthrust mobilization in patients with primary complaints of neck pain.[113–117] Currently, there is Level B evidence supporting its use in this population. The majority of these studies have utilized thoracic thrust manipulation, as this has shown significantly greater short-term benefits than nonthrust mobilization in improving pain and disability.[114] Thoracic thrust manipulation has been advocated as an integral component in the multimodal management of patients with mechanical neck pain.[114,118]

Evidence for Cervical Traction

There is Level C evidence regarding the use of cervical traction for patients with mechanical neck disorders with or without radicular symptoms.[113,118–120] Few studies have found traction to exhibit useful outcomes in samples of patients with cervical radiculopathy. Joghataei et al.[121] reported that when traction was combined with electrotherapy and exercise there were improvements in upper extremity grip strength. Shakoor et al.[83] found a trend toward significance when traction was used in conjunction with neck strengthening exercises when compared to a control group, which received nonsteroidal inflammatory medications only. Other studies have reported benefit from combining cervical traction with a multimodal treatment regimen.[113,122] However, a study by Young et al.[118] demonstrated no significant difference in short-term outcome of pain, disability, and function in patients with cervical radiculopathy receiving multimodal care with or without intermittent cervical mechanical traction.

Summary

- Overall, there is substantial evidence that a treatment approach that consists of some element of orthopedic manual therapy is associated with a positive outcome.
- Patient outcomes after treatment based on mobilization and manipulation are equally beneficial.
- When performed alone, mobilization and manipulation both provide some benefit; however, when combined with exercise, both methods of treatment were beneficial for pain reduction and functional improvements in patients with or without cervicogenic headaches.

Chapter Questions

1. Describe the responsibilities of the cervical intervertebral disc, the uncovertebral joints, and the zygopophyseal joints in stability and movement of the cervical spine.

2. Define the directional coupling pattern of the cervical spine and the importance of initiation of movement.

3. Indicate which spinal segments are most commonly associated with cervicogenic headaches and outline a treatment regimen.

4. Describe the subjective symptoms and patient examination findings associated with cervical instability, CAD, and whiplash.

5. Describe how combined movements of the cervical spine place greater force upon the elastic and/or inelastic aspects of a segment.

Patient Cases

Case 5.1: Mary Johnson (26-year-old female)

Diagnosis: Whiplash-associated disorder

Observation: She exhibits forward head posture and a noticeable fear of movement and diminished range during active assessment.

Mechanism: Was involved in a motor vehicle accident approximately 2 days ago.

Concordant Sign: Most concordant pain involves extension of the neck.

Nature of the Condition: She is unable to work because of pain (she is an accountant). Her concentration and ability to sit for long periods is affected. Simple movements trigger symptoms and increase pain dramatically. She requires use of pain medication to decrease symptoms.

Behavior of the Symptoms: Pain originates at the base of the occiput and radiates bilaterally to the upper trapezius muscles.

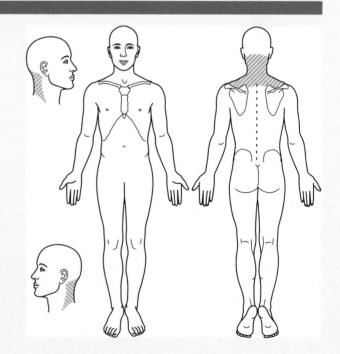

Pertinent Patient History: Diagnosed with Ehlers-Danlos syndrome 4 years prior.

Patient Goals: She would like to decrease her current pain and return to work.

Baseline: At rest 4/10 NAS for pain, when worst 7/10 pain.

Examination Findings: All active movements are limited and painful, extension is concordant and limited. Passive physiological findings are similar. The patient guards during passive movement. The majority of the pain is isolated at the upper C-spine; most concordant with UPAs to C2–C3 and C1–C2.

1. Based on these findings, what else would you like to examine?
2. Is this patient a good candidate for manual therapy?
3. What is the expected prognosis of this patient?
4. What treatments do you feel presented in this book may be beneficial for this patient?

Case 5.2: John Smith (58-year-old male)

Diagnosis: Spondylosis of the cervical spine

Observation: He exhibits forward head posture with slight side flexion away from the right side. The posterior neck posture is flattened. There is a visible Dowager's hump in upper thoracic spine.

Mechanism: Insidious onset. Symptoms have been present for well over 8 months.

Concordant Sign: Right side flexion reproduces right arm pain. Extension reproduces neck pain.

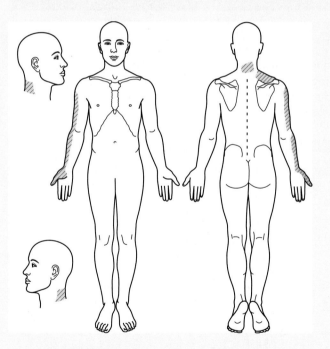

Nature of the Condition: He considers the symptoms a nuisance. He is able to work all day (he places cable for phone companies) without too much pain. He is able to drive and do anything he wants. He takes ibuprofen only to control symptoms.

Behavior of the Symptoms: Pain in arm is worse in the morning and during right side flexion. Pain in neck is worse during aggressive lifting or when he sleeps on a bad pillow.

Pertinent Patient History: Diagnosed with osteoarthritis 10 years ago.

Patient Goals: He is concerned about the arm pain and would like to resolve that aspect of his problem. He feels the neck pain is age-related and that there is little to do for that.

Baseline: Pain in the arm is 4/10 whereas pain in the neck is 2/10. When worse, the pain is 5/10 for the arm and 3/10 for the neck.

Examination Findings: Extension reproduces arm pain (slightly) but primarily neck pain. Side flexion to the right reproduces the right arm pain. Upper thoracic mobility assessed with PAs is lacking considerably. Reflexes, manual muscle testing, and sensibility testing is all normal in the right arm.

1. Based on these findings, what else would you like to examine?
2. Is this patient a good candidate for manual therapy?
3. What is the expected prognosis of this patient?
4. What treatments do you feel presented in this book may be beneficial for this patient?

Case 5.3: Carla Robertson (79-year-old female)

Diagnosis: Cervical strain

Observation: She holds her head very still and exhibits very poor posture (forward head) and thoracic kyphosis.

Mechanism: Insidious onset. She reports symptoms of pain and a general lack of wellness for over 20 years.

Concordant Sign: She indicates that quick movements of her head make her feel unsteady.

Nature of the Condition: The condition is very stable and does not appear to exhibit easy flare-ups. She indicates that she has stopped driving, shopping, and socializing because of the lack of wellness.

Behavior of the Symptoms: Lack of wellness and unsteadiness is worse at the end of the day or when fatigued. She indicates that when her neck bothers her she feels clumsiness in her legs and hands.

Pertinent Patient History: Multiple medical problems unrelated to her current condition; long-term history of hyperthyroid syndrome.

Patient Goals: She is interested in addressing the general lack of wellness and unsteadiness.

Baseline: Pain is only 1/10.

Examination Findings: Range of motion is limited throughout but not concordant to symptoms. Extension of the neck is concordant to feelings of gait clumsiness. None of the active or passive findings reproduce pain.

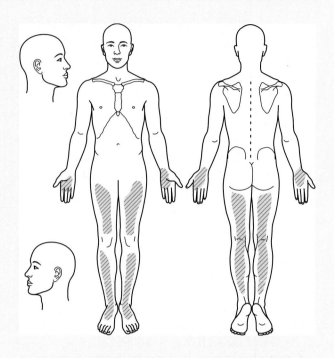

1. Based on these findings, what else would you like to examine?
2. Is this patient a good candidate for manual therapy?
3. What is the expected prognosis of this patient?
4. What treatments do you feel presented in this book may be beneficial for this patient?

PEARSON
myhealthprofessionskit™

Use this address to access the Companion Website created for this textbook. Simply select "Physical Therapy" from the choice of disciplines. Find this book and log in using your username and password to access video clips demonstrating various techniques and the anatomy and arthrological information for this chapter.

References

1. Cattrysse E, Swinkels RA, Oostendorp RA, Duquet W. Upper cervical instability: are clinical tests reliable? *Man Ther.* 1997;2(2):91–97.

2. Cook C, Hegedus E. *Orthopedic physical examination tests: An evidence-based approach.* Upper Saddle River, NJ; Prentice Hall: 2008.

3. Kerry R, Taylor AJ, Mitchell J, McCarthy C, Brew J. Manual therapy and cervical arterial dysfunction, directions for the future: a clinical perspective. *J Man Manip Ther.* 2008;16(1):39–48.

4. Kerry R, Taylor A, Mitchell J, Brew J, Kiely R, McCarthy C. Cervical artery dysfunction assessment framework. Manipulation Association of Chartered Physiotherapists. 2005.

5. Kerry R, Taylor AJ. Cervical arterial dysfunction: knowledge and reasoning for manual physical therapists. *J Orthop Sports Phys Ther.* 2009;39(5):378–387.

6. Barker WH, Howard VJ, Howard G, Toole JF. Effect of contralateral occlusion on long-term efficacy of endarterectomy in the asymptomatic carotid atherosclerosis study (ACAS). ACAS Investigators. *Stroke.* 2000;10:2330–2334.

7. Gross AR, Kay T, Hondras M, et al. Manual therapy for mechanical neck disorders: A systematic review. *Man Ther.* 2002;7(3):131–149.

8. Di Fabio RP. Manipulation of the cervical spine: Risks and benefits. *Phys Ther.* 1999;79(1):50–65.

9. Mann T, Refshauge KM. Causes of complications from cervical spine manipulation. *Aust J Physiother.* 2001;47(4):255–266.

10. Johnson C, Grant R, Dansie B, Taylor J, Spyropolous P. Measurement of blood flow in the vertebral artery using colour duplex Doppler ultrasound: establishment of the reliability of selected parameters. *Man Ther.* 2000;5(1):21–29.

11. Schneider PA, Rossman ME, Bernstein EF, Ringelstein EB, Torem S, Otis SM. Noninvasive evaluation of vertebrobasilar insufficiency. *J Ultrasound Med.* 1991;10(7):373–379.

12. Licht PB, Christensen HW, Hojgaard P, Marving J. Vertebral artery flow and spinal manipulation: A randomized, controlled and observer-blinded study. *J Manipulative Physiol Ther.* 1998; 21(3):141–144.

13. Refshauge KM. Rotation: A valid premanipulative dizziness test? Does it predict safe manipulation? *J Manipulative Physiol Ther.* 1994;17(1):15–19.

14. Rivett DA, Sharples KJ, Milburn PD. Effect of prema-nipulative tests on vertebral artery and internal carotid artery blood flow: A pilot study. *J Manipulative Physiol Ther.* 1999;22(6):368–375.

15. Maitland GD. *Maitland's vertebral manipulation.* 6th ed. London; Butterworth-Heinemann: 2001.

16. Grant R. Vertebral artery testing: The Australian Physiotherapy Association Protocol after 6 years. *Man Ther.* 1996;1(3):149–153.

17. Zaina C, Grant R, Johnson C, Dansie B, Taylor J, Spyropolous P. The effect of cervical rotation on blood flow in the contralateral vertebral artery. *Man Ther.* 2003;8(2):103–109.

18. Grant R. *Physical therapy of the cervical and thoracic spine.* 3rd ed. New York; Churchill Livingstone: 2002.

19. Magarey ME, Rebbeck T, Coughlan B, Grimmer K, Rivett DA, Refshauge K. Pre-manipulative testing of the cervical spine review, revision and new clinical guidelines. *Man Ther.* 2004;9(2):95–108.

20. Dvorak J, Antinnes JA, Panjabi M, Loustalot D, Bonomo M. Age and gender related normal motion of the cervical spine. *Spine.* 1992;17(10 Suppl):S393–298.

21. Fischer RP. Cervical radiographic evaluation of alert patients following blunt trauma. *Ann Emerg Med.* 1984;13:905–907.

22. Makofsky H. The influence of forward head posture on dental occlusion. *Cranio.* 2000;18:30–39.

23. Visscher C, De Boer W, Lobbezoo F, Habets L, Naeije M. Is there a relationship between head posture and craniomandibular pain? *J Oral Rehabilitation.* 2002;29:1030–1036.

24. Nicolakis P, Nicolakis M, Piehslinger E, et al. Relationship between craniomandibular disorders and poor posture. *Cranio.* 2000;18:106–112.

25. Santander H, Miralles R, Perez J, et al. Effects of head and neck inclination on bilateral sternocleidomastiod EMG activity in healthy subjects and in patients with myogenic cranio-cervical mandibular dysfunction. *Cranio.* 2000;18:181–191.

26. Wright E, Domenech M, Fischer J. Usefulness of posture training for patients with temporomandibular disorders. *J Am Dent Assoc.* 2000;131:202–210.

27. Watson DH, Trott PH. Cervical headache: An investigation of natural head posture and upper cervical flexor muscle performance. *Cephalalgia.* 1993;13(4):272–284.

28. Marcus D, Scharff L, Mercer S, Turk D. Musculoskeletal abnormalities in chronic headache: A controlled comparison of headache diagnostic groups. *Headache.* 1998;39:21–27.

29. Niere KR, Torney SK. Clinicians' perceptions of minor cervical instability. *Man Ther.* 2004;9(3):144–150.

30. Paley D, Gillespie R. Chronic repetitive unrecognized flexion injury of the cervical spine (high jumper's neck). *Am J Sports Med.* 1986;14:92–95.

31. Olsen K, Joder D. Diagnosis and treatment of cervical spine clinical instability. *J Orthop Sports Phys Ther.* 2001;31(4):194–206.

32. Jull G, Barrett C, Magee R, Ho P. Further clinical clarification of the muscle dysfunction in cervical headache. *Cephalalgia.* 1999;19(3):179–185.

33. Lestini W, Wiesel S. The pathogenesis of cervical spondylosis. *Clin Orthop.* 1989;239:69–93.

34. Montazem A. Secondary tinnitus as a symptom of instability of the upper cervical spine: Operative management. *Int Tinnitus J.* 2000;6(2):130–133.

35. Niere K, Selvaratnam P. The cervical region. In Zuluaga et al. (eds.) *Sports physiotherapy: Applied science and practice.* Melbourne; Churchill Livingstone: 1995.

36. O'Sullivan P, Burnett A, Alexander F, Gadsdon K, Logiudice J, Miller D. Quirke H. Lumbar repositioning deficit in specific a low back pain population. *Spine.* 2003;28:1074–1079.

37. Klein G, Mannion A, Panjabi M, Dvorak J. Trapped in the neutral zone: another symptom of whiplash-associated disorder? *Eur Spine J.* 2001;10(2):141–148.

38. Emery SE. Cervical spondylotic myelopathy: Diagnosis and treatment. *J Am Acad Orthop Surg.* 2001;9(6):376–388.

39. McNamara RM, Heine E, Esposito B. Cervical spine injury and radiography in alert, high-risk patients. *J Emerg Med.* 1990;8:177–182.

40. McKee TR, Tinkoff G, Rhodes M. Asymptomatic occult cervical spine fracture: Case report and review of the literature. *J Trauma.* 1990;30:623–626.

41. Bayless P, Ray VG. Incidence of cervical spine injuries in association with blunt head trauma. *Am J Emerg Med.* 1989;7:139–142.

42. Vandemark RM. Radiology of the cervical spine in trauma patients: Practice pitfalls and recommendations for improving efficiency and communication. *AJR.* 1990;155:465–472.

43. Bandiera G, Stiell C, Wells G, et al. Canadian C-Spine and CT Head Study Group, The Canadian C-Spine rule performs better than unstructured physician judgment, *Ann Emerg Med.* 2003;42:395–402.

44. Grieve G. *Common vertebral joint problems.* 2nd ed. Edinburgh; Churchill Livingstone: 1988.

45. Reiter MF, Boden SD. Inflammatory disorders of the cervical spine. *Spine.* 1998;23:2755–2766.

46. Cook C, Brismee JM, Sizer P. Suggested factors associated with clinical cervical spine instability: A Delphi study of physical therapists. *Phys Ther.* 2005;85:895–906.

47. Cook C, Roman M, Stewart KM, Leithe LG, Isaacs R. Reliability and diagnostic accuracy of clinical special tests for myelopathy in patients seen for cervical dysfunction. *J Orthop Sports Phys Ther.* 2009;39(3):172–178.

48. Coronado R, Hudson B, Sheets C, et al. Correlation of magnetic resonance imaging findings and reported symptoms in patients with chronic cervical dysfunction. *J Man Manip Ther.* 2009;17:148–153.

49. Dvorak J. Epidemiology, physical examination, and neurodiagnostics. *Spine.* 1998;23:2663–2672.

50. Sandmark H, Nisell R. Validity of five common manual neck pain provoking tests. *Scand J Rehabil Med.* 1995;27(3):131–136.

51. Lee RY, McGregor AH, Bull AM, Wragg P. Dynamic response of the cervical spine to posteroanterior mobilisation. *Clin Biomech.* 2005;20(2):228–231.

52. Sterling M, Jull G, Carlsson Y, Crommert L. Are cervical physical outcome measures influenced by the presence of symptomatology? *Physiother Res Int.* 2002;7(3):113–121.

53. Yelland M. Back, chest and abdominal pain: How good are spinal signs at identifying musculoskeletal causes of back, chest or abdominal pain? *Aust Fam Physician.* 2001;30:980–912.

54. Patla C, Paris S. Reliability of interpretation of the Paris classification of normal end feel for elbow flexion and extension. *J Man Manip Ther.* 1993;1:60–66.

55. Chesworth B, MacDermid J, Roth J, Patterson SD. Movement diagram and "end-feel" reliability when measuring passive lateral rotation of the shoulder in patients with shoulder pathology. *Phys Ther.* 1998;78:593–601.

56. Cooperman J, Riddle D, Rothstein J. Reliability and validity of judgments of the integrity of the anterior cruciate ligament of the knee using the Lachman's test. *Phys Ther.* 1990;70:225–233.

57. Petersen C, Hayes K. Construct validity of Cyriax's selective tension examination: Association of end-feels with pain at the knee and shoulder. *J Orthop Sports Phys Ther.* 2000;30:512–527.

58. White A, Panjabi M. *Clinical biomechanics of the spine.* Philadelphia; J.B. Lippincott: 1990.

59. Penning L, Tondury G (Abstract). Enststehung, Bau and Funktion der meniskoiden Strukturen in den Halswirbelgelenken. *Z Orthop.* 1964;1:14.

60. Tong HC, Haig AJ, Yamakawa K. The Spurling test and cervical radiculopathy. *Spine.* 2002;27(2):156–159.

61. Fjellner A, Bexander C, Faleij R, Strender LE. Interexaminer reliability in physical examination of the cervical spine. *J Manipulative Physiol Ther.* 1999;22(8):511–516.

62. Haas M, Groupp E, Panzer D, Partna L, Lumsden S, Aickin M. Efficacy of cervical endplay assessment as an indicator for spinal manipulation. *Spine.* 2003;28(11):1091–1096.

63. Aquino RL, Caires PS, Furtado FC, Loureiro AV, Ferreira PH, Ferreira M. Applying joint mobilization at different cervical vertebral levels does not influence immediate pain reduction in patients with chronic neck pain: A randomized clinical trial. *J Man Manipulative Ther.* 2009;17:95–100.

64. Schomacher J. The effect of an analgesic mobilization technique when applied at symptomatic or asymptomatic levels of the cervical spine in subjects with neck pain: A randomized controlled trial. *J Man Manipulative Ther.* 2009;17:101–108.

65. McLean S, Naish R, Reed L, Urry S, Vicenzino B. A pilot study of the manual force levels required to produce manipulation induced hypoalgesia. *Clin Biomech (Bristol, Avon).* 2002;17(4):304–308.

66. Schmid A, Brunner F, Wright A, Bachmann LM. Paradigm shift in manual therapy?: Evidence for a central nervous system component in the response to passive cervical joint mobilisation. *Man Ther.* 2008;13(5):387–396.

67. Jull G, Bogduk N, Marsland A. The accuracy of manual diagnosis for cervical zygopophyseal joint pain syndromes. *Med J Aust.* 1988;148(5):233–236.

68. Jull G, Treleaven J, Versace G. Manual examination: Is pain provocation a major cue for spinal dysfunction? *Aust J Physiotherapy.* 1994;40(3):159–165.

69. Matyas T, Bach T. The reliability of selected techniques in clinical arthrometrics. *Aust J Physiotherapy.* 1985;31:175–199.

70. Cook C, Wright A. Motion palpation of the spine: Doomed to failure? *Orthopedic Division Review.* Nov/Dec, 2007.

71. Maher C, Latimer J. Pain or resistance: The manual therapists' dilemma. *Aust J Physiotherapy.* 1992;38:257–260.

72. Wright A, Vicenzino B. Cervical mobilization techniques, sympathetic nervous system effects, and their relationship to analgesia. In: Shacklock M (ed). *Moving in on pain.* Melbourne; Butterworth Heinemann: 1995.

73. Travell J, Simons D. Myofascial pain and dysfunction. In: *The trigger point manual;* Vol. 2., The lower extremities. Baltimore; Williams & Wilkins: 1992.

74. Alvarez DJ, Rockwell PG. Trigger points: Diagnosis and management. *Am Fam Physician.* 2002;65(4):653–660.

75. Fernandez-de-las-Penas C. Interaction between trigger points and joint hypomobility: A clinical perspective. *J Man Manipulative Ther.* 2009;17:74–77.

76. Uthaikhup S, Sterling M, Jull G. Cervical musculoskeletal impairment is common in elders with headache. *Man Ther.* 2009;14(6):636–641.

77. O'Leary S, Jull G, Kim M, Vicenzino B. Specificity in retraining craniocervical flexor muscle performance. *J Orthop Sports Phys Ther.* 2007;37(1):3–9.

78. Lee H, Nicholson LL, Adams RD. Cervical range of motion associations with subclinical neck pain. *Spine.* 2003; 29:33–40.

79. Maitland GD. *Peripheral manipulation.* 3rd ed. London; Butterworth-Heinemann: 1986.

80. Edmondston SJ, Allison GT, Gregg CD, Purden SM, Svansson GR, Watson AE. Effect of position on the posteroanterior stiffness of the lumbar spine. *Man Ther.* 1998;3(1):21–26.

81. Trott P. Management of selected cervical syndromes. In: Grant R (ed). *Physical therapy of the cervical and thoracic spine.* 3rd ed. New York; Churchill Livingstone: 2002.

82. Childs J, Fritz J, Piva S, Whitman J. Proposal of a classification system for patients with neck pain. *J Orthop Sports Phys Ther.* 2004;34:686–700.

83. Shakoor M, Ahmed M, Kibria G, et al. (abstract). Effects of cervical traction and exercise therapy in cervical spondylosis. *Bangladesh Med Res Counc Bull.* 2002;28:61–69.

84. Harrison D, Cailliet R, Betz J, et al. Conservative methods of reducing lateral translation postures of the head: A nonrandomized clinical control trial. *J Rehabil Res Dev.* 2004;41:631–639.

85. Grant R, Jull G, Spencer T. Active stabilizing training for screen based keyboard operators: A single case study. *Aust J Physiotherapy.* 1997;43:235–242.

86. Jull G, Trott P, Potter H, et al. A randomized controlled trial of exercise and manipulative therapy for cervicogenic headache. *Spine.* 2002;27:1835–1843.

87. Abdulwahab S, Sabbahi M. Neck retractions, cervical root decompression, and radicular pain. *J Orthop Sports Phys Ther.* 2000;30:4–12.

88. Swank A, Funk D, Durham M, Roberts S. Adding weights to stretching exercise increases passive range of motion for healthy elderly. *J Strength Cond Res.* 2003;17:374–378.

89. Vicenzino B, Collins D, Wright A. An investigation of the interrelationship between manipulative therapy-induced hypoalgesia and sympathoexcitation. *J Manipulative Physiol Ther.* 1998;21:448–453.

90. Vicenzino B, Collins D, Wright A. Sudomotor changes induced by neural mobilization techniques in asymptomatic subjects. *J Man Manipulative Ther.* 1994;2:66–74.

91. Simon R, Vicenzino B, Wright A. The influence of an anteroposterior accessory glide of the glenohumeral joint on measures of peripheral sympathetic nervous system function in the upper limb. *Man Ther.* 1997;2(1):18–23.

92. Solly S. Cervical postero–anterior mobilization: A brief review of evidence of physiological and pain relieving effects. *Phys Ther Rev.* 2004;9:182–187.

93. Vicenzino B, Paungmali A, Buratowski S, Wright A. Specific manipulative therapy treatment for chronic lateral epicondylalgia produces uniquely characteristic hypoalgesia. *Man Ther.* 2001;6:205–212.

94. Lovick T. Interactions between descending pathways from the dorsal and ventrolateral periaqueductal gray matter in the rat. In: Depaulis A, Bandler R (eds). *The midbrain periaqueductal gray matter.* New York; Plenum Press: 1991.

95. Magarey ME, Rebbeck T, Coughlan B, Grimmer K, Rivett DA, Refshauge K. Pre-manipulative testing of the cervical spine review, revision and new clinical guidelines. *Man Ther.* 2004;9(2):95–108.

96. Jull G, Zito G, Trott P, Potter H, Shirley D. Inter-examiner reliability to detect painful cervical joint dysfunction. *Aust J Physiotherapy.* 1997;43:125–129.

97. Lee R, Evans J. An in-vivo study of the intervertebral movements produced by posteroanterior mobilisation. *Clin Biomech.* 1997;12:400–408.

98. McGregor A, Wragg P, Gedroyc W, Can interventional MRI provide an insight into the mechanics of a posterior–anterior mobilisation? *Clin Biomech.* 2001;16, 926–929.

99. Reid SA, Rivett DA, Katekar MG, Callister R. Sustained natural apophysial glides (SNAGS) are an effective treatment for cervicogenic dizziness. *Man Ther.* 2008;13:357–366.

100. Hall T, Chan HT, Christensen L, Odenthal B, Wells C, Robinson K. Efficacy of a C1–C2 self-sustained natural apophyseal glide (SNAGs) in the management of cervicogenic headache. *J Orthop Sports Phys Ther* 2007;37(3):100–107.

101. Ferber R, Osternig L, Gravelle D. Effect of PNF stretch techniques on knee flexor muscle EMG activity in older adults. *J Electromyography Kinesi.* 2002;12:391–397.

102. Triano JJ, Rogers CM, Combs S, Potts D, Sorrels K. Quantitative feedback versus standard training for cervical and thoracic manipulation. *J Manipulative Physiol Ther.* 2003;26(3):131–138.

103. Sarigiovannis P, Hollins B. Effectiveness of manual therapy in the treatment of non-specific neck pain: A review. *Phys Ther Rev.* 2005;10:35–50.

104. Gross AR, Hoving JL, Haines TA, Goldsmith CH, Kay T, Aker P, Bronfort G. A Cochrane review of manipulation and mobilization for mechanical neck disorders. *Spine.* 2004;29(14):1541–1548.

105. Hurwitz EL, Morgenstern H, Harber P, Kominski GF, Belin TR, Yu F, Adams AH. A randomized trial of medical care with and without physical therapy and chiropractic care with and without physical modalities for patients with low back pain: 6-month follow-up outcomes from the UCLA low back pain study. *Spine.* 2002;27(20):2193–2204.

106. Cleland JA, Whitman JM, Fritz JM. Effectiveness of manual physical therapy to the cervical spine in the management of lateral epicondylalgia: a retrospective analysis. *J Orthop Sports Phys Ther.* 2004;34(11):713–722.

107. Giles LG, Muller R. Chronic spinal pain: A randomized clinical trial comparing medication, acupuncture, and spinal manipulation. *Spine.* 2003;28(14):1490–1502.

108. Hurwitz EL, Morgenstern H, Vassilaki M, Chiang LM. Frequency and clinical predictors of adverse reactions to chiropractic care in the UCLA neck pain study. *Spine* (Phila. Pa. 1976). 2005;30(13):1477–1484.

109. Gross AR, Hoving JL, Haines TA, et al. Cervical Overview Group. A Cochrane review of manipulation and mobilization for mechanical neck disorders. *Spine* (Phila. Pa. 1976). 2004;29(14):1541–1548.

110. Hurwitz EL, Aker PD, Adams AH, Meeker WC, Shekelle PG. Manipulation and mobilization of the cervical spine. A systematic review of the literature. *Spine.* 1996;21(15):1746–1759.

111. Allison GT, Nagy BM, Hall T. A randomized clinical trial of manual therapy for cervico-brachial pain syndrome: A pilot study. *Man Ther.* 2002;7(2):95–102.

112. Harris K, Heer D, Roy T, Santos D, Whitman J, Wainner R. Reliability of a measurement of neck flexor muscle endurance. *Phys Ther.* 2005;85:1349–1355.

113. Cleland JA, Fritz JD, Whitman JM, Heath R. Predictors of short-term outcomes in people with a clinical diagnosis of cervical radiculopathy. *Phys Ther.* 2007;87:1619–1632.

114. Cleland JA, Glynn P, Whitman JM, Eberhart Sl, MacDonald C, Childs JD. Short-term effects of thrust versus nonthrust mobilization/manipulation directed at the thoracic spine in patients with neck pain: A randomized controlled trial. *Phys Ther.* 2007;87(4):431–440.

115. Cleland JA, Childs JD, Fritz, JM, Whitman JM, Eberhart SL. Development of a clinical prediction rule for guiding treatment of a subgroup of patients with neck pain: Use of thoracic spine manipulation, exercise, and patient education. *Phys Ther.* 2007;87(1):9–23.

116. Gonzalez-Iglesias J, Fernandez-de-las-Penas C, Cleland JA, Alburqueque-Sendin, F, Palomeque-del-Cerro L, Mendez-Sanchez R. Inclusion of thoracic spine manipulation into an electro-therapy/thermal program for the management of patients with acute mechanical neck pain: a randomized clinical trial. *Man Ther.* 2009;14(3):306–313.

117. Gonzalez-Iglesias J, Fernandez-de-las-Penas C, Cleland JA, Gutierrez-Vega MR. Thoracic spine manipulation for the management of patients with neck pain: A randomized clinical trial. *J Orthop Sports Phys Ther.* 2009;39(1):20–27.

118. Young IA, Michener LA, Cleland JA, Aguilera AJ, Snyder AR. Manual therapy, exercise, and traction for patients with cervical radiculopathy: A randomized clinical trial. *Phys Ther.* 2009;89(7):632–642.

119. Graham N, Gross AR, Goldsmith C. Mechanical traction for mechanical neck disorders: A systematic review. *J Rehabil Med.* 2006;38:145–152.

120. Graham N, Gross A, Goldsmith CH, et al. Mechanical traction for neck pain with or without radiculopathy. *Cochrane Database of Systematic Reviews* 2008;3. Art. No: CD006408. DOI:10.1002/14651858.CD006408.pub2.

121. Joghataei MT, Arab AM, Khaksar H. The effect of cervical traction combined with conventional therapy on grip strength on patients with cervical radiculopathy. *Clin Rehabil.* 2004;18(8):879–887.

122. Cleland JA, Whitman JM, Fritz JM, Palmer JA. Manual physical therapy, cervical traction, and strengthening exercises in patients with cervical radiculopathy: A case series. *J Orthop Sports Phys Ther.* 2005;35:802–811.

Manual Therapy of the Temporomandibular Joint

Chad E. Cook

Objectives

- Understand the normal and pathological kinematics associated with temporomandibular joint movement.
- Recognize the patient subjective characteristics associated with temporomandibular disorders.
- Understand the pertinent cervical and temporomandibular joint clinical examination features.
- Recognize the techniques of treatment that have yielded the highest success in the literature.

Clinical Examination

Observation

Posture   Several studies have suggested a causative relationship between posture and temporomandibular disorders (TMD).[1-4] Others have suggested no or poor association between posture and TMD.[5,6] Most postural dysfunctions are associated with concurrent forward head and elevated trapezius tension.[7,8] Forward head and corresponding muscle activity negatively influences masticatory function,[1] thus potentially placing subjects at risk for muscle strain and tension to the masticatory system. Friction and colleagues[9] identified 85% of subjects with TMD to have forward head posture, thus elevating the risk of masticatory dysfunction.

Resting Position of the Teeth   During observation, assessment of the resting position of the teeth may assist the clinician in determining if the patient is predisposed to TMD. Conditions such as overbites, underbites, and other dental abnormalities may alter the bite and function of the temporomandibular joint (TMJ). The normal resting position of the teeth is slight opening with the tongue placed near the roof of the mouth (Figure 6.1 ■).

Symmetry of Movement   Observation of symmetry of jaw movement, bite, and facial muscle composition may also provide useful information. Most individuals with TMD have overactive muscles

of mastication and may demonstrate hypertrophy of the masseter. Asymmetric bites may alarm the clinician to internal derangements during moving of the jaw.

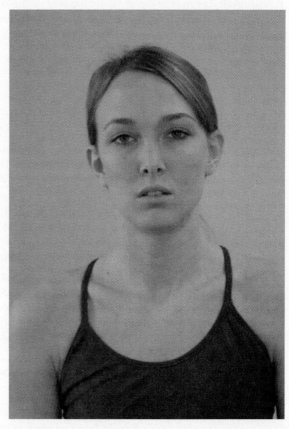

■ **Figure 6.1**   Normal Resting Position of the Teeth

Summary

- Observations such as asymmetries of teeth, jaw movement, muscle hypertrophy, and posture may yield useful information when examining TMD.
- The normal resting position of the teeth is slight opening with the tongue placed near the roof of the mouth.

Summary

- Common patient history complaints associated with TMD include joint sounds, limitation of jaw movement, muscle tenderness, pain in the periauricular region, bruxism, sensitive teeth, and burning mouth.
- Several psychosocial co-contributors are present in TMD including anxiety, depression, personality disorders, and stress.

Patient History

The primary patient subjective complaints associated with TMD include one or more of the following: joint sounds, limitation of jaw movement, muscle tenderness, or pain in the periauricular region.[10] Others have reported symptoms such as bruxism (teeth grinding), sensitive teeth, and burning mouth associated with TMD.[11] Any of these findings should be evaluated during a carefully constructed patient history.

Because concurrent symptoms with pain of cervical spine origin may exist with TMD, further questioning should reflect pain provocations associated with the cervical spine.[12] Conditions such as radiculopathy and myelopathy are of cervical spine origin since each is associated with nerve root or spinal cord compression. Additionally, pain that occurs near the end of the day, during sleep, or during cervical movements may be associated with the cervical spine and should be carefully evaluated.

Psychosocial Factors

Since psychosocial factors are considered common covariates in the cause and contribution of TMD, a careful examination of selected psychosocial factors is suggested. Wright et al.[13] reported that high-risk patients with TMD were more likely to have anxiety disorders and were four times more likely to exhibit a personality disorder such as avoidant, dependent, or obsessive–compulsive traits. Those with high-risk TMD also were more depressed and reported higher pain levels than controlled subjects. Rantala et al.[14] acknowledged the influence of somatization in patients with TMD, noting the concurrence of TMD symptoms and myofascial complaints of pain. Lastly, Ahlberg et al.[15] reported that smoking and high stress levels were associated with concurrent higher report of pain compared to controls, thus necessitating smoking cessation and stress rehabilitation.

Physical Examination

Active Physiological Movements

Ruling out the Cervical Spine   There is significant overlap between pain associated with TMD and cervicogenic pain.[3,16] Because of this, it is necessary to perform a cervical screen to identify the potential contribution of pain in isolation of the cervical spine. Cervicogenic pain may arise from a number of causes, including trauma,[1] posture,[7] and degenerative changes. Since posture of the cervical spine and related muscular spasm can increase the risk for muscle strain and tension to the masticatory system, it is essential to rule out the presence of a cervical disorder prior to evaluation of the temporomandibular joint.

The reader is suggested to refer back to Chapter 5, specifically the active physiological examination of the cervical spine. Of the cervical physiological movements, cervical rotation may yield the most influential findings during examination. Braun and Schiffman[17] reported that cervical rotation and flexion and extension measures of mobility were useful predictors to determine masticatory muscle tenderness. In addition to rotation, active physiological movements such as extension, flexion, and side flexion with overpressure are necessary to determine the contribution of the cervical spine to the presenting patient symptoms.

Summary

- An appropriate examination of the cervical spine is necessary to "rule out" cervical involvement and to determine if contribution from the cervical spine is prominent.
- The movements of active physiological rotation and to a lesser extent flexion and extension are associated with increased pain in the masseter.

Examination of the Temporomandibular Joint   The clinical examination is the most important diagnostic component of evaluation of TMJ pain.[18] The clinical examination is directed toward assessment of symmetry of motion and reproduction of pain during the movement cycle. Pain with active and passive movements may identify retrodiscal structures as the source of symptoms since these structures are tensioned or compressed during movement. Selection of the appropriate treatment modality (i.e., stretching, strengthening, or physical agents) hedges on the findings of the clinical evaluation.[18]

Active Movements of a Nondisplaced Disc   All four active movements of depression, protrusion, and medial and lateral translation may stress the posterior–superior ligamentous structures. These motions should be assessed for pain production and asymmetry of movement.

Active Movements of a Displaced Disc   With an anteriorly displaced disc, the superior–posterior structures and the sphenomandibular ligament are compressed or stretched by the condyle during movement.[21] Because of this, active and passive movement may yield differences in findings. Protraction will stretch retrodiscal tissue and may reproduce pain similar to end-range pain. During full mouth opening an audible repositioning is generally noticeable as the condyle slips posteriorly to the disc.[21] Decreasing cranial compression reduces the likelihood of repositioning and can be accomplished by placing a device such as a gauge between the molars of the patient prior to mouth opening.[21] This primarily reduces cranial compression during opening.

Summary

- Several TMJ-specific movements require examination to determine which movement may be contributing to TMD.

- Measurement of maximal mouth opening, protrusion, and retrusion may be a useful method to determine dysfunction and to measure progress.

- The presence of a displaced disc may yield different active examination findings and warrant careful attention. Typically, disc displacement is associated with pain during full mouth opening and a clicking noise.

Depression (Mouth closing) Measurement of Deviation

Depression involves the closing of the mouth, incorporating contact between the upper and lower teeth (if present) of the patient.

1. To test depression, the clinician instructs the patient to bite down hard (Figure 6.2 ■).

2. If necessary, with a gloved hand, the clinician views the bite formation for symmetry.

3. The patient is queried regarding production of concordant symptoms.

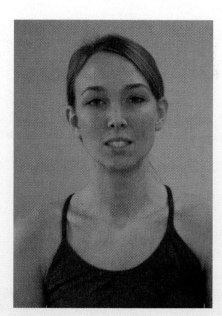

■ Figure 6.2   TMJ Depression

Protrusion

Protrusion involves the anterior displacement of the lower jaw and subsequent unloading of retrodiscal tissues.

1. The clinician instructs the patient to stick his or her chin outward as far as he or she can (Figure 6.3 ■). The clinician may be required to demonstrate the movement for the patient.

2. The clinician views the bite formation for symmetry.

3. The patient is queried regarding production of concordant symptoms.

4. With a gloved hand and a tape measure, the clinician measures the protrusive displacement of the patient.

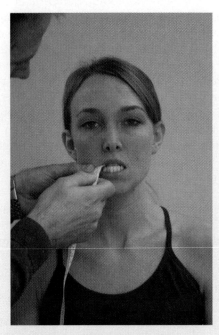

■ **Figure 6.3** TMJ Protrusion: Measurement

Medial Translation and Lateral Translation

Medial and lateral translation involves the medial and lateral movement of the lower jaw with respect to the maxilla.

1. Resting symptoms are assessed.

2. The clinician instructs the patient to translate his or her jaw as far as he or she can to the left (Figure 6.4 ■).

3. The clinician views the bite formation for symmetry.

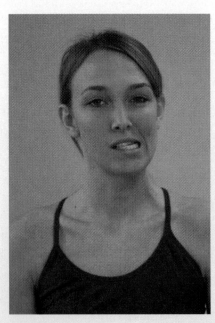

■ **Figure 6.4** TMJ Medial and Lateral Translation

④ The patient is queried regarding production of concordant symptoms.

⑤ Using a gloved hand and a tape measure, the clinician measures the translation using the landmarks of the front two bottom and top teeth.

⑥ The process is repeated in the opposite direction (Figure 6.5 ■).

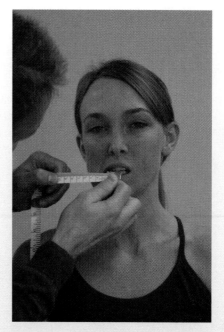

■ **Figure 6.5** TMJ Medial and Lateral Translation: Measurement

Mouth Opening (Measurement)

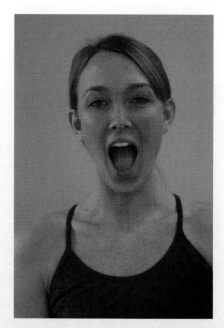

Masumi et al.[19] reported that differences in mouth opening were not discriminatory enough to identify a selected type of TMD, indicating that all forms of TMD demonstrate restrictions in maximal mouth opening. The sphenomandibular ligament provides the necessary mechanism for stability of the jaw and may be painful at end ranges of mouth opening (without disc involvement) or during forced retrusion.[20]

① Resting symptoms are assessed.

② The clinician instructs the patient to open his or her mouth as wide as possible.

③ With a gloved hand, the clinician may view the bite formation for symmetry by moving the lips away from the teeth (Figure 6.6 ■).

■ **Figure 6.6** TMJ Maximal Mouth Opening

④ The patient is queried regarding production of concordant symptoms.

(Continued)

⑤ The patient is evaluated for symmetry during opening.

⑥ Using a gloved hand and a tape measure, the clinician measures the distance of mouth opening by using the bottom of the top teeth and the top of the bottom teeth as the landmarks (Figure 6.7 ■).

⑦ If the movement reproduces the patient's symptoms, auscultation of the TMJ is beneficial to determine the presence of a click (Figure 6.8 ■).

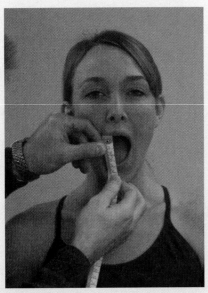

■ **Figure 6.7**   TMJ Maximal Mouth Opening: Measurement

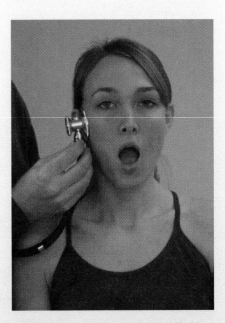

■ **Figure 6.8**   Auscultation of the TMJ

Lower Jaw Retrusion

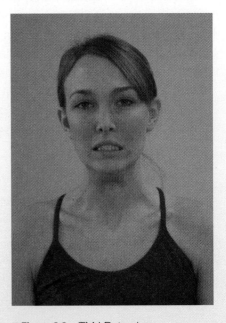

Retrusion involves an anterior to posterior movement of the lower jaw with respect to the stationary maxilla and can compress retrodiscal tissues.

① Resting symptoms are assessed.

② The clinician instructs the patient to retract his or her lower jaw as posteriorly as possible (Figure 6.9 ■).

③ The clinician views the bite formation for symmetry and queries the patient regarding production of concordant symptoms.

■ **Figure 6.9**   TMJ Retrusion

④ Using a gloved hand, the clinician measures the retrusion by using the bottom of the top teeth and the top of the bottom teeth as the landmarks (Figure 6.10 ■).

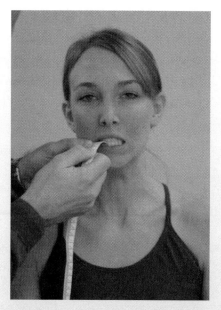

■ **Figure 6.10**   Measurement of Retrusion

Passive Movements

All four passive movements of depression, protrusion, and medial and lateral translation may stress the posterior–superior ligamentous structures. In most cases, the findings associated with passive range of movement will replicate the findings of the active examination.[21] Conditions associated with myofascial pain may be less painful and demonstrate less articular dysfunction during passive movement than active. Truelove et al.[22] suggest that differences of 5 millimeters between active and passive movements are indicative of muscular dysfunction and may represent a myofascial disorder.

Passive Accessory Tests   Although the movement of the TMJ is not purely linear, passive accessory movements may be helpful in identifying that the TMJ is the origin of the pain.[23]

Caudal Glide

A caudal glide may place tension on contractile and noncontractile tissues and is a purported treatment method for contractile relaxation and pain control.

① With the use of a gloved hand (after symptoms are assessed), the clinician places his or her thumb inside the mouth of the patient. The thumb lies parallel on the top of the teeth and flush to the posterior–inferior molars of the patient (Figure 6.11 ■). This technique should not be performed if the patient has false teeth or no molars.

② The clinician applies a caudal distraction and repeats the movement several times to examine whether the movement is concordant.

③ The patient is queried for reproduction of the concordant sign and the behavior of the reproduction.

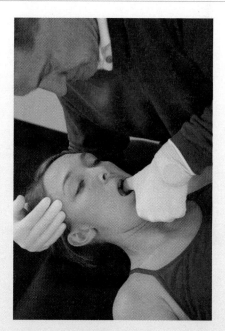

■ **Figure 6.11**   Caudal Glide

Anterior Glide

As with a caudal glide, an anterior glide may be useful to determine if a treatment consisting of repeated anterior movements is useful in reducing contractile tension and myofascial pain.

1. Using a gloved hand, the clinician places his or her thumb inside the mouth of the patient, hooking the bottom teeth at the incisor and four front teeth and the jaw caudally with the lateral border of the index finger (Figure 6.12 ■).

2. The clinician applies an anterior distraction and repeats the movement several times to examine if the movements are concordant.

3. The patient is queried for reproduction of the concordant sign and the behavior of the reproduction.

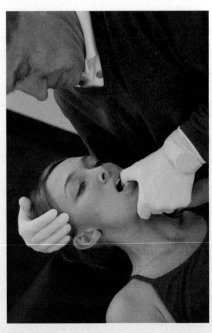

■ **Figure 6.12**   Anterior Glide

Combined Movements Hesse and Naeije[24] reported that joint play movements are beneficial in identifying the presence of a TMJ dysfunction. The following techniques allow joint play assessment and concurrent palpation near the auricular canal, outside the mouth. The examination is required bilaterally for comparison of mobility.

Posterior–Anterior Mobilization

1. The patient assumes a sidelying position.

2. With a tip-to-tip thumb contact, the clinician palpates the posterior aspect of the condyle of the mandible (Figure 6.13 ■).

3. Using a light to progressively more heavy force the clinician applies a posterior to anterior movement to the condyle. The patient may actively open his or her jaw during the movement to enhance the assessment.

4. The patient is queried for reproduction of the concordant sign and the behavior of the reproduction.

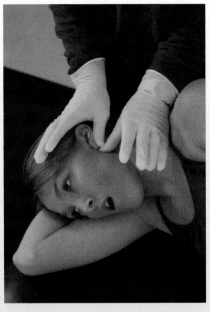

■ **Figure 6.13**   PA of Condyle on Temporal Bone–Sidelying

Anterior–Posterior Mobilization

1. The patient assumes a sidelying position.

2. With a tip-to-tip thumb contact, the clinician palpates the anterior aspect of the condyle of the mandible (Figure 6.14 ■).

3. Using a light to progressively more heavy force the clinician applies an anterior to posterior movement to the condyle. The patient may open or close his or her jaw to enhance the assessment of this technique.

4. The patient is queried for reproduction of the concordant sign and the behavior of the reproduction.

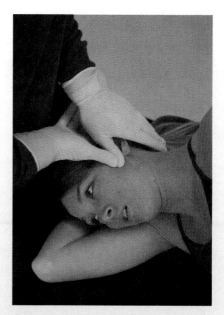

■ **Figure 6.14** AP of Condyle on Temporal Bone–Sidelying

During passive opening of the dysfunctional jaw, the condyles are often displaced superiorly, placing both tension and compression forces on the ligamentous structures and retrodiscal region. Combining a caudal displacement by placing an inferior force as closely to the TMJ as possible reduces the risk of compressing and abnormally tensioning these structures. This requires a combined passive movement in order to adequately examine the passive physiological and accessory movements of the jaw.

Ventrocaudal Translation

A ventrocaudal translation more accurately mimics the actual movement of the TMJ and may reduce the compression of selected tissues that was present during a passive accessory and was not relieved during repeated movements. The posterior–superior structures are stressed during ventrocaudal translation.

1. The patient is placed in a supine position.

2. Using a gloved hand the clinician places his or her thumb inside the mouth of the patient. The thumb lies parallel and on top of the teeth and flush to the posterior–inferior molars of the patient. In Figure 6.15 ■, the clinician is assessing the left TMJ. This technique should not be performed if the patient has false teeth or no molars.

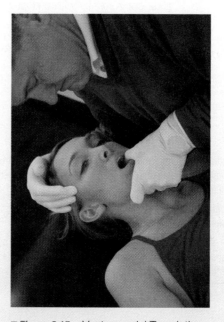

■ **Figure 6.15** Ventrocaudal Translation

(Continued)

③ The ventrocaudal translation requires a combined caudal glide concurrently with a ventral or anterior glide. The movement creates a decompressive force of the condyle to the temporal bone.

④ The patient is queried for reproduction of the concordant sign and the behavior of the reproduction.

Caudal–Retrusive Glide

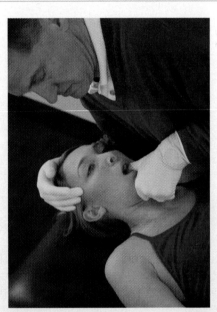

Performing a concurrent caudal and retrusion glide (AP) is warranted if symptoms were reproduced slightly during active retrusion. If caudal glide and retrusion are painful, both the superior–posterior structures and the sphenomandibular ligament are compressed.[21]

① The patient assumes a supine position.

② Using a gloved hand the clinician places his or her thumb inside the mouth of the patient. The thumb lies parallel and on top of the teeth and flush to the posterior–inferior molars of the patient. In Figure 6.16 ■, the left TMJ is the treated side. This technique should not be performed if the patient has false teeth or no molars.

■ **Figure 6.16** Caudal Glide and Retrusion

③ The caudal–retrusive glide requires a combined caudal glide concurrently with a posterior glide or retrusion movement. The movement provides a decompressive force of the superior–anterior structures in the retrodiscal region.

④ The patient is queried for reproduction of the concordant sign and the behavior of the reproduction.

Summary

- Selected passive movements place tension on targeted structures and may be useful in identifying the origin of the movement dysfunction.
- Combined passive movements are effective in provoking tissues in a biomechanically normal position.
- Some of the other passive movements may cause pain by placing tension or compression on tissues by moving into a plane that doesn't normally occur during jaw excursion.

Special Clinical Tests

Palpation   Palpation of the TMD muscles should involve assessment of the temporalis, masseter, lateral and medial pteryoideus, and platysma, digastricus, mylohyoideus, and geniohyoideus. (See Figures 6.17 ■–6.20 ■.)

Palpation has been advocated as a useful diagnostic tool for the presence of myofascial, internal derangement, and/or osteoarthritis[23,25] (Table 6.1 ■). However, palpation does not have the capacity to differentially identify disparate conditions.[26]

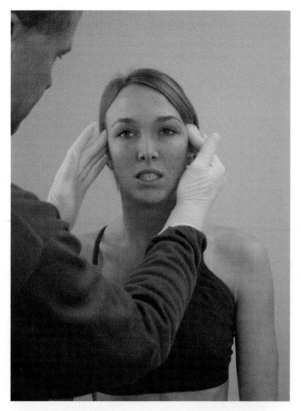

■ **Figure 6.17**   Palpation of the Temporalis Muscles

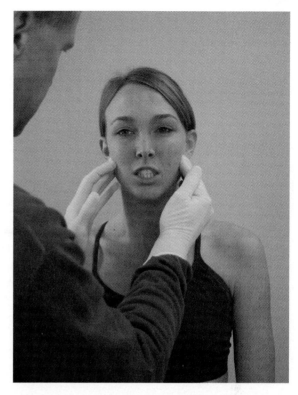

■ **Figure 6.18**   Palpation of the Masseter Muscles

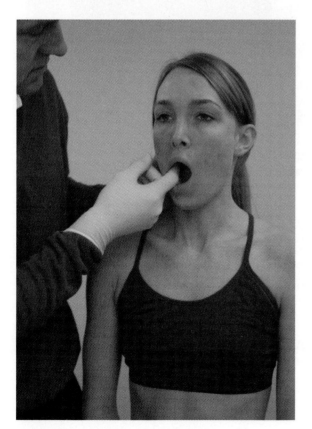

■ **Figure 6.19**   Palpation of the Lateral Pteryoideus Muscles

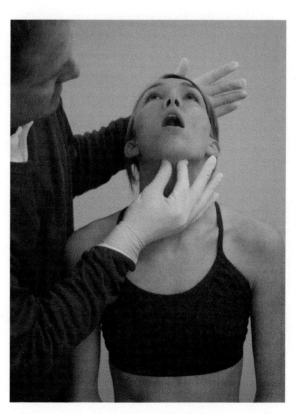

■ **Figure 6.20**   Palpation of the Submandibular Muscles

■ TABLE 6.1 Diagnostic Accuracy Values of Palpatory Testing of the TMD

Author	Reliability	Sensitivity	Specificity	LR+	LR−
de Wijer et al.[27] (muscle)	0.51 (kappa)	NT	NT	NT	NT
de Wijer et al.[27] (joint)	0.33 (kappa)	NT	NT	NT	NT
Manfredini et al.[28] (lateral joint)	NT	83	69	2.7	0.2
Manfredini et al.[28] (posterior joint)	NT	85	62	2.2	0.2
Visscher et al.[29] (full region)	NT	75	67	2.3	0.4
Lobbezoo-Scholte et al.[30] (full region)	NT	86	64	2.4	0.2

Manual Muscle Testing Contractile structures are often painful during conditions associated with myofascial pain.[22] By testing the selected muscular actions, the examiner may be able to identify painful movements or coordination problems during activation.

Resisted Opening

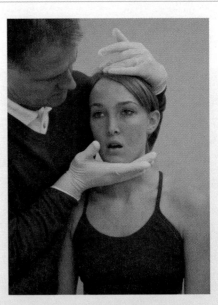

1. The patient is placed in a sitting position.

2. The head is carefully positioned in proper alignment. The mouth is prepositioned in a closed or mostly closed position, with neutral protrusion or retrusion.

3. The clinician places a comfortable but firm grip in the mandible of the patient.

4. The patient is instructed to open his or her mouth against the resistance of the clinician (Figure 6.21 ■).

5. Symptoms are reassessed.

■ Figure 6.21 Resisted Opening

Resisted Closing

1. The patient is placed in a sitting position.

2. The head is carefully positioned in proper alignment and the mouth is prepositioned in opening.

3. The clinician places a comfortable but firm grip in the mandible of the patient.

4. The patient is instructed to bite downward against the resistance of the clinician (Figure 6.22 ■).

5. Symptoms are reassessed.

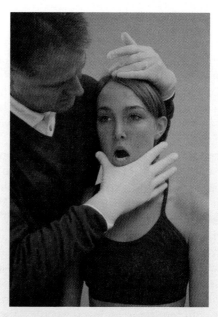

■ **Figure 6.22**   Resisted Closing

Resisted Medial and Lateral Excursion

1. The patient is placed in a sitting position.

2. The head is carefully positioned in proper alignment and resting symptoms are assessed.

3. The clinician places a comfortable but firm grip in the mandible of the patient.

4. The patient is instructed to perform a lateral excursion (Figure 6.23 ■) to a directed side (the left side in Figure 6.23).

5. To test medial excursion, resistance would be placed on the opposite side of the targeted side.

6. The process is repeated for the opposite side.

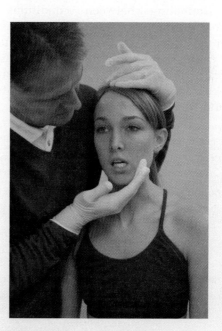

■ **Figure 6.23**   Resisted Medial and Lateral Excursion

Treatment Techniques

Treatment Philosophy

At present there is no true undeniable "criterion standard" for detection of TMD.[31] Comparison with magnetic resonance imaging (MRI) is purportedly the most accurate method for identification of disc impairments[32] and osteoarthritis, but yields little value in detecting pain of myofascial origin.

Selected clinical tests have shown merit in identifying patients with significant symptoms associated with TMD. Four tests—passive maximal mouth opening, palpation of the TMJ and masticatory muscles, TMJ joint play, and TMJ compression—were significantly associated with patient report of pain in the TMD.[21] Others have advocated the use of palpation but suggest that active maximal mouth opening yields comparable value with passive movements.[31] Including joint noises with the previously suggested categories may improve the capability of identifying an intra-articular disorder.[33] All the clinical criteria exhibit similar "fair to moderate" reliability whether performed by a physical therapist, dentist, or surgeon.[34] TMD can be both extra-articular and intra-articular and no one test stands out as a significantly strong predictor for TMD.

Roberts et al.[35] suggests that clinical findings are not discriminatory enough to identify patients with a variety of dysfunctions associated with TMD. Others agree, indicating that clinicians are poor at discriminating between conditions such as osteoarthritis and internal derangement and whether the presence of an anteriorly translated disc exists.[36,37] The trend within the literature suggests that clinicians are effective in identifying the presence of TMD but lack the discrimination to identify the origin and type of dysfunction.

The treatment philosophy for TMD is no different from that advocated within this book. The patient response-based model requires a careful evaluation of pain-provoking movements and a diligent understanding of the cause and effect of repeated movements, positions, or stability exercises. As with shoulder pathology, TMD may exhibit unidirectional hypermobility. Mobilizing in the appropriate direction may reduce the tendency of the jaw to displace during mouth opening and may further promote normalized movement. When assessing TMD it is imperative that the clinician distill what "form" of dysfunction he or she is treating in order to more effectively target the concordant sign. Careful examination is necessary because it is apparent that patients with TMD do not spontaneously recover over time and multiple forms of treatments have demonstrated improvement over no intervention.[38]

As discussed with cervical disorders, TMD may best be categorized into classification groups. Truelove et al.[22] offer a classification system consisting of three major categories: (1) internal derangement, (2) degenerative and or inflammatory conditions, and (3) myofascial conditions. (See Table 6.2 ■.)

Internal Derangement The term internal disc derangement is often used to describe the altered biomechanics of the TMJ. Traditionally, internal disc derangement is diagnosed when clicking is prevalent, intermittent bouts of locking occur, and a reduction in mouth opening is prominent during passive and active assessment.[22] Early conditions of internal disc derangement involve disc displacement with reduction. A disc displacement occurs when the normally superior disc displaces, typically anterior, so that the concave aspect of the disc is anterior and no longer congruent with the convex aspect of the condyle.

■ TABLE 6.2 Characteristics of TMD Classifications

Classification	Included Diagnoses	Clinical Symptoms
Myofascial pain	1. Myalgia type I 2. Myalgia type II 3. Myofascial pain dysfunction	• Orofacial pain • Muscle pain with palpation • Greater pain with active opening and closing than with passive opening and closing
Internal derangement	1. Disc displacement with reduction 2. Disc displacement without reduction 3. Perforation of the posterior ligament or disc	• Click in the TMJ during range of motion • Click in the TMJ during lateral excursion • <35 mm of mouth opening • No significant difference between active and passive opening
Degenerative and/or inflammatory conditions	1. Capsulitis 2. Synovitis 3. Sprain/strain 4. Arthritis 5. Arthralgia	• Pain in the joint during palpation • Pain in the joint during function • Pain in the joint during assisted opening • Possible history of trauma (sprain/strain) • Pain on right and left excursions

Adapted from Truelove et al.[22].

A disc displacement with reduction refers to a disc that is displaced in the closed mouth position but assumes a normal position relative to the condyle with jaw opening. A disc displacement without reduction refers to a disc that is displaced at all mandibular positions and does not reduce during opening or closing of the jaw. It has been suggested that a disc displacement without reduction is a consequential condition associated with long-term disc displacement with reduction.[39] Contradictory evidence is provided by Sener and Akganlu,[40] who found that there were no differences in MRI characteristics between an anterior disc displacement with and without reduction or the degenerative tendencies between the two disorders.

A disc displacement with perforation refers to a disc that is displaced and damaged. Disc perforation may occur from abnormal stress and poor articulation during movement that can lead to degeneration and break down over time. There are no distinctive criteria associated with disc perforation.[22]

Degenerative and/or Inflammatory Conditions

Degenerative conditions include symptoms such as pain in the joint during palpation, function, and passive opening.[22] Several different categories may fall within the realm of degeneration including capsulitis/synovitis, sprain/strain, degenerative joint disease, and arthritis.[22]

Myofascial Conditions

Myofascial conditions are associated with orofacial pain and are typically quantified during palpation of the muscle sites (two or more sites) and greater movement during passive movement than active movement.

Differentiation of Pain from Cervical Contribution

In normal conditions, the resting position of the jaw requires minimal muscular contraction and places little stress in intra-articular structures.[19] This relaxed position is associated with normal postural positioning of the head, neck, and jaw. Krause[19] suggests that the

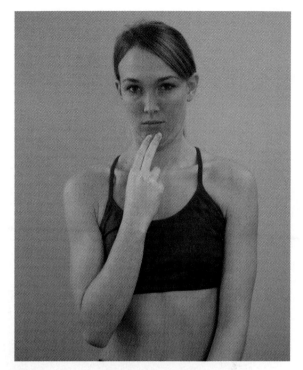

■ **Figure 6.24**   Sitting Chin Retractions

amount of time spent in this position is therapeutic to the patient and should be sought as an intervention. Since forward head and abnormal cervical position can affect the resting activity of the TMJ, postural training has merit during treatment of TMD, specifically when reduction of mouth opening is an issue.[41]

In the cervical chapter, several postural exercises were presented. These exercises were both actively and passively oriented and involved techniques to enhance normal posture. Studies have shown some degree of successful outcome with implementation of an active exercise program,[42] specifically those that focus on postural exercises[43,44] or strengthening.[42] One common postural exercise is the prone cervical retraction technique (Figure 6.25 ■), which is designed to incorporate a passive stretch during an active strengthening movement.

Repeated sitting chin retractions (Figure 6.24 ■) have demonstrated improvement in resting posture

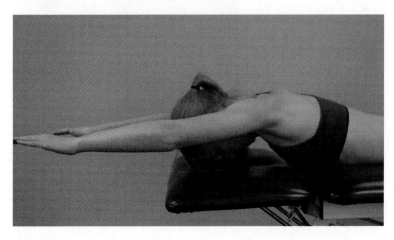

■ **Figure 6.25**   Prone Chin Retractions with Arm Lifts

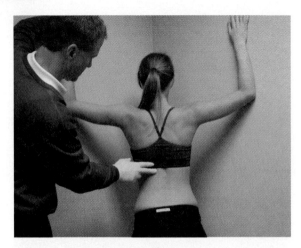

■ **Figure 6.26**   Thoracic Corner Stretch

in asymptomatic subjects.[44] Additionally, postural exercises such as those discussed in Chapter 7 may be useful for postural improvement. The following exercises (Figures 6.25–6.27 ■) are analogous to those presented by Wright et al.[1] in their successful active intervention program for TMD.

Treating Internal Derangement   Internal derangement often refers to a nonhomogenous set of symptoms that are associated with improper TMJ movement. Treatment of internal derangement, specifically with the use of mobilization, has been successful in reducing the anterior displacement of a disc[43,44] and yields higher outcomes than no intervention.[45]

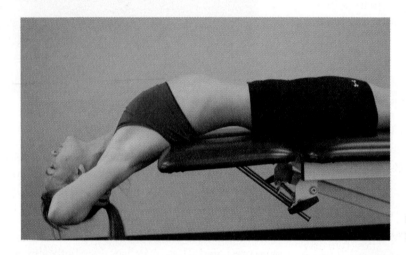

■ **Figure 6.27**   Supine Upper Back Stretches

Caudal Glide

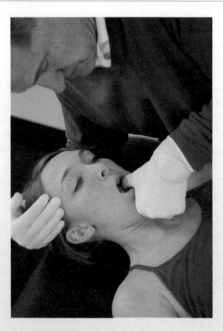

① The clinician places his or her thumb (of a gloved hand) inside the mouth of the patient. The thumb lies parallel to the top of the teeth and flush to the posterior–inferior molars of the patient. This technique should not be performed if the patient has false teeth or no molars. In Figure 6.28 ■, the left TMJ is the treated side.

② The clinician applies a caudal distraction and repeats the movement several times to examine a trend if concordant.

③ The patient is queried for reproduction of the concordant sign and the behavior of the reproduction.

■ **Figure 6.28**   Caudal Glide

Anterior Glide

1. The patient assumes the supine position.

2. Using a gloved hand the clinician places his or her thumb inside the mouth of the patient. The thumb hooks the bottom teeth at the incisor and four front teeth. In Figure 6.29 ■, the left TMJ is the treated side.

3. The clinician applies an anterior distraction and repeats the movement several times to examine a trend if concordant.

4. The patient is queried for reproduction of the concordant sign and the behavior of the reproduction.

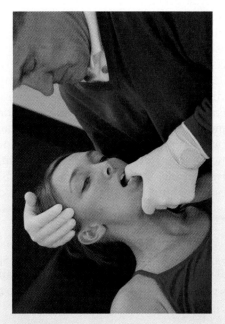

■ **Figure 6.29**   Anterior Glide

Ventrocaudal Translation

1. The patient assumes the supine position.

2. Using a gloved hand the clinician places his or her thumb inside the mouth of the patient. The thumb lies parallel to the top of the teeth and flush to the posterior–inferior molars of the patient (Figure 6.30 ■). This technique should not be performed if the patient has false teeth or no molars.

3. The ventrocaudal translation requires a combined caudal glide concurrently with a ventral or anterior glide. The movement promotes a decompressive force of the condyle to the temporal bone.

4. The patient is queried for reproduction of the concordant sign and the behavior of the reproduction.

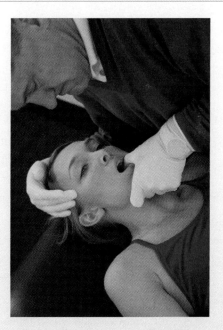

■ **Figure 6.30**   Ventrocaudal Translation

Therapeutic exercise has shown benefit on a patient population of anterior disc displacement with reduction. Yoda et al.[46] demonstrated that exercise, which also consisted of selected mobilization and stretching, was successful enough to reduce the risk of surgery and lowered the requirement for splint therapy. Similar findings have also been recorded for internal derangement conditions treated by mobilization, posture, and exercises post-operatively.[47] Pain-free strengthening and coordination exercises should be performed with careful attention for prevention of clicking and displacement. Both isometric and isotonic exercises are helpful in building coordination during movement.

Treating Myofascial Pain Treating myofascial pain is generally performed with night splints, postural improvements, rest, and modalities.[48] However, mobilization techniques designed to reduce

pain may be appropriate[49] when this dysfunction is encountered, specifically those designed to assist in allowing a nonpainful resting position.[50] Physical therapy treatment of myofascial conditions, which consisted of massage, ultrasound, and muscle stretching, was as effective as counseling.[51] In another study, some patients reported complete abolishment of pain with improvement levels higher than those reported in the no-treatment control group.[52]

Treating Inflammation Inflammation may be present specifically if movements such as passive and active opening at full range or retrusion reproduce symptoms. Passive movements during mobilization and repetitive stretching have been associated with chemical changes that reduce pain and improve appropriate collagen remodeling.[53] Long-term results demonstrated the positive outcomes continued comparatively even after 3 years removed from care.[54]

Lateral Glide with Mobilization: Mobilization with Movement

Mobilization with movement may also be useful in treating this population. Mobilization with movement involves active movement of the jaw by the patient during passive mobilization by the clinician.

1. The patient assumes a sitting position.

2. The patient is instructed to actively glide the jaw toward the restricted direction (to the left in Figure 6.31 ▪) while the clinician applies an anterior glide of the condyle using a light to progressively more heavy force.

3. To enhance left excursion, the clinician should apply an anterior force on the right condyle. The contact force is externally at the posterior aspect of the condyle.

4. The patient is queried for reproduction of the concordant sign and the behavior of the reproduction.

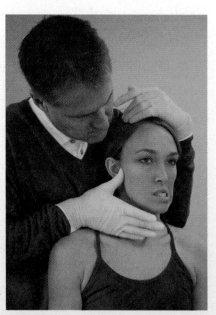

▪ **Figure 6.31** Active Lateral Glide with Mobilization: Mobilization with Movement

Protrusion with Mobilization: Mobilization with Movement

1. The patient assumes a sitting position.

2. The patient is instructed to actively protrude the jaw while the clinician applies an anterior glide of the condyle using a light to progressively more heavy force. The set-up for this procedure is similar to that in Figure 6.31 with the exception of the active movement of the patient.

3. The contact force is externally at the posterior aspect of the condyle.

4. The patient is queried for reproduction of the concordant sign and the behavior of the reproduction.

Summary

- Treatment of TMD follows the patient response-based method format but may benefit from further subcategorization into classification models.

- Manual therapy methods may be helpful when performed in conjunction with other rehabilitative methods.

- Mobilization with movement can involve active movement of the patient and passive movement by the clinician.

Treatment Outcomes

The Evidence

There is a paucity of well-designed clinical trials that report the benefit of a manual therapy rehabilitative intervention for TMD. The majority of trials have reported the outcomes of pharmacological or splint-related interventions. Although physical therapy has been commonly associated with significantly better outcomes than a pragmatic intervention, the physical therapy intervention has varied widely among studies.

Frequently, interventions have included the use of ultrasound, exercise, diathermy, home education, and stretching.[55] Of these interventions, exercise with the addition of selected mobilization and stretching methods has the most documented merit, having demonstrated the ability to reduce the risk of surgery and intensity of need for splint therapy.[46,47] In most cases, manual therapy was combined with other interventions such as exercise. In all cases, the outcomes were only short term.[56]

Of the manual therapy–oriented studies, there are a number of weak randomized controlled trials in which manual therapy was an embedded intervention. There are also case-series designs and several pre- and post-test designs. Findings suggest that the use of manual therapy in combination with active exercise or manual therapy alone as an intervention is beneficial in improving maximal mouth opening.[57–64] There is less evidence to support the reduction of pain with manual therapy. Because of the limited quality of the studies, the findings are at best Level B.

Level B evidence for the benefit of an upper quarter postural treatment is present as well. Wright et al.[7] performed general posture stretching exercises that targeted the thoracic and cervical spine on a group of 60 patients with TMD. After 4 weeks, the patients were re-examined for changes in symptoms and found statistically significant improvements when compared to the normal intervention control group.

Summary

- Numerous studies advocate the use of manual therapy, postural exercises, stretching, and modalities in the treatment of various forms of TMD. The majority of these studies are case reports.

- Exercise combined with mobilization and stretching yields positive outcomes for TMD. Postural exercise targeted to the upper quarter has demonstrated clinical utility as well.

Chapter Questions

1. Describe the role of the retrodiscal tissue toward the pathology of the temporomandibular joint.

2. Describe the documented relationship between cervical posture, cervical impairment, and the presence of TMD.

3. Describe the three primary classifications of TMD and outline how treatment varies between each classification.

4. Outline the mechanism of which the patient response-based method is applied for assessment and treatment of patients with applicable TMD.

Patient Cases

Case 6.1: Gretchan Leon (19-year-old female)

Diagnosis: TMD
Observation: She exhibits forward head posture, noticeable hypertrophy of the muscle of mastication, and appears anxious during the evaluation.
Mechanism: Insidious onset of jaw pain that initiated over 7 years ago.

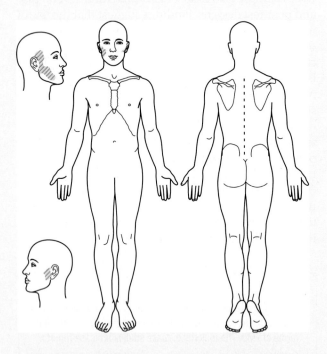

Concordant Sign: Her most painful movement involves wide opening of her mouth.
Nature of the Condition: She indicates that she has recently dropped out of college because the pain was so debilitating. Her anxiety and stress levels were worse during school and she found herself grinding her teeth as a stress-relieving mechanism. She indicates that once her pain flares up it takes several hours for the symptoms to subside.
Behavior of the Symptoms: The pain is isolated to the anterior aspect of the jaw.
Pertinent Patient History: Was diagnosed with social anxiety disorder approximately 4 years ago. She currently takes medication for this condition.
Patient Goals: She is concerned that her jaw pain will lead to surgical intervention.
Baseline: At rest, 4/10 NAS for pain; when worst, 6/10 pain.
Examination Findings: All active movements are limited. Maximal mouth opening is 32 millimeters and lateral excursion to the left is painful on the right. Palpation of the temporalis muscle is painful and there is a click during opening and subsequent closing of the jaw.

1. Based on these findings, what else would you like to examine?
2. Is this patient a good candidate for manual therapy?
3. What is the expected prognosis of this patient?
4. What treatments presented in this book may be beneficial for this patient?

Case 6.2: Chris Halliwell (25-year-old male)

Diagnosis: TMD
Observation: He exhibits forward head posture with a posterior neck posture that is flattened. There is a visible Dowager's hump in upper thoracic spine.
Mechanism: He reports symptoms that initiated 6 months ago after putting in a new faucet under a sink within a very crowded space.

Concordant Sign: He claims his concordant pain occurs during cervical extension.
Nature of the Condition: He considers the symptoms a nuisance. He is a plumber and is able to work through the pain but feels it does affect his productivity at work.
Behavior of the Symptoms: The symptoms are localized at the side of his neck and bilaterally on his face/jaw.

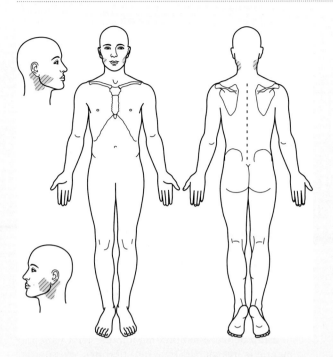

Pertinent Patient History: Nothing that is of concern.

Patient Goals: He is concerned the symptoms will worsen. He had never heard of TMD prior to his diagnosis and is concerned about what he has read on the Internet.

Baseline: His current symptoms are at 3/10; when worse, 5/10.

Examination Findings: He has no pain during jaw movements with the exception of resisted testing of the jaw. Maximal mouth opening is 46 millimeters. He has no clicking or grinding with any movements.

1. Based on these findings, what else would you like to examine?
2. Is this patient a good candidate for manual therapy?
3. What is the expected prognosis of this patient?
4. What treatments do you feel presented in this book may be beneficial for this patient?

PEARSON
myhealthprofessionskit™

Use this address to access the Companion Website created for this textbook. Simply select "Physical Therapy" from the choice of disciplines. Find this book and log in using your username and password to access video clips and the anatomy and arthrological information.

References

1. Wright E, Domenech M, Fischer J. Usefulness of posture training for patients with temporomandibular disorders. *JADA.* 2000;131:202–210.
2. Gonzalez H, Manns A. Forward head posture: Its structural and functional influence on the stomatognathic system, a conceptual study. *Cranio.* 1996;14:71–80.
3. Austin D. Special considerations in orofacial pain and headache. *Dent Clin North Am.* 1997;41:325–339.
4. Braun B. Postural differences between asymptomatic men and women and craniofacial pain patients. *Arch Phys Med Rehabil.* 1991;72:653–656.
5. Hackney J, Bade D, Clawson A. Relationship between forward head posture and diagnosed internal derangement of the temporomandibular joint. *J Orofac Pain.* 1993;7:386–390.
6. Darlow L, Pesco J, Greenberg M. The relationship of posture to myofascial pain dysfunction syndrome. *J Am Dent Assoc.* 1987;114:73–75.
7. Enwemeka C, Bonet I, Ingle J, Prudhithumrong S, Ogbahon F, Gbenedio N. Postural correction in persons with neck pain. Part II. Integrated electromyography of the upper trapezius in three simulated neck positions. *J Orthop Sports Phys Ther.* 1986;8:240–242.
8. Schuldt K, Ekholm J, Harms-Ringdahl K, Nemeth G, Arborelius U. Effects of changes in sitting work posture on static neck and shoulder muscle activity. *Ergonomics.* 1986;29:1525–1537.
9. Friction JR, Hathaway KM, Bromaghim C. Interdisciplinary management of patients with TMJ and craniofacial pain: Characteristics and outcome. *J Craniomandib Disord.* 1987;1(2):115–122.
10. Benoit P. History and physical examination for TMD. In: Krause S. (ed). *Clinics in physical therapy: Temporomandibular disorders.* New York; Churchill Livingstone: 1994.
11. Johansson A, Unell L, Carlsson GE, Söderfeldt B, Halling A. Differences in four reported symptoms related to temporomandibular disorders in a cohort of 50-year-old subjects followed up after 10 years. *Acta Odontol Scand.* 2008;66(1):50–57.
12. Visscher CM, Lobbezoo F, de Boer W, van der Zaag J, Naeije M. Prevalence of cervical spinal pain in craniomandibular pain patients. *Eur J Oral Sci.* 2001;109: 76–80.
13. Wright AR, Gatchel RJ, Wildenstein L, Riggs R, Buschang P, Ellis E III. Biopsychosocial differences between high-risk and low-risk patients with acute TMD-related pain. *J Am Dent Assoc.* 2004;135(4):474–483.

14. Rantala M, Ahlberg J, Suvinen T, Savolainen A, Kononen M. Chronic myofascial pain, disk displacement with reduction and psychosocial factors in Finnish non-patients. *Acta Odontol Scand.* 2004;62: 293–297.

15. Ahlberg J, Savolainen A, Rantala M, Lindholm H, Kononen M. Reported bruxism and biopsychosocial symptoms: A longitudinal study. *Community Dent Oral Epidemiol.* 2004;32:307–311.

16. Evcik D, Aksoy O. Correlation of temporomandibular joint pathologies, neck pain, and postural differences. *J Phys Ther Sci.* 2000;12:97–100.

17. Braun B, Schiffman E. The validity and predictive value of four assessment instruments for evaluation of the cervical and stomatognathic systems. *J Craniomandib Disord.* 1991;5:239–244.

18. Katzburg R, Westesson PL. *Diagnosis of the temporomandibular joint.* Philadelphia; WB Saunders: 1993.

19. Masumi S, Kim Y, Clark G. The value of maximum jaw motion measurements for distinguishing between common temporomandibular disorder subgroups. *Oral Surg Med Oral Pathol Oral Radiol Endod.* 2002;93:552–559.

20. Langendoen J, Muller J, Jull G. Retrodiscal tissue of the temporomandibular joint: clinical anatomy and its role in diagnosis and treatment of arthropathies. *Man Ther.* 1997;2:191–198.

21. Krause S. Physical therapy management of TMD. In: Krause S. (ed). *Clinics in physical therapy: Temporomandibular disorders.* New York; Churchill Livingstone: 1994.

22. Truelove E, Sommers E, LeReshce L, Dworkin S, von Korff M. Clinical diagnostic criteria for TMD. New classification permits multiple diagnoses. *J Am Dent Assoc.* 1992;123:47–54.

23. Hesse J, van Loon L, Maeije M. Subjective pain report and the outcome of several orthopaedic tests in craniomandibular disorder patients with recent pain complaints. *J Oral Rehabil.* 1997;24:483–489.

24. Hesse J, Naeije M. Biomechanics of the TMJ. In: Krause S. (ed). *Clinics in physical therapy: Temporomandibular disorders.* New York; Churchill Livingstone: 1994.

25. Kirveskari P. Prediction for demand for treatment of temporomandibular disorders. *J Oral Rehabil.* 2001;28: 572–575.

26. van der Weele L, Dibbets J. Helkimo's index: A scale or just a set of symptoms? *J Oral Rehabil.* 1987;14:229–237.

27. de Wijer A, Lobbezoo-Scholte AM, Steenks MH, Bosman F. Reliability of clinical findings in temporomandibular disorders. *J Orofac Pain.* 1995;9(2):181–191.

28. Manfredini D, Segù M, Bertacci A, Binotti G, Bosco M. Diagnosis of temporomandibular disorders according to RDC/TMD axis I findings: A multicenter Italian study. *Minerva Stomatol.* 2004;53(7–8):429–438.

29. Visscher CM, Naeije M, De Laat A, et al. Diagnostic accuracy of temporomandibular disorder pain tests: A multicenter study. *J Orofac Pain.* 2009;23(2):108–114.

30. Lobbezoo-Scholte AM, Steenks MH, Faber JA, Bosman F. Diagnostic value of orthopedic tests in patients with temporomandibular disorders. *J Dent Res.* 1993;72(10): 1443–1453.

31. Emshoff R, Brandlmaier I, Bosch R, Gerhard S, Rudisch A, Bertram S. Validation of the clinical diagnostic criteria for temporomandibular disorders for the diagnostic subgroup: Disc derangement with reduction. *J Oral Rehabil.* 2002;29(12):1139–1145.

32. Tasaki MM, Westesson PL. Temporomandibular joint: diagnostic accuracy with sagittal and coronal MR imaging. *Radiology.* 1993;186(3):723–729.

33. Lobbezoo-Scholte AM, de Wijer A, Steenks MH, Bosman F. Inter-examiner reliability of six orthopaedic tests in diagnostic subgroups of craniomandibular disorders. *J Oral Rehabil.* 1994;21(3):273–285.

34. de Wijer A, Lobbezoo-Scholte AM, Steenks MH, Bosman F. Reliability of clinical findings in temporomandibular disorders. *J Orofac Pain.* 1995;9(2): 181–191.

35. Roberts C, Katzberg RW, Tallents RH, Espeland MA, Handelman SL. The clinical predictability of internal derangements of the temporomandibular joint. *Oral Surg Oral Med Oral Pathol.* 1991;71(4):412–414.

36. Emshoff R, Innerhofer K, Rudisch A, Bertram S. Relationship between temporomandibular joint pain and magnetic resonance imaging findings of internal derangement. *Int J Oral Maxillofac Surg.* 2001;30(2): 118–122.

37. Yatani H, Minakuchi H, Matsuka Y, Fujisawa T, Yamashita A. The long-term effect of occlusal therapy on self-administered treatment outcomes of TMD. *J Orofac Pain.* 1998;12(1):75–88.

38. Brown D, Gaudet E. Temporomandibular disorder treatment outcomes: Second report of a large-scale prospective clinical study. *Cranio.* 2002;20:244–253.

39. Nitzan DW, Dolwick MF. An alternative explanation for the genesis of closed-lock symptoms in the internal derangement process. *J Oral Maxillofac Surg.* 1991;49(8): 810–815.

40. Sener S, Akganlu F. MRI characteristics of anterior disc displacement with and without reduction. *Dentomaxillofac Radiol.* 2004;33(4):245–252.

41. Komiyama O, Kawara M, Arai M, Asano T, Kobayashi K. Posture correction as part of behavioral therapy in treatment of myofascial pain with limited opening. *J Oral Rehabil.* 1999;26(5):428–435.

42. Shakoor M, Ahmed M, Kibria G, et al. (abstract). Effects of cervical traction and exercise therapy in cervical spondylosis. *Bangladesh Med Res Counc Bull.* 2002; 28:61–69.

43. Harrison D, Cailliet R, Betz J, et al. Conservative methods of reducing lateral translation postures of the head: A nonrandomized clinical control trial. *J Rehabil Res Dev.* 2004;41:631–639.

44. Grant R, Jull G, Spencer T. Active stabilizing training for screen based keyboard operators: A single case study. *Aust J Physiotherapy.* 1997;43:235–242.

45. Nicolakis P, Erdogmus B, Kopf A, et al. Effectiveness of exercise therapy in patients with internal derangement of the temporomandibular joint. *J Oral Rehabil.* 2001;28:1158–1164.

46. Yoda T, Sakamoto I, Imai H, et al. A randomized controlled trial of therapeutic exercise for clicking due

to disk anterior displacement with reduction in the temporomandibular joint. *Cranio.* 2003;21:10–16.

47. Oh D, Kim K, Lee G. The effect of physiotherapy on post-temporomandibular joint surgery patients. *J Oral Rehabil.* 2002;29:441–446.

48. Nicolakis P, Erdogmus B, Kropf A, Nicolakis M, Piehslinger E, Fialka-Moser V. Effectiveness of exercise therapy in patients with myofascial pain dysfunction syndrome. *J Oral Rehabil.* 2002;29:362–368.

49. Friedman MH. The hypomobile temporomandibular joint. *Gen Dent.* 1997;45(3):282–285.

50. Deodata F, Cristiano S, Trusendi R, Giorgetti R. A functional approach to the TMJ disorders. *Prog Orthod.* 2003;4:20–37.

51. De Laat A, Stappaerts K, Papy S. Counseling and physical therapy as treatment for myofascial pain of the masticatory system. *J Orofac Pain.* 2003;17:42–49.

52. Nicolakis P, Burak E, Kollmitzer J, et al. An investigation of the effectiveness of exercise and manual therapy in treating symptoms of TMJ osteoarthritis. *Cranio.* 2001;19:26–32.

53. Sambajon V, Cillo J, Gassner R, Buckley M. The effects of mechanical strain on synovial fibroblasts. *J Oral Maxillofac Surg.* 2003;61:707–712.

54. Nicolakis P, Erdogmus CB, Kollmitzer J, et al. Long-term outcome after treatment of temporomandibular joint osteoarthritis with exercise and manual therapy. *Cranio.* 2002;20(1):23–27.

55. Gray R, Quayle AA, Hall CA, Schofield MA. Physiotherapy in the treatment of temporomandibular joint disorders: A comparative study of four treatment methods. *Br Dent J.* 1994;176:257–261.

56. Medlicott M, Harris S. A systematic review of the effectiveness of exercise, manual therapy, electrotherapy, relaxation training, and biofeedback in the management of temporomandibular disorder. *Phys Ther.* 2006;86: 955–973.

57. De Laat A, Stappaerts K, Papy S. Counseling and physical therapy as treatment for myofascial pain of the masticatory system. *J Orofac Pain.*2003;17(1):42–49.

58. Jagger RG. Mandibular manipulation of anterior disc displacement without reduction. *J Oral Rehabil.* 1991; 18:497–500.

59. Magnusson T, Syren M. Therapeutic jaw exercises and interocclusal appliance therapy. *Swed Dent.* 1999;23: 27–37.

60. Michelotti A, Steenks MH, Farella M, et al. The additional value of a home physical therapy regimen versus patient education only for the short-term treatment of myofascial pain of the jaw muscles: Short-term results of a randomized clinical trial. *J Orofac Pain.* 2004;18(2):114–125.

61. Minagi S, Nozaki S, Sato T, Tsuru H. A manipulation technique for treatment of anterior disk displacement with reduction. *J Prosthet Dent.*1991;65:686–691.

62. Nicolakis P, Erdogmus CB, Koff A, et al. Effectiveness of exercise therapy in patients with myofascial pain dysfunction syndrome. *J Oral Rehabil.* 2002;29:362–368.

63. Monaco A, Cozzolino V, Cattaneo R, Cutilli T, Spadaro A. Osteopathic manipulative treatment (OMT) effects on mandibular kinestics: Kinesiographic studies. *Eur J Paediatr Dent.* 2008;9:37–42.

64. Ismail F, Demling A, Hessling K, Fink M, Stiesch-Scholz M. Short-term efficacy of physical therapy compared to splint therapy in treatment of arthrogenous TMD. *J Oral Rehabil.* 2007;34:807–813.

Manual Therapy of the Thoracic Spine

Chad E. Cook

Objectives

- Identify pertinent structure and biomechanics of the thoracic spine.
- Demonstrate the appropriate and valid thoracic spine examination sequence.
- Identify plausible mobilization and manual therapy treatment techniques for the thoracic spine and rib cage.
- Discuss the evidence of the effect of mobilization and manual therapy on recovery for patients with thoracic impairments in randomized trials.

Clinical Examination

Differential Diagnosis

Differentiation of musculoskeletal pain from that of visceral origin is necessary for proper treatment selection.[1] There are several potential pain generators within the thoracic spine, including the vertebral disc, the vertebrae, dura mater, longitudinal ligaments, the posterior thoracic muscles, the costotransverse joints, and the zygopophyseal joints.[2] Testicular pain has been linked to lower thoracic dysfunction,[3] headaches have been associated with a dysfunction to T4,[4] and **costochondral** deformities may mimic a submucosal gastric tumor.[5] Furthermore, the lower thoracic segments often refer pain that mimics symptoms associated with the lumbar spine.[6]

The thoracic region houses numerous visceral organs that can refer pain that mimics musculoskeletal origin.[1] Chest pain can be from the heart, abdominal organs, musculoskeletal tissue, psychogenic generators, or selected disease processes.[7-9] In addition, musculoskeletal structures can mimic pain of visceral origin as well. Hypertonic saline injections in normal volunteers into the thoracic interspinous muscles and ligaments can produce local or referred pain to the anterior aspect of the chest that mimics heart pain[2] (Table 7.1 ■).

Differentiation is necessary to avoid misdiagnosis of an individual during the initial screen. Many patients with noncardiac chest pain have anterior chest tenderness to palpation that is absent in control groups without chest pain; however, reproduction of the pain by palpation alone is only found in some of the patients.[10] The location of the complaint of pain cannot with certainty be used as a guide to determine the location of the source since the thoracic pain generators can refer pain to multiple areas of the body.[2] Adler[11] suggests the use of pain reproduction methods to differentiate musculoskeletal and psychogenic phenomena based on two principles: (1) the ability to reproduce or reduce the pain and (2) selective change in the motoric action of the subject.

Summary

- Pain generators of the thoracic spine include both musculoskeletal and visceral origins.
- Differentiation of pain is necessary. It is recommended that pain reproduction is mandatory prior to treatment secondary to the risks of underlying pain of visceral origin.

Observation

Posture In standing posture, the line of gravity passes anteriorly to the thoracic spine, creating a moment that increases thoracic kyphosis.[12] Both passive and active forces are necessary to prevent excessive kyphosis; the deep paraspinal musculature is constantly active, thus functioning to stabilize the posture.[13] Nonetheless, the morphology of the thoracic spine is highly related to the resting length of an individual's

■ **TABLE 7.1** Dermatomal Regions for Referred Visceral Pain

Affected Viscera	Painful Region
Heart	C8–T4 (T4–7 is a common source of pseudo-anginal pain)
Bronchioles, lungs	T2–4
Esophagus	T5–6
Stomach	T6–10
Liver, gallbladder	T7–9
Spleen	T6–10
Pancreas	T6–10
Kidney	T10–11
Ureter	T11–12
Appendix	T11–12

posture and most likely contributes more to postural parameters than any other component.[14]

Increased thoracic kyphosis is a common finding among the general population and is a finding that purportedly may lead to musculature weakness, arthrological pain, and stiffness, as well as alteration of mechanoreceptors.[14,15] Janda described a postural phenomenon called "upper crossed syndrome," which is a sequence of adaptive changes associated with forward head posture, thoracic kyphosis, shortened pectoralis major and minor muscles, upper trapezius muscles, levator scapula muscles, and sternocleidomastoid musculature in addition to lengthened middle and lower trapezius, serratus anterior, rhomboids, and deep neck musculature.[16] Forward head and thoracic kyphosis are directly related and may contribute to myofascial pain syndromes and decreased pain thresholds.[17] Ironically, although postural abnormalities are often treated as a cause of thoracic pain, little quantitative evidence exists to directly correlate pain and postural dysfunction.[12,18]

Postural changes are common in patients with osteoporosis, often contributing to vertebral compression fractures, which exhibit wedging upon compression of the vertebrae.[19] Compression fractures can lead to physiological changes in posture, most commonly kyphosis and potentially scoliosis.[19] Postural kyphosis alters the shape and function of the rib cage by increasing the anterior–posterior diameter, thus altering the respiratory capacity of the individual.[19] Two studies have suggested that thoracic kyphosis of 50 degrees or greater may be associated with balance disturbances.[20,21]

Scoliosis may be functional or structural and is common in younger individuals or individuals who have experienced a trauma.[22] Structural scoliosis is considered a loss of flexibility in the thoracic spine that does not resolve passively or actively.[23] Functional scoliosis retains a functionally normal range but exhibits lateral curvature that is adaptive or "functionally acquired" for external commands.[23] Younger individuals and older patients, specifically after degenerative changes, may exhibit structural scoliosis.[24] Shoulder dysfunction may be associated with posture or weak scapular muscles.[25]

Summary

- Postural problems, typically associated with kyphosis, are common dysfunctions within the postural spine.
- Poor posture is not directly correlated with thoracic spine pain.
- Scoliosis is typically associated with younger individuals but may be present in older patients.

Patient History

Psychosocial Factors   Similar to the psychosocial factors associated with lumbar spine pain, comparable factors may contribute to recovery for the thoracic spine. These psychosocial factors include abnormalities in pain perception, job-related intricacies, psychological dysfunction, social support challenges, and disability perceptions. It is imperative to note that factors that increase one's risk for injury may not increase one's risk for poor prognosis.[26] A challenge to the rehabilitation clinician is that many thoracolumbar injuries that are intrinsically similar pathologically involving similar treatment interventions often result in a wide range of outcomes.[26]

Report of pain location is also inconsistent in the thoracic spine because sympathetic responses may elicit visceral or musculoskeletal influences, yielding variability in pain location. Consequently, pain from the heart, gall bladder, kidneys, and other organs can refer as thoracic pain and should be ruled out for patients with suspicion of these findings.[27]

Summary

- Patients with pain from the thoracic spine are expected to be affected from similar psychosocial factors as patients with lumbar spine origin.
- Pain from the heart, gall bladder, kidneys, and other organs can refer as thoracic pain and should be ruled out for patients with suspicion of these findings.

Physical Examination

Active Physiological Movements

Isolating active physiological movement specifically to the thoracic spine is challenging. In all forms of movement, the cervical and lumbar spines will contribute to the motion and may require clearing. Within the following descriptions, subtle tips regarding positioning may best emphasize movements to improve the focus on the thoracic spine.

Active Flexion

Because many elderly patients assume a slightly flexed thoracic posture as a position of comfort, end-range active movements may be beneficial to assess. If a patient exhibits pertinent pretest signs of a potential compression fracture, the performance of active flexion and specifically flexion with overpressure are contraindicated. A careful history and assessment of risk factors may helpfully outline the risk of this procedure.

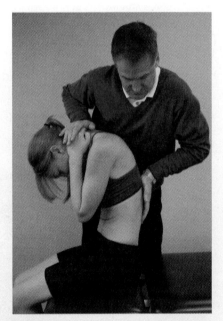

■ **Figure 7.1**   Overpressure of Flexion of the Thoracic Spine

1. The patient is seated in a straddled position to stabilize the pelvis.

2. The patient is instructed to move toward flexion by pulling his or her elbows toward the groin.

3. The patient is instructed to move only to the first point of pain. Pain is assessed to determine if concordant.

4. The patient is instructed to move beyond the first point of pain toward end range. After a sustained hold or repeated movements, the concordant movement is again reassessed.

5. If the patient demonstrates pain-free movement, an overpressure (Figure 7.1 ■) is applied by pulling the elbows into flexion and placing the lumbar region into flexion.

Active Extension

Individuals lose extension for a number of reasons, including associative degenerative changes. Subsequently, it is important to determine the outcome of repeated movements near end range of extension or a sustained hold prior to administering this approach as a home- or clinic-based program.

1. The patient is seated in a straddled position to stabilize the pelvis.

2. The hands of the patient are laced behind his or her head.

3. The patient is instructed to lift his or her elbows up toward the sky, promoting extension of the thoracic spine (Figure 7.2 ■) but only to the first point of pain. Pain is assessed to determine if concordant.

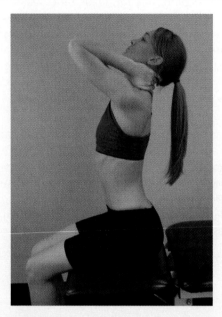

■ **Figure 7.2** Active Extension of the Thoracic Spine

4. The patient is instructed to move beyond the first point of pain toward end range.

5. After a sustained hold or repeated movements, the concordant movement is again reassessed.

6. If the patient demonstrates pain-free movement, an overpressure is applied by pulling up on the elbows toward the ceiling while stabilizing the thoracic spine into extension with the opposite hand (Figure 7.3 ■).

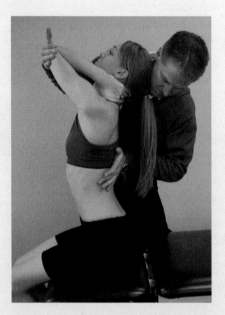

■ **Figure 7.3** Overpressure of Extension of the Thoracic Spine

Active Side Flexion

Active side flexion is generally coupled (which means it involves a number of different planes of movement) in the upper and lower thoracic regions but is often isolated in the mid-thoracic region. It is helpful to view the side flexion from the anterior and posterior of the patient to determine the curvature of side flexion, especially in the mid-thoracic region.

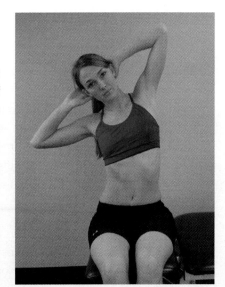

■ **Figure 7.4** Active Side Flexion of the Thoracic Spine

1. The patient is seated and the elbows of the patient are flexed to his or her side (the fingers are laced and placed behind the head).

2. The patient is instructed to move toward side flexion by moving one elbow toward his or her pelvis in a curvilinear movement (Figure 7.4 ■).

3. The patient is instructed to move only to the first point of pain and if pain is present it is assessed to determine if concordant.

4. The patient is then instructed to move beyond the first point of pain toward end range. After a sustained hold or repeated movements, the concordant movement is again reassessed.

5. If the patient demonstrates pain-free movement, an overpressure is applied by pulling the patient into further side flexion using a handgrip near the axilla or upper arm of the patient (Figure 7.5 ■).

6. The procedure is repeated on the opposite side.

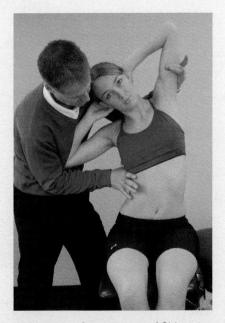

■ **Figure 7.5** Overpressure of Side Flexion of the Thoracic Spine

Active Rotation

Rotation in the upper and lower thoracic spine is also coupled but often is not in the mid-thoracic region. In order to promote full rotation of the upper thoracic spine, cervical rotation toward end range is sometimes necessary. If the movement demonstrates pain, it is important to differentiate the cervical and thoracic spine using isolated rotation tests for each segment.

1. The patient is seated and the arms are crossed over his or her chest. The thoracic spine should remain in slight flexion to lessen the contribution of the lumbar spine.

2. The patient is instructed to rotate in a horizontal plane, with or without cervical spine rotation, depending on the targeted region. In Figure 7.6 ■, the patient does not incorporate cervical rotation.

3. The patient is instructed to move only to the first point of pain. Pain is assessed to determine if concordant.

4. The patient is instructed to move beyond the first point of pain toward end range. After a sustained hold or repeated movements, the concordant movement is again reassessed.

5. If the patient demonstrates pain-free movement, an overpressure is applied by pulling the shoulders into further rotation and by blocking the knees of the patient to prevent compensation (Figure 7.7 ■).

6. The procedure is repeated on the opposite side.

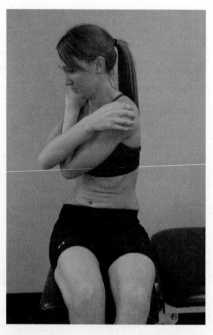

■ **Figure 7.6** Active Rotation of the Thoracic Spine

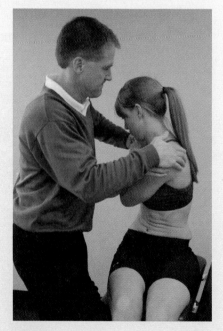

■ **Figure 7.7** Overpressure of Rotation of the Thoracic Spine

Central Posterior Anterior (CPA)

Assessment of a CPA is a common component of a thoracic examination[12] and is a provocation-based movement. Stiffness of a CPA is affected by many factors including the level of the assessed vertebra (cephalic segments have greater stiffness than caudal segments)[12] and the rigidity of the rib cage.[31] Because the spinous processes of the thoracic spine are angled inferiorly, a posterior to anterior motion to the thoracic spine may promote extension of the specific segments.

1. The patient assumes a prone lying position and resting symptoms are assessed.

2. The clinician palpates the targeted level feeling for the first thoracic spinous processes. This segment is localized first by finding C6 and working caudally. C6 disappears (moves posterior to anterior) during active extension while C7 stays pronounced.

3. The clinician applies a PA force using a pisiform contact to the first point of reported pain (Figure 7.15 ■). Pain is assessed to determine if concordant. This process is continued at all thoracic segments or is focused on those segments based on the detailed history. Movement and force is applied beyond the first point of pain toward end range.

4. Sustained holds or repeated movements that affect the concordant sign are utilized to determine potential treatment selection.

Changes of angle of pressure may alter the report of symptoms of the patient. By aiming the movements more caudally, cranially, medially, or laterally, the clinician may more effectively reproduce the symptoms of the patient.

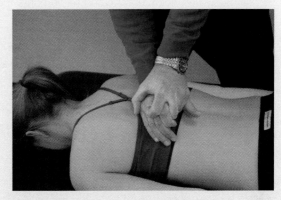

■ Figure 7.15   Central Posterior–Anterior to the Facet

Unilateral Posterior Anterior (UPA)   Assessment of a UPA is part of a normal thoracic examination.[12] A UPA is a provocation-based movement and is applied perpendicular to the facet planes. The facets lie just laterally to the spinous processes (albeit at different levels). The facets can be palpated in thin-framed individuals as a valley or deficit within the boney architecture.

Combined Passive Movements   The size of the thoracic spine and the complexity of movements of the region often require the use of combined passive movements to fully distinguish the actual concordant sign. Potentially combined movements may include a combination of the isolated movement of any of the active physiological motions and passive physiological movements concurrently during passive accessory, provocation, or plane-based glides.

Unilateral Posterior Anterior to the Facet

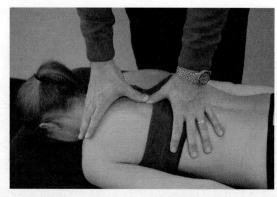

■ **Figure 7.16** Unilateral Posterior–Anterior to the Facet

1. The patient assumes a prone lying position.

2. The clinician palpates the targeted level feeling for the deficit just lateral to the spinous processes. The clinician may use a thumb to thumb contact point since the facets are not as pronounced as the spinous processes.

3. The clinician applies a PA force to the first point of reported pain and pain is assessed to determine if concordant (Figure 7.16 ■). This process is continued at all thoracic segments or is focused on those segments based on the detailed history. Movement and force is applied beyond the first point of pain toward end range.

4. Sustained holds or repeated movements that influence the concordant sign are utilized to determine potential treatment selection.

Changes of angle of pressure may alter the report of symptoms of the patient. By aiming movements more caudally, cranially, medially, or laterally, the clinician may more effectively reproduce the symptoms of the patient.

5. The process is generally repeated on the opposite side.

Unilateral Posterior Anterior (UPA) to the Costotransverse Joint

A unilateral PA of the costotransverse joint requires the identification of the joint articulation lateral to the midline of the thoracic spine. The articulation is both inferior and superior to the rib attachment. The elevated portion laterally is the distal end of the transverse process.

1. The patient assumes a prone lying position.

2. The clinician palpates the targeted level feeling for the raised region approximately two thumbs-width lateral to the spinous processes.

3. The clinician applies a PA force to the first point of reported pain and pain is assessed to determine if concordant (Figure 7.17 ■). This process is continued at all thoracic segments or is focused on those segments based on the detailed history. Movement and force is applied beyond the first point of pain toward end range.

4. Sustained holds or repeated movements that affect the concordant sign are utilized to determine potential treatment selection.

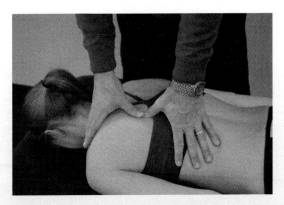

■ **Figure 7.17**   Unilateral Posterior–Anterior to the Costotransverse Joint

Changes of angle of pressure may alter the report of symptoms of the patient. By aiming movements more caudally, cranially, medially, or laterally, the clinician may more effectively reproduce the symptoms of the patient.

⑤ The process is repeated on the opposite side.

Transverse Glides

Transverse glides are a form of assessment technique that applies a lateral glide to the spinous processes of the spine. The technique is also a provocation-based procedure and has been well studied for its neurophysiological affects.[32,33]

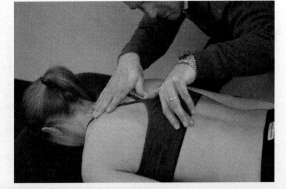

■ **Figure 7.18**   Transverse Glide of Thoracic Spinous Process

① The patient is positioned in prone or side-lying, and the neck is placed in neutral.

② The clinician palpates the targeted spinous process using the tips of the thumb.

③ Using one thumb pad, the clinician applies a very broad and deep contact to the side of the spinous process, applying more force on the base of the spinous process than the posterior tip (Figure 7.18 ■).

④ The clinician then aligns the forearm so that it is parallel to the force to the spinous process and pushes to the first point of reported pain.

⑤ The clinician then pushes beyond the first point of pain toward end range, reassesses pain and quality of movement, and checks for splinting or muscle spasm. Passive repeated movements are performed at end range and assessment of changes in pain level and determination if the pain is concordant are performed.

Anterior–Posterior (AP) Mobilizations

An AP mobilization is a provocation-based examination technique. The assessment of an anterior–posterior accessory motion at the sternum routinely demonstrates greater mobility than a similar PA assessment performed posteriorly to the facets or costovertebral joints.[12] Isolated rib movement is opposite of the movement posterior to the spine with extension producing cephalic rotation of the joint and flexion producing caudal rotation.[34]

A condition known as costochondritis may produce isolated pain directed at the two rib–sternal attachments. This is a common cause of chest-wall pain that mimics a cardiac response. This condition is also called Tietze's syndrome when the findings are present in the superior-most joints and occurs most frequently at the fourth to sixth ribs.[35]

1. The patient assumes a supine position.

2. The clinician palpates the targeted level and gathers a baseline of pain.

3. To assess the connection of the sternum to the cartilage the clinician should palpate joint line just lateral to the sternum on ribs 3 to 8 (Figure 7.19 ■).

4. To assess the ribs' connection to the cartilage the clinician may need to palpate lateral, approximately 2 inches from the sternum toward the angular connection of the rib (Figure 7.20 ■).

5. The clinician applies an AP force to the first point of reported pain, determining whether the pain is concordant. Movement and force is applied beyond the first point of pain toward end range. Sustained holds or repeated movements that affect the concordant sign are utilized to determine potential treatment selection. As with the posterior–anterior movements, changes of angle of pressure may alter the report of symptoms of the patient.

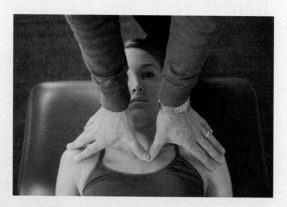

■ **Figure 7.19** UAP of the Sternum to Cartilage

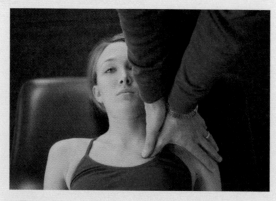

■ **Figure 7.20** UAP of the Ribs to Cartilage

Transverse Glide with Rotation

1. The patient sits at the edge of the plinth and resting symptoms are assessed.

2. The clinician rotates the patient into rotation while loading. Special effort should be made not to engage end-range rotation.

3. At the desired rotation (concordant position), the clinician applies a transverse glide into the rotation to the first point of reported pain (Figure 7.21 ■). Pain is assessed to determine if concordant. The clinician may also choose to apply a posterior–anterior force, central or unilateral (Figure 7.22 ■).

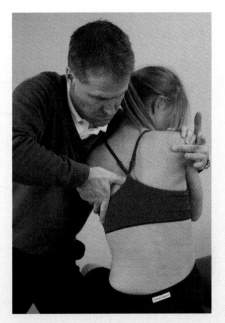

■ **Figure 7.21**   Transverse Glide with Rotation

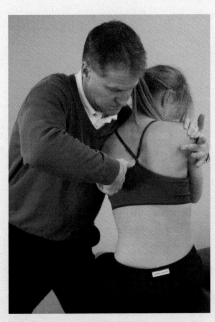

■ **Figure 7.22**   Physiological Rotation with PA Glide

Rotation and Side Flexion

Rotation and side flexion can be integrated for a combined procedural assessment.

1. The patient sits at the edge of the plinth and the clinician puts the patient into rotation. Special effort should be made not to engage end-range rotation.

2. At the desired rotation (concordant position), the clinician applies a passive physiological side flexion force in the opposite direction of the rotation to the first point of reported pain (Figure 7.23 ■).

3. Movement and force is applied beyond the first point of pain toward end range.

4. Sustained holds or repeated movements that influence the concordant sign are examined to determine potential treatment selection.

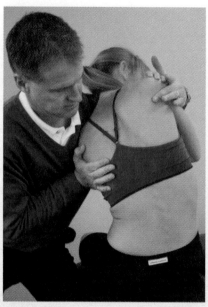

■ **Figure 7.23** Combined Physiological Rotation and Side Flexion

Extension with a Posterior–Anterior Mobilization

Extension and a posterior–anterior force may be useful in identifying patients who may benefit from postural treatment.

1. The patient sits at the edge of the plinth.

2. The clinician extends the patient into the desired pre-extension position.

3. At the desired preposition of extension (concordant position), the clinician can apply either a superiorly based (Figure 7.24 ■) or an inferiorly based force to the ribs and facets.

4. The clinician must modulate the force with the first point of reported pain. Movement and force is applied beyond the first point of pain toward end range.

5. Sustained holds or repeated movements that influence the concordant sign are utilized to determine potential treatment selection.

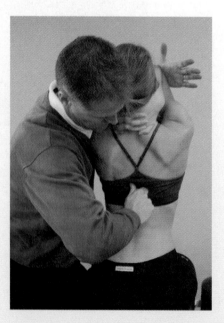

■ **Figure 7.24** Passive Physiological Extension with a PA Force

Summary

- Passive physiological movements are often integrated with active physiological movements of the thoracic spine.
- Passive accessory movements require the careful separate examination of the facet joints and the costotransverse joints, both of which may be the pain generator of the thoracic spine.
- Combined movements can be used to further isolate a movement dysfunction.

Special Clinical Tests

Palpation   Christensen et al.[36] reported the reliability of motion palpation in sitting and prone and paraspinal palpation for tenderness. Using an expanded and more liberal definition of agreement, the pooled kappa values were 0.59 to 0.77 overall, which is considered fair to good. Love and Brodeur[37] found poor interrater reliability but good intrarater reliability by chiropractic students in detecting hypomobility of the thoracic spine. Expanding a segment's range to include the segment above or below improved the reliability of thoracic palpation significantly, although caution must be taken in interpretation of these results as the study was performed on asymptomatic subjects.[38]

Haas et al.[39] advocated the use of end-range palpation for detection of rotation stiffness as a decision-making tool for a manipulative procedure. Their study outlined the clinical effectiveness after isolating the restricted movement during palpation and subsequent manipulation. Lewis et al.[40] reported the benefit of surface palpation for location of the scapula as well as the use of the position of the scapula to determine thoracic landmarks such as the lower border of the scapula (T12).

Manual Muscle Testing   Frese et al. reported low interrater reliability when testing middle and inferior trapezius strength.[41] Paraspinal strength testing is also poorly quantified and has been presented numerous ways within the literature. Empirically, strength assessment of the paraspinal muscles *should* yield useful information since passive and active stabilization forces are required to prevent excessive kyphosis. Within the thoracic spine, the deep paraspinal musculature function actively to stabilize the posture—a process that differs from the lumbar spine.[13]

Summary

- Palpation for stiffness, when an expanded definition is used, is more useful than isolation of a single segment.
- Although manual muscle testing provides poor interrater reliability, the procedure may be useful in assigning exercises for stabilization.

Treatment Techniques

Postural

Renno et al.[19] have demonstrated improvements in thoracic posture in a mixed treatment program that consisted of stretching, strengthening, and respiratory work. Mostly, however, conservative postural treatment consisting of similar treatments to the above-mentioned has included populations of patients with thoracic outlet syndrome or other characterized disorders. Although understudied, there does seem to be a consistency toward the benefit of stretching and strengthening exercises for the thoracic spine. These techniques may be passive or therapist facilitated.

Passive Stretches   The following passive approaches in Figures 7.25 ■–7.27 ■ adopt the same principle for pain reduction and postural improvement associated with stretching. Stretches should be limited to patient tolerance with hold times of 15–20 seconds.

Therapist Facilitated   Therapist-facilitated techniques (Figures 7.28 ■ and 7.29 ■) are useful if the patient does not tolerate mobilization or manipulation and serve as a strong adjunct to strengthening exercises.

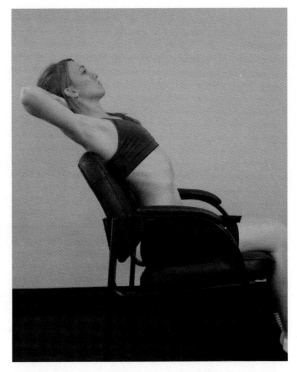

■ **Figure 7.25**   Thoracic Extension in Sitting

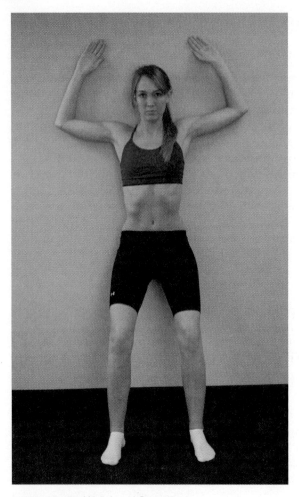

■ **Figure 7.26**   Wall Angel Stretches

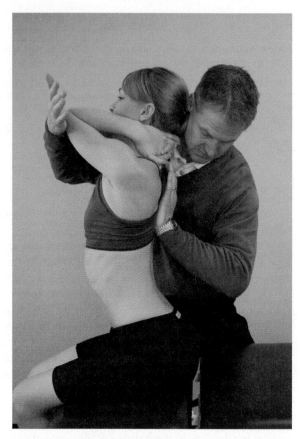

■ **Figure 7.28**   Seated Mid-Thoracic Stretch

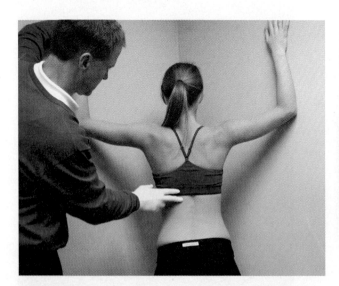

■ **Figure 7.27**   Corner Stretches for Upper Thoracic Mobility

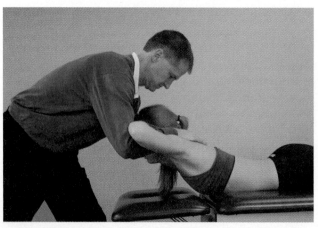

■ **Figure 7.29**   Prone Mid-Thoracic Stretch

Traction Techniques

Sitting Traction

Traction of the thoracic region may be useful when radicular symptoms are suspected or when postural improvement and enhanced mobility are goals.

1. Sitting traction is performed by placing the patient near the back of the plinth, adjacent to the clinician. The plinth height should be at a level where the clinician has to squat to reach the patient.

2. A belt is used to stabilize the pelvis of the patient to the table.

3. The patient is placed in a slumped (flexed) position and his or her arms are crossed and cradled at the elbows.

4. The right arm of the clinician reaches around the front of the patient and scoops the left arm of the patient, followed by the same procedure (left on right) for the opposite arm.

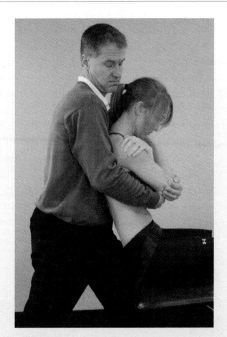

■ **Figure 7.30**   Sitting Traction Technique

5. While maintaining flexion, the patient is scooped into traction by the clinician extending his or her knees (Figure 7.30 ■). The technique is held as long as possible.

Supine Traction

Supine traction is an easier technique to perform when patients are large or if the clinician is small in stature.

1. Prior to the patient lying supine, a belt is placed horizontally across the table at the site where the clinician is interested in mobilization into traction.

2. Once the patient lies supine and places his or her hands behind the head, the clinician fastens and snugs the belt around his or her back.

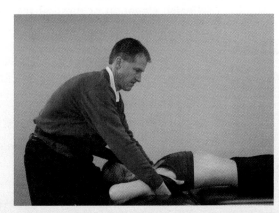

■ **Figure 7.31**   Supine Traction Technique

3. By pulling backward, the clinician can apply a traction force through his or her body (with the belt producing the majority of the pull), which reduces the load placed upon the arms (Figure 7.31 ■).

4. The position is held as long as possible.

Of the two techniques, the supine traction technique is best for postural gains whereas the sitting traction technique is likely better for treatment of radicular symptoms.

Mobilization

The ability to determine the true stiffness of joints in the thoracic region is significantly altered by the mobility of the rib cage during a PA.[31] Additionally, if the patient has a variable amount of air within the lungs, a technique that has an element of compression such as a PA can be altered. This necessitates the importance of assessment of pain response as well as detection of stiffness.

As discussed in Chapter 1, there is also moderate evidence to support that manual therapy provides an excitatory effect on sympathetic nervous system activity,[32,33,42,43] findings that are supported within the thoracic spine. An excitatory effect on the sympathetic nervous system occurs concurrently with a reduction of hypoalgesia and may parallel the effects of stimulation of the dorsal periaqueductal gray matter of the midbrain, a process that has occurred in animal research.[44,45] Documented evidence supports the benefit of modulation of pain and has a nonlocalized effect. Wright[46] outlines that hypoalgesia and sympathoexcitation are correlated, suggesting that individuals who exhibit the most change in pain perception also exhibit the most change in sympathetic nervous system function.

As with cervical spine mobilizations, those used and found concordant during the examination may yield potential treatment choices if positive results were found with sustained or repeated movements. The techniques of the PA, AP (of the costo-sternal joints), the transverse glide, and the UPA may be effective in modulating pain and stiffness.

Mobilization of the First Rib

Although controversial and lacking in appropriate investigation, the first rib may be a culprit in thoracic outlet syndrome. Thoracic outlet syndrome is a combination of symptoms in which cervico–brachial nerve–related pain occurs because of compression or traction. Theoretically, elevation of the first rib may lead to entrapment or injury of the nerve.

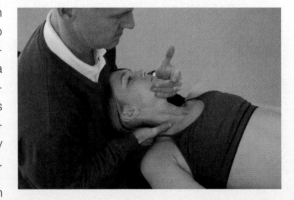

■ **Figure 7.32** Mobilization of the First Rib in Supine

1 The patient is placed in a supine position and resting symptoms are assessed.

2 The first rib is palpated posteriorly (the right first rib is targeted in Figure 7.32 ■).

3 The clinician places the patient's head in side flexion to the same side and rotation away, which reduces the stress of the scalene muscles on the first rib and allows the rib to "drop" during mobilization. The force of the mobilization is toward the anterior, contralateral hip anterior superior iliac spine (ASIS).

The technique can also be performed in a sitting position.

1 The patient sits and leans posteriorly against the clinician.

2 The clinician places the opposite arm of the first rib over the leg for support of the patient.

3. The first rib (the right first rib is targeted in Figure 7.33 ■) is palpated posteriorly and the clinician places the patient's head in side flexion to the same side and rotation away.

4. The clinician glides the movement at an angle toward the opposite hip of the patient.

5. Concurrently, the clinician may move the patient into side flexion of the trunk to enhance the movement of the technique.

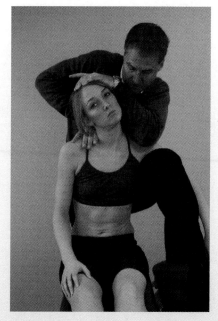

■ **Figure 7.33**   Mobilization of the First Rib in Sitting

Combined Movements

Combined movements are often required to move within the plane of the facet. Because the thoracic segments face inferiorly and anteriorly, facet movement is curvilinear and slide occurs during opening and closing. In contrast, gapping occurs when both the joint is opened using a perpendicular-directed force.

Facet Joint Gapping, Mobilization with Movement

The mobilization of a locked thoracic facet using a postural mobilization along the axis and plane of the facet may open the facet and decrease the impingement of the meniscoid.

1. The patient assumes a sitting position.

2. The patient's arms are crossed in front of the body so that the clinician may use the arms as a lever to position the thoracic spine into further flexion or rotation.

3. The clinician pulls the arms into flexion and rotation to the opposite side of the facet dysfunction and encourages the patient to actively move into this position. This movement serves to "open" the thoracic facet on the targeted side (the right side in Figure 7.34 ■).

(Continued)

④ The clinician then applies a superior to anterior directed force along the plane of the facet. This motion theoretically creates traction to the facet to enhance an opening moment.

⑤ The clinician may apply a static hold, a muscle energy technique, or oscillations in this position.

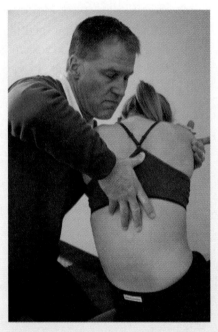

■ **Figure 7.34**   Mobilization of a Locked Thoracic Facet

Rotation and Side Flexion, Mobilization with Movement

Rotation and side flexion combines two passive physiological techniques for assessment.

① The patient sits at the edge of the plinth.

② The patient actively moves into rotation, toward the concordant position of pain.

③ Concurrently with active rotation, the clinician applies a passive physiological side flexion force to the first point of reported pain (Figure 7.35 ■).

④ Movement and force is applied beyond the first point of pain toward end range.

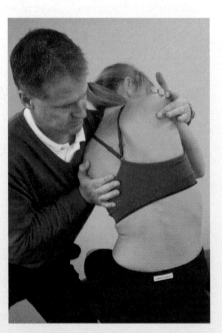

■ **Figure 7.35**   Combined Physiological Rotation and Side Flexion: Mobilization with Movement

Extension with a Posterior–Anterior Mobilization, Mobilization with Movement Extension and a posterior–anterior force may be useful in identifying patients who may benefit from postural treatment. During extension, the ribs rotate caudally during facet closure. The clinician may choose to work opposite of the rib movement or with the rib movement caudally to enhance extension motion. To perform the technique, the patient sits at the edge of the plinth. The clinician extends the patient into the desired pre-extension position. At the desired preposition of extension (concordant position), the clinician can apply either a superiorly based or an inferiorly based force to the ribs and/or facets. The clinician must modulate the force with the first point of reported pain. The clinician may instruct the patient to move into extension as well. Movement and force is applied beyond the first point of pain toward end range. Sustained holds or repeated movements that affect the concordant sign are utilized to determine potential treatment selection.

Rib Mobilization with Movement

A rib mobilization with movement technique involves an upward glide of the rib during an opening procedure involving side flexion away from the guilty region or a downward glide of the rib during a closing procedure of side flexion toward the targeted rib. Hooking the lateral aspect of the first metacarpal below or above the rib enhances the targeted movement. When rotation is desired, the movement of the rib mobilization should be targeted cephalically for rotation away (Figure 7.36 ■) and caudally during rotation toward (Figure 7.37 ■) the targeted rib.

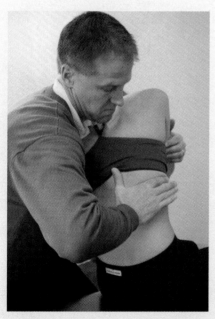

■ **Figure 7.36**   Rib Mobilization with Movement, Side Flexion Away from the Targeted Rib: Rib Upward Glide

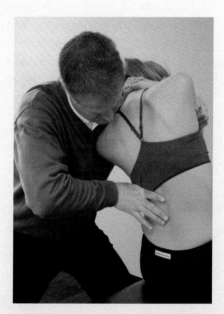

■ **Figure 7.37**   Rib Mobilization with Movement, Side Flexion toward the Targeted Rib: Rib Downward Glide

Manipulation

General Techniques Ross and colleagues[47] reported that the accuracy of a thoracic manipulation is less specific than previously assumed. Slightly over 50% of thoracic joint manipulations resulted in a cavitation at the targeted level. Typical errors in segmental manipulation of nearly 3.5 cm from the desired target were recorded. Bereznick et al.[48] acknowledged a similar problem during the use of a "screw" manipulation identifying that the skin friction tension was not helpful in allowing a clinician to target the manipulation at a selected vector.

Selection of thrust manipulation over nonthrust manipulation should be based on sound clinical reasoning. Thrust manipulation may be effective for those patients who are not irritable, have limited relative or no absolute contraindications, and for those that have demonstrated benefit in the past. Since thrust manipulation does not have the luxury of an examination-based outcome (i.e., use of repeated or sustained holds to outline the potential response), the ability to know the expected outcome is less than with nonthrust manipulation.

Targeted Specific Techniques

Targeted specific techniques are designed to focus on a specific area and to create a minimal amount of movement to adjacent segments.

Distraction Manipulation of the Upper Thoracic Segments

The cervico–thoracic junction is a stable region solidified by the connection of the ribs to the cervical-like upper thoracic segments. The upper thoracic facets tilt anteriorly, decreasing the likelihood of a gapping during an AP manipulation procedure. Consequently, an effective technique that produces facet sliding can be performed in sitting if the flexion of the upper thoracic region is maintained throughout the process.

1. The patient sits at the edge of the plinth; the arms are wrapped behind the head and the fingers are interlaced.

2. The clinician stands behind the patient and inserts his or her forearms anteriorly to the humerus and posterior to the forearm of the patient.

3. The clinician then grips the thumbs of the patient with his or her hands.

4. The patient is placed in further flexion and encouraged to relax.

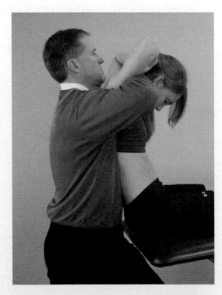

■ **Figure 7.38** Distraction Manipulation of the Upper Thoracic Segments

5. The clinician increases the stability of the arm-to-arm grip by pulling outward into external rotation at the shoulders (Figure 7.38 ■). Gently rocking the patient side to side may also assist in relaxing the patient.

6. The manipulation force is anterior and upward. Careful attention is required to avoid an extension movement of the patient's thoracic spine.

Prone Cervico–Thoracic (CT) Junction Manipulation

The prone CT junction manipulation is a method that is effective in targeting segments C7 to T2. Less force is required for the manipulation and for smaller clinicians, the prone CT junction manipulation is relatively easy to administer.

1. The patient is positioned in prone and the head is rotated away from the targeted side of the manipulation.

2. The arm that is on the side that the head is rotated is placed in shoulder abduction and elbow flexion.

3. The clinician leans over the patient caudal to the head.

4. Using the thumb, the clinician blocks the spinous process caudal to the targeted joint (Figure 7.39 ■).

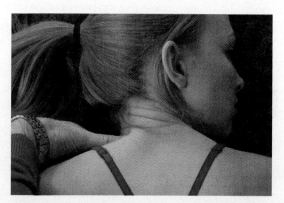

5. The clinician then places the palm of his or her hand on the patient's zygomatic arch and applies a superior diagonal force into side flexion and extension.

6. At the perceived end point, the clinician applies a thrust into the extended side flexion position (Figure 7.40 ■).

■ **Figure 7.39**   The Spinous Process Blocking Method

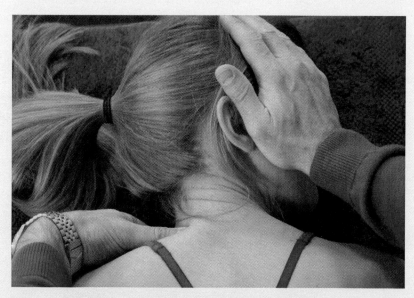

■ **Figure 7.40**   Prone Cervico–Thoracic Junction Manipulation

The Pistol Manipulation

Cleland et al.[49] also found strength gains of the inferior trapezius with thoracic manipulation versus a sham technique. The pistol technique used may be responsible for improvement of thoracic extension a physiological movement that has been linked to short-term improvements in shoulder flexion.[50]

The supine technique is often termed the "pistol."

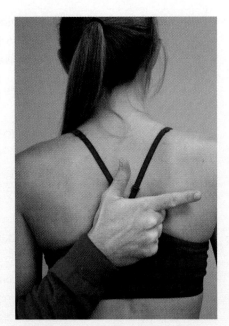

■ **Figure 7.41**   The Pistol Grip

1 The pistol requires that the patient place their arms in an over- and undercrossing technique (not crossing the arms) while firmly gripping his or her own thoracic region with the hands.

2 The clinician stands to the opposite side of the targeted segment (right side to treat the left side, Figure 7.41 ■).

3 Using the arm furthest from the targeted side, the clinician gently pulls the patient into sidelying position.

4 The clinician then leans over the patient and places the hand behind the patient's back just caudal to the targeted segment. The pistol grip allows the transverse processes to articulate with the thenar eminence and the folded digits of the clinician's hand (Figure 7.41).

5 The patient is then "scooped" into flexion (using his or her arms as a lever) and is gently placed over the pistol hand of the clinician (careful effort is made to keep the patient in thoracic flexion) (Figure 7.42 ■).

6 The clinician may further enhance the contact point on the patient's transverse process by pronating the wrist or through ulnar deviation of the forearm. The clinician's thrust should be through the shaft of the humeri while careful attention toward keeping the flexed thoracic position of the patient. The force of the thrust should go through the chest of the clinician to ensure enough vigor is applied.

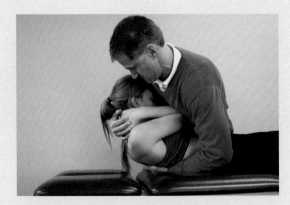

■ **Figure 7.42**   The Pistol Manipulation

The Screw Manipulation

The "screw" manipulation is a fairly aggressive manipulative technique in which the transverse processes are forced into a posterior to anterior direction. Chiropractors averaged 462–482 Newtons of force during a thoracic screw manipulation technique, producing this peak force in approximately 120 milliseconds.[51] Others have reported peak thrust values of over 1100 Newtons with a thoracic screw, albeit during shorter periods of peak output.[52]

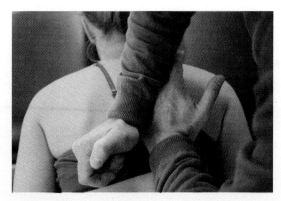

■ **Figure 7.43**   Hand Placement for the Screw Manipulation

1. The patient lies in a prone position.

2. The clinician identifies the targeted guilty segment with the concordant application of a UPA.

3. The clinician identifies the direction of the manipulation by applying a lateral stress (transverse force) to the adjacent spinous process to determine the painful and stiff segment (Figure 7.43 ■). For example, if a UPA of the T5 facet on the right produced the concordant sign, and a lateral glide of the spinous process of T5 to the right and a lateral glide of the spinous process of T6 to the left caused similar pain, then the hand placement by the clinician would be one pisiform on the right facet of T5 and one pisiform on the left facet of T6.

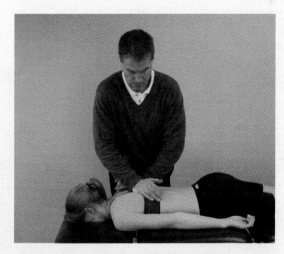

■ **Figure 7.44**   The Screw Manipulation

4. The clinician then preloads the tissue and takes up the slack (Figure 7.44 ■). The thrust occurs directly toward the patient once the patient completely exhales his or her respiratory volume.

5. The clinician can target the costo-transverse joints by slightly further laterally to the facets (Figure 7.45 ■).

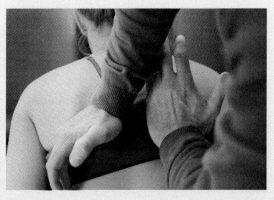

■ **Figure 7.45**   The Screw Manipulation on the Costo-Transverse Joints

The Costotransverse Manipulation

The costotransverse manipulation is a general manipulation that is often effective on the lower costotransverse joints of the thoracic spine.

1. The patient lies in a prone position and the clinician stabilizes the costotransverse joint with the palm of one hand while lifting upward on the ASIS of the ipsilateral side.

2. The clinician rotates the ASIS upward until movement is felt at the stabilized costotransverse joint.

3. The ASIS is pulled further upward (into contralateral rotation) until a posteriorly directed force is felt by the clinician at the costotransverse joint. At that point, a downward thrust is applied to the costotransverse joint.

The Adjusted Pistol

The pistol is considered an opening technique, thus theoretically the method should improve flexion. Using targeted specific objectives, clinicians can further the opening of the desired segments (facet or ribs) by performing one of three methods.

Two adjustments can be made with the pistol manipulation to target the upper and lower thoracic spines. For the upper thoracic spine, pulling the thoracic spine into extension (by pulling caudally on the transverse processes) rearranges the facet planes horizontally and improves the likelihood of a manipulation (Figure 7.46 ■).

For the lower thoracic spine, pushing the thoracic spine into flexion (by pushing cranially on the transverse processes) rearranges the facet planes horizontally and improves the likelihood of a successful manipulation (Figure 7.47 ■).

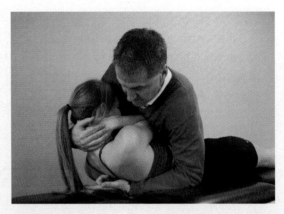

■ **Figure 7.46** Adjustment for the Upper Thoracic Spine

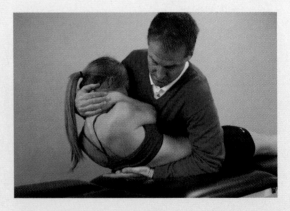

■ **Figure 7.47** Adjustment for the Lower Thoracic Spine

The clinician can also focus on a specific side using the pistol. One method used to open the segments further involves passive side flexion away from the targeted side. The clinician may further enhance the contact point on the targeted transverse process by pronating the wrist and/or ulnar deviation of the hand. The manipulation is performed similar to the general method in this targeted specific preposition.

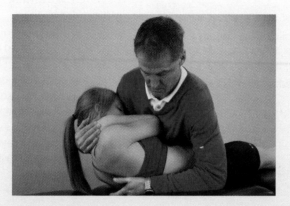

■ **Figure 7.48** Further Adjustment of the Pistol to Target One Side

The Adjusted Screw

The screw is considered a closing technique and may be beneficial to gain extension. To adjust, the clinician can preposition the patient into side flexion toward the side that is restricted (the right side in Figure 7.49 ■). In other words, during examination the patient demonstrated pain while moving into extension or side flexion. The technique is performed in a similar manner in this prepositioned posture.

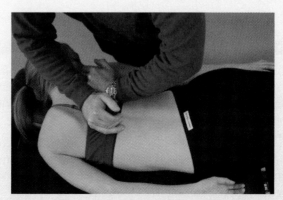

■ **Figure 7.49** Adjusted Screw by Prepositioning in Side Flexion

Summary

- Passive stretches may be beneficial for postural correction or as an adjunct for pain modulation techniques.
- Passive mobilization techniques are selected based on patient response.
- Mobilization of the first rib is designed to decrease pain associated with thoracic outlet syndrome.
- Manipulation may be effective for reduction of pain and stiffness.
- Manipulation is selected based on clinical reasoning. At present, no clinical prediction rules are present to determine when to select manipulation versus mobilization for the thoracic spine.
- Combined techniques may be necessary for mobilization along the plane of the facet.

Treatment Outcomes

The Evidence

Overall, few studies have investigated the benefits of manual therapy on the thoracic spine. Studies have outlined the effectiveness of mobilization for treatment of thoracic disorders in case studies[1,53-55] (Level D) and have reported positive benefit. Others have reported that mobilization and manipulation leads to increases in lower thoracic strength when compared to controls such as sham manipulation[14,49] (Level C). At this time, no studies had evaluated the effectiveness of mobilization of the thoracic spine in a well-designed randomized clinical trial.

As with mobilization, few studies have investigated the benefit of treating the thoracic spine with manipulation. Schiller[56] performed a small, randomized controlled trial including 30 subjects and found benefit over subtherapeutic ultrasound. However, this trial was very small and used subjects that were younger and were followed for only a short period of time (Level C). Additionally, subjects were not classified into similar groups.

A growing body of evidence is accumulating that suggests that thoracic manipulation (thrust technique) (Level B) leads to a short-term reduction of pain in patients with neck or shoulder disorders.[50,57-60] In nearly all cases, the studies suggest that patients with mechanical neck or shoulder pain that is not severe or related to radicular symptoms may have short-term improvements in report of pain, hypoalgesia, and pressure pain thresholds.

Summary

- Thoracic mobilization and manipulation are advocated in single case study designs.
- There appears to be merit and benefit in treating the cervical spine and/or shoulder with thoracic manipulation.
- Only one study has been performed that randomized patients with a thoracic spine injury into comparison groups. More research is needed to determine the benefit of manual therapy of the thoracic spine.

Chapter Questions

1. Describe the facet orientation of the thoracic spine. How does the facet orientation and the contribution of the rib cage influence the stability of the thoracic spine?

2. Describe the coupling pattern of the thoracic spine. Does this coupling pattern change throughout the thoracic spine?

3. Identify the specific characteristics of the thoracic spine examination that are unique. How does fine-tuning selected movement in the thoracic spine assist in improving data collection during treatment? Describe the methods of this process.

4. Compare and contrast the biomechanical constructs behind mobilization and manipulation of the thoracic spine.

5. Describe the literature associated with thoracic spine outcomes with manual therapy.

Patient Cases

Case 7.1: Larry Goldman (53-year-old male)

Diagnosis: Thoracic strain

Observation: He exhibits significant kyphosis in mid-thoracic region and is obese and appears in ill health.

Mechanism: Last week, after a flight to Australia in which he sat for up to 30 hours, he started to notice sharp pain in his mid-thoracic region.

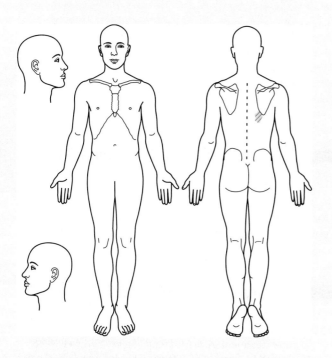

Concordant Sign: Thoracic extension.

Nature of the Condition: He indicates the problem is a nuisance but it is painful during deep breathing and he is worried he may have "tore a muscle." The pain is transient only and does not last when instigated.

Behavior of the Symptoms: The pain is localized on the right side, near the mid-thoracic region, at T7.

Pertinent Patient History: He has a heart murmur and takes medications for high cholesterol.

Patient Goals: He would like to rid himself of the pain during deep breathing or during active extension.

Baseline: At rest, 1/10 NAS for pain; when worst, 6/10 pain.

Examination Findings: Active extension is the most painful movement. PAs to T7 are reproductive of the concordant pain but UPAs to the right costotransverse segment are even more provocative.

1. Based on these findings, what else would you like to examine?
2. Is this patient a good candidate for manual therapy?
3. What is the expected prognosis of this patient?
4. What treatments do you feel presented in this book may be beneficial for this patient?

Case 7.2: Mabel Knowles (62-year-old female)

Diagnosis: Thoracic strain

Observation: She exhibits significant kyphosis in mid-thoracic region and appears frail. There is a visible Dowager's hump in upper thoracic spine.

Mechanism: Insidious onset. Symptoms have been present for well over 12 months.

Concordant Sign: Long-term flexion causes a bruising sensation in the mid-thoracic region, whereas extension is sharp and painful in the same area.

Nature of the Condition: The pain is really affecting her lifestyle. She used to walk for exercise but has stopped recently because of the pain. When the pain is triggered it typically takes about 30 minutes for it to subside. She takes naproxen to reduce the symptoms.

Behavior of the Symptoms: Pain in arm is worse as the day progresses. She sleeps in a recliner because lying supine is too painful to tolerate.

Pertinent Patient History: Diagnosed with osteoarthritis 17 years ago and has an inguinal hernia.

Patient Goals: She is concerned that she significantly injured her back.

Baseline: The pain in her thoracic spine is 4/10 at rest and can increase to 8/10 when really provoked.

Examination Findings: Active extension reproduces the sharp thoracic pain, whereas flexion, carrying objects, driving, and walking all reproduce

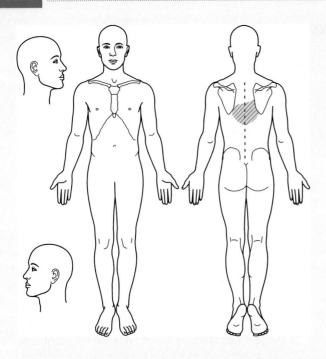

the ache in her thoracic spine that she calls a "bruise." PAs all reproduce similar symptoms at T6 and T7, especially CPAs.

1. Based on these findings, what else would you like to examine?
2. Is this patient a good candidate for manual therapy?
3. What is the expected prognosis of this patient?
4. What treatments do you feel presented in this book may be beneficial for this patient?

PEARSON
myhealthprofessionskit™

Use this address to access the Companion Website created for this textbook. Simply select "Physical Therapy" from the choice of disciplines. Find this book and log in using your username and password to access video clips and the anatomy and arthrological information.

References

1. McRae M, Cleland J. Differential diagnosis and treatment of upper thoracic pain: A case study. *J Man Manip Ther.* 2003;11:43–48.
2. Bogduk N. Innervation and pain patterns of the cervical spine. In: Grant R (ed). *Physical therapy of the cervical and thoracic spine.* 3rd edition. New York; Churchill Livingstone: 2002.
3. Doubleday KL, Kulig K, Landel R. Treatment of testicular pain using conservative management of the thoracolumbar spine: A case report. *Arch Phys Med Rehabil.* 2003;84(12):1903–1905.
4. DeFranca GG, Levine LJ. The T4 syndrome. *J Manipulative Physiol Ther.* 1995;18(1):34–37.
5. Mergener K, Brandabur JJ. Costochondral deformity masquerading as a submucosal gastric tumor. *Endoscopy.* 2003;35(3):255.
6. Feinstein B, Langton JBK, Jameson RM, Schiller F. Experiments on referred pain from deep somatic tissues. *J Bone Jnt Surg.* 1954;36:981–987.
7. Jinno T, Tago M, Yoshida H, Yamane M. (abstract). Case of thoracoabdominal aortic aneurysm complicated with Buerger's disease. *Kyobu Geka.* 2001;54:1121–1124.
8. Hubbard J. The differential diagnosis of chest pain. *Nurs Times.* 2002;98(50):30–31.
9. Hamberg J, Lindahl O. Angina pectoris symptoms caused by thoracic spine disorders: Clinical examination and treatment. *Acta Med Scand Suppl.* 1981;644:84–86.
10. Wise CM, Semble EL, Dalton CB. Musculoskeletal chest wall syndromes in patients with noncardiac chest pain: A study of 100 patients. *Arch Phys Med Rehabil.* 1992; 73(2):147–149.
11. Adler R. The differentiation of organic and psychogenic pain. *Pain.* 1981;10(2):249–252.
12. Edmondston SJ, Singer KP. Thoracic spine: Anatomical and biomechanical considerations for manual therapy. *Man Ther.* 1997;2(3):132–143.
13. Moore KL. Muscles and ligaments of the back. In Singer KP, Giles LF (eds). *Clinical anatomy and management of low back pain.* Oxford; Butterworth-Heinemann: 1997.
14. Liebler E, Tufano-Coors L, Douris P, et al. The effect of thoracic spine mobilization on lower trapezius strength testing. *J Man Manip Ther.* 2001;9:207–212.
15. Claus AP, Hides JA, Moseley GL, Hodges PW. Different ways to balance the spine: Subtle changes in sagittal spinal curves affect regional muscle activity. *Spine.* 2009;34(6):E208–14.
16. Janda V. Muscles and motor control in cervicogenic disorders: assessment and management. In: Grant R (ed). *Physical therapy of the cervical and thoracic spine.* 3rd ed. New York; Churchill Livingstone: 2002.

17. Christie HJ, Kumar S, Warren SA. Postural aberrations in low back pain. *Arch Phys Med Rehabil.* 1995;76: 218–224.

18. Refshauge KM, Goodsell M, Lee M. The relationship between surface contour and vertebral body measures of upper spine curvature. *Spine.* 1994;19(19):2180–2185.

19. Renno A, Granito R, Driusso P, Costa D, Oishi J. Effects of an exercise program on respiratory function, posture, and on quality of life in osteoporotic women: A pilot study. *Physiother.* 2005;91:113–118.

20. Cook C. The relationship between posture and balance disturbances in women with osteoporosis. *Phys Occupation Ther Geriatrics.*2003;20(3):37–50.

21. Woodhull-McNeal AP. Changes in posture and balance with age. *Aging* (Milano). 1992;4(3):219–225.

22. White AA III, Panjabi MM. The clinical biomechanics of scoliosis. *Clin Orthop Relat Res.* 1976;(118):100–112.

23. Hawes M. The use of exercises in the treatment of scoliosis: An evidence-based critical review of the literature. *Ped Rehabilitation.* 2003;6:171–182.

24. Schwab F, Dubey A, Gamez L, et al. Adult scoliosis: Prevalence, SF-36, and nutritional parameters in an elderly volunteer population. *Spine.* 2005;30(9): 1082–1085.

25. Voight ML, Thomson BC. The role of the scapula in the rehabilitation of shoulder injuries. *J Athl Train.* 2000;35(3):364–372.

26. Crook J, Milner R, Schultz IZ, Stringer B. Determinants of occupational disability following a low back injury: A critical review of the literature. *J Occup Rehabil.* 2002;12(4):277–295.

27. Janing W. Systemic and specific authonomic reactions in pain: Efferent, afferent, and endocrine components. *Eur J Anaesthesiol.* 1985;2:319–346.

28. Theodoridis D, Ruston S. The effect of shoulder movements on thoracic spine 3D motion. *Clin Biomech* (Bristol, Avon). 2002;17(5):418–421.

29. Lee D. Rotational instability of the mid thoracic spine: assessment and management. *Man Ther.* 1996;1: 234–241.

30. Brismee JM, Gipson D, Ivie D, et al. Interrater reliability of a passive physiological intervertebral motion test in the mid-thoracic spine. *J Manipulative Physiol Ther.* 2006;29:368–373.

31. Chansirinukor W, Lee M, Latimer J. Contribution of ribcage movement to thoracolumbar posteroanterior stiffness. *J Manipulative Physiol Ther.* 2003;26(3):176–183.

32. Vicenzino B, Paungmali A, Buratowski S, Wright A. Specific manipulative therapy treatment for chronic lateral epicondylalgia produces uniquely characteristic hypoalgesia. *Man Ther.* 2001;6:205–212.

33. Simon R, Vicenzino B, Wright A. The influence of an anteroposterior accessory glide of the glenohumeral joint on measures of peripheral sympathetic nervous system function in the upper limb. *Man Ther.* 1997;2(1):18–23.

34. Lee D. Biomechanics of the thorax. In: Grant R (ed). *Physical therapy of the cervical and thoracic spine.* 3rd ed. New York; Churchill Livingstone: 2002.

35. Freeston J, Karim Z, Lindsay K, Gough A. Can early diagnosis and management of costochondritis reduce acute chest pain admissions? *J Rheumatol.* 2004;31(11): 2269–2271.

36. Christensen HW, Vach W, Vach K, Manniche C, Haghfelt T, Hartvigsen L, Hoilund-Carlsen PF. Palpation of the upper thoracic spine: An observer reliability study. *J Manipulative Physiol Ther.* 2002;25(5):285–292.

37. Love RM, Brodeur RR. Inter- and intra-examiner reliability of motion palpation for the thoracolumbar spine. *J Manipulative Physiol Ther.* 1987;10(1):1–4.

38. Heiderscheit B, Boissonnault W. Reliability of joint mobility and pain assessment of the thoracic spine and rib cage in asymptomatic individuals. *J Man Manip Ther.* 2008;16:210–216.

39. Haas M, Panzer D, Peterson D, Raphael R. Short-term responsiveness of manual thoracic end-play assessment to spinal manipulation: A randomized controlled trial of construct validity. *J Manip Physiol Ther.* 1995;18:582–589.

40. Lewis J, Green A, Reichard Z, Wright C. Scapular position: The validity of skin surface palpation. *Man Ther.* 2002;7(1):26–30.

41. Frese E, Brown M, Norton BJ. Clinical reliability of manual muscle testing: Middle trapezius and gluteus medius muscles. *Phys Ther.* 1987;67(7):1072–1076.

42. Vicenzino B, Collins D, Wright A. Sudomotor changes induced by neural mobilization techniques in asymptomatic subjects. *J Manual Manip Ther.* 1994;2:66–74.

43. Vicenzino B, Collins D, Wright A. An investigation of the interrelationship between manipulative therapy–induced hypoalgesia and sympathoexcitation. *J Manipulative Physiol Ther.* 1998;21:448–453.

44. Wright A. Pain-relieving effects of cervical manual therapy. In: Grant R (ed). *Physical therapy of the cervical and thoracic spine.* 3rd ed. New York; Churchill Livingston: 2002.

45. Lovick T. Interactions between descending pathways from the dorsal and ventrolateral periaqueductal gray matter in the rat. In: Depaulis A, Bandler R (eds). *The midbrain periaqueductal gray matter.* New York; Plenum Press: 1991.

46. Wright A. Recent concepts in the neurophysiology of pain. *Man Ther.* 1999;4:196–202.

47. Ross JK, Bereznick D, McGill S. Determining cavitation location during lumbar and thoracic spinal manipulation. *Spine.* 2004;29:1452–1457.

48. Bereznick DE, Ross JK, McGill SM. The frictional properties at the thoracic skin–fascia interface: implications in spine manipulation. *Clin Biomech* (Bristol, Avon). 2002;17(4):297–303.

49. Cleland J, Selleck B, Stowell T, et al. Short-term effect of thoracic manipulation on lower trapezius muscle strength. *J Man Manip Ther.* 2004;12(2):82–90.

50. Crawford HJ, Jull GA. The influence of thoracic posture and movement of range of arm elevation. *Physiother Theory Pract.* 1993;9:143–149.

51. Forand D, Drover J, Suleman Z, Symons B, Herzog W. The forces applied by female and male chiropractors during thoracic spinal manipulation. *J Manipulative Physiol Ther.* 2004;27(1):49–56.

52. Kirstukas SJ, Backman JA. Physician-applied contact pressure and table force response during unilateral

thoracic manipulation. *J Manipulative Physiol Ther.* 1999;22(5):269–279.

53. Horton SJ. Acute locked thoracic spine: treatment with a modified SNAG. *Man Ther.* 2002;7:103–107.

54. Fruth SJ. Differential diagnosis and treatment in a patient with posterior upper thoracic pain. *Phys Ther.* 2006;86:254–268.

55. Kelley JL, Whitney SL. The use of nonthrust manipulation in an adolescent for the treatment of thoracic pain and rib dysfunction: A case report. *J Orthop Sports Phys Ther.* 2006;36:887–892.

56. Schiller L. Effectiveness of spinal manipulative therapy in the treatment of mechanical thoracic spine pain: A pilot randomized clinical trial. *J Manipulative Physiol Ther.* 2001;24(6):394–401.

57. González-Iglesias J, Fernández-de-las-Peñas C, Cleland JA, Gutiérrez-Vega Mdel R. Thoracic spine manipulation for the management of patients with neck pain: A randomized clinical trial. *J Orthop Sports Phys Ther.* 2009;39(1):20–27.

58. González-Iglesias J, Fernández-de-las-Peñas C, Cleland JA, Alburquerque-Sendín F, Palomeque-del-Cerro L, Méndez-Sánchez R. Inclusion of thoracic spine thrust manipulation into an electro-therapy/thermal program for the management of patients with acute mechanical neck pain: A randomized clinical trial. *Man Ther.* 2009;14(3):306–313.

59. Fernández-de-Las-Peñas C, Alonso-Blanco C, Cleland JA, Rodríguez-Blanco C, Alburquerque-Sendín F. Changes in pressure pain thresholds over C5–C6 zygapophyseal joint after a cervicothoracic junction manipulation in healthy subjects. *J Manipulative Physiol Ther.* 2008;31(5):332–337.

60. Cleland JA, Glynn P, Whitman JM, Eberhart SL, MacDonald C, Childs JD. Short-term effects of thrust versus nonthrust mobilization/manipulation directed at the thoracic spine in patients with neck pain: A randomized clinical trial. *Phys Ther.* 2007;87(4):431–440.

Manual Therapy of the Shoulder Complex

Chad E. Cook

Chapter 8

Objectives

- Identify the pertinent structures and biomechanics of the shoulder complex.
- Demonstrate an appropriate and valid shoulder examination sequence.
- Identify plausible mobilization and manual therapy treatment techniques for the shoulder complex.
- Discuss the influence of manual therapy on recovery for shoulder-related dysfunction.

Clinical Examination

Differential Diagnosis

A careful patient history will improve the identification of red flags that masquerade as dysfunction of the shoulder (Table 8.1 ■). The presence of red flags requires further investigation and differential assessment.

Multiple structures throughout the upper quarter and abdominal cavity can refer pain to the shoulder region.[1-3] Most commonly, cervical spine lesions can cause secondary shoulder symptoms or referred pain to the shoulder.[4] Additionally, it is common to see misdiagnoses of cervical pain from shoulder lesions that refer pain proximally to the cervical region.[5] It is essential to rule out the contribution of the cervical spine for shoulder pain by using overpressures or a brief active and provocative cervical examination.

A number of serious pathologies of the shoulder can initially present with nonspecific shoulder pain

■ TABLE 8.1 Red Flags for Shoulder Impairment

Red Flag	Relationship
Age > 50	Increased risk of rotator cuff tear and other serious pathologies
Night pain	Increased risk of serious pathology such as tumor
Weight loss	Increased risk of cancer or auto-immune dysfunction
Fever	Increased risk for systemic infection
Pain unrelated to activity	Increased risk for referred pain from a visceral source
Pain not relieved by rest	Increased risk for referred pain from a visceral source
History of smoking	Increased risk for lung cancer and referred pain associated with cancer
Previous history of cancer	Increased risk for referral of pain and/or metastasis
Cardiac risk factors	Myocardial infarction may refer pain to the left shoulder
Pleuritic pain	Increased risk for Pancoast tumor

■ TABLE 8.2 Extrinsic Causes of Shoulder Pain

Type	Source
Neurological	Cervical radiculopathy
	Upper trunk brachial plexopathy
	Neurologic amyotrophy
	Focal mononeuropathy
	Muscular dystrophy
Cardiovascular	Cardiac ischemia
	Thoracic outlet syndrome
	Aortic disease
	Axillary thrombosis
Pulmonary	Upper lobe pneumonia
	Pulmonary embolism
	Pneumothorax
	Pneumoperitoneum
Malignancy	Pancoast tumor
	Metastatic cancer
Abdominal	Biliary disease
	Hepatic disease
	Pacreatitis
	Splenic injury
	Perforated viscus

(Table 8.2 ■). Disease or injury to the lungs, pancreas, aortic artery, and/or liver may refer pain to the shoulder. Pain associated with these structures is not reproduced during mechanical movements, may not decrease with appropriate rest,[6] and may initiate with an insidious onset.

In some cases, loss of function secondary to shoulder impairments outweighs pain as the most concordant problem. Thus, it is beneficial to identify movement-related dysfunctions that may assist in identifying a particular shoulder disorder.[7] If scapular winging is prominent during arm elevation, a serratus anterior or trapezius dysfunction should be expected. Recent trauma or a viral illness may contribute to dysfunction of the long thoracic nerve. If the patient demonstrates early breaking during movements and the inability to externally rotate the arm upon command, one should suspect the possibility of a rotator cuff tear or suprascapular nerve entrapment.

When pain radiates below the elbow the clinician should always clear the cervical spine, although referred pain from the rotator cuff is not abnormal. If pain occurs during throwing or if a "dead arm" is present after using the arm, one should suspect instability. If pain occurs with clicking, the labrum may be involved. Lastly, if pain is worse while lying on the shoulder during sleeping, impingement may be present.

Summary

- The cervical spine may refer pain to the shoulder and structures such as the lung, pancreas, aortic artery, and liver may refer pain to the shoulder.
- Recognizable impairments during shoulder movement may assist in isolating certain structures (e.g., the rotator cuff) or conditions (e.g., impingement).

Observation

Asymmetry of shoulder heights (e.g., right side is higher than the left side), size, and muscle build is often used erroneously to determine pathology in a shoulder. Some degree of asymmetry in a shoulder is normal and does not indicate the presence of pathology.[6] Priest and Nagel[8] found that hand dominance often leads to a lower (depressed) dominant shoulder and hypertrophy of the musculature on the ipsilateral side. While minor variations often mean little, gross atrophy of the shoulder musculature may be an indicator of spinal accessory nerve or long thoracic nerve entrapment and is essential to evaluate.

Altered humeral head position, specifically anterior displacement, may predispose an individual to shoulder pain and dysfunction.[9,10] This is often observed as a predominance of the humeral head anteriorly during a resting position. Anterior displacement of the humeral head is a common problem and is generally associated with a tight posterior capsule.[11]

Posture

Chronic rounded shoulders posture can also foster anterior translation of the humeral head. Weiser et al.[12] demonstrated an increase in anterior translation of the humeral head resulting in excessive strain on the inferior glenohumeral ligament in simulated scapular protraction. The authors believed that chronic protraction results in an anterior glenohumeral instability due to overstretching of the anterior capsule.

Taping for posture does not increase the muscle activity for scapular muscles but is effective in reducing a passive load on the anterior structures that are impinged.[13] However, taping can cause skin breakdown in an elderly population and should be used cautiously. Increasing the mobility of the anterior and posterior shoulder structures, a consequence of taping, may improve the resting position of the scapula, potentially improving the scapular and glenohumeral kinematics.[14]

Cervicothoracic posture can significantly influence the position and mobility of the scapula. Forward head posture may reduce the available range of motion of shoulder flexion,[15] whereas upper thoracic flexion may limit unilateral upper shoulder abduction and flexion.[16] Thoracic kyphosis is also associated with decreased shoulder flexion[17,18] and a reduction of the amount of force one can generate at the glenohumeral joint.[17]

Summary

- Asymmetry of the two shoulders is often erroneously used to determine pathology in a shoulder, specifically since some degree of asymmetry is normal.
- An anteriorly translated humeral head is common during shoulder pathology.
- Although treatment for postural abnormalities may not be directly related to shoulder recovery, improvements in shoulder range of motion and scapular position are common when posture is addressed.

Patient History

Mechanism of Injury

A careful examination of the mechanism of injury may be helpful in identifying the type of shoulder dysfunction. For example, pain during a fall may be associated with acromioclavicular joint (AC), specifically if the patient reports a concordant pain during movement of the arm across the body or after wearing a heavy backpack. Pain from a labral tear is often associated with trauma. Pain during overhead activity may implicate the rotator cuff just as pain during selected arm postures that encourage impingement may warrant investigation of flexibility and strength assessment. Lastly, patients that report a "dead arm" sensation in the acceleration phase of throwing may have instability.[6] A combination of pathologies may be present as well, specifically in situations where trauma precipitated symptoms.

The age of the individual may prove noteworthy as well. Older patients are more likely to experience rotator cuff injuries[19] just as younger patients are more likely to experience instability.[4] Restrictions associated with capsulitis are more common in middle-aged females and less common in younger individuals.[4] Nonshoulder structures that refer pain into the shoulder region such as pain associated with cervical are more common in patients age 45 and older and less common in younger individuals.[4]

Psychosocial Issues

A relationship between selected psychosocial factors and shoulder pain among workers has been suggested in several studies.[20–22] Common psychosocial factors associated with shoulder pain include burnout,[20] mild and severe depression,[20] inability to express one's symptoms well,[20] high job demands or stress,[21–23] and low pain threshold.[21] Others have reported that the influence of psychosocial factors are not near as prevalent as physiological requirements such as repetitive work.[24,25]

Summary

- The mechanism of injury may help distill the type of pathology of the shoulder.
- Trauma is generally associated with a rotator cuff tear, a acromio-clavicular injury, or a labral tear. Degeneration is associated with impingement, rotator cuff weakness, and capsulitis.
- Although likely not as significant as physiological factors, psychosocial factors may affect the recovery rate of patients with a shoulder-related injury.

Clinical Examination

Active Physiological Movements

Range-of-motion losses of the shoulder associated with pathology can occur in all planes of motion.[26] Cyriax[27] initially promoted the concept of a pattern of loss (by ratio) in patients with capsuloligamentous dysfunction, a concept identified as a "capsular pattern." Cyriax[27] proposed that the shoulder capsular pattern losses of external rotation (mostly), followed by abduction, then internal rotation (the least loss), were predictable in the shoulder and should prompt a clinician to target the capsuloligamentous components for treatment.

Rundquist and Ludewig[28] reported that significant variability in capsular patterns were present in patients with idiopathic loss of range of motion, a pattern that changed when shoulder abduction was incorporated. Others[29,30] have identified variability in the capsular pattern in patients diagnosed with adhesive capsulitis of the shoulder and suggested that the theory of a single capsular pattern lacks evidence.

Most likely, the variability of a capsular pattern is explained by the different contributions of the capsule and ligaments during movement of the shoulder. As discussed in the biomechanics section, movements such as abduction can alter the contribution of the shoulder ligaments toward stability of the shoulder and may place selective tension on disparate aspects of the capsule. Since damage or injury of the shoulder can be isolated to a specific aspect of the capsule, it is intuitive to assume that different injuries may yield variations in range-of-motion restrictions. During the active range of motions of flexion and abduction, restrictions within the capsule may result in a "drift" toward the plane of the scaption.[31]

Bilateral Shoulder Flexion

Examining bilateral shoulder flexion is beneficial in determining symmetry of movement and assessing scapulohumeral rhythm. Symmetrical movement requires a balance of active muscular control and compliance of passive structures.[11] The primary contributors to symmetrical movement include the force-coupled movements of the rotator cuff at the glenohumeral joint, and the force-coupled control of the serratus anterior and appropriate stabilization and movement contributions from the trapezius for the scapulothoracic joint.[32,33]

Pain intensity is important to identify during active movement because pain has been shown to inhibit the contribution of the serratus anterior and the lower fibers of the trapezius. With inhibition of these two critical muscles, movements near and above 90 degrees of elevation are significantly altered. The scapula should move congruently with the thorax, with slight internal rotation and a medial glide.[34] Pain might cause abnormal scapular elevation, lateral translation, and AC joint separation.

1. The patient should stand in the targeted posture (typically standing).

2. The patient is requested to raise both arms together.

3. The clinician should carefully evaluate movement for symmetry and appropriate sequencing.

4. The patient is requested to lower both arms together, the clinician carefully evaluating movement for symmetry and appropriate sequencing.

Unilateral Shoulder Flexion

With active range of movements, the noninvolved shoulder is evaluated first.

1. The patient should stand and raise his or her arm to the first point of pain (if present) (Figure 8.1 ■). Movement height and quality are evaluated.

2. The patient is requested to raise the arm past the first point of pain (if present) toward end range. Pain is again evaluated and compared to the initial point of pain.

3. The patient is then requested to perform repeated movements near the end range to determine the behavior of the pain.

4. If no pain was reproduced during the movement, an overpressure is performed to the patient.

5. The motion is repeated on the other side.

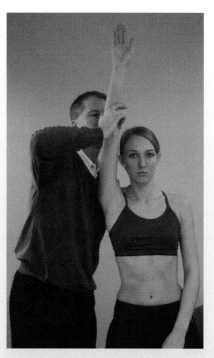

■ **Figure 8.1** Unilateral Active Physiological Shoulder Flexion with Overpressure

Bilateral Shoulder Abduction

Bilateral shoulder abduction is beneficial to analyze. As with shoulder flexion, the appropriate force-coupled contractions of the shoulder musculature are required for symmetry and stability. One common problem seen during pain and/or rotator cuff dysfunction is the rapid dropping of the arm during 70–110 degrees of shoulder abduction. At this position, control of the drop of the humerus requires use of a strong eccentric contraction and if weakness or pain is present during this position the arm will rapidly drop.

1. The patient should stand in the targeted posture.

2. The patient is requested to raise both arms together.

3. The clinician should carefully evaluate movement for symmetry and appropriate sequencing.

4. The patient is requested to lower both arms together.

5. The clinician should carefully evaluate movement for symmetry and appropriate sequencing.

Unilateral Shoulder Abduction

1. The patient stands in the targeted posture.

2. The patient is requested to raise the arm to his or her side, to the first point of pain (if present); movement height and quality are evaluated (Figure 8.2 ■).

3. The patient is requested to raise the arm to his or her side past the first point of pain (if present) toward end range. Pain is again evaluated and compared to the initial point of pain.

4. The patient is requested to perform repeated movements near the end range to determine the behavior of the pain.

5. If no pain was reproduced during the movement, an overpressure is performed by taking the humerus further into abduction, sometimes requiring movement behind the patient's neck (Figure 8.3 ■).

6. The motion is repeated on the other side.

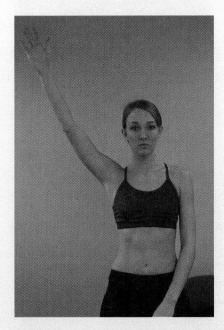

■ **Figure 8.2** Active Physiological Shoulder Abduction

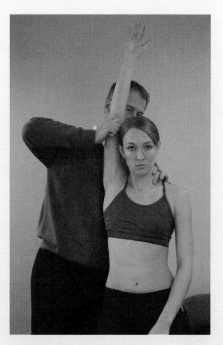

■ **Figure 8.3** Active Physiological Shoulder Abduction with Overpressure

Extension

Isolated active extension is an effective method to determine the passive mobility of the biceps tendon and may be useful in determining if the humerus has shifted anteriorly in the joint cavity (range will be limited and pain will be located anteriorly at the shoulder).

1. The patient stands in the targeted posture and baseline symptoms are evaluated.

2. The patient is requested to move his or her arm backward to the first point of pain (if present). Movement distance and quality are evaluated.

3. The patient is requested to move beyond the first point of pain near end range with repeated movements.

4. If no pain is present, an overpressure is applied to clear the movement. The complete procedure is repeated on the opposite side.

Horizontal Adduction

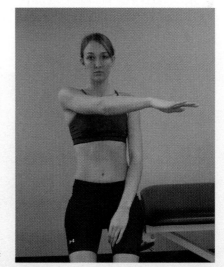

Isolated horizontal adduction is an effective movement to test the flexibility of the posterior capsule. To engage the posterior capsule further, internal rotation can be added as a combined movement.

1. The patient stands in the targeted posture and baseline symptoms are evaluated.

2. The patient is requested to move his or her arm across the body in an attempt to place the hand on the opposite shoulder (Figure 8.4 ▪).

3. The patient is instructed to identify the first point of pain (if present) and movement distance and quality are evaluated.

▪ **Figure 8.4** Active Physiological Shoulder Horizontal Adduction

4. The patient is requested to move beyond the first point of pain near end range with repeated movements.

5. If no pain is present an overpressure is applied to clear the joint.

6. The complete procedure is repeated on the opposite side.

Functional Active Shoulder Movements Functional active shoulder movements differ from plane-based motions in that the movements incorporate a number of different patterns of plane-based movements simultaneously.

Bilateral External Rotation

Bilateral external rotation at 90 degrees of abduction places a greater stress on the inferior capsular structures than an external rotation movement with the arm placed at the side.[35] It may be conducive to measure external rotation in both positions (at 90 degrees and at 0 degrees at the side), although a passive physiological assessment will provide more specific information as to the position of the impairment.

1 The patient stands in the targeted posture.

2 Baseline symptoms are evaluated.

3 The patient is directed to raise both arms and lace the hands behind the head (Figure 8.5 ■).

4 If no pain is present during the movements, the patient may require overpressure, which is applied by gently pulling back on the elbows while behind the patient. Overpressure can occur to one or both arms at the same time.

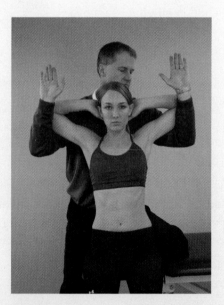

■ **Figure 8.5** Functional Abduction and External Rotation with and without Overpressure

Bilateral Internal Rotation/Extension and Adduction

The combined movement of internal rotation, extension, and adduction examines the mobility of numerous structures of the shoulder. Limitations of range may be associated with tightness of the posterior capsule, irritation of the biceps tendon, capsulitis and tenderness of the anterior capsule, or a number of other causes. It is essential to further examine a positive finding during active movements using passive movements to better isolate tightness or lack of stability.

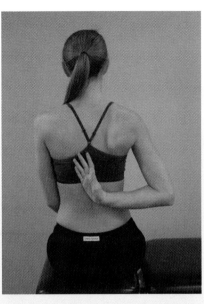

■ **Figure 8.6** Internal Rotation, Extension, and Adduction

1 The patient stands in the targeted posture and baseline symptoms are evaluated.

2 Starting with the uninvolved side first, the patient is instructed to lift his or her arm behind the back as high as he or she can reach (Figure 8.6 ■). The clinician uses his or her finger to identify the height reached.

3 The patient is instructed to perform the activity on the opposite symptomatic side.

4 The maximum heights between the symptomatic and asymptomatic side are compared for symmetry.

Apley's Scratch Test

Apley's Scratch Test is useful in assessing functional shoulder range of motion in the combined movements of abduction and external rotation and abduction and internal rotation.[36] The test is functional because the movements are required during daily activities such as donning and doffing shirts and undergarments, combing the hair, and hygiene activities.

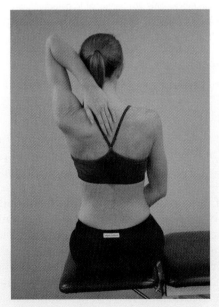

1 To assess this sequence of movements, the patient stands in the targeted posture.

2 Starting with the uninvolved side first, the patient is instructed to reach behind his or her head and touch as low as possible on the spine (Figure 8.7 ■).

■ **Figure 8.7** Abduction and External Rotation

(Continued)

③ The patient is then instructed to reach behind his or her back and reach the same aspect of the opposite shoulder blade now moving with the involved side.

④ The patient is prompted to try and touch the fingers of both hands during the combined movements of abduction and external rotation with one arm and adduction and internal rotation of the other (Figure 8.8 ■).

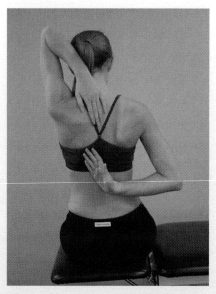

■ **Figure 8.8** Apley's Scratch Test

Summary

• Active physiological patterns of motion such as those associated with a theoretical capsular pattern fail to demonstrate validity at the shoulder. Shoulder impairments often demonstrate variable patterns of range of motion loss.

• Functional movements are beneficial to determine where in the active range of motion individuals report concordant signs.

Passive Movements

Passive Physiological Movements Passive physiological movement examination is beneficial in determining plane-based range of motion and articular-based translation of the glenohumeral joint. Passive movement patterns may or may not provide beneficial information in isolating causal structures. Selected movements such as decreases in internal range of motion are indicative of isolated pathology (typically impingement), although the ability to classify these pathologies is only fair to moderate.[37]

The use of combined movements is useful in the shoulder since there are a variety of ranges and hundreds of potential combinations of movements with the joint. Additionally, selected standards of the shoulder such as the loose-packed and close-packed position are variable and questionable.[38] The following procedures are recommended for assessment of passive physiological movements of the shoulder. Any modification of these positions is warranted if the modification finds the concordant movement of that patient.

Passive End-Feel for the Shoulder Cyriax proposed a verbal classification scheme called "end-feel" to describe the passive resistance of end range passive movement in a joint.[27] End feel is described in terms of resistance and pain expressed by the patient. For the shoulder, physical therapists who have evaluated end-feel have demonstrated moderate agreement for resistance and substantial agreement for report of pain by the patient.[39] Hayes and Peterson[40] reported substantial intra- and interrater reliability for shoulder abduction, adduction, and internal and external rotation.[41] Abnormal end-feels are more likely to be associated with a pain response than normal end feels.[41] Since a capsular pattern demonstrates variability and because clinicians often make decisions associated with mobilization or stretching based on end-feel assessment, agreement is an essential aspect for treatment decision making.

Shoulder Flexion

Passive shoulder flexion movements may be painful on patients with anterior impingement or in isolated cases of capsulitis or shoulder restriction associated with a rotator cuff tear. Shoulder flexion is most limited by the medial glenohumeral ligament.

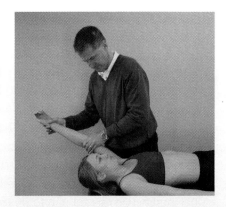

■ **Figure 8.9**   Passive Shoulder Flexion

1 The patient is placed at 0 degrees of shoulder flexion and internal/external rotation.

2 The clinician first addresses the noninvolved extremity and the patient is instructed to report the first incidence of pain during passive movement.

3 Slowly, the clinician elevates the upper extremity into flexion (Figure 8.9 ■). The range of motion (ROM) is recorded at the first reported incidence of pain and pain is evaluated to determine if concordant.

4 The clinician passively moves the shoulder beyond the first point of pain (if present) toward end range. End-feel of the shoulder end range is evaluated and the process is repeated for the opposite involved side.

Shoulder Abduction

Passive shoulder abduction movement may implicate restrictions of the capsule or impingement of the subacromial space. Additionally, significant capsular restrictions may be present if scapular movement occurs concurrently with glenohumeral movement during the first 30 degrees of abduction.

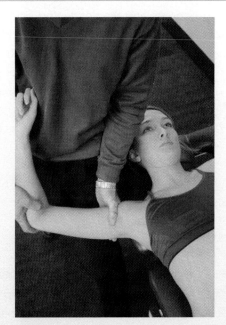

1 The patient is placed at 0 degrees of shoulder abduction and internal/external rotation and resting symptoms are evaluated.

2 The clinician first addresses the noninvolved extremity. Slowly, the clinician elevates the upper extremity into abduction (Figure 8.10 ■).

3 The patient is instructed to report the first incidence of pain during passive movement and the ROM is recorded at that range. Pain is evaluated to determine if concordant.

■ **Figure 8.10**   Passive Shoulder Abduction

4 Then, the clinician passively moves the shoulder beyond the first point of pain (if present) toward end range. End-feel of the shoulder's terminal range is evaluated and the process is repeated for the opposite involved side.

Shoulder External Rotation

Passive assessment of external rotation (ER) requires examination during different degrees of abduction to investigate fully the capsuloligamentous complex of the shoulder. The superior glenohumeral ligament is tensioned during external rotation at 0 degrees of abduction, the middle glenohumeral ligament is tensioned during the gradual increase in ranges of 0 to 90 degrees of abduction, and the inferior glenohumeral ligament is tensioned during passive external rotation at 90 degrees or more of abduction. A contextual relationship between passive external rotation and translatory glide and vice versa is well supported in the literature. Mihata et al.[42] found that external rotation stretching led to improvements in anterior, inferior, and anterior–posterior glide on cadaveric specimens. Excessive stretching leads to elongation of the anterior band of the inferior glenohumeral ligament. For careful evaluation of external rotation, the movement should be tested at 0, 45, and 90 degrees and the unaffected side should always be evaluated prior to the affected side.

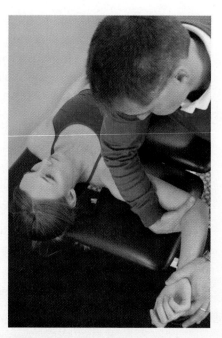

■ **Figure 8.11**   Stabilization Procedure for External Rotation

Typically, the movements of internal rotation (IR) and ER require stabilization of the anterior shoulder to reduce compensatory movements and false range of motion. This is accomplished by the clinician using his or her forearm to block the anterior aspect of the shoulder. The hand of the same arm cups the elbow to provide a pivot point for shoulder rotation (Figure 8.11 ■). The hand of the clinician may substitute for their forearm if the patient is small or if the clinician's arm is too long to function as a stabilizing and pivot source.

1. The patient is placed in supine.

2. When the involved extremity is tested, the shoulder is first placed in zero degrees of abduction. The hand of the clinician can stabilize the patient's anterior shoulder to reduce compensation (Figure 8.12 ■).

3. Slowly, the clinician passively rotates the upper extremity into external rotation.

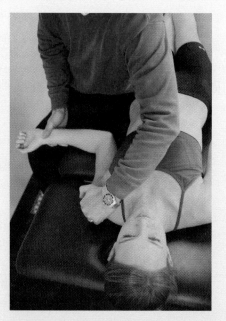

■ **Figure 8.12**   External Rotation at 0 Degrees of Abduction

④ The patient is instructed to report the first incidence of pain during passive movement and the ROM is recorded at that level. Pain is evaluated to determine if concordant.

⑤ The clinician passively moves the affected shoulder beyond the first point of pain (if present) toward end range and end-feel of the shoulder is evaluated.

⑥ To further examine external rotation the shoulder is moved to approximately 45 degrees of abduction.

⑦ Using his or her forearm, the clinician blocks the anterior aspect of the shoulder to prevent compensatory movement.

⑧ The hand of the same arm cups the elbow to provide a pivot point.

⑨ Baseline symptoms are evaluated.

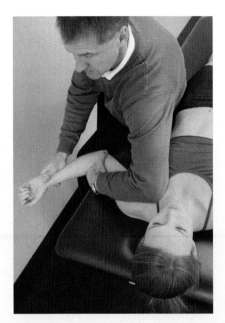

■ **Figure 8.13**   External Rotation at 45 Degrees of Abduction

⑩ Slowly, the clinician passively rotates the upper extremity into external rotation (Figure 8.13 ■) and the patient is instructed to report the first incidence of pain during passive movement. The ROM is recorded at the first reported incidence of pain and the pain is evaluated to determine if concordant.

⑪ The clinician passively moves the shoulder beyond the first point of pain (if present) toward end range and end-feel of the shoulder is evaluated.

⑫ Lastly, the shoulder is placed in abduction at 90 degrees.

⑬ Using his or her forearm, the clinician blocks the anterior aspect of the shoulder to prevent compensatory movement.

⑭ The hand of the same arm cups the elbow to provide a pivot point.

⑮ Baseline symptoms are evaluated.

⑯ Slowly, the clinician passively rotates the upper extremity into external rotation.

⑰ The patient is instructed to report the first incidence of pain during passive movement and the ROM is recorded at that level; pain is evaluated to determine if concordant.

⑱ The clinician passively moves the shoulder beyond the first point of pain (if present) toward end range (Figure 8.14 ■) and end-feel of the shoulder is evaluated.

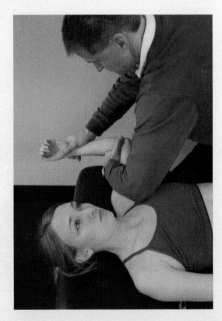

■ **Figure 8.14**   External Rotation at 90 Degrees of Abduction

Shoulder Passive Physiological Internal Rotation

Passive internal rotation movements should be assessed with the arm at the side (0 degrees) or at 70–90 degrees of abduction or flexion. In all cases, the posterior capsule contributes toward limiting movement but other structures may be indicted if pain is concordant in one movement and not another. Internal rotation during shoulder flexion places stress on the anterior structures of the shoulder and may be painful in asymptomatic shoulders. At 70–90 degrees, the inferior glenohumeral ligament and the inferior posterior capsule are tensioned and if restricted, may limit movement. For careful evaluation, the unaffected side should always be tested prior to the affected side.

Internal Rotation at 0 Degrees of Abduction

1. The patient is placed in supine position and the elbow is flexed to 90 degrees.

2. Using his or her hand, the clinician blocks the anterior aspect of the shoulder to prevent compensatory movement.

3. Slowly, the clinician passively rotates the upper extremity into internal rotation (Figure 8.15 ■).

4. The patient is instructed to report the first incidence of pain during passive movement and the ROM is recorded at that level; pain is evaluated to determine if concordant.

5. The clinician passively moves the shoulder beyond the first point of pain (if present) toward end range and end-feel of the shoulder is evaluated.

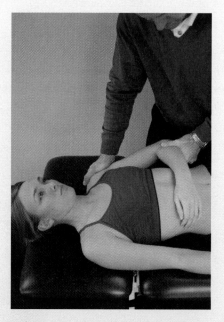

■ **Figure 8.15**   Internal Rotation at 0 Degrees of Abduction

Internal Rotation at 70–90 Degrees of Abduction

1. The patient is placed in supine position and the elbow is flexed to 90 degrees.

2. Using his or her forearm, the clinician blocks the anterior aspect of the shoulder to prevent compensatory movement.

3. The hand of the same arm cups the elbow to provide a pivot point; baseline symptoms are evaluated.

4. Slowly, the clinician passively rotates the upper extremity into internal rotation (Figure 8.16 ■).

5. The patient is instructed to report the first incidence of pain during passive movement and the ROM is recorded at level; pain is evaluated to determine if concordant.

6. The clinician passively moves the shoulder beyond the first point of pain (if present) toward end range and end-feel of the shoulder is evaluated.

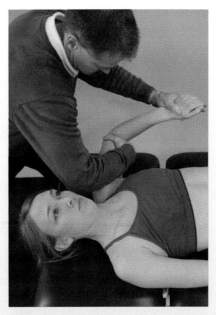

■ **Figure 8.16**   Internal Rotation at 70–90 Degrees of Abduction

Shoulder Horizontal Adduction

The passive movements into horizontal adduction may be limited because of tightness in the posterior capsule, pain in the anterior structures of the glenohumeral joint (anterior impingement syndrome), or secondary to pain in the acromioclavicular joint. Passive horizontal adduction with internal rotation of the glenohumeral joint may further engage the posterior capsule and may be necessary to ascertain fully the limitation (if present). It is essential to query the patient regarding the location of the pain, whether the pain is concordant, and to determine the potential reasons why the movement is painful.

Horizontal Adduction with Neutral Rotation

1. The patient is placed in supine position.

2. The clinician first addresses the noninvolved extremity.

3. The clinician stands to the side of the extremity evaluated.

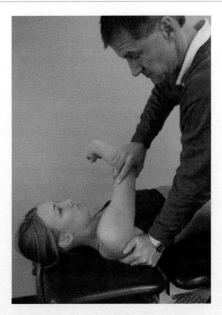

■ **Figure 8.17**   Horizontal Adduction at Neutral

(Continued)

④ Using the cephalic hand (left hand in Figure 8.17 ■), the clinician stabilizes the lateral border of the scapula. The opposite hand holds the elbow and functions to move the patient's extremity.

⑤ The patient is instructed to report the first incidence of pain during passive movement and the ROM is recorded at that level; pain is evaluated to determine if concordant.

⑥ The clinician passively moves the shoulder beyond the first point of pain (if present) toward end range.

Horizontal Adduction with Internal Rotation

① The patient is placed in supine position.

② The clinician stands to the side of the extremity evaluated.

③ Using the cephalic hand, the clinician stabilizes the lateral border of the scapula, while the opposite hand holds the elbow and functions to move the patient's extremity.

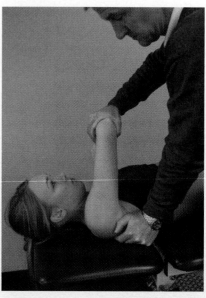

■ **Figure 8.18** Horizontal Adduction with Prepositioned Internal Rotation

④ The clinician passively internally rotates the extremity using the elbow as a lever. (Figure 8.18 ■).

⑤ The patient is instructed to report the first incidence of pain during passive movement and the ROM is recorded at that level; pain is evaluated to determine if concordant.

⑥ Then, the clinician passively moves the shoulder beyond the first point of pain (if present) toward end range.

Shoulder Passive Extension

Passive shoulder extension may be limited if the anterior structures of the glenohumeral capsule are restricted.

① The clinician first addresses the noninvolved extremity after placing the patient in supine.

② The patient is placed lateral to the edge of the table to allow the shoulder to clear the side of the table during extension and the patient is instructed to report the first incidence of pain during passive movement.

3 The clinician passively moves the shoulder into extension (Figure 8.19 ■) and the ROM is recorded at the first reported incidence of pain. Pain is evaluated to determine if concordant.

4 Then, the clinician passively moves the shoulder beyond the first point of pain (if present) toward end range.

5 The process is repeated on the involved, opposite side.

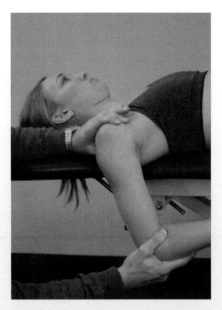

■ **Figure 8.19** Passive Physiological Extension

Summary

- The findings associated with end-feel and first point of resistance at the shoulder are reliable among clinicians.
- Because different capsuloligamentous components are responsible for resisting movements at different ranges, it is important to test movements such as internal and external rotation at varying degrees of flexion and abduction.
- Combining movements to increase the tension within the capsuloligamentous region may be necessary to isolate the concordant sign.

Passive Accessory Movements During pathology to the shoulder a prepositioning of the humeral head, either anteriorly or posteriorly in the joint, is common. Harryman et al.[43] suggested that this phenomenon is associated with asymmetric tightening of the capsule, a phenomenon that leads to translation of the humeral head in the opposite direction of the limited capsule. Subsequently, a tight posterior capsule would lead to a prepositioning of anterior translation at the glenohumeral joint, vice versa for a tight anterior capsule.

Joint mobilization techniques are beneficial for patients with shoulder restrictions and occasionally preferable to physiological stretching because the movements provide a precise stretch to the restricted aspect of the capsule (when prepositioned in the restricted position). This precision can typically occur with less infliction of pain, less required force, and less compression on painful structures.[44-46] Conroy and Hayes outline that joint mobilizations are effective in reducing pain and edema, through selective stretching of causative structures.[46] Selective stretching requires the administration of the appropriate force, in the targeted and appropriate direction, performed over a period of time.[47]

Mobilizations performed at end range have long been advocated for improvement of range of motion by many authors.[48,49] However, end ranges of motion do limit the amount of available translation of the humeral head.[50,51] Most notably, posterior-anterior (PA) translation decreases during prepositioning into external rotation of the shoulder. In contrast, anterior-posterior (AP) translation is not decreased during preposition of internal rotation of the shoulder.[50] Hsu and colleagues[51] reported that more displacement occurs during a PA glide than AP glide during prepositioning of abduction. Mobilizations at end range do lead to multidirectional improvements in range of motion for patients with adhesive capsulitis[52] and are appropriate for patients in which stiffness is their cardinal finding.

Glenohumeral Posterior Anterior (PA) Glide

A PA glide in a loose-packed position may not be helpful in improving range of motion for restricted abduction and/or external rotation.[51] A PA glide is equally effective for improving abduction as an AP when the humerus is placed in an end-range position.[51] A PA glide does lead to neurophysiological changes, including increased conductivity for the complete upper limb.[53]

PA for Pain Control

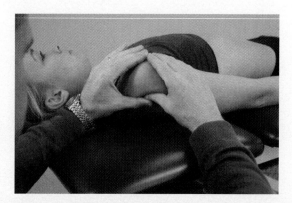

① The patient is placed in supine and their hands are draped across their stomach (not shown in Figure 8.20).

② The clinician uses both thumbs to contact the posterior aspect of the humeral head of the patient, whereas the fingers rest gently on the anterior surface of the patient's shoulder.

③ Using the side of the plinth as a lever, the clinician gently applies a force posterior to anterior first, then pulls downward on the humeral head to reposition the shoulder (Figure 8.20 ■). This technique is performed well within the tolerance of the patient and is repeated a number of times in order to incorporate pain reduction.

■ **Figure 8.20**   PA for Pain Relief

PA for Range-of-Motion Gains

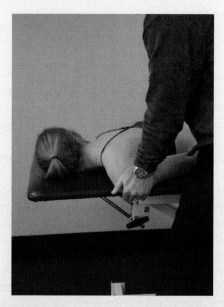

① The patient is placed in prone and resting symptoms are assessed.

② The clinician uses the palm of his or her hand to contact the posterior aspect of the shoulder (Figure 8.21 ■). To enhance the vigor of the mobilization the shoulder can be elevated (flexion or abduction) to the concordant limit of the patient.

③ Then, the clinician performs a PA mobilization at the range limitation of the patient. The use of external or internal rotation prepositioning furthers the effect of the end-range mobilization.

■ **Figure 8.21**   Prone PA for Range-of-Motion Gains

Glenohumeral Anterior–Posterior (AP) Glide

An AP glide in a loose-packed position may not be helpful in improving range of motion for abduction and/or internal rotation, specifically if internal rotation is limited toward the end of normal available range.[51] In a neutral position the middle posterior capsule limits AP translation whereas in a preposition of abduction, the middle and inferior posterior capsule limits movement.[54,55]

Mobilization, designed to improve shoulder flexion or abduction, is most appropriately performed at end range,[51] and since the majority of shoulder pathologies lead to anterior migration of the humeral head, an anterior to posterior glide may be the best selection. Conroy and Hayes[46] performed mobilizations at mid-range and theorized the lack of benefit may be associated with the inability to engage the capsule appropriately while in a loose-packed position.

1. The patient is placed in supine and resting symptoms are assessed.

2. The clinician glides the patient's shoulder to the first point of pain (Figure 8.22 ■).

3. If pain occurs before the onset of stiffness, the mobilization should be performed at that range using less intense force.

4. If stiffness is encountered concurrently or before pain, a more aggressive mobilization at that range or in preposition of shoulder flexion (Figure 8.23 ■) or abduction is beneficial.

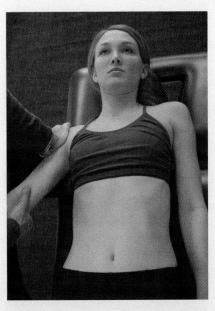

■ **Figure 8.22** Mobilization at Early AP Ranges

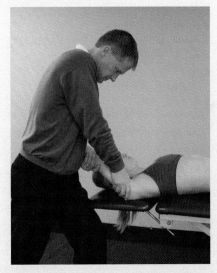

■ **Figure 8.23** End-Range AP Mobilization in Preposition of Flexion

Glenohumeral Shoulder Traction

A glenohumeral shoulder traction technique has not shown to lead to joint separation with the arm placed at the side near the loose-packed position or during a close-packed position.[38] Subsequently, a traction-based mobilization will primarily demonstrate neurophysiological benefits, specifically useful for patients with pain as the primary disorder.

1. The patient is placed in supine and resting symptoms are assessed.

2. The clinician may use his or her forearm to stabilize the anterior aspect of the shoulder. Placing the patient's forearm in pronation helps concentrate the traction force to the shoulder (Figure 8.24 ■).

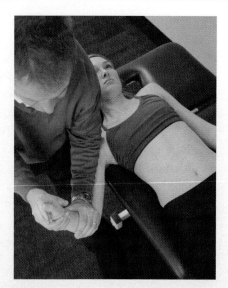

■ **Figure 8.24** Traction Mobilization for Pain Reduction

3. The clinician moves the patient's shoulder to the first point of pain by performing a long axis distraction force. The appropriate response of the mobilization is pain reduction.

Glenohumeral Inferior (Caudal) Glide

Hsu and colleagues[56] reported improvements in the mobility of cadaveric tissue when an inferior glide was applied to the shoulder at the end, or near end range, of abduction. The techniques used in the cadaveric study were effective for abduction mobility gains and were more effective than similar mobilization performed at 40 degrees of abduction (non–end range).

1. With the patient in a supine position the clinician prepositions the shoulder in neutral or slight abduction.

2. The clinician then glides the humeral head inferiorly to the first point of pain (Figure 8.25 ■). If pain occurs before the onset of stiffness, the mobilization should be performed at that range using less intense force.

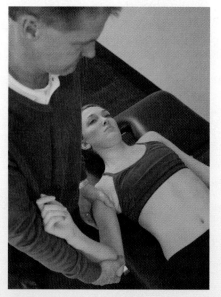

■ **Figure 8.25** Mobilization at Early Ranges of Inferior Glide

3 If stiffness is encountered concurrently or before pain, or if the pain of the patient only occurs at mid- or end-range abduction, an aggressive mobilization at those ranges is beneficial (Figure 8.26 ■).

4 Upon completion, the clinician should reassess the movement restriction of the patient.

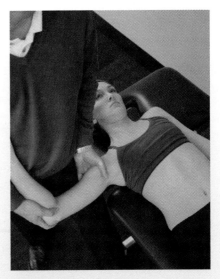

■ Figure 8.26   End-Range Inferior Glide Mobilization

Acromioclavicular PA Glide

The acromioclavicular joint translates posterior to anterior during scapular retraction.

1 To perform a similar movement of posterior to anterior translation, the patient should be placed in a supine position.

2 The clinician places his or her thumb in the posterior "V" notch (just posterior to the medial aspect of the AC joint). The contact point of the thumbs is on the posterior clavicle.

3 The clinician applies a PA glide to the AC (Figure 8.27 ■) in an attempt to reproduce symptoms. If concordant, the clinician may apply treatment using this technique and can adjust the position of the scapular to sensitize the movement.

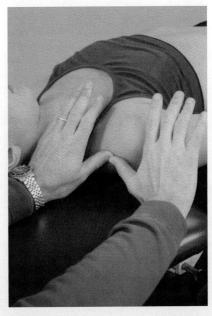

■ Figure 8.27   Acromioclavicular PA Mobilization

Acromioclavicular Inferior Glide

The clavicle moves inferiorly on the scapular (acromion) contact during arm elevation.

1. To perform a similar assessment technique, the patient assumes a supine position.

2. For inferior glide, the clinician places his or her thumb on the superior surface just medial to the AC joint (clavicular contact).

3. The clinician applies an inferior glide to the AC (Figure 8.28 ■) in an attempt to reproduce symptoms.

4. If concordant, the clinician may apply treatment using this technique, and can adjust the position of the scapula by moving the arm into flexion or abduction to further sensitize the movement (Figure 8.29 ■). The patient who responds best to this assessment/treatment is one that encounters pain only during end ranges of movements that are across the body or over his or her head.

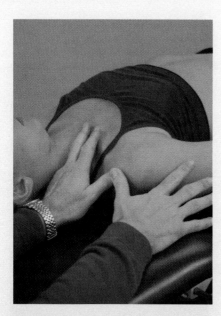

■ **Figure 8.28** Acromioclavicular Inferior Mobilization

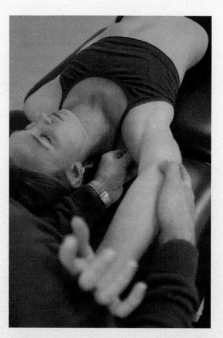

■ **Figure 8.29** Preposition of the Shoulder in Flexion to Enhance the Inferior Glide of the AC Joint

Acromioclavicular AP Glide

The clavicle moves posteriorly on the acromion during protraction and abduction of the scapula.

1. To assess a motion similar to this passively, the patient should be placed in a supine position.

2. The clinician places his or her thumb anterior on the "V" notch (just anterior to the medial aspect of the AC joint with a clavicular contact).

3. The clinician applies an AP glide to the AC (Figure 8.30 ■) in an attempt to reproduce symptoms. If concordant, the clinician may apply treatment using this technique and can adjust the position of the scapula through arm movements (such as flexion, abduction, or horizontal adduction) to sensitize the movement.

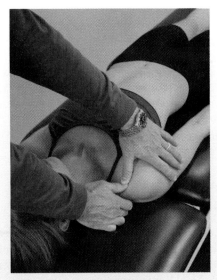

■ **Figure 8.30** Anterior–Posterior Mobilization of the AC Joint

Sternoclavicular (SC) Inferior Glide

The clavicle moves inferiorly with respect to the sternum during arm elevation. The motion involves both inferior translation of the medial clavicle and an upward rotation of the lateral aspect of the clavicle.

1. To test this movement, the patient assumes a supine position.

2. The clinician places his or her thumb superior to the SC joint, lateral to the actual joint space (clavicular contact).

3. The clinician applies an inferior glide to the medial clavicle (Figure 8.31 ■) in an attempt to reproduce symptoms. If concordant, the clinician may apply treatment using this technique and can adjust the position arm (greater or less arm elevation) to sensitize the movement.

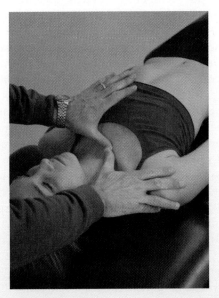

■ **Figure 8.31** Inferior Glide of the Sternoclavicular Joint

Summary

- Passive accessory movements are most appropriately assessed at early, mid, and end ranges of arm movement.

- Because most pathologies cause an anterior migration of the humeral head, an AP force may exhibit the most sensitivity as the concordant sign. However, this does not mean that this directional force is useful during treatment. A PA force may be most useful in normalizing movement.

- End-range accessory motions may be more beneficial in improving range of motion at the shoulder.

Special Clinical Tests

A useful special clinical test should help the examiner distinguish between disorders with symptoms that closely mimic one another. The tests are performed to shed additional light when the examiner is still unsure of the diagnosis after taking a thorough history and after performance of active physiological motions, passive physiological motions, and passive accessory motions. Palpation, muscle strength assessment, and physical examination tests (special tests) can be helpful in this elucidating role. Essentially, the special clinical test should be confirmatory in nature.

Palpation   Numerous authors have reported the benefit of palpation of the shoulder during differential diagnosis. Wolf and Agrawal[57] and Lyons and Tomlinson[58] described the accuracy of transdeltoid palpation (the Rent Test) in detecting full thickness rotator cuff tears. Palpation over the acromioclavicular (AC) joint was found to be highly sensitive though not specific in detecting AC joint pathology.[59] Palpation over the cervical spine may reproduce shoulder symptoms if the cause of the shoulder pain is actually cervical radiculopathy.[4] Subacromial impingement often hurts superiorly at the shoulder joint at the connection of the C4–5 dermatome.[4] Osteoarthritis is typically painful directly on the joint line of the patient, either anterior or posterior. Anterior impingement is often painful directly over the acromion but caution must be used during this assessment because any condition that causes anterior migration of the humeral head (and most conditions do cause this) will place pressure on the anterior soft-tissue structures and will be painful. A patient with rotator cuff weakness will often report pain over the upper trapezius but not the posterior cervical spine.[4]

Muscle Testing   Kelly et al.[60] used electromyography to determine the optimal test to isolate each rotator cuff muscle during the motions of elevation, internal rotation, and external rotation. They defined an optimal test as one with good test–retest reliability with maximum muscle activation while minimizing synergist activation and positional pain. The optimal supraspinatus test was the "full can," with the arms elevated to 90 degrees in the scapular plane with thumbs facing up. Testing the supraspinatus in the "empty can" position, which is 90 degrees of elevation in the scapular plane with full internal shoulder rotation, is a specific but not a sensitive test, useful only in ruling in subacromial impingement.

Although less investigated, selected positions may also improve the contractile capacity of the infraspinatus. According to Kelly et al.,[60] the infraspinatus was best tested with the patient's elbow at the side and flexed to 90 degrees, and the shoulder in 45 degrees of internal rotation.

"Giving way" due to weakness or pain was a specific but not sensitive test, useful in ruling in subacromial impingement.[60,61] The subscapularis was tested optimally, with the patient's arm behind his or her low back and lifted off of the low back (lift-off sign). The optimal test position of the teres minor muscle has not been as rigorously studied but the suggested position to isolate this muscle is with the patient in supine resisting an internal rotation force.[62] The best position in which to evaluate rotator cuff co-contraction is performed during placement of the fibers of the relevant muscles in optimal alignment to achieve relocation of the humeral head in the scapular plane.[63] The position that most closely reflects this is scaption.

Treatment Techniques

Previously, Winters and colleagues[64] classified variant forms of "shoulder pain" as (1) synovial in origin (glenohumeral joint); (2) shoulder girdle (may involve the cervical spine, thoracic spine, or other nonsynovial categories); and (3) combinations (both synovial and nonsynovial). Treatment benefit depended on the classification. For example, patients without a synovial component benefited from manipulative procedures more so than those with synovial problems. Consequently, careful attention and a comprehensive examination consisting of isolation of the concordant sign are crucial to classify the origin of the pain generator.

Similar to the interventions associated with the cervical and thoracic spine and all other regions of the body, treatment selection is predicated upon the findings of the examination. However, the complexities involved in the biomechanical variability of the shoulder require the clinician to understand the influences of the active structures of the shoulder and the benefit associated with targeting these structures during treatment. Subsequently, the clinician should always consider the potential merits associated with rotator cuff and upper quarter strengthening in addition to any form of intervention.

Active Physiological Movements   The majority of active physiological treatment interventions will take the form of active strengthening. A strengthening approach will depend on the form of impairment displayed by the patient and the level of recovery that patient exhibits. For example, for post-surgical patients, active physiological movements may consist of gentle pain-free movements or subthreshold isometric exercises versus a nonsurgical patient with impingement who may receive exercises that are more aggressive.

Active physiological movements to treat the shoulder in absence of strengthening may be less beneficial in the shoulder. The repeated movements or sustained positions of the concordant pain that are found during the shoulder examination will rarely reduce symptoms, specifically if the patient demonstrates impingement. The reader is suggested to explore additional books or articles that focus on the most efficient methods of shoulder strengthening.

One form of treatment that does not focus exclusively on shoulder movements is a postural-based intervention. This treatment may consist of active exercises (Figures 8.32 ■ and 8.33 ■) designed to target the cervical and thoracic posture, which indirectly

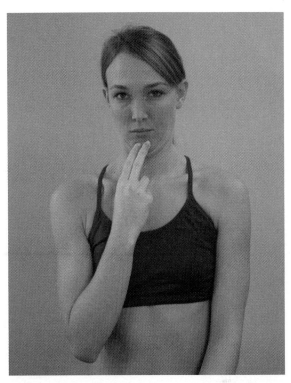

■ **Figure 8.33**   Repeated Neck Retraction for Improvement of Shoulder Range of Motion

improves the range of motion of the shoulder. Although a postural approach may not lead to reduction of pain in the shoulder, this approach has been shown to improve the overall range of motion of the shoulder or the total range available before pain is encountered.[65]

Passive Physiological Movements   Several methods of passive physiological stretching may be beneficial for treatment of the stiff shoulder. Since the findings of the examination will drive the treatment selection, repeated or sustained passive movements toward end range of a restricted or painful plane-based movement will identify the correct selection of the physiological stretch. Manually assisted movements such as contract–relax or hold–relax techniques (Figures 8.34 ■–8.38 ■) may prove beneficial and are often tolerated better during application. Because posterior capsule tightness is common in shoulder dysfunction and often corresponds with internal rotation restriction, hold–relax stretching of the internal rotators is of specific benefit.

Passive Accessory Movements/Mobilization   The biomechanics of the capsule of the shoulder allow for a significant amount of joint play when the humerus assumes early range of motions. Because of this, mobilization procedures to increase range of motion are generally more beneficial at end ranges (at the

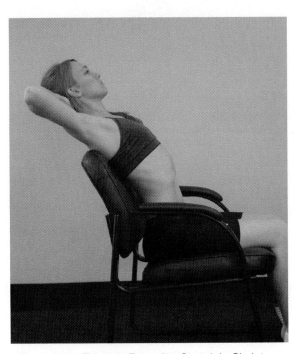

■ **Figure 8.32**   Thoracic Extension Stretch in Chair to Improve Shoulder Range of Motion

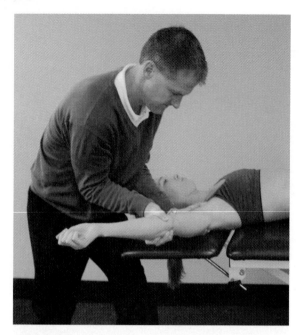

■ **Figure 8.34** Hold–Relax Stretching of Shoulder Abduction

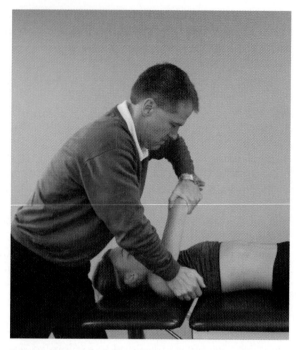

■ **Figure 8.36** Hold–Relax Stretching of Horizontal Adduction

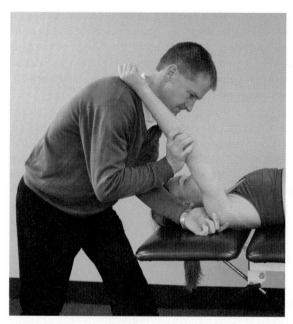

■ **Figure 8.35** Hold–Relax Stretching of Shoulder Flexion

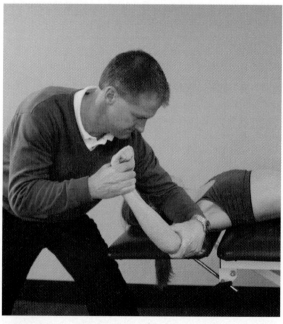

■ **Figure 8.37** Hold–Relax Stretching of External Rotation

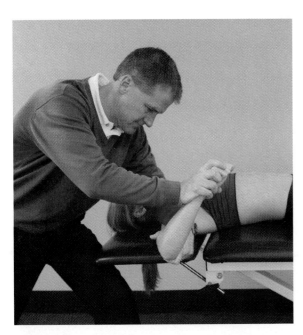

■ **Figure 8.38** Hold–Relax Stretching of Internal Rotation

range of motion restriction),[51] whereas early range of motions are more appropriate for patients who exhibit pain dominance and cannot tolerate aggressive mobilization at end range.

As with active and passive physiological applications, passive accessory techniques are borne from the examination. Applications that reproduce the concordant sign and subsequently reduce pain or increase range of motion after repeated movements or sustained holds are appropriate selections for treatment. Consequently, the passive accessory examination methods are all potential treatment selections for the glenohumeral, acromioclavicular, and sternoclavicular joints.

There are two instances in which subtle variations from the examination procedures are necessary and appropriate: (1) when the capsule would benefit from further tightening and (2) when the joints would benefit from a traction technique for pain control. Since these are not typically components of the examination (traction is sometimes used during the examination), the procedures require careful consideration.

Acromioclavicular (AC) and Sternoclavicular (SC) Traction

AC and SC traction may be beneficial when treating a patient whose primary problem is pain or when treating conditions associated with poor posture. Both joints can be targeted during the same application if the clinician makes minor adjustments in hand position.

1 The clinician places a rolled towel longitudinally on the treatment plinth parallel with the patient's spine.

2 The clinician stands to the side of the treatment plinth, opposite to the targeted joint.

3 The clinician stabilizes the side of the patient (nonaffected side) that is closest to him or her by placing his or her forearm on the sternum of the patient and by using his or her ulnar border to compress the clavicle downward toward the table.

4 To target the SC, the clinician places his or her nonstabilizing hand on the clavicle of the opposite side (left SC is being treated in Figure 8.39 ■) and places a traction force parallel with the clavicle.

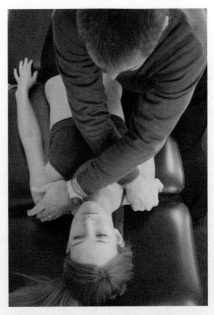

■ **Figure 8.39** Traction of the SC Joint

(Continued)

⑤ To target the AC and SC, the clinician places his or her nonstabilizing hand (left hand in Figure 8.40 ■) on the anterior head of the humerus and places a traction force away from the shoulder.

⑥ Treatment techniques may consist of a sustained hold or repeated movements.

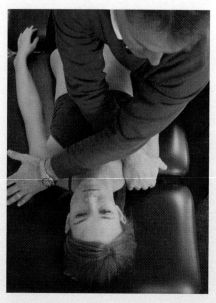

■ **Figure 8.40** Traction of the AC Joint

AC Mobilization in Preposition

The majority of the movement of the AC is required near end-range positions of glenohumeral flexion or abduction. Consequently, it is beneficial to mobilize the AC joint when the glenohumeral joint is prepositioned near end range.

① The patient assumes a supine position and the clinician elevates the patient's arm into flexion or abduction (requesting the patient's assistance in holding the extremity in place).

② The clinician then applies an inferior or anterior glide (whichever is concordant) in this preposition. In Figure 8.41 ■, a PA is demonstrated and the force from the clinician is from the lateral border of the index finger.

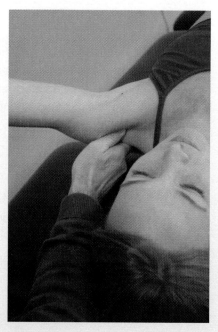

■ **Figure 8.41** AC Mobilization in Preposition

Posterior Capsule Mobilization in a Preposition of Internal Rotation and Adduction

A restriction of the posterior capsule frequently contributes to range-of-motion losses and impairment at the shoulder.[43,66] Because the capsule is difficult to isolate during a planar mobilization, prepositioning of the glenohumeral joint may improve the likelihood of isolating the structure.

1. The procedure is performed with the patient in the supine position.

2. The clinician stabilizes the shoulder blade with his or her arm that is cephalad to the patient (right hand in Figure 8.42 ■) while standing at the side of the involved extremity of the patient.

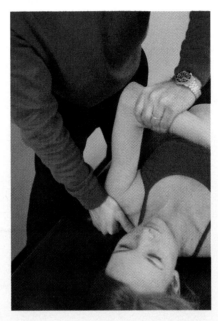

■ **Figure 8.42** Preposition and Stabilization of the Shoulder

3. The clinician then internally rotates (to end range), adducts (just past midline), and flexes (to approximately 90 degrees) the targeted shoulder to "wind up" the posterior capsule. The cephalad arm stabilizes the patient's shoulder blade to prevent the migration toward the patient's head.

4. While maintaining the stabilization and preposition the clinician then applies an inferior force along the shaft of the humerus (Figure 8.43 ■). The patient reports the feeling of a sharp sensation on the posterior capsule, not the medial aspect of the humerus. If pain is felt medially, structures are likely impinged, and the clinician should readjust the position.

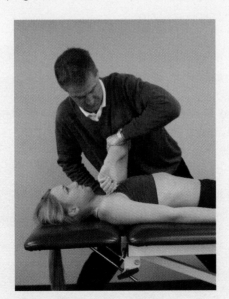

■ **Figure 8.43** Posterior Capsule Mobilization

A posterior glide has been shown to be a more effective mobilization method in improving external rotation than a posterior–anterior approach, an approach that is advocated by the convex-concave rule.[67] In addition, mobilization methods at end range (mobilization at the limit or at pain)[51] and high-grade (stronger) mobilizations both lead to better outcomes.[52]

Compression and Distraction in the Shoulder Quadrant

Maitland[68] advocated the use of compression and distraction procedures in the quadrant position to target joint and capsular structures. The quadrant position involves several combined movements of (1) internal rotation, abduction, and extension and (2) external rotation, flexion, and abduction. Theoretically, the movements engage the tension of the capsule throughout the available combined ranges of the glenohumeral joint and may demonstrate significant reproduction of symptoms from the patient.

① The technique is performed with the patient in a supine position.

② To initiate the quadrant, the clinician moves the patient's shoulder toward the combined movement of internal rotation, abduction, and extension (Figure 8.44 ■).

③ During treatment, clinicians may apply either traction or compressive forces if these forces elicit further symptoms. A more detailed description of the quadrant technique and all of the facets associated with these maneuvers is available in Maitland's book on peripheral manipulation.[68]

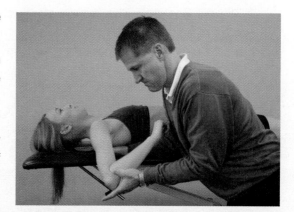

■ **Figure 8.44** The Combined Movement of Internal Rotation, Abduction, and Extension

④ To complete the full movement of the quadrant, the clinician then slowly moves the shoulder throughout the ranges of abduction by allowing external rotation to replace the prepositioning of internal rotation (Figure 8.45 ■).

⑤ The shoulder is slowly moved toward the patient's head, in search of a position that targets the concordant sign of the patient.

⑥ Once the concordant position is found, the clinician can apply a compressive or distractive force. As with all techniques, repeated movements or sustained holds should result in a reduction of symptoms for the treatment to be considered beneficial and appropriate.

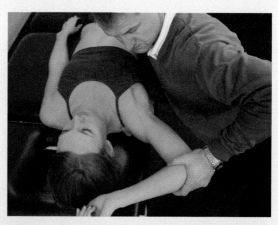

■ **Figure 8.45** Compressive or Distractive Force During Preposition of External Rotation, Abduction, and Flexion

Mobilization with Movement Mobilization with movement techniques incorporate a passive application by the clinician with an active movement by the patient.

Active End-Range Flexion with Downward Glide

Techniques performed at end range designed to promote the final degrees of flexion are typically incorporated in the final stages of an intervention.

1. One method, designed to promote end-range gains, is performed in supine position.

2. The clinician places his or her hand posteriorly to the shoulder and provides a caudal (and slide anterior) glide to the shoulder while the patient moves actively into shoulder flexion. The clinician may use his or her other hand to enhance the movement of active flexion (Figure 8.46 ■).

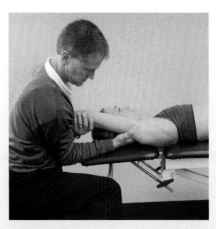

■ **Figure 8.46**   Active End-Range Flexion with Downward Glide

Active End-Range Abduction with Downward Glide

A mobilization with movement technique to promote the final degrees of abduction is also performed in supine.

1. The patient assumes the supine position.

2. The clinician places his or her hand superiorly to the shoulder and provides a caudal glide to the shoulder while the patient

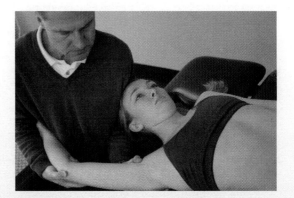

■ **Figure 8.47**   Active End-Range Abduction with Downward Glide

moves actively into shoulder abduction. The clinician may use his or her other hand to enhance the active abduction (Figure 8.47 ■).

Active Internal Rotation with Anterior to Posterior Glide

Often, patients with limited shoulder internal rotation will have tightness in his or her posterior capsule. An AP glide and active movement into internal rotation are both designed to stretch the posterior capsule.

The technique is performed in supine and the clinician places his or her hand anteriorly to the shoulder and provides an AP glide while the patient moves actively into internal rotation (Figure 8.48 ■). The clinician may use his or her other hand to enhance the active internal rotation.

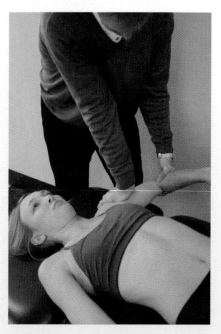

■ **Figure 8.48** Active Internal Rotation with Anterior to Posterior Glide

Active Shoulder Flexion or Abduction with AC Joint Anterior Glide

A mobilization with movement technique that engages end-range flexion and/or abduction involves an anterior and caudal glide of the AC. The technique is performed in supine and is performed near end range of flexion or abduction. Active movement is critical to improve the outcome of the treatment and may consist of either flexion or abduction (Figure 8.49 ■).

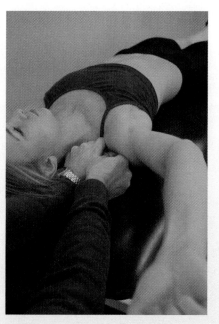

■ **Figure 8.49** Active Shoulder Flexion/Abduction with AC Joint Anterior Glide

Shoulder Manipulation

For a patient that primarily demonstrates stiffness with no signs of instability, a manipulative procedure may be beneficial to improve range of motion.[64] Generally, the manipulative procedure involves a posterior force applied to the humerus upon a fixed scapula, and because the procedure is very vigorous, it should only be considered for a select patient population. A patient who demonstrates instability, frailty, or is fearful of the technique is not a candidate for the procedure.

1. The technique is performed in a supine position.

2. Similar to the set-up and preposition of the mobilization to the posterior capsule described earlier, the clinician internally rotates, adducts, and flexes the shoulder.

3. Instead of singularly blocking the shoulder from superior migration, the clinician also elevates the scapula from the treatment table by placing his or hand under the scapula (Figure 8.50 ■). By blocking the spine of the scapula superiorly, the clinician prevents the superior migration.

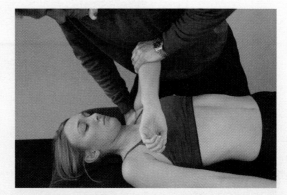

■ **Figure 8.50** The Glenohumeral Manipulation

4. The clinician applies a load through the humerus to take up the capsular slack. Once the slack of the capsule has been taken up, the clinician applies a series of quick thrusts through the humerus. Occasionally, an audible will accompany the manipulation.

Posterior Capsule Stretching

There are number of methods available to stretch the posterior capsule as a component of a home program. One of the most common, referred to as the "sleeper stretch,"

1. The clinician places the patient on his or her side and abducts the shoulder to 90 degrees.

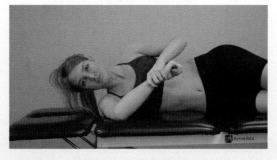

■ **Figure 8.51** The Sleeper Stretch

2. The shoulder is internally rotated to tension and held in that position (Figure 8.51 ■). The tension is held for 15–30 seconds.

(Continued)

Izumi et al.[69] suggest a modification to target the upper and lower capsule. The authors recommend 30 degrees of extension followed by internal rotation. The position is tensioned and held for 15–30 seconds (Figure 8.52 ■).

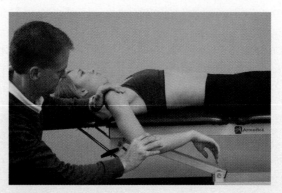

■ **Figure 8.52** Posterior Capsule (Upper and Lower Capsule) Stretch

Scapulothoracic Mobilization/Stretching

In some instances, scapulothoracic mobilization or stretching is beneficial for improving mobility of the upper quadrant. The procedure may lead to postural improvements and is generally very relaxing to a patient who has high levels of pain.

1. The patient assumes a sidelying position, facing the clinician.

2. The non-plinth-sided arm of the patient is secured to the clinician by placing the thumb of the patient in a belt loop or by having the patient relax his or hand on the clinician's hip.

3. The clinician secures the inferior border of the scapula with his or her caudal-most hand and does the same for the spine of the scapula with the cephalad-most hand (Figure 8.53 ■).

4. The clinician can apply a downward, medial, lateral, or upward force of the scapula and may combine the movements if desired.

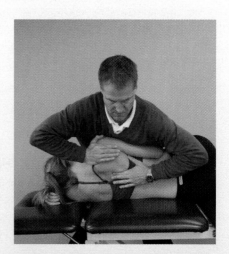

■ **Figure 8.53** Multidirectional Mobilization of the Scapulothoracic Joint

The technique selected should depend on patient tolerance, the restriction identified, and the concordant findings of the patient.

Summary

- Active physiological movements associated with strengthening should be a part of most manual therapy shoulder-related interventions.

- Some postural exercises may assist in improving range of motion in the shoulder, but will not likely reduce the pain associated with the shoulder impairment.

- The most effective and sensitive passive physiological movements are commonly associated with combined movements.

- Hold–relax stretching is helpful in allowing the patient to control the force of the stretch targeted at the guilty structure.

- Selection of the passive accessory mobilization method is based on the findings of the examination or careful assessment of dominance of pain versus stiffness.

- Compression and distraction techniques may further improve or isolate the structure targeted during the treatment application.

Treatment Outcomes

The Evidence

Mobilization with Movement   There appears to be Level B evidence that mobilization with movement and massage improve pain and active elevation in the scapular plane in patients with mechanical shoulder pain[70] and that mobilization with movement increases overall range of motion of the shoulder.[71]

Mobilization   There is Level B evidence that massage, manual therapy (mobilization), and exercise is more beneficial than exercise alone in patients with subacromial impingement syndrome.[72] Beyond these applications, there is predominantly Level C evidence that manual therapy is no more effective than other interventions when treating pain or lost motion and conflicting evidence about the effect of manual therapy with regard to the restoration of function.[73]

There is less evidence that manual therapy is beneficial for patients with adhesive capsulitis. Mobilization has been shown to be less effective than steroid injections[74] and benefits may depend on the prognostic phase during which the shoulder is encountered. One study, which claimed the comparison of joint mobilization with patients exhibiting adhesive capsulitis, provided very liberal inclusion criteria that most likely included patients with stiffness but not actual adhesive capsulitis.[75] The author reported significant improvement in passive shoulder abduction in patients that received various inferior, anterior, and posterior glide-based joint mobilization techniques but no reduction in pain.[75] In general, the evidence seems to support that higher grades of mobilization are superior to lower grades with respect to improvements in function in patients with adhesive capsulitis.[73]

Function may improve in the short term in patients with subacromial impingement syndrome who receive manual therapy[71,76] along with strengthening. In a high-quality study, Conroy and Hayes[77] found that soft-tissue mobilization was no less effective than joint mobilization in patients with impingement. Senbursa and colleagues[78] found improvements using a multimodal manual therapy technique (mobilization and soft-tissue mobilization) over strengthening alone.

Not surprisingly, in patients given the generic diagnosis of shoulder pain or dysfunction (a group composed of heterogeneous subgroups), there is Level C (conflicting evidence from strong randomized controlled studies) evidence that manual therapy is beneficial in the short term when compared to other usual physical therapy interventions.[73] In the long term, there is Level C evidence that manual therapy is no more effective than usual care for pain or functional improvement, but that manual therapy does improve active shoulder range of motion.[73] In many cases, the lack of effectiveness of manual therapy may be attributed to widely varying definitions of manual therapy and the heterogeneous nature of the patient population under study.

Manipulation   Mobilization and manipulation were found to be superior to modalities and/or steroid injections in the treatment of classified shoulder girdle patients.[64] The authors classified patients based on complaints that were: (1) isolated to the shoulder, (2) were referred from other structures such as the cervical or thoracic spine, and (3) were a mixture of both regions. Although this finding does not profoundly implicate the use of manipulation for the shoulder, it does support the use of manipulation for pain-referring structures that mimic shoulder conditions. Patients who demonstrated "synovial pain" that was associated with the shoulder actually improved quicker using injection therapy than forms of manual therapy and modalities.

Stretching   Posterior capsule stretching has been shown to improve shoulder movements.[79] Of the many that exist, the cross-body stretch has demonstrated the greatest improvement in treatment of a tight posterior capsule.[80] Unfortunately, there are no studies that have investigated the long-term benefits (Level D).

Manipulation of Regions Outside the Direct Intervention of the Shoulder Boyles and colleagues[81] demonstrated immediate and short-term (48-hour) benefits using thoracic spine manipulation on patients with impingement syndrome of the shoulder. The study demonstrated changes in both pain and disability scores. McClatchie et al.[82] provided mobilization to asymptomatic cervical spines of 21 subjects with shoulder pain and found immediate effects of pain reduction and improved range of motion of the shoulder. Others have suggested that mobilizing the upper quarter in addition to the shoulder is beneficial.[64,72] At this point, Level B evidence suggests a conjunctive program may provide short-term benefits.

Summary

- Moderate evidence exists that demonstrates the benefits of mobilization with movement and massage for patients with nonspecific shoulder pain/dysfunction
- Evidence exists that demonstrates the benefits of mobilization, exercise, and massage for patients with impingement syndrome while Level B evidence suggests mobilization is no more helpful for adhesive capsulitis than usual care.
- Patients with synovial pain may benefit from a cortisone injection versus mobilization or manipulation.
- Studies in this area may suffer from widely varying definitions of manual therapy and the use of heterogeneous patient populations.

Chapter Questions

1. Describe the clinical utility and validity of selected theoretical constructs such as the capsular pattern and convex–concave rule, and the benefit of these constructs to treatment intervention.

2. Describe the biomechanical relationship between the clavicle, the scapula, and the humerus during shoulder movements.

3. Describe how posture can affect shoulder range of motion.

4. Outline which of the concurrent movements of the spine are necessary for shoulder elevation.

5. Identify why combined movements are often beneficial and necessary to target capsuloligamentous tissues of the shoulder.

6. Outline the evidence associated with manual therapy treatment of the shoulder.

Patient Cases

Case 8.1: Kyle Sistrunk (43-year-old male)

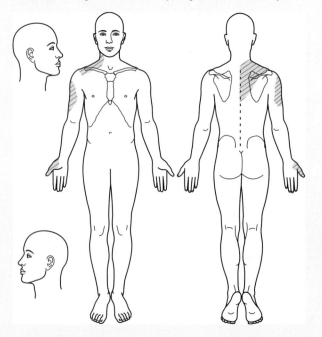

Diagnosis: Impingement syndrome

Observation: He exhibits significant kyphosis, rounded shoulders, and a flattened neck. There is no visual atrophy of the shoulder.

Mechanism: He notes an insidious onset.

Concordant Sign: His worst pain occurs while working on projects in front of him.

Nature of the Condition: He indicates he tolerates the condition fine and it does not impede his work. Once his shoulder and arm symptoms are flared up, it takes several hours to calm these down.

Behavior of the Symptoms: The pain in the shoulder migrates toward the thumb when symptoms are at their worst.

Pertinent Patient History: He reports a history of chronic low back pain.

Patient Goals: He is concerned he is losing strength in his right arm and would like to address the shoulder problem and the loss of strength he is experiencing.

Baseline: At rest, 3/10 NAS for pain; when worst, 4/10 pain.

Examination Findings: Arm and shoulder pain are worse during shoulder abduction and external rotation during both active and passive activities. Passive accessory movements do not reproduce his shoulder or arm pain.

1. Based on these findings, what else would you like to examine?
2. Is this patient a good candidate for manual therapy?
3. What is the expected prognosis of this patient?
4. What treatments do you feel presented in this book may be beneficial for this patient?

Case 8.2: Mindy Sims (14-year-old female)

Diagnosis: Impingement syndrome

Observation: Mindy exhibits forward head posture with rounded shoulders. Her posture is characteristic of a competitive swimmer.

Mechanism: Mindy indicated that she started experiencing soreness in her shoulders well over 12 months ago.

Concordant Sign: As a butterfly specialist (swim stroke), Mindy indicates her pain is worse during the active abduction and external rotation phase of the stroke.

Nature of the Condition: Her symptoms are manageable but have increased over the last 6 months. She swims well over 5,000 meters per day and manages to tolerate the pain despite this. She takes naproxen to reduce the symptoms.

Behavior of the Symptoms: The pain is isolated in the shoulder most of the time but when flared up will refer down into the elbow and into the middle finger.

Pertinent Patient History: Nothing pertinent.

Patient Goals: She is concerned about the chronicity of her pain and how it will impact her swim career.

Baseline: The pain in her shoulder at rest is 2/10; when flared up, 6/10.

Examination Findings: She exhibits pain during active flexion and abduction, demonstrated pain during APs, and has weakness of the scapular muscles and external rotators. She

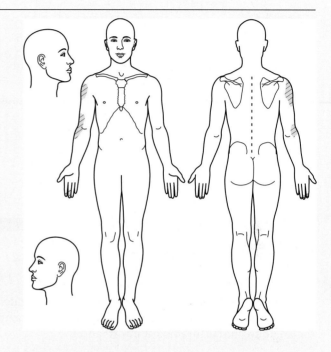

exhibits significant stiffness during internal rotation, flexion, and adduction.

1. Based on these findings, what else would you like to examine?
2. Is this patient a good candidate for manual therapy?
3. What is the expected prognosis of this patient?
4. What treatments do you feel presented in this book may be beneficial for this patient?

Case 8.3: Lilly Ardent (45-year-old female)

Diagnosis: Adhesive capsulitis

Observation: She exhibits significant kyphosis in mid-thoracic region and upper thoracic spine.

Mechanism: Insidious onset. Symptoms have been present for well over 12 months.

Concordant Sign: Trying to fasten her bra or reach in her back pocket.

Nature of the Condition: Her symptoms were much worse 6 months ago, so much so that it substantially impacted her activities of daily living. Her condition has improved and now tolerates self-stretching and strengthening without long periods of pain afterward. She takes ibuprofen to reduce the symptoms.

Behavior of the Symptoms: The pain is isolated in the shoulder region. During aggressive stretching she reports pain in the scapular region as well.

Pertinent Patient History: Diagnosed with lung cancer 4 years ago and is currently in remission.

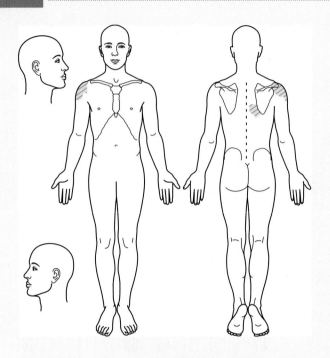

Patient Goals: She is interested in increasing the mobility and function of her arm.

Baseline: Her baseline pain at rest is 3/10; 6/10 when heavily provoked.

Examination Findings: All active and passive physiological findings demonstrate a full one-third loss of range in all planes. Passive accessory movements are all restricted and concordant.

1. Based on these findings, what else would you like to examine?
2. Is this patient a good candidate for manual therapy?
3. What is the expected prognosis of this patient?
4. What treatments do you feel presented in this book may be beneficial for this patient?

PEARSON
myhealthprofessionskit

Use this address to access the Companion Website created for this textbook. Simply select "Physical Therapy" from the choice of disciplines. Find this book and log in using your username and password to access video clips and the anatomy and arthrological information.

References

1. Walsh RM, Sadowski GE. Systemic disease mimicking musculoskeletal dysfunction: A case report involving referred shoulder pain. *J Orthop Sports Phys Ther.* 2001;31(12):696–701.

2. Petchkrua W, Harris SA. Shoulder pain as an unusual presentation of pneumonia in a stroke patient: A case report. *Arch Phys Med Rehabil.* 2000;81(6):827–829.

3. Khaw PY, Ball DL. Relief of non-metastatic shoulder pain with mediastinal radiotherapy in patients with lung cancer. *Lung Cancer.* 2000;28(1):51–54.

4. Manifold SG, McCann PD. Cervical radiculitis and shoulder disorders. *Clin Orthop Relat Res.* 1999;368:105–113.

5. Gorski JM, Schwartz LH. Shoulder impingement presenting as neck pain. *J Bone Joint Surg Am.* 2003; 85-A(4):635–638.

6. Baquie P. Sports medicine. Dead arm. *Aust Fam Physician.* 1997;26(11):1336–1337.

7. Woodward T, Best T. The painful shoulder: Part I. Clinical evaluation. *Am Fam Physician.* 2000;61:3079–3088.

8. Priest J, Nagel D. Tennis shoulder. *Am J Sports Med.* 1976;4(1):28–42.

9. Bak K, Fauno P. Clinical findings in competitive swimmers with shoulder pain. *Am J Sports Med.* 1997;25(2):254–260.

10. Ludewig P, Cook T. Translations of the humerus in persons with shoulder impingement syndrome. *J Orthop Sports Phys Ther.* 2002;32(6):248–259.

11. Hess S. Functional stability of the glenohumeral joint. *Man Ther.* 2000;5(2):63–71.

12. Weiser WM, Lee TQ, McMaster WC, McMahon PJ. Effects of simulated scapular protraction on anterior glenohumeral stability. *Am J Sports Med.* 1999;27(6):801–805.

13. Cools AM, Witvrouw EE, Danneels LA, Cambier DC. Does taping influence electromyographic muscle activity in the scapular rotators in healthy shoulders? *Man Ther.* 2002;7(3):154–162.

14. Michener L, McClure P, Karduna A. Anatomical and biomechanical mechanisms of subacromial impingement syndrome. *Clin Biomech.* 2003;18:369–379.

15. Crawford H, Jull G. The influence of thoracic posture and movement on the range of arm elevation. *Physiother Theory Pract.* 1993;9:143–148.

16. Solem-Bertoft E, Thuomas KA, Westerberg CE. The influence of scapular retraction and protraction on the width of the subacromial space. An MRI study. *Clin Orthop Relat Res.* 1993;(296):99–103.

17. Bullock MP, Foster NE, Wright CC. Shoulder impingement: The effect of sitting posture on shoulder pain and range of motion. *Man Ther.* 2005;10(1):28–37.

18. Culham E, Peat M. Functional anatomy of the shoulder complex. *J Orthop Sports Phys Ther.* 1993;18(1):342–350.

19. Litaker D, Pioro M, El Bilbeisi H, Brems J. Returning to the bedside: Using the history and physical examination to identify rotator cuff tears. *J Am Geriatr Soc.* 2000;48:1633–1637.

20. Miranda H, Viikari-Juntura E, Heistaro S, Heliovaara M, Riihimaki H. A population study on differences in the determinants of a specific shoulder disorder versus nonspecific shoulder pain without clinical findings. *Am J Epidemiol.* 2005;161:847–855.

21. Ostergren PO, Hanson BS, Balogh I, et al. Incidence of shoulder and neck pain in a working population: Effect modification between mechanical and psychosocial exposures at work? Results from a one year follow up of the Malmo shoulder and neck study cohort. *J Epidemiol Comm Health.* 2005;59(9):721–728.

22. Nahit ES, Pritchard CM, Cherry NM, Silman AJ, Macfarlane GJ. The influence of work related psychosocial factors and psychological distress on regional musculoskeletal pain: A study of newly employed workers. *J Rheumatol.* 2001;28:1378–1384.

23. Vasseljen O, Holte KA, Westgaard RH. Shoulder and neck complaints in customer relations: individual risk factors and perceived exposures at work. *Ergonomics.* 2001;44(4):355–372.

24. Jull-Kristensen B, Sogaard K, Stroyer J, Jensen C. Computer users' risk factors for developing shoulder, elbow and back symptoms. *Scand J Work Environ Health.* 2004;30:390–398.

25. van der Windt DA, Thomas E, Pope DP, et al. Occupational risk factors for shoulder pain: a systematic review. *Occup Environ Med.* 2000;57:433–442.

26. Reeves B. The natural history of the frozen shoulder syndrome. *Scand J Rheumatol.* 1975;4(4):193–196.

27. Cyriax J. *Textbook of orthopedic medicine. Vol 1: Diagnosis of soft tissue lesions.* 7th ed. New York; Macmillan: 1978.

28. Rundquist P, Ludewig P. Patterns of motion loss in subjects with idiopathic loss of shoulder range of motion. *Clin Biomech.* 2004;19:810–818.

29. Rundquist PJ, Anderson DD, Guanche CA, Ludewig PM. Shoulder kinematics in subjects with frozen shoulder. *Arch Phys Med Rehabil.* 2003;84:1473–1479.

30. Mitsch J, Casey J, McKinnis R, Kegerreis S, Stikeleather J. Investigation of a consistent pattern of motion restriction in patients with adhesive capsulitis. *J Man Manip Ther.* 2004;12:153–159.

31. Magrarey M, Jones M. Clinical evaluation, diagnosis and passive management of the shoulder complex. *New Zealand J Physiother.* 2004;32:55–66.

32. Poppen HK, Walker PS. Normal and abnormal motion of the shoulder. *J Bone Joint Surg.* 1976;58A:195–201.

33. Magarey ME, Jones MA. Specific evaluation of the function of force couples relevant for stabilization of the glenohumeral joint. *Man Ther.* 2003;8(4):247–253.

34. Mulligan BR. The painful dysfunctional shoulder: A new treatment approach using 'Mobilisation with Movement'. *New Zealand J Physiother.* 2003;31:140–142.

35. Terry GC, Hammon D, France P, Norwood LA. The stabilizing function of passive shoulder restraints. *Am J Sports Med.* 1991;19:26–34.

36. Woodward T, Best T. The painful shoulder: Part II. Acute and chronic disorders. *Am Fam Physician.* 2000;61(11):3291–3300.

37. de Winter A, Jans M, Scholten R, Deville W, van Schaardenburg D, Bouter L. Diagnostic classification of shoulder disorders: Interobserver agreement and determinants of disagreement. *Ann Rheum Dis.* 199;58:272–277.

38. Gokeler A, Paridon-Edauw GH, DeClercq S, Matthijs O, Dijkstra PU. Quantitative analysis of traction in the glenohumeral joint: In vivo radiographic measurements. *Man Ther.* 2003;8:97–102.

39. Chesworth B, MacDermid J, Roth J, Patterson S. Movement diagram and "end feel" reliability when measuring passive lateral rotation of the shoulder in patients with shoulder pathology. *Phys Ther.* 1998;78:593–601.

40. Hayes K, Peterson C. Reliability of assessing end-feel and pain and resistance sequence in subjects with painful shoulders and knees. *J Orthop Sports Phys Ther.* 2001;31:432–445.

41. Peterson CM, Hayes W. Construct validity of Cyriax's selective tension examination: Association of end-feels with pain at the knee and shoulder. *J Orthop Sports Phys Ther.* 2000;30:512–527.

42. Mihata T, Lee Y, McGarry MH, Abe M, Lee TQ. Excessive humeral external rotation results in increased shoulder laxity. *Am J Sports Med.* 2004;32(5):1278–1285.

43. Harryman DT, Sidles JA, Harris SL, et al. Translation of the humeral head on the glenoid with passive glenohumeral motion. *J Bone Jnt Surg.* 1990;79A(9):1334–1343.

44. Johns R, Wright V. Relative importance of various tissues in joint stiffness. *J Appl Physiol.* 1962;17:824–830.

45. Lundberg J. The frozen shoulder. Clinical and radiographical observations. The effect of manipulation under general anesthesia. Structure and glycosaminoglycan content of the joint capsule. Local bone metabolism. *Acta Orthop Scand.* 1969;Suppl 119:1–59.

46. Conroy D, Hayes K. The effect of joint mobilization as a component of comprehensive treatment for primary shoulder impingement syndrome. *J Orthop Sports Phys Ther.* 1998;28(1):3–14.

47. Warren J, Micheli L, Arslanian L, Kennedy J, Kennedy R. Scapulothoracic motion in normal shoulders and shoulders with glenohumeral instability and impingement syndrome. *Clin Orthop.* 1971;285:191–199.

48. Edmond SL. *Manipulation and mobilization: Extremities and spinal techniques.* St Louis, Mo; Mosby: 1993.

49. Wadsworth CT. Frozen shoulder. *Phys Ther.* 1986;66(12): 1878–1883.

50. Moore SM, Musahl V, McMahon PJ, Debski RE. Multidirectional kinematics of the glenohumeral joint during simulated simple translation tests: Impact on clinical diagnoses. *J Orthop Res.* 2004;22(4):889–894.

51. Hsu AT, Hedman T, Chang JH, Vo C, Ho L, Ho S, Chang GL. Changes in abduction and rotation range of motion in response to simulated dorsal and ventral translational mobilization of the glenohumeral joint. *Phys Ther.* 2002;82(6):544–556.

52. Vermeulen HM, Obermann WR, Burger BJ, Kok GJ, Rozing PM, van den Ende CH. End range mobilization techniques in adhesive capsulitis of the should joint: A multiple subject case report. *Phys Ther.* 2000;80:1204–1213.

53. Simon R, Vicenzino B, Wright A. The influence of an anteroposterior accessory glide of the glenohumeral joint on measures of peripheral sympathetic nervous system function in the upper limb. *Man Ther.* 1997; 2(1):18–23.

54. O'Brien SJ, Schwartz RS, Warren RF, Torzilli PA. Capsular restraints to anterior–posterior motion of the abducted shoulder: A biomechanical study. *J Shoulder Elbow Surg.* 1995;4:298–308.

55. Brenneke SL, Reid J, Ching RP, Wheeler DL. Glenohumeral kinematics and capsulo-ligamentous strain resulting from laxity exams. *Clin Biomech.* 2000;15: 735–742.

56. Hsu A, Ho L, Hedman T. Joint position during anterior–posterior glide mobilization: Its effect on glenohumeral abduction range of motion. *Arch Phys Med Rehabil.* 2000;81:210–214.

57. Wolf EM, Agrawal V. Transdeltoid palpation (the rent test) in the diagnosis of rotator cuff tears. *J Shld Elb Surg.* 2001;10(5)470–473.

58. Lyons AR, Tomlinson JE. Clinical diagnosis of tears of the rotator cuff. *J Bone Joint Surg.* 1992;74-B (3):414–415.

59. Walton J, Mahajan S, Paxinos A, et al. Diagnostic values of tests for acromioclavicular joint pain. *J Bone Joint Surg.* 2004;86-A(4):807–812.

60. Kelly BT, Kadrmas WR, Speer KP. The manual muscle examination for rotator cuff strength. *Am J Sports Med.* 1996;24(5):581–588.

61. Park HB, Yokota A, Gill HS, El Rassi G, McFarland EG. Diagnostic accuracy of clinical tests for the different degrees of subacromial impingement syndrome. *J Bone Joint Surg.* 2005;87-A (7):1446–1455.

62. Kendall F, McCreary EK, Provance PG. *Muscles testing and function.* Baltimore; Williams and Wilkins: 1993.

63. Wilk KE, Andrews JR, Arrigo CA, Keirns MA, Erber DJ. The strength characteristics of internal and external rotator muscles in professional baseball pitchers. *Am J Sports Med.* 1993;21(1):61–66.

64. Winters JC, Groenier KH, Sobel JS, Arendzen HH, Meyboom-de Jongh B. Classification of shoulder complaints in general practice by means of cluster analysis. *Arch Phys Med Rehabil.* 1997;78:1369–1374.

65. Lewis JS, Wright C, Green A. Subacromial impingement syndrome: The effect of changing posture on shoulder range of movement. *J Orthop Sports Phys Ther.* 2005;35(2):72–87.

66. Brossmann J, Preidler KW, Pedowitz RA, White LM, Trudell D, Resnick D. Shoulder impingement syndrome: Influence of shoulder position on rotator cuff impingement: An anatomic study. *AJR Am J Roentgenol.* 1996;167(6):1511–1515.

67. Johnson AJ, Godges JJ, Zimmerman GJ, Ounanian LL. The effect of anterior versus posterior glide joint mobilization on external rotation range of motion in patients with shoulder adhesive capsulitis. *J Orthop Sports Phys Ther.* 2007;37(3):88–99.

68. Maitland GD. *Peripheral manipulation.* London; Butterworth Heinemann: 1986.

69. Izumi T, Aoki M, Muraki T, Hidaka E, Miyamoto S. Stretching positions for the posterior capsule of the glenohumeral joint: Strain measurement using cadaver specimens. *Am J Sports Med.* 2008;36:2014–22.

70. Teys P, Bisset L, Vicenzino B. The initial effects of a Mulligan's mobilization with movement technique on range of movement and pressure pain threshold in pain-limited shoulders. *Man Ther.* 2008;13:37–42.

71. Kachingwe A, Phillips B, Sletten E, Plunkett S. Comparison of manual therapy techniques with therapeutic exercise in the treatment of shoulder impingement: A randomized controlled trial. *J Man Manip Ther.* 2008;16:238–247.

72. Bang M, Deyle G. Comparison of supervised exercise with and without manual physical therapy for patients with shoulder impingement syndrome. *J Orthop Sports Phys Ther.* 2000;30(3):126–137.

73. Ho CY, Sole G, Munn J. The effectiveness of manual therapy in the management of musculoskeletal disorders of the shoulder: A systematic review. *Man Ther.* 2009;14(5):463–474.

74. Dacre JE, Beeney N, Scott DL. Injections and physiotherapy for the painful stiff shoulder. *Ann Rheum Dis.* 1989;48(4):322–325.

75. Nicholson G. The effects of passive joint mobilization on pain and hypomobility associated with adhesive capsulitis of the shoulder. *J Orthop Sports Phys Ther.* 1985;6:238–246.

76. Jonsson P, Wahlström P, Ohberg L, Alfredson H. Eccentric training in chronic painful impingement syndrome of the shoulder: Results of a pilot study. *Knee Surg Sports Traumatol Arthrosc.* 2006;14:76–81.

77. Conroy D, Hayes K. The effect of joint mobilization as a component of comprehensive treatment for primary shoulder impingement syndrome. *J Orthop Sports Phys Ther.* 1998;28(1):3–14.

78. Senbursa G, Baltaci G, Atay A. Comparison of conservative treatment with and without manual physical therapy for patients with shoulder impingement syndrome: A prospective, randomized clinical trial. *Knee Surg Sports Traumatol Arthrosc.* 2007;15(7): 915–921.

79. Laudner KG, Sipes RC, Wilson JT. The acute effects of sleeper stretches on shoulder range of motion. *J Athl Train.* 2008;43(4):359–363.

80. McClure P, Balaicuis J, Heiland D, Broersma ME, Thorndike CK, Wood A. A randomized controlled comparison of stretching procedures for posterior shoulder tightness. *J Orthop Sports Phys Ther.* 2007;37(3): 108–114.

81. Boyles RE, Flynn TW, Whitman JM. Manipulation following regional interscalene anesthetic block for shoulder adhesive capsulitis: A case series. *Man Ther.* 2005;10:164–171.

82. McClatchie L, Laprade J, Martin S, Jaglal SB, Richardson D, Agur A. Mobilizations of the asymptomatic cervical spine can reduce signs of shoulder dysfunction in adults. *Man Ther.* 2009;14(4):369–374.

Manual Therapy of the Elbow–Wrist–Hand

Chad E. Cook and Amy Cook

Objectives

- Understand the normal and pathological kinematics associated with each elbow, wrist, or hand movement.
- Recognize the patient history characteristics associated with elbow, wrist, or hand injuries.
- Recognize the techniques of treatment that have yielded the highest success in the literature.
- Identify the level of evidence for manual therapy approaches of the elbow–wrist–hand region.

Clinical Examination

Observation

The utility of location of pain for differential diagnosis does exhibit some merit. Conditions such as lateral epicondylitis use location of pain for two or three diagnostic criteria: pain over the lateral epicondyle, tenderness over the same area, and exacerbation of pain by resisted wrist extension.[1,2] Medial epicondylitis is less investigated but for diagnosis also requires pain exhibition over the medial elbow (which may radiate distally or proximally), local tenderness, and pain aggravated by resisted wrist flexion when the forearm is extended.[3]

A **hand diagram** has been frequently used for the diagnosis of carpal tunnel syndrome (CTS). Typically, this method of assessment demonstrates high sensitivity and very good specificity.[4–7] Symptom patterns from a hand diagram identified preoperatively are effective in predicting the outcome of carpal tunnel release and are independent of psychosocial covariates that may influence outcome.[8,9] Tenosynovitis of the first dorsal compartment is characterized by pain on the radial side of the wrist, impairment of thumb function, and thickening of the ligamentous structure covering the tendons in the first dorsal compartment of the wrist.[3]

An individual with significant elbow effusion often holds his or her arm in a position of 70–80 degrees of flexion.[10] Additionally, swelling often increases joint fullness just distally to the lateral epicondyle of the humerus. Dislocations of the elbow present with prominence of the olecranon of the ulna or radial head since most elbow dislocations are posterior or posterior–lateral.[10] Olecranon bursitis is visible during extreme swelling and should be noted.

Observation may be useful in identifying hand dysfunction associated with resting position.[11] The resting attitude of the normal quiescent hand may identify an underlying pathology.[12] At rest, the hand demonstrates approximately 20–30 degrees of extension and 10–15 degrees of ulnar deviation.[13] The fingers and the thumb are slightly flexed and the palm demonstrates an arch that is progressively more flexed from radial to ulnar. Additionally, the fingers are more flexed as the digits progress ulnarly. Ulnar palsy is occasionally termed "bishop's hand" because the second and third digits maintain an extended posture while digits 4 and 5 are significantly flexed secondary to lack of intrinsic muscle innervation.[14] Flexor or extensor tendon ruptures generally result in a resting position of extension or flexion, respectively.[11] Radial nerve palsy results in the inability to actively extend the wrist and a resting position of slight wrist flexion.[14] Medial nerve palsy results in weakness of the flexor pollicus longus and flexor digitorum profundus. During pinch tests the patient will exhibit pad to pad pinching and an inability to distally flex the interphalangeal joint.

Hand texture including color, moisture, edema, and atrophy require careful assessment. Absence of moisture on the distal phalanx may indicate a digital nerve injury.[11] Additionally, differences in skin color (blanched or hyperemic) or the inability to appropriately sweat at a localized region may also be related to a digital nerve dysfunction.[11] Edema may be associated with soft tissue–related injuries or a fracture and significant atrophy may be associated with an upper motor neuron lesion.[15,16]

Introspection

It is intuitive to assume that most elbow, wrist, and hand injuries are associated with some form of trauma or overuse. Subsequently, careful attention to the lifestyle, occupation, and activities of the patient is required in order to fully comprehend the likely outcome for the patient. Effective orthopedic manual therapy may require strengthening, activity modification, and bracing as well as diligent assessment of potential proximal contributors such as the shoulder and cervical and thoracic spine.

Summary

- The use of a pain diagram to outline the location of symptoms may be more useful for the hand than for the elbow.
- When examining a patient with elbow–wrist–hand injuries, it is imperative to evaluate the work performance requirements of the patient.
- Hand texture may assist in diagnosis of nerve-related impairments or fractures.

Patient History

Elbow Symptoms

A number of tests may assist in identifying selected elbow impairments. To improve the ability to isolate the disorder, it is best to categorize elbow impairments by location. Lateral elbow pain is commonly associated with lateral epicondalgia but requires differentiation from less common disorders such as radial tunnel syndrome or posterolateral rotary instability.[17] Additionally, patients who report a history of trauma require diagnostic work-up to determine the presence of a radial head fracture, an injury that typically occurs during a fall on an outstretched forearm. Medial impairments of the elbow include golfer's elbow, little leaguer's elbow, and cubital tunnel syndrome. Anterior problems at the elbow may include biceps bursitis or tumor. Lastly, posterior elbow pain may include olecranon bursitis, olecranon fracture, or triceps tendonitis.

It is critical that a thorough patient history is performed to outline the potential causes and contributions to the elbow-related pain.[18] Cervical radiculopathy can masquerade as an impairment of the elbow. Selected elbow conditions can refer pain to the forearm and wrist/hand. Lateral epicondylitis may refer pain to the proximal forearm extensor muscle mass.[19] Additionally, in some fractures such as a humerus fracture, it is common to see radial and medial nerve trauma in adults more so than children.[20]

Wrist/Hand Symptoms

Patient report of wrist and hand symptoms provides the examiner with useful information, specifically in the capacity to differentiate selected forms of wrist/hand dysfunction. Wrist fractures are relatively common and are generally associated with trauma. The most common fracture of the wrist is a scaphoid fracture, which involves an injury either by a fall on an outstretched hand or by a direct blow to the palm. A lunate fracture is relatively uncommon, often is reported as weakness of the wrist, and generally involves hyperextension of the wrist or impact to the heel of the hand during a fall. A triquetrum fracture occurs from forced hyperextension with the wrist typically in ulnar deviation versus the injury associated with radial deviation (scaphoid). A capitate fracture may occur during a fall on an outstretched hand with forced dorsiflexion and a degree of radial deviation of the wrist or during direct impact or a crush injury to the dorsum of the wrist.[21] Because of the difficulty with identifying the number of possible wrist-related fractures the use of a radiograph is essential when a traumatic history is present with poor improvement or reduction of symptoms over time.[22]

Inflammatory processes are common in patients with osteoarthritis or rheumatoid arthritis. Patients with these conditions often exhibit morning stiffness, disuse pain, and pain with extreme overuse.[20] Commonly, patients may complain of heat with erythema of selected joints. Complaints of pain with passive movement may be present during a number of dysfunctions including tenosynovitis, wrist instability, and arthritic conditions. Motor weakness is generally associated with muscular atrophy (if chronic) and may be a consequence of an upper motor neuron dysfunction or CTS.[12]

Symptoms associated with CTS and other focal peripheral neuropathy include pain, numbness, and tingling in the distribution of the median nerve in at least two of the digits 1, 2, or 3, and the palm or dorsum of the hand.[23,24] These symptoms are generally present with or without pain and may radiate to the forearm, elbow, and shoulder.[24] CTS symptoms are usually worse at night and can awaken patients from sleep.[24-26]

Instability is associated with pain during or shortly after a recent injury to the wrist. Pain is frequently present during grasping wide objects, shaking hands, handling work tools, and other activities that require a power grip.[12] Often, the wrist will exhibit popping and cracking noises during movements.

Psychosocial Factors

Psychosocial factors such as work stress, poor locus of control, poor social support, and elevated perceptions of work-related stress have been associated with increased patient complaints of the upper extremity.[27] Henderson et al.[28] identified the prevalence of high pain intensity scores, depression, and helplessness covariates with the likelihood of reported CTS. Several studies have found common covariate traits among occupationally related elbow, wrist, and hand injuries and have found that individuals who indicated they had poor social support and limited peer contact were more likely to report elbow, wrist, and hand pain;[29-32] job situations in which perceived high work demand was prevalent were also linked to report of wrist and hand symptoms;[30-32] and lastly, some report lack of control, specifically during work-related demands, was also related to an increased risk of reporting hand-, elbow-, and wrist-related symptoms.[31]

Summary

- Conditions at the elbow are frequently described by location. Lateral elbow pain is commonly associated with lateral epicondalgia, radial tunnel syndrome, or posterolateral rotary instability. Medial impairments of the elbow include golfer's elbow, little leaguer's elbow, and cubital tunnel syndrome. Anterior problems at the elbow may include biceps bursitis or tumor. Lastly, posterior elbow pain may include olecranon bursitis, olecranon fracture, or triceps tendonitis.
- Conditions at the wrist may include fractures (most common), instability, or inflammatory responses.
- Covariate psychosocial conditions have been associated with lateral elbow pain and carpal tunnel syndrome.

Physical Examination

Active Physiological Movements

Active movements at the elbow may be limited by a number of pathological structures. Full ranges of extension are often limited by abnormalities in the olecranon process after a fracture, loose bodies associated with degeneration or trauma, edema, or by damage or compensatory changes in the anterior ligaments of the elbow. Full ranges of flexion can be limited by damage to the coronoid process of the elbow, edema, excessive soft tissue of the anterior forearm and biceps, and specifically selected damage to the posterior and anterior ligaments.

The active movements at the wrist and hand are extremely complex and rarely involve isolated planar movements. It is necessary to watch for deviations during movements, substitution patterns, and recruitment of the elbow joint during limitations in active motion. It is also important to address wrist motions in patients with elbow pain since both joints house two joint muscle systems that can influence symptom reproduction.

Several nonmechanical pathologies can cause wrist and hand pain and must be differentiated during the clinical examination process. Pain may be associated with disease processes that affect the bone, cartilage, synovium, nerves, blood vessels, muscle, or connective tissue.[12] Neoplasms in the hand may arise insidiously, thereby causing local swelling, pain, and dysfunction. A rare disorder, Reiter's syndrome, may cause symptoms associated with arthritis acutely, and can progress to fever, weight loss, and anorexia.[12] Lupis is more common than Reiter's syndrome and may cause swan neck deformities and ulnar deviation similar to rheumatoid arthritis. Scleroderma, a connective tissue disorder, may exhibit skin thickening or symptoms similar to arthritis. Disorders such as vasculitis, polychondritis, and septic infections are differentiated with careful history and clinical examinations.

Values involving goniometric range of motion are important to consider at the elbow and the wrist/hand and have demonstrated reliability.[33-35] These measures generally involve single planar movements that are not necessarily the functional ranges of the elbow, wrist, and hand; however, loss of these movements has been associated with decline in perceived function.[36]

As many structures contribute concurrently to elbow and wrist/hand pain, it is useful to perform the elbow wrist/hand examination at the same time. Throughout this chapter, elbow wrist/hand examination is performed concurrently, although isolating the examination to target the elbow or wrist/hand exclusively is often warranted.

Active Elbow and Wrist Flexion

Normal values for active range of elbow flexion arc range from 0 degrees of extension to 140 degrees of flexion.[37–39] The carrying angle changes from valgus to varus, substantially altering the ability to assess resting carrying angle in patients with significant swelling.[40]

Active wrist flexion allows assessment of the proximal, mid, and distal carpal joints, although it is hypothesized that the radiocarpal joint moves more substantially than the others.[41] Active restriction with pain may be associated with capsular restriction, a volar intercalated segmental instability, or pain in the extensor structures of the forearm.

1. To assess active elbow and wrist flexion, the patient sits or stands. It is beneficial to perform the movements bilaterally for observational assessment.

2. The patient is instructed to abduct the shoulder to approximately 90 degrees bilaterally.

3. The patient is instructed to flex the elbow and wrist to the first point of pain. Pain is assessed for the concordant sign. The patient is instructed to move beyond the first point of pain toward end range. Pain is assessed to determine the influence on the concordant sign.

Active Elbow and Wrist Extension

Active extension normally allows full extension or functional hyperextension.[37] The presence of joint edema, heterotrophic ossification, osteophytes, or medial elbow tightness may limit the ability to move into full extension. Nearly 50 percent of baseball players exhibit limitations in the ability to achieve full extension secondary to hypertrophy of the medial structures of the elbow.[37]

Active wrist extension also involves assessment of the proximal, mid-, and distal carpal joints and again it is hypothesized that the radiocarpal joint substantially moves more than the others.[41] This emphasis of movement is most likely associated with the biomechanical variability and complexity of the mid-carpal joint and the relative stability of the carpo–metacarpal complex.

1. To assess active elbow or wrist extension, the patient sits or stands. It is beneficial to perform the movements bilaterally for observational assessment.

2. The patient is instructed to flex the shoulder to approximately 90 degrees bilaterally.

3. The patient is instructed to extend the elbow and wrist to the first point of pain. Pain is assessed for the concordant sign.

4. The patient is instructed to move beyond the first point of pain toward end range. Pain is assessed to determine the effect on the concordant sign.

Active Elbow and Wrist Supination and Pronation

Normal values of supination and pronation are 80–90 degrees when the elbow is held at 90 degrees of flexion.[37–39] Variations will occur with significant swelling at the elbow secondary to the shared capsule. Additionally, the inability to achieve 90 degrees of flexion may reduce the capacity to fully translate the radius with respect to the ulna, further altering movement.

Some degree of radial–ulnar supination is a product of wrist movement. Noticeable reductions of movement are associated with individual carpal bone fractures or dysfunction associated with carpal to carpal ligamentous groups. McGee[42] suggests that up to 20 degrees of the available supination range of motion is associated with wrist movement.

Since pronation requires lateral translation of the radius with respect to the ulna, a fair degree of mobility is required within the shared capsule and within the radial head. Like supination, some degree of radial–ulnar pronation is a product of wrist movement. McGee[42] suggests that up to 15 degrees of the available pronation range of motion is associated with wrist movement.

1. To assess these movements, the patient sits or stands. It is beneficial to perform the movements bilaterally for observational assessment.

2. The patient is instructed to first flex the elbow to 90 degrees or the maximum available range of motion up to 90 degrees.

3. The patient is then instructed to supinate the elbow to the first point of pain. Pain is assessed for the concordant sign.

4. The patient is instructed to move beyond the first point of pain toward end range. Pain is assessed to determine the effect on the concordant sign.

5. The patient is then instructed to pronate the elbow to the first point of pain. Pain is assessed for the concordant sign.

6. The patient is instructed to move beyond the first point of pain toward end range. Pain is assessed to determine the effect on the concordant sign.

Active Wrist Radial and Ulnar Deviation

Wrist radial and ulnar deviation is in some fashion a product of concurrent flexion and extension of the wrist. Radial deviation tends to couple with wrist extension and the end-feel is generally restricted by the osseoligamentous structures of the carpal bones. Ulnar deviation tends to couple with wrist flexion. Like radial deviation the end-feel associated with wrist ulnar deviation is generally restricted by the osseoligamentous structures of the carpal bones.

1. To assess active wrist radial and ulnar deviation, the patient sits or stands.
2. The patient is instructed to flex the elbow for prepositioning.
3. The patient is instructed to move in radial deviation to the first point of pain. The pain is assessed to determine if concordant.
4. The patient is then instructed to move beyond the first point of pain toward end range. Pain is assessed to determine the effect on the concordant sign.
5. The patient is then instructed to move in ulnar deviation to the first point of pain. The pain is assessed to determine if concordant.
6. The patient is then instructed to move beyond the first point of pain toward end range. Pain is assessed to determine the effect on the concordant sign. It is beneficial to perform these motions bilaterally.

The full active physiological elbow, wrist, and hand sequence can be performed in six quick and easy movements. Figure 9.1 ■ demonstrates these movements collectively as one sequence.

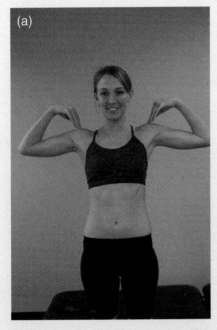
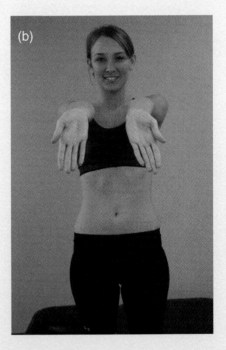

■ **Figure 9.1**   The Active Physiological Elbow and Wrist Sequence

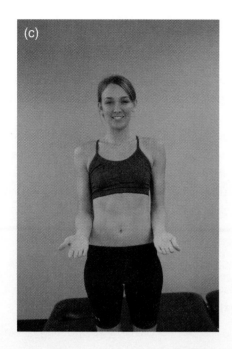

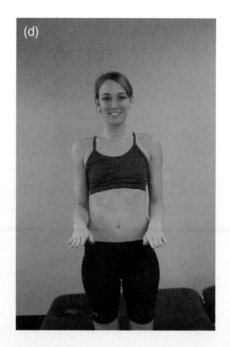

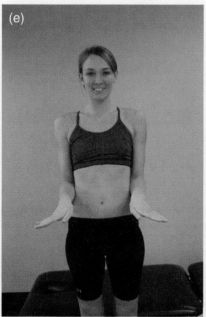

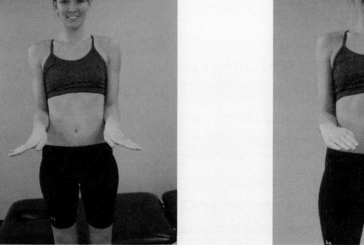

■ **Figure 9.1** (Continued)

Active Group Finger Flexion and Extension

Finger flexion requires the passive engagement of the finger extensors and the active engagement of the finger flexors (primarily the superficialis and profundus). Finger flexion should be symmetric and pain free in the undamaged hand.

The extensor mechanism of the fingers is a complex system of intercrossed fibers from the extensor digitorum communis, the extensor indicis, the lumbricals, and the first volar interosseous muscles. The fibers work in concert to create a hood structure over the dorsum of the finger that collectively extends the middle and distal interphalangeal joints.[43] Failure of the extensor mechanism may be the result of tightness in ligaments, disruption of the extensor tendon, or other phenomena.

1. To assess active group finger flexion and extension, the patient sits or stands.

2. The patient is instructed to extend the wrist and elbow to neutral for prepositioning.

3. For finger flexion, the patient is instructed to concurrently flex the fingers to the first point of pain. The pain is assessed to determine if concordant.

4. The patient is then instructed to move beyond the first point of pain toward end range. Pain is assessed to determine the influence on the concordant sign.

5. For finger extension, the patient is instructed to concurrently extend the fingers to the first point of pain. The pain is assessed to determine if concordant.

6. The patient is then instructed to move beyond the first point of pain toward end range. Pain is assessed to determine the influence on the concordant sign. It is beneficial to perform these motions bilaterally.

Active Group Finger Adduction and Abduction

Abduction at the thumb is produced by the abductor pollicis longus and abductor pollicis brevis. Finger abduction is produced by the dorsal interossei and the abductor digiti minimi. Thumb adduction is provided by the adductor pollicis while finger adduction is a product of palmar interossei contraction.

1. The patient sits or stands and resting symptoms are assessed.

2. The patient is instructed to extend the wrist to neutral for prepositioning.

3. For finger adduction, the patient is instructed to concurrently adduct the fingers against the adjacent fingers to the first point of pain; the pain is assessed to determine if concordant.

4. The patient is then instructed to move into further adduction beyond the first point of pain toward end range. Pain is assessed to determine the effect on the concordant sign.

5. The patient is instructed to extend the wrist to neutral for prepositioning (for finger abduction) and is instructed to concurrently abduct the fingers to the first point of pain.

6. The patient is then instructed to move into further abduction beyond the first point of pain toward end range. Pain is assessed to determine the effect on the concordant sign. It is beneficial to perform these motions bilaterally.

Functional Active Movements

Conventional wrist and hand assessment evaluates movements in single planes in isolated directions.[44] Actual movement of the wrist/hand involves coupled movements in multiple planes. These movements are generally considered more functional than single plane excursions.

Several studies have evaluated and proposed range-of-motion parameters for "functional" range at the wrist. Range-of-motion parameters are important measurement features of the wrist and have been associated with disability both functionally and through patient perception.[36] Generally, functional range-of-motion values of the wrist include 5–10 degrees of flexion, 15–30 degrees of extension,[45,46] 10 degrees of radial deviation, and 15 degrees of ulnar deviation.[45]

Functional movements of the wrist involve coupled motion. Coupled functional movement of the wrist include flexion/ulnar deviation (Figure 9.2 ■) and extension/radial deviation (Figure 9.3 ■). These coupled movements are often called the dart thrower's positions.

Hand movements involve a complex set of functional patterns to accomplish tasks such as grip, manipulation, and tasks that require dexterity. The inability to accomplish the following functional tasks, if associated with joint or soft-tissue restrictions, may be an indication to attempt range-of-motion gains for the patient. The clinician is encouraged to evaluate tip to tip and pad to pad movements as well as two different forms of gripping methods: (1) power grip (Figure 9.4 ■) and (2) narrow grip (Figure 9.5 ■).

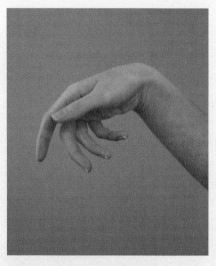

■ **Figure 9.2**   Coupled Flexion and Ulnar Deviation

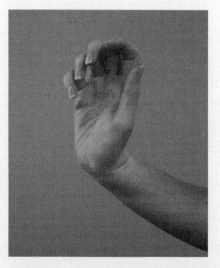

■ **Figure 9.3**   Coupled Extension and Radial Deviation

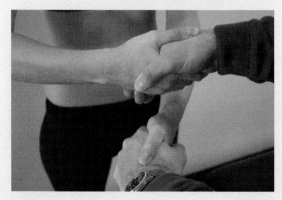

■ **Figure 9.4**   Power Grip Shake

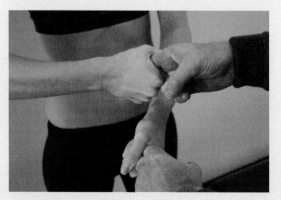

■ **Figure 9.5**   Narrow Grip Shake

Summary

- Because of the multiple planes of movement associated with the elbow–wrist–hand, a general screen that examines general planar active movement is a quick method to identify movement dysfunction.

- Most wrist motion is coupled as is the elbow to a minor degree. When a movement is isolated as pathological to a specific joint, the coupled movements may benefit from assessment.

- Functional movements such as finite finger motions and power movements such as a grip or hand shake provide the clinician with additional active assessment features.

are presented in concert. The concerted presentation allows for a smoother examination and the ability to compare similar movements that may demonstrate concordant findings.

There are a myriad of potential causal structures for an elbow–wrist–hand dysfunction. Consequently, it is imperative that the clinician isolate the findings to a selected region, in order to more comprehensively passively examine the region. The most effective method of selection involves the judicious use of overpressure and the results of the overpressure in identifying the concordant pain of the patient.

Passive Movements

Passive and Combined Physiological Movements of the Elbow Because combined movements are such a critical aspect of the elbow,[47] the passive examination procedures

Passive Elbow Flexion

1. The patient is placed in a supine position.

2. The forearm is prepositioned in a supinated posture.

3. The clinician stabilizes the humerus of the patient by cupping the posterior aspect of the upper arm in the hand and supporting the upper arm on the plinth.

4. The clinician passively flexes the elbow to the first point of pain and the pain is assessed to determine if concordant (Figure 9.6 ■).

5. The clinician passively flexes the elbow past the first point of pain and the pain is reassessed to determine if worse, better, or the same.

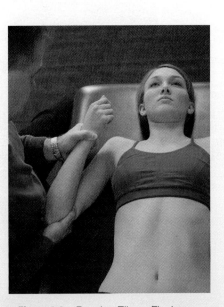

■ Figure 9.6   Passive Elbow Flexion

Passive Elbow Flexion with Overpressure

Overpressure into flexion is necessary to rule out flexion as a contributor to the dysfunction. End-feel in terminal flexion is generally soft, an associative finding with compression of soft tissues.

1. At the limit of active elbow flexion, the clinician passively supplies an end-range movement.

2. At the passive end range, a quick overpressure of sustained and/or repeated movements is supplied. Adjustments of force are appropriate, specifically if prepositioning of valgus or varus is desired. Pain is assessed to determine the effect on the concordant sign.

3. Compression through the long axis of the lower arm is another potential tool used to sensitize the overpressure procedure.

Passive Elbow Flexion with Varus and Valgus Force

A significant amount of valgus to varus conversion occurs during extension to flexion movement.[47] Passive elbow flexion with varus is the motion required during the combined movements of flexion and supination of the wrist. Passive elbow flexion with a valgus force is the motion required during the combined movements of flexion and pronation of the wrist.

1. The patient is placed in a supine position.

2. The forearm is prepositioned in a supinated posture and the clinician stabilizes the humerus of the patient by cupping the posterior aspect of the upper arm in the hand and supporting the upper arm on the plinth.

3. To reduce potential internal rotation at the shoulder, the arm is prepositioned in slight external rotation (Figure 9.7 ■).

4. The clinician passively and concurrently flexes and places a varus force at the elbow to the first point of pain; the pain is assessed to determine if concordant.

5. After repeated movements the pain is reassessed to determine if worse, better, or the same.

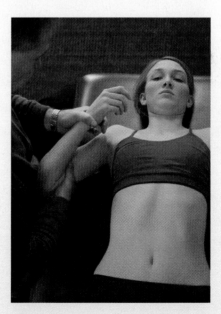

■ **Figure 9.7**   Passive Elbow Flexion with a Varus Force

(Continued)

6 To reduce potential external rotation at the shoulder during flexion and a valgus force, the arm is prepositioned in slight internal rotation.

7 The clinician passively and concurrently flexes and places a valgus force at the elbow to the first point of pain; the pain is assessed to determine if concordant.

8 The clinician passively and concurrently flexes and places a valgus force at the elbow past the first point of pain (Figure 9.8 ■).

9 After repeated movements the pain is reassessed to determine if worse, better, or the same.

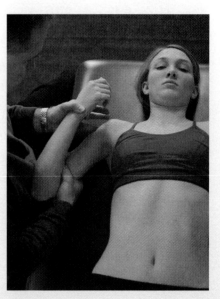

■ **Figure 9.8** Passive Elbow Flexion with a Valgus Force

Passive Elbow Extension

Passive elbow extension may be limited by the presence of heterotrophic ossification, edema, osteophytes, or medial elbow tightness.

1 The patient is positioned in supine.

2 The clinician places the forearm over the anterior aspect of the patient's shoulder and loops the wrist around the posterior aspect of the patient (Figure 9.9 ■). This creates a stable support at the elbow joint and reduces the tendency of the shoulder to rise during elbow extension.

3 The clinician then passively moves the elbow into extension to the first point of pain; the pain is assessed to determine if concordant.

4 The clinician then passively moves the elbow beyond the first point of pain to determine the effect of further range of motion on the symptoms.

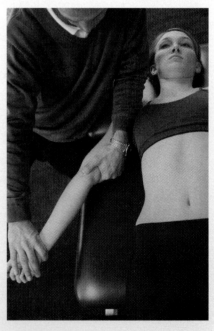

■ **Figure 9.9** Passive Elbow Extension

Passive Elbow Extension with Overpressure

Overpressure is necessary to rule out the presence of pain during extension. A bony end-feel is associated with the olecranon block; a softer end-feel generally means a ligamentous block; an empty end-feel may be associated with pain, fear, or significant swelling.

1. At the limit of passive physiological elbow extension, the clinician passively supplies an end-range movement.

2. At the passive end range, a quick overpressure of sustained and/or repeated movements is supplied. Adjustments of force are appropriate, specifically if prepositioning of valgus or varus is desired. Pain is assessed to determine the effect on the concordant sign.

3. Compression through the long axis of the lower arm is another potential tool used to sensitize the overpressure procedure.

Passive Elbow Extension with a Varus and Valgus Force

Passive elbow extension with a varus force is the motion required for the combined movements of extension and pronation.[47] Passive elbow extension with a valgus force is the motion required for the combined movements of extension and supination.

1. Passive elbow extension with a varus and valgus force is assessed with the patient in a supine position.

2. The clinician places the forearm over the anterior aspect of the patient's shoulder and loops the wrist around the posterior aspect of the patient (Figure 9.10 ■).

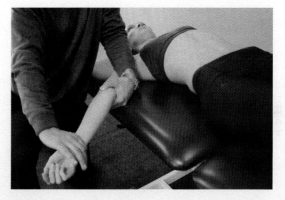

■ **Figure 9.10** Elbow Extension with Varus

3. This creates a stable support at the elbow joint and reduces the tendency of the shoulder to rise during elbow extension. To reduce the tendency of shoulder internal rotation, the upper arm is prepositioned into slight external rotation.

4. The clinician then passively moves the elbow into extension and a varus force to the first point of pain; the pain is assessed to determine if concordant.

5. The clinician then passively moves the elbow beyond the first point of pain to determine the influence of further range of motion on the symptoms.

(Continued)

1. For a varus the patient is placed in a similar position. The clinician places the forearm over the anterior aspect of the patient's shoulder and loops the wrist around the posterior upper arm of the patient. This creates a stable support at the elbow joint and reduces the tendency of the shoulder to rise during elbow extension.

2. To reduce the tendency of shoulder external rotation, the upper arm is prepositioned into slight internal rotation.

3. The clinician then passively moves the elbow into extension and a valgus force to the first point of pain (Figure 9.11 ■). The pain is assessed to determine if concordant.

4. The clinician then passively moves the elbow beyond the first point of pain to determine the influence of further range of motion on the symptoms.

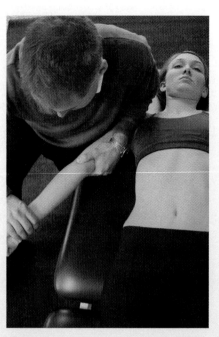

■ **Figure 9.11**   Elbow Extension with Valgus

Passive Physiological Supination

Both supination and pronation involve movement at the proximal and distal radioulnar joint and movement within the wrist carpals. To ensure specific assessment of the proximal and distal radioulnar joint, the contact point for the clinician is proximal to the radiocarpal row.

1. The patient is positioned in a supine position. The clinician flexes the elbow to 90 degrees and stabilizes the distal wrist using an adduction grasp between the thumb and index finger.

2. The clinician then slowly rotates the radioulnar joint into supination to the first point of pain; pain is assessed to determine if concordant.

3. The clinician then slowly rotates past the first point of pain into further supination. If painful, the clinician may provide repeated motions or sustained holds to determine the outcome (Figure 9.12 ■).

4. The movement is repeated for pronation.

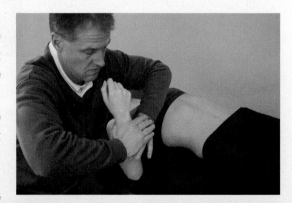

■ **Figure 9.12**   Proximal and Distal Radioulnar Supination

Passive Wrist Supination and Pronation

Up to 20–30% of forearm supination is a product of carpal joint movements. The movements may occur at the proximal row (predominantly), mid-carpal row (less predominant), or carpometacarpal junctions (even less predominant). To differentiate between carpal contributions it is essential to assess each row individually if supination and/or pronation are concordant during active movements.

Proximal Row Supination and Pronation

Supination of the proximal row requires the stabilization of the radius and ulna while performing supination of the proximal carpal row.

1. The patient is positioned in supine.

2. The clinician flexes the elbow to 90 degrees and stabilizes the radius and ulna by using an adduction grasp between the thumb and index finger of one hand and placing the other hand around the proximal carpal row of the wrist.

3. The clinician passively moves the proximal carpal row into supination while stabilizing the radius and the ulna. Movement is stopped at the first point of pain and pain is assessed to determine if concordant (Figure 9.13).

4. The clinician then passively moves the proximal row further into supination to determine the effect on pain.

5. The clinician may apply repeated movements or a sustained hold to determine the effect.

6. If the passive movement is not painful, overpressure is applied to the movement.

7. Isolated pronation of the proximal row requires the stabilization of the radius and ulna while the clinician passively moves the proximal carpal row into pronation while stabilizing the radius.

8. Movement is stopped at the first point of pain. Pain is assessed to determine if concordant.

9. The clinician then passively moves the proximal row further into pronation on the radius to determine the effect on pain. The clinician may apply repeated movements or a sustained hold to determine the effect.

10. If the passive movement is not painful, overpressure is applied to the movement.

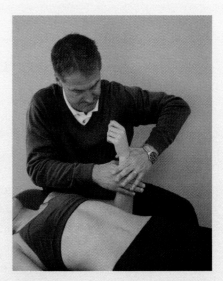

■ **Figure 9.13**   Proximal Row Supination

Mid-Carpal Joint Supination

Assessment of the mid-carpal row requires the stabilization of the proximal carpal row during subsequent movement of the distal row into supination.

1. The patient is positioned in supine.

2. The clinician flexes the elbow to 90 degrees and stabilizes the proximal carpal bones using an adduction grasp between the thumb and index finger of one hand and placing the other hand around the distal carpal row of the wrist.

3. The clinician passively moves the distal carpal row into supination while stabilizing the proximal carpal row. Movement is stopped at the first point of pain and pain is assessed to determine if concordant.

4. The clinician then passively moves the distal row further into supination to determine the effect on pain. The clinician may apply repeated movements or a sustained hold to determine the effect. If the passive movement is not painful, overpressure is applied to the movement.

5. To assess pronation, the clinician passively moves the distal carpal row into pronation while stabilizing the proximal carpal row (Figure 9.14 ■). Movement is stopped at the first point of pain and pain is assessed to determine if concordant.

6. The clinician then passively moves the distal row further into pronation to determine the effect on pain. The clinician may apply repeated movements or a sustained hold to determine the effect. If the passive movement is not painful, overpressure is applied to the movement.

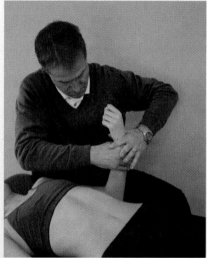

■ **Figure 9.14** Mid-Carpal Row Supination

Passive Carpometacarpal Joint Supination and Pronation

The carpometacarpal joint, which also contributes to supination, must be isolated for appropriate assessment.

1. To assess this region, the patient is positioned in supine and resting symptoms are assessed.

2. The clinician flexes the elbow to 90 degrees and stabilizes the proximal and distal carpal bones using an adduction grasp between the thumb and index finger of one hand and placing the other hand around the metacarpals of the patient's hand.

3. The clinician passively moves the metacarpals of the hand into supination while stabilizing the proximal and distal carpals. Movement is stopped at the first point of pain and pain is assessed to determine if concordant.

④ The clinician then passively moves the metacarpals further into supination to determine the effect on pain (Figure 9.15 ■). The clinician may apply repeated movements or a sustained hold to determine the effect. If the passive movement is not painful, overpressure is applied to the movement.

⑤ To assess pronation, the clinician passively moves the metacarpals of the hand into pronation while stabilizing the proximal and distal carpals. Movement is stopped at the first point of pain and pain is assessed to determine if concordant. The clinician then passively moves the metacarpals further into pronation to determine the effect on pain. The clinician may apply repeated movements or a sustained hold to determine the effect. If the passive movement is not painful, overpressure is applied to the movement.

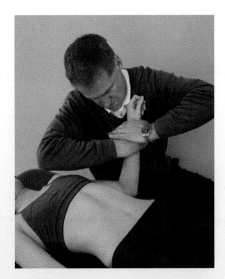

■ **Figure 9.15**   Carpometacarpal Joint Pronation

Passive and Combined Physiological Movements of the Wrist and Hand   Because combined movements are such a critical aspect of the wrist and hand, the passive examination procedures are presented in concert. The concerted presentation allows for a smoother examination and the ability to compare similar movements that may demonstrate concordant findings.

Passive Physiological Wrist Flexion

Pain associated with wrist instability such as a ventral intercalated segmental instability (VISI) is typically reproduced during passive flexion or extension of the wrist throughout focused movements of the metacarpals.[12] Wrist flexion often involves the combined movements of flexion, ulnar deviation, and supination. Single plane movements such as isolated flexion, extension and ulnar and radial deviation may require advanced assessment of combined movements if the single movements are concordant.

Because of the elasticity of the forearm extensor muscles and the contribution of these muscles to the mobility of wrist flexion, significant diligence should be used to ensure end-range overpressure assessment. Resistance is encountered early in wrist flexion and overpressure at midranges may fail to implicate actual pathology isolated at this junction.

① The patient is positioned in supine.

② The clinician flexes the elbow to 90 degrees and stabilizes the radius on the palmar aspect of the wrist with one hand while the other secures the dorsal aspect of the hand.

(Continued)

③ The clinician passively moves the wrist into flexion. Movement is stopped at the first point of pain and pain is assessed to determine if concordant.

④ The clinician then passively moves the wrist further into flexion to determine the influence on pain (Figure 9.16 ■). The clinician may apply repeated movements or a sustained hold to determine the effect.

⑤ At the limit of active wrist flexion, the clinician passively supplies an end-range movement of overpressure into further flexion.

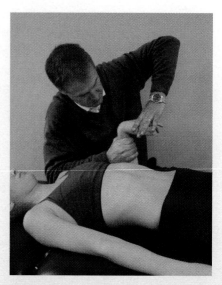

■ **Figure 9.16**   Passive Physiological Wrist Flexion

Passive Wrist Extension

Pain associated with wrist instability such as a dorsal intercalated segmental instability (DISI) is typically reproduced during passive flexion or extension of the wrist during focused movements of the metacarpals.[12] Wrist extension promotes the combined movements of extension, pronation, and radial deviation. Painful single plane movements of extension may require advanced assessment of combined movements if concordant. As with wrist flexion overpressure assessment, the end range of wrist extension encounters significant resistance, providing false suggestions of actual end-feel.

① The patient is positioned in supine.

② The clinician flexes the elbow to 90 degrees and stabilizes the radius on the dorsal aspect of the wrist with one hand while the other secures the palmar aspect of the hand.

③ The clinician passively moves the wrist into extension. Movement is stopped at the first point of pain and pain is assessed to determine if concordant.

④ The clinician then passively moves the wrist further into extension to determine the influence on pain (Figure 9.17 ■). The clinician may apply repeated movements or a sustained hold to determine the effect.

⑤ At the limit of active wrist extension, the clinician passively supplies an end-range movement of overpressure into further extension.

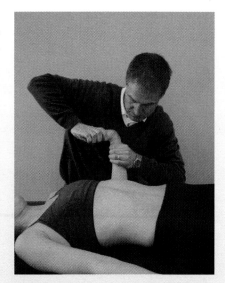

■ **Figure 9.17** Passive Physiological Wrist Extension

Passive Ulnar and Radial Deviation

Limitation of ulnar and radial deviation is commonly associated with intercarpal restrictions, fractures, or other capsular injuries. Overpressure into ulnar deviation is required to clear this planar movement and because ulnar movement is frequently coupled with flexion, it is common to see concurrent discomfort with flexion and ulnar deviation. Because radial movement is frequently coupled with extension, it is common to see concurrent discomfort with extension and radial deviation.

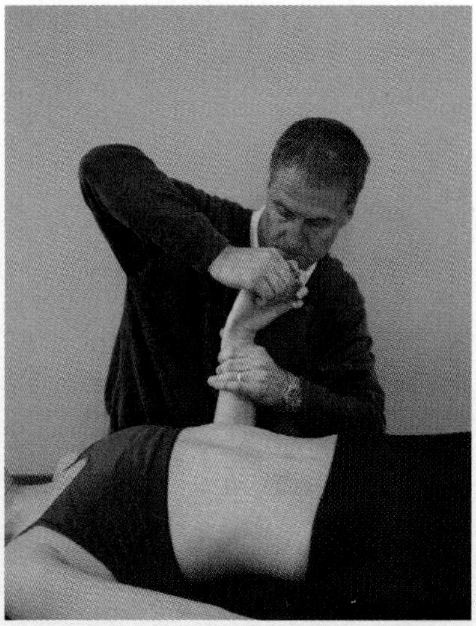

① The patient is positioned in supine.

② The clinician flexes the elbow to 90 degrees and stabilizes the wrist on the ulnar aspect with one hand while the other secures the radial aspect of the wrist and hand.

③ The clinician passively moves the wrist into ulnar deviation. Movement is stopped at the first point of pain and pain is assessed to determine if concordant.

④ The clinician then passively moves the wrist further into ulnar deviation to determine the effect on pain (Figure 9.18 ■). The clinician may apply repeated movements or a sustained hold to determine the effect.

■ **Figure 9.18** Passive Physiological Ulnar Deviation of the Wrist

(Continued)

⑤ At the limit of active wrist ulnar deviation and if the passive movement does not produce pain, the clinician passively supplies an end-range movement of overpressure.

⑥ For radial deviation, the clinician flexes the elbow to 90 degrees and stabilizes the wrist on the radial aspect with one hand while the other secures the ulnar aspect of the wrist and hand.

⑦ The clinician passively moves the wrist into radial deviation. Movement is stopped at the first point of pain and pain is assessed to determine if concordant.

⑧ The clinician then passively moves the wrist further into radial deviation to determine the effect on pain (Figure 9.19 ■). The clinician may apply repeated movements or a sustained hold to determine the effect.

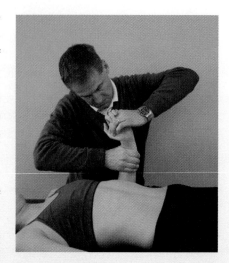

■ **Figure 9.19** Passive Physiological Radial Deviation of the Wrist

⑨ At the limit of active wrist radial deviation and if the passive movement does not produce pain, the clinician passively supplies an end-range movement of overpressure.

Passive Carpometacarpal Joint Extension and Flexion

The movements associated with the carpometacarpal joints of the second through fifth digits are minimal but necessary. Along with the previous assessments of pronation and supination of this region, flexion and extension may provide further isolation of the concordant impairment of the wrist/hand.

Because the joint is inherently stable and is difficult to isolate, a counterpoint procedure is necessary for passive physiological assessment.

① To assess this movement the patient is positioned in supine.

② The clinician flexes the elbow to 90 degrees and stabilizes the wrist in neutral at the proximal and mid-carpal joints.

③ Using the other hand the clinician applies a counterpoint procedure by applying an extension movement at the carpometacarpal (CMC) joint.

④ For CMC extension, the clinician's thumb applies a palmar movement just distal to the CMC while the hand applies a dorsal movement at the distal aspect of the metacarpal.

⑤ The procedure is repeated at digits 2–5 using appropriate repeated motions and overpressure if warranted.

⑥ For CMC flexion, the clinician's thumbs apply a dorsal movement just distal to the CMC while the hand applies a palmar movement at the distal aspect of the metacarpal.

⑦ The procedure is repeated at digits 2–5 using appropriate repeated motions and overpressure if warranted.

Passive Physiological Flexion and Adduction of the Thumb

The articular complex of the first CMC joint (the thumb) allows multiple variations of physiological movements. The movements of flexion and adduction, although different, share a common end point just adjacent and flush to the second metacarpal. It is uncommon to see physiological restrictions of these movements.

1 To assess these movements the patient is positioned in supine.

2 Using one hand, the clinician can stabilize the trapezium of the wrist to isolate movement to the CMC and distal joints of the thumb.

3 If physiological movement without stabilization is solicited, no stabilization of the trapezium is necessary.

4 From a starting point of thumb extension or abduction, the thumb is passively moved medially toward the second metacarpal (Figure 9.20 ■). Movement is stopped at the first point of pain. The pain is assessed to determine if concordant.

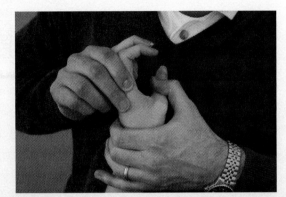

■ **Figure 9.20** Passive Physiological Flexion/Adduction of the Thumb

5 As with the previous assessments, repeated or end-range movements are used to determine if this movement is a treatment option.

Passive Physiological Extension and Abduction of the Thumb

Passive extension of the thumb is limited by the volar and radial structures of the hand. Passive extension occurs in the coronal plane while passive abduction occurs in the sagittal plane. Proximal interphalangeal joint (PIP) extension and abduction may be limited during disease processes such as arthritis or sepsis.

1 The patient is positioned in supine.

2 Using one hand, the clinician stabilizes the trapezium (if desired) of the wrist to isolate movement to the CMC and distal joints of the thumb.

3 If movement specific to the distal segments is desired the stabilization force should move to the proximal aspects of the PIP and the distal interphalangeal joint (DIP).

(Continued)

④ For thumb extension the starting point is thumb flexion. The thumb is passively moved within the coronal plane toward extension. Movement is stopped at the first complaint of pain. If painful the complaint is assessed to determine if concordant (Figure 9.21 ■).

⑤ As with the previous assessments, repeated or end-range movements are used to determine if this movement is a treatment option.

⑥ Overpressures are required to rule out the joints of the thumb and the opposite side should be tested if appropriate.

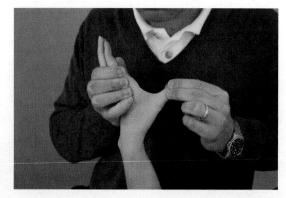

■ **Figure 9.21** Passive Physiological Extension of the Thumb

⑦ For thumb abduction the starting point for motion is thumb adduction. Using one hand, the clinician stabilizes the trapezium (if desired) of the wrist to isolate movement to the CMC and distal joints of the thumb.

⑧ If movement specific to the distal segments is desired the stabilization force should move to the proximal aspects of the PIP and the DIP.

⑨ From a starting point of thumb flexion, the thumb is passively moved within the sagittal plane toward abduction (Figure 9.22 ■). Movement is stopped at the first complaint of pain. The pain is assessed to determine if concordant.

⑩ As with the previous assessments, repeated or end range movements are used to determine if this movement is a treatment option.

⑪ Overpressures are required to rule out the joints of the thumb and the opposite side should be tested if appropriate.

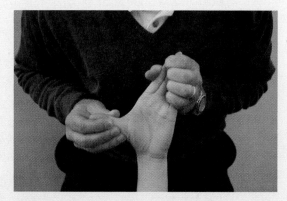

■ **Figure 9.22** Passive Physiological Abduction of the Thumb

Passive Physiological Metacarpophalangeal Joint Flexion and Extension

Manipulation of small objects requires the coupled movements of metacarpophalangeal (MCP) joint flexion/extension, rotation, and abduction/adduction. Rotation occurs primarily in extension but assessment in selected degrees of flexion may also be beneficial.

Flexion of the MCP joints of digits 2–5 reduces the simultaneous movements of abduction/adduction and rotation of the same joint. "Joint play" subsequently is greater during MCP extension, introducing an increased frequency of MCP flexion restrictions versus extension restrictions.

Passive Physiological Flexion of the Metacarpophalangeal Joint

1. The patient is positioned in supine.

2. Using one hand, the clinician individually grasps the distal aspect of the metacarpal of digits 2–5 depending on where the desired movement is required.

3. From a starting point of extension, the proximal phalange (and subsequent middle and distal phalange) is moved into flexion while concurrently stabilizing the articulating metacarpal. Movement is stopped upon the first point of pain. Any pain is assessed to determine if concordant.

4. As with the previous assessments, repeated or end-range movements are used to determine if this movement is a treatment option.

5. Overpressures are required to rule out the movement.

6. For MCP extension the MCP is prepositioned into flexion. From a starting point of flexion, the proximal phalange (and subsequent middle and distal phalange) is moved into extension while concurrently stabilizing the distal metacarpal. Movement is stopped upon the first point of pain. Any pain is assessed to determine if concordant.

7. As with the previous assessments, repeated or end-range movements are used to determine if this movement is a helpful treatment option.

8. Overpressures are required to rule out the guilt of the movement.

Metacarpophalangeal Joint Rotation (in Extension)

1. The patient is positioned in supine.

2. Using one hand, the clinician individually grasps the distal aspect of the metacarpal of digits 2–5 depending on where the desired movement is required. The metacarpal is stabilized distally.

3. The PIP is prepositioned into flexion, allowing a sturdy structure for grasp by the clinician.

4. Rotation into both directions is applied to the first point of pain and pain is assessed to determine if concordant (Figure 9.23 ■).

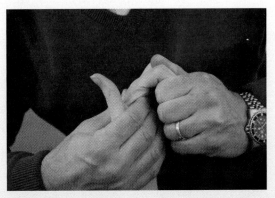

■ **Figure 9.23** Passive Physiological Rotation of the Metacarpophalangeal Joint

Metacarpophalangeal Joint Abduction and Adduction

1. Using one hand, the clinician individually grasps the distal aspect of the metacarpal of digits 2–5 depending on where the desired movement is required.

2. The PIP may be prepositioned into flexion, allowing a sturdy structure for grasp by the clinician, although maintaining extension will not affect the abduction or adduction.

3. Abduction and subsequent adduction is applied to the first point of pain and pain is assessed to determine if concordant.

4. Repeated and end-range movements and overpressures may be necessary to further distal information regarding the joint.

Proximal Interphalangeal and Distal Interphalangeal Joint Flexion and Extension

Restriction may occur into PIP flexion secondary to tightness in the lateral and dorsal structures of the second through fifth digits. Restrictions may occur into extension associated with tightness of the volar plate of the finger or tightness in the oblique lateral ligaments of the finger.

1. The patient is positioned in supine.

2. Using one hand, the clinician individually grasps the distal aspect of the proximal phalange, just proximal to the PIP.

3. Using the opposite hand, the clinician grasps the middle phalange.

4. For the DIP, the clinician individually grasps the distal aspect of the middle phalange, just proximal to the DIP.

5. Using the opposite hand, the clinician grasps the distal phalange just distal to the DIP.

6. Flexion and subsequent extension are performed to the PIP and DIP. Movement is restricted to the first point of pain and pain is assessed to determine if concordant.

7. Repeated and end-range movements and overpressures may be necessary to further distal information regarding the joint.

Passive Accessory Movements of the Elbow

Passive accessory motions of the elbow are useful for identifying directional stiffness and the concordant sign of the patient.

Passive Accessory Movements of the Wrist

Passive accessory movements are useful in identifying concordant findings of arthrological nature.

Posterior–Anterior of the Humeroulnar Joint

A posterior–anterior (PA) of the humeroulnar joint (HUJ) most likely is a combination of physiological and slight accessory movement. The congruence of the HUJ reduces the plausibility of a direct PA motion because the olecranon will compress against the humerus.

1 The patient is positioned in prone.

2 The arm is prepositioned into extension at the side of the patient.

3 The anterior aspect of the arm is cradled by the fingers of the clinician. The thumbs are placed on the posterior aspect of the olecranon using a pad to pad placement (Figure 9.24 ■).

4 The clinician applies a combined movement of lifting the anterior aspect of the arm while applying a PA force to the olecranon of the elbow.

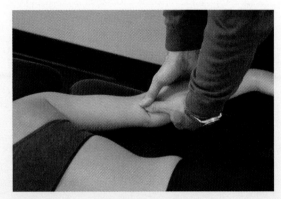

■ **Figure 9.24**   Posterior–Anterior of the Humeroulnar Joint

5 The clinician pushes to the first point of pain, and pain is assessed to determine if concordant.

6 The clinician then applies a PA force beyond the first point of pain toward end range.

7 Sustained holds or repeated movements are performed to determine the influence on the patient's condition.

8 The opposite side is assessed if appropriate.

Posterior–Anterior of the Humeroradial Joint

Though less common, an isolated impairment to the humeroradial joint (HRJ) can restrict full extension. Additionally, a PA to the HRJ may be beneficial if the patient exhibits complaints during the combined movements of extension and supination.

1 The patient is positioned in prone.

2 The anterior aspect of the arm is cradled by the fingers of the clinician.

(Continued)

③ The thumbs are placed on the posterior–lateral aspect of the radial head using a pad to pad placement (Figure 9.25 ■).

④ The clinician applies a combined movement of lifting the anterior aspect of the arm while applying a PA force to the elbow.

⑤ The clinician pushes to the first point of pain. Pain is assessed to determine if concordant.

⑥ The clinician then applies a PA force beyond the first point of pain toward end range.

⑦ Sustained holds or repeated movements are performed to determine the influence on the patient's condition.

⑧ The opposite side is assessed if appropriate.

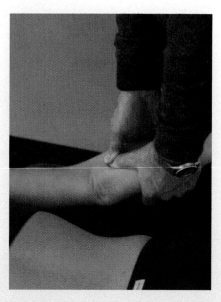

■ **Figure 9.25** Posterior–Anterior of the Humeroradial Joint

Anterior–Posterior of the Humeroulnar Joint

The congruent articular arrangement of the HUJ reduces the amount of passive joint play. Essentially, the majority of the movement at this joint is a traction-based movement where the ulna is distracted from the convex humerus.

① The patient is positioned in supine.

② The elbow is prepositioned in slight flexion at the side of the patient.

③ The posterior aspect of the forearm is cradled by the fingers of the clinician.

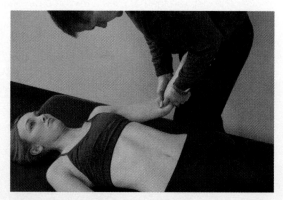

■ **Figure 9.26** Anterior–Posterior of the Humeroulnar Joint

④ The thumbs are placed on the anterior aspect of the ulna through the soft tissue of the brachium (Figure 9.26 ■).

⑤ The clinician applies a combined movement of lifting the posterior aspect of the forearm while applying an AP force to the anterior aspect of the ulna.

⑥ The clinician pushes to the first point of pain. Pain is assessed to determine if concordant.

⑦ The clinician then applies an AP force beyond the first point of pain toward end range.

⑧ Sustained holds or repeated movements are performed to determine the influence on the patient's condition.

⑨ The opposite side is assessed if appropriate.

Anterior–Posterior of the Humeroradial Joint

An AP of the HRJ may be effective if the patient exhibits restrictions in the combined movements of flexion and pronation.

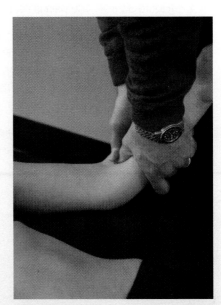

■ **Figure 9.27**   Anterior–Posterior of the Humeroradial Joint

1. The patient is positioned in supine.

2. The elbow is prepositioned in slight flexion at the side of the patient.

3. The posterior aspect of the forearm is cradled by the fingers of the clinician.

4. The thumbs are placed on the anterior aspect of the radial head through the soft tissue of the anterior aspect of the extensor group.

5. The clinician applies a combined movement of lifting the posterior aspect of the arm while applying an AP force to the elbow (Figure 9.27 ■).

6. The clinician pushes to the first point of pain; pain is assessed to determine if concordant.

7. The clinician then applies an AP force beyond the first point of pain toward end range.

8. Sustained holds or repeated movements are performed to determine the influence on the patient's condition.

9. The opposite side is assessed if appropriate.

Posterior–Anterior of the Radioulnar Joint (Medial Glide of the Radial Head)

During supination the ulna exhibits external rotation while the radius moves distally and medially. Prepositioning of the elbow in supination alters the axis of the proximal radioulnar joint (PRUJ) which increases the intensity of force that is translated through the joint.[48]

1. The patient assumes a sitting position.

2. The patient assists in stabilizing the distal wrist using the opposite hand.

(Continued)

③ The clinician applies a PA force to the first point of pain to the posterior–lateral aspect of the radial head (Figure 9.28 ■). The pain is assessed to determine if concordant.

④ The movement is repeated, pushing beyond the first point of pain toward end range. Repeated movements or sustained holds may be helpful to determine the influence of movement on the joint.

⑤ The patient may enhance the intensity of the movement by passively supinating the wrist.

⑥ The opposite side is assessed if appropriate.

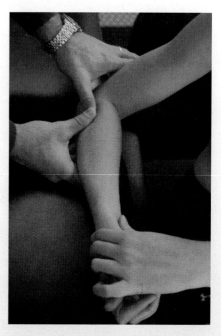

■ **Figure 9.28** Posterior–Anterior of the Radioulnar Joint

Anterior–Posterior of the Radioulnar Joint (Lateral Glide of the Radial Head)

During pronation, the radius moves both proximally and laterally while the ulna concurrently internally rotates. By altering pronation or supination prepositions the clinician can adjust the intensity of force and implicate different aspects of the capsule and ligaments.[48]

① The patient assumes a sitting position.

② The patient assists in stabilizing the distal wrist using the opposite hand.

③ The clinician applies an AP force to the first point of pain to the anterior–medial aspect of the radial head (Figure 9.29 ■). The pain is assessed to determine if concordant.

④ The movement is repeated pushing beyond the first point of pain toward end range. Repeated movements or sustained holds may be helpful to determine the influence of movement on the joint.

⑤ The patient may enhance the intensity of the movement by passively pronating the wrist.

⑥ The opposite side is assessed if appropriate.

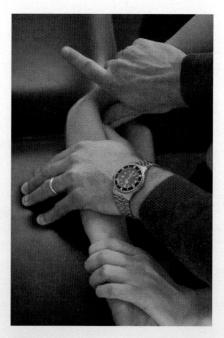

■ **Figure 9.29** Anterior–Posterior of the Radioulnar Joint

Posterior–Anterior and Anterior–Posterior Glide of the Proximal Carpal Row

A PA and an AP glide of the proximal carpal row may benefit movement such as extension and flexion and may indirectly improve restrictions in pronation and supination.

1. The patient assumes a sitting position.

2. For a PA glide, the patient's forearm is pronated. For an AP glide the patient's forearm is supinated.

3. The clinician stabilizes the proximal wrist by firmly grasping the radius and ulna.

4. With the other hand the clinician grasps the patient's carpal bones just distal to the proximal carpal row.

5. The clinician applies an AP force to the first point of pain to the proximal carpal row (Figure 9.30 ■). The pain is assessed to determine if concordant.

6. The movement is repeated, pushing beyond the first point of pain toward end range.

7. Repeated movements or sustained holds may be helpful to determine the influence of movement on the joint.

8. The patient's wrist is pronated for the PA glide.

9. The clinician applies a PA force to the first point of pain to the proximal carpal row (Figure 9.31 ■). The pain is assessed to determine if concordant.

10. The movement is repeated, pushing beyond the first point of pain toward end range.

11. Repeated movements or sustained holds may be helpful to determine the influence of movement on the joint.

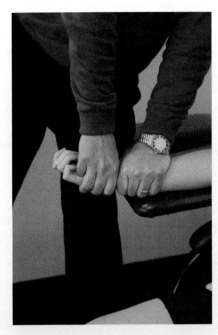

■ Figure 9.30 Anterior–Posterior Glide of the Proximal Carpal Row

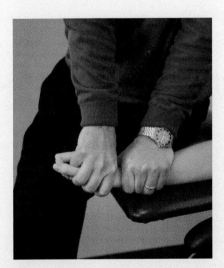

■ Figure 9.31 Posterior–Anterior Glide of the Proximal Carpal Row

Posterior–Anterior and Anterior–Posterior Glide of the Mid-Carpal Row

Although less mobile than the proximal row, a PA and an AP of the mid-carpal row may also improve movements such as flexion and extension as well as indirectly improving the movements of pronation and supination.

1. The patient assumes a sitting position.
2. The positioning and set-up is identical to the proximal carpal row.
3. The clinician stabilizes the proximal carpal row by firmly grasping the proximal carpal bones.
4. With the other hand the clinician grasps the carpal bones just distal to the proximal carpals or mid-carpal joint.
5. The clinician applies an AP force to the first point of pain to the mid-carpal row. The pain is assessed to determine if concordant.
6. The movement is repeated, pushing beyond the first point of pain toward end range.
7. Repeated movements or sustained holds may be helpful to determine the influence of movement on the joint.
8. The patient's wrist is pronated for the PA glide.
9. The clinician applies a PA force to the first point of pain to the mid-carpal row; the pain is assessed to determine if concordant.
10. The movement is repeated, pushing beyond the first point of pain toward end range.
11. Repeated movements or sustained holds may be helpful to determine the influence of movement on the joint.
12. To isolate the CMC joint the clinician follows the same procedures outlined for the proximal and mid-carpal rows but stabilizes the distal carpal bones and moves the metacarpals in an AP or PA fashion.

Radial and Ulnar Glide of the Wrist

In theory, radial and ulnar glide of the wrist should improve the movements of ulnar and radial deviation.

1. The patient assumes a sitting position.

2. The clinician stabilizes the proximal wrist by firmly grasping the radius and ulna.

3. With the other hand the clinician grasps the carpal bones just distal to the proximal carpal row.

4. The clinician applies an ulnar glide to the first point of pain to the proximal carpal row (Figure 9.32 ■). The pain is assessed to determine if concordant.

5. The movement is repeated, pushing beyond the first point of pain toward end range.

6. Repeated movements or sustained holds may be helpful to determine the influence of movement on the joint.

7. The clinician alters his or her position to apply a radial glide.

8. The clinician applies a radial glide to the first point of pain to the proximal carpal row (Figure 9.33 ■). The pain is assessed to determine if concordant.

9. The movement is repeated, pushing beyond the first point of pain toward end range.

10. Repeated movements or sustained holds may be helpful to determine the influence of movement on the joint.

The ulnar and radial glide can be repeated using the same landmarks as the AP and PA glide to target the mid-carpal and CMC rows.

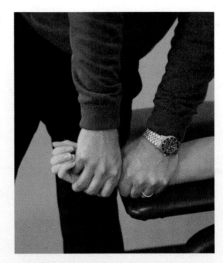

■ **Figure 9.32** Ulnar Glide of the Proximal Carpal Row

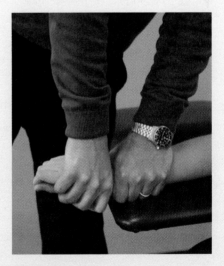

■ **Figure 9.33** Radial Glide of the Proximal Carpal Row

Medial Glide (Extension and Abduction) of the First Carpometacarpal Joint or Metacarpophalangeal Joint

Injury to the thumb often leads to a reduction of abduction and extension at the carpometacarpal (CMC) and metacarpophalangeal (MCP) joint. Tightness in the medial structures and stretching of the lateral structures result in an imbalance in tissues. The medial glide technique is designed to improve the mobility of the soft-tissue structures, thus normalizing motion.

1. A medial glide is performed in a sitting position.

2. The thumb is prepositioned into slight extension or abduction, whichever the focus of motion that is desired.

3. The clinician places one thumb distal and one thumb proximal to the MCP (Figure 9.34 ■).

4. The fingers of the clinician are laced around the medial aspect of the thumb and hand as a counterforce.

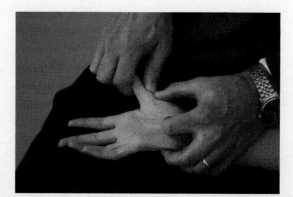

■ **Figure 9.34** Metacarpophalangeal Joint Medial Glide

5. The clinician applies a medial glide to the first point of pain; the pain is assessed to determine if concordant.

6. The movement is repeated, pushing beyond the first point of pain toward end range.

7. Repeated movements or sustained holds may be helpful to determine the influence of movement on the joint.

Anterior–Posterior and Posterior–Anterior Glides of the Metacarpophalangeal Joint, Proximal Interphalangeal Joint, and Distal Interphalangeal Joint

AP and PA glides of the MCP, PIP, and DIP are designed to improve the range of motion of flexion and extension of the fingers.

1. The patient assumes a sitting position.

2. Resting symptoms are assessed.

3. For a PA glide, the patient's forearm is pronated. For an AP glide the patient's forearm is supinated.

4. Using a pincer grasp the clinician stabilizes the joint (MCP, PIP, or DIP) just proximal to the joint line and grasps the joint with the other hand just distal to the joint line (Figure 9.35 ■).

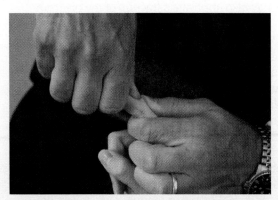

■ Figure 9.35 Posterior–Anterior Glide of the PIP

5. The clinician applies an AP or PA glide to the first point of pain. The pain is assessed to determine if concordant.

6. The movement is repeated, pushing beyond the first point of pain toward end range.

7. Repeated movements or sustained holds may be helpful to determine the effect of movement on the joint.

Summary

- Because of the multiple planes of movement associated with the elbow–wrist–hand, a general screen that examines general planar passive movement is a quick method to identify movement dysfunction.

- Most wrist motion is coupled. When a passive or an accessory movement is isolated as pathological to a specific joint, assessment of the coupled movements may be beneficial.

- The primary purpose as assessment of passive motion is to determine whether the passive movement may be beneficial as a treatment mechanism. Subsequently, it is imperative to determine the effect of sustained holds or repeated movements during a passive or accessory movement.

Special Clinical Tests

Palpation   Palpation at the elbow includes both bony and soft-tissue palpation. Bony palpation should include the medial and lateral epicondyles of the humerus, the olecranon process of the humerus, and the radial head of the radius, specifically at the contact point of the capitulum.

Soft-tissue palpation should include the lateral, posterior, and medial musculature, the biceps tendon anteriorly, the ulnar nerve medially, and the ulnar collateral ligament medially. The medial collateral ligaments are easier to expose and palpate when the arm is supinated and flexed to approximately 90 degrees.

Sucher[49] advocates the benefit of palpation for CTS of the hand. Others have reported that isolated tenderness to the snuff-box may be indicative of a scaphoid fracture, pain directly on the scaphoid tubercle may indicate instability, and tenderness to the hook of the hamate may indicate a hamate fracture.[11] Isolated tenderness to the pisiform may also implicate a fracture of the pisiform.[11]

Muscle Testing   Manual muscle testing at the elbow using a dynamometer has been shown to demonstrate comparable validity to pain report in patients with medial elbow pain.[50] It has been suggested that isolating the middle finger of the extensor digitorum communis is beneficial in isolating pain associated with lateral epicondylitis.[51] This suggestion lacks investigation and may yield imprecise findings. Nonetheless, this method, identified as the Maudsley Test, is described further in the special clinical tests section. Additional forms of manual muscle testing of the wrist and hand are less discriminative and therefore should be used in concert with other examination methods.[52]

Summary

- The use of palpation may be helpful to localize symptoms in the elbow–wrist–hand.
- Manual muscle testing of the elbow may be a valid method of determining strength loss.

Treatment Techniques

Active Physiological Movements

The propensity for elbow stiffness following a trauma is very high.[53,54] Large amounts of range-of-motion loss are common, often in the extensors greater than in the flexors.[53] Both intrinsic and extrinsic factors are related to range-of-motion losses[55] and both may benefit from active plane-based movements.

An exercise program of wrist glides has been advocated by Akalin and colleagues for treatment of carpal tunnel syndrome[56] (Figure 9.36 ■). The five discrete movements involved finger positions that were (1) straight, (2) hooked, (3) tabletop, and (4) a fist. The movements are designed to provide tendon gliding without significant discomfort to the patient.

Passive Physiological Movements

Many of the same passive physiological assessment movements and hand holds used within the examination process are plausible treatment techniques,

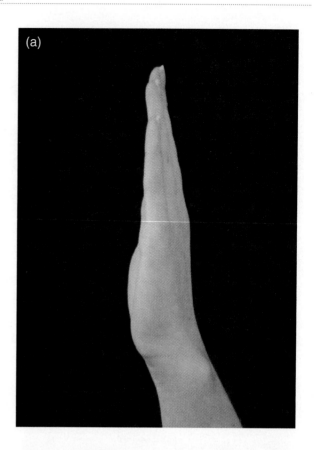

(a)

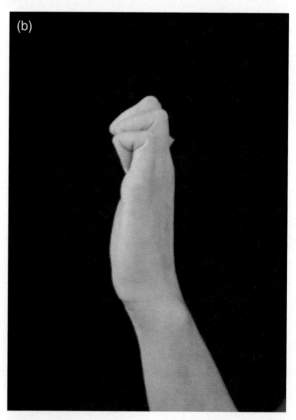

(b)

■ **Figure 9.36**   Wrist Glide Techniques Used as a Home Program

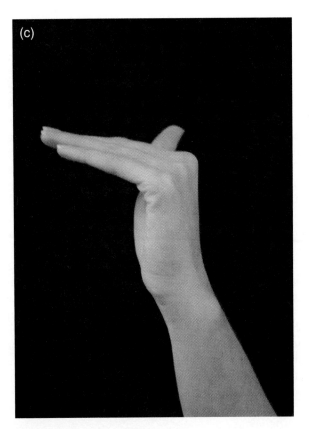

(c)

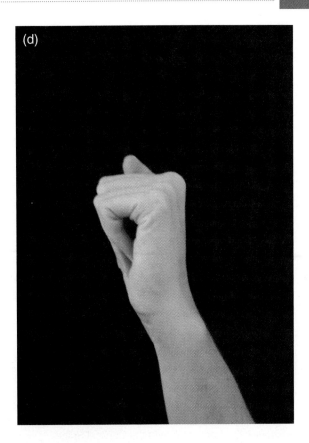

(d)

■ **Figure 9.36**   (Continued)

specifically if sustained holds or repeated movements lead to a reduction of pain. For the elbow, it is useful to incorporate the coupled movements of elbow extension and flexion with varus and valgus forces.

Passive Accessory Movements

Like passive physiological techniques, the crux behind patient-based indices of assessment suggests that treatment methods are selected based on concordant examination findings. Subsequently, many of the passive accessory treatments reflect the same position and stabilization demonstrated during the examination section of this chapter. However, some alterations are plausible during passive accessory treatment that may improve the outcome of the intervention.

Cervical Mobilization or Manipulation for Elbow Pain

There is also moderate evidence to support that manual therapy provides an excitatory effect on sympathetic nervous system activity.[57–59] Specially, the manual therapy mobilization techniques associated with AP and lateral glides have been well documented.[60] An excitatory effect on the sympathetic nervous system occurs concurrently with a reduction of hypoanalgesia and may parallel the effects of stimulation of the

dorsal periaqueductal gray area of the mid-brain, a process that has occurred in animal research.[61] Documented evidence supports the benefit of modulation of pain and remarkably has a nonlocalized effect. Stimulation of the cervical spine has demonstrated upper extremity changes in pain response (pressure pain) and a measurable sympathoexcitatory effect.[61–63] Techniques include a lateral glide of the cervical spine (Figure 9.37 ■) and AP and PA glides, which are both described in Chapter 5.

The Use of a Belt during Elbow Distraction

Stabilization during elbow distraction can be challenging, specifically during prepositioning of elbow flexion. The judicious use of a mobilization belt can improve the stabilization of the humerus to allow a more vigorous mobilization of the HUJ or HRJ [64] (Figure 9.38 ■). When using a belt, pay careful attention to the friction and pressure the belt places on human tissue.

Mobilizations with Movements

The Elbow   Paungmali et al.[65] and Vicenzino et al.[62] describe a mobilization technique for lateral epicondylalgia in which a lateral glide is performed at the elbow. This technique is performed by stabilizing

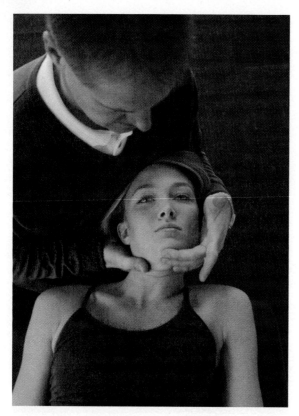

■ **Figure 9.37** Lateral Glide of the Cervical Spine

the internally rotated shoulder at the distal humerus, while concurrently performing a lateral glide at the ulna by contact on the medial side using a belt. The patient performs a gripping procedure during the mobilization in order to reproduce the patient's pain, albeit only to threshold levels (Figure 9.39 ■). Their findings suggest that the mobilization with movement technique yielded physiological effects similar to those produced with spinal manipulation. Abbott[66] and Abbott et al.[67] describe a similar technique that involves repeated wrist extension by the patient versus gripping an object.

The technique can also be performed without the use of a belt, as pictured in Figure 9.40 ■.

Lateral Glide of Radius and Ulna during Wrist Grip   For patients who complain of lateral elbow pain during flexion, a mobilization with movement technique can be performed in supine. The patient is given an object to grip. The clinician stabilizes the humerus while providing a concurrent lateral glide to the radius and ulna (Figure 9.41 ■). The patient grips the object the same time the lateral glide is administered. The patient is instructed to move the elbow actively into flexion.

The Wrist

Mobilization with Movement of the Proximal Row of the Wrist (Radial Glide)   In a single case study, Backstrom[68] describes a mobilization with movement to the wrist for the treatment of De Quervain's

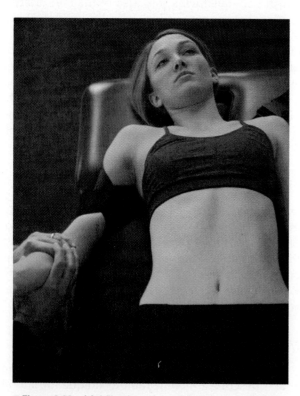

■ **Figure 9.38** Mobilization of the Elbow Using a Belt to Brace the Humerus

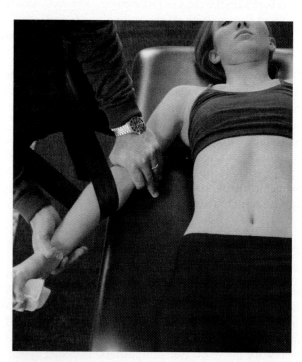

■ **Figure 9.39** Lateral Glide with a Belt and an Active Gripping Procedure

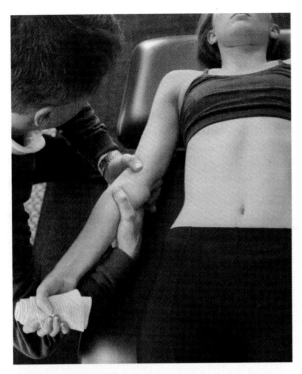

■ **Figure 9.40**   Lateral Glide of Radius and Ulna during Wrist Grip with Active Elbow Extension

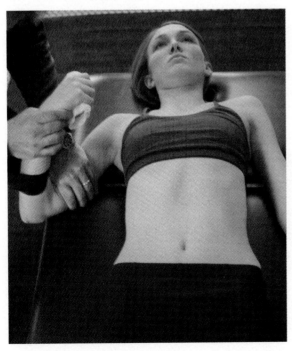

■ **Figure 9.41**   Lateral Glide of Radius and Ulnar during Wrist Grip with Active Elbow Flexion

tenosynovitis. This technique uses pain-free radial glides from the clinician during concurrent thumb extension by the patient (Figure 9.42 ■).

Mobilization with Movement using a Radial Glide and Active Flexion   The following technique may be useful in patients with limited and painful flexion. The clinician stabilizes the distal radius and ulna and provides a radial glide to the carpal rows. Biomechanically, a radial glide is coupled with flexion (Figure 9.43 ■). The patient is instructed to perform an active wrist flexion movement.

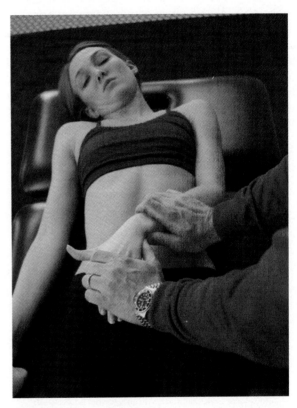

■ **Figure 9.42**   Mobilization with Movement of the Proximal Row of the Wrist; Radial Glide

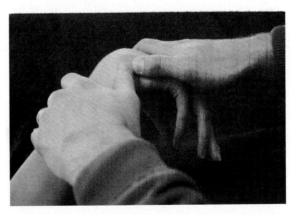

■ **Figure 9.43**   Mobilization with Movement of the Wrist using Radial Glide and Active Wrist Flexion

Mobilization with Movement using an Ulnar Glide and Active Extension The following technique may be useful in patients with limited and painful extension. The clinician stabilizes the distal radius and ulna and provides an ulnar glide to the carpal rows. Biomechanically, an ulnar glide is coupled with extension (Figure 9.44 ■). The patient is instructed to perform an active extension movement.

Ulnar Glide of Wrist during Closed-Chain Active Extension For patients with painful and limited extension, a closed-chain active extension approach may be useful. The patient is instructed to weight bear on the wrist while in extension. The clinician stabilizes the distal radius and ulna and performs an ulnar glide to the wrist. The patient is instructed to weight bear through the wrist and move into further extension (while maintaining the closed-chain position) (Figure 9.45 ■).

Manually Assisted Posterior–Anterior to the Wrist Maitland[69] promoted the use of passive physiological movement of the wrist during concurrent passive accessory motion at the carpal bones. These column mobilizations are designed to improve the AP or PA movement of the carpal bones during physiological flexion and extension at the wrist. If the wrist is divided into three theoretical columns (medial, middle, and lateral), the pressure from the thumb can promote an AP or PA movement on the adjacent columns (Figure 9.46 ■).

Manipulation

Manipulation of the Elbow Kaufman[70] described the use of the manipulation method in the treatment of lateral epicondylitis of the elbow. The technique, sometimes termed "Mill's manipulation," is performed by rapidly driving the elbow into extension, after a prepositioning of pronation and wrist flexion (Figure 9.47 ■). The clinician's thumb applies a PA force on the humeral head, which enhances the distraction at the humeral–radial joint.

Watson's Manipulation of the Wrist A technique designed to manipulate the carpal bones was used as a treatment technique for lateral epicondylitis. The technique involves a prepositioning of the patient with the forearm of the affected side on a table with the palmar side of the hand facing down. The clinician grasps the patient's scaphoid bone between the clinician's thumb and index finger and extends the wrist dorsally at the same time the scaphoid bone was manipulated ventrally (Figure 9.48 ■). The authors repeated this procedure 20 times and alternated by either forced passive extension of the wrist or extension against resistance.

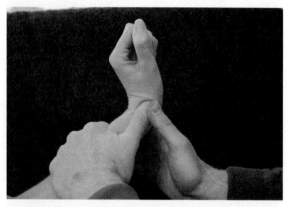

■ **Figure 9.44** Mobilization with Movement Using an Ulnar Glide and Active Extension

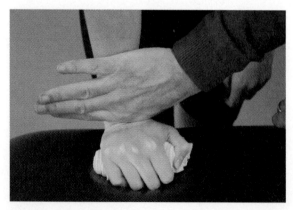

■ **Figure 9.45** Ulnar Glide of Wrist during Closed-Chain Active Extension

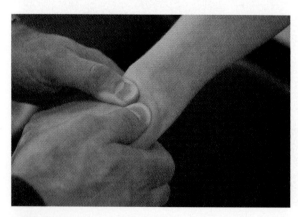

■ **Figure 9.46** Manually Assisted Mobilization PA of the Columns

Manipulation of the Carpal Joints of the Wrist
Kaufman and Bird[71] describe a series of radiocarpal wrist manipulations used in the treatment of a patient with chronic dysfunction associated with a Colles' fracture (Figures 9.49 ■ and 9.50 ■). Their isolated, single case findings advocate the use of manipulation for an increase in range of motion and grip strength.

Summary

- The majority of the treatment techniques used for the elbow–wrist–hand is borne from the examination methods.
- Selected treatment methods may be enhanced by using the coupled movements of the elbow and wrist and by incorporating patient assistance during movements.

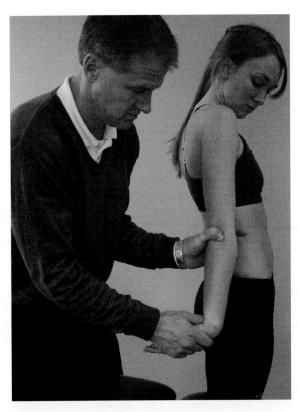

■ **Figure 9.47**   Manipulation of the Elbow

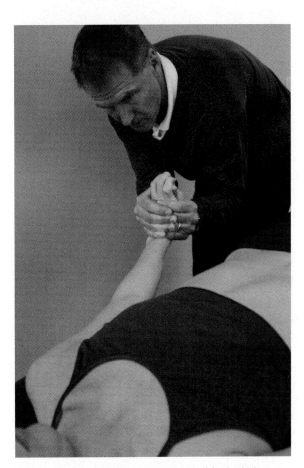

■ **Figure 9.49**   Longitudinal Distraction Manipulation Preposition of Extension

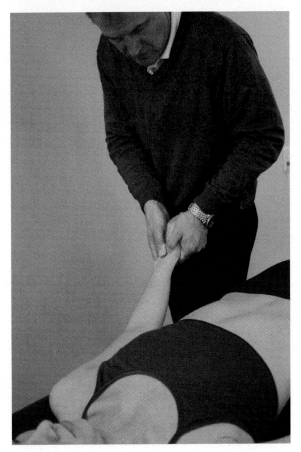

■ **Figure 9.48**   The End Position of the Manipulation Technique

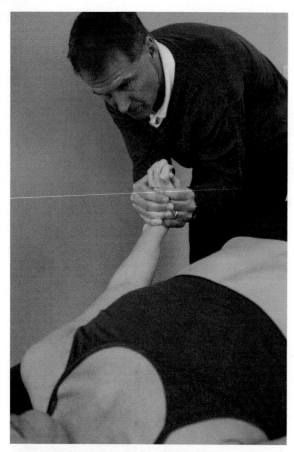

■ **Figure 9.50** Longitudinal Distraction Manipulation Preposition of Flexion

Treatment Outcomes

The Evidence

Active Range-of-Motion Exercises Early elbow movement may help reduce the losses; however, it is common to see degenerative changes, fibrous tissue adhesions, musculotendinous structures, ectopic ossification, loose bodies, and/or osteophytes.[54,55] Lastly, age (> 70 years) is a more significant factor in active and passive range-of-motion loss versus gender[72] most likely associated with the biomechanical changes of degeneration.

Active movement for the treatment of the wrist/hand has a well-documented benefit. Early movement, focusing on separate exercises of the wrist and hand after surgical treatment of CTS, has been associated with better outcomes versus immobilization.[73] Others have reported the benefit of an active range-of-motion treatment in the intervention of uncomplicated distal radius fractures[74] (Level C).

Passive Physiological Movements Few studies have examined the benefits of passive physiological movements of the elbow or wrist. Coyle and Robertson[75] reported improvement in radiocarpal range of motion in a small trial of patients who had encountered a distal radius fracture, although oscillations resulted in a better overall outcome and were more effective in reducing pain. Clinically, elbow extension is generally the most difficult range of motion to improve with treatment. Although Cyriax and Cyriax[76] reported that the capsular pattern of the elbow is flexion loss greater than extension, although there have been no studies that have substantiated or refuted this finding. The movements associated with passive physiological stretching and oscillatory glides may be beneficial in the treatment of elbow, wrist, and hand pain. As with the patient response-based guidelines, treatment methods selected based on concordant examination findings are warranted. Treatments such as passive elbow flexion with and without varus and valgus forces and passive elbow extension with and without varus and valgus forces may improve the outcome of a manual therapy intervention. By using the stabilization methods discussed earlier the clinician improves the dosage of the force applied through the elbow, wrist, and hand (Level D).

Nerve Glides Radial nerve glides and radial head mobilization for elbow pain has demonstrated better outcomes than a standard approach that included ultrasound, strengthening, and friction massage.[77] Case studies have reported the benefit of nerve gliding exercises in patients with cubital tunnel syndrome.[78] More studies have investigated the benefit in wrist- and hand-related regions. Median nerve gliding exercise relieved pain and improved range of motion for patients more so than patients who received no treatment, but demonstrated comparable outcomes to joint mobilization in patients with CTS.[79] In another population of patients with CTS, splinting performed with nerve glides demonstrated a reduction of pain and an improvement in grip strength; however, the effect was not significantly better than splinting alone.[56] Lastly, adding nerve glides to standard care in treatment of CTS has not shown significant long-term benefit[80] (Level B, no benefit).

Passive Accessory Mobilizations A significant amount of literature has been dedicated to the outcome associated with passive accessory movements. Coyle and Robertson[75] demonstrated improvements in pain and function using a treatment approach of passive accessory glides in patients' after Colles' fracture. Their findings suggested that oscillatory mobilization was more effective (specifically on pain) than static stretching. Randall et al.[81] reported that joint mobilization was more effective than a home exercise program of general exercises. The techniques utilized were standard carpal joint glides to patient tolerance.

Mobilization of the wrist may be useful for patients with CTS,[82] although a direct comparative trial against a control has yet to be performed (Level D). In a comprehensive literature review, Bisset et al.[83] and Herd and Meserve[84] reported benefits associated with elbow pain using cervical mobilizations. Variations in application have included the use of compression versus distraction, prepositioning in a restriction versus the use of a "loose-packed" mobilization, and other nuances. Ishikawa et al.[85] reported that the use of wrist distraction during carpal mobilization may reduce the amount of carpal excursion during mobilization. The authors suggest that the nonuse of traction is associated with greater physiological, coupled, and intercarpal movement. Tal-Akabi and Rushton[79] advocate that joint mobilization leads to improvements in pain and range of motion more so than no treatment and lead to a reduction in surgical intervention.[79] Mobilization with movement appears to be more beneficial than a wait-and-see approach or a cortisone injection for patients with tennis elbow[83] (Level B).

Manipulation Procedures   For treatment of the elbow, manipulation of the carpal bones has shown benefit in a randomized controlled trial investigating patients with lateral epicondylitis. Those who received "conventional" care and wrist manipulation performed better than those who just received conventional care for treatment of lateral epicondylitis.[86] The Mills manipulation demonstrated significant short- and long-term improvements in patients with lateral epicondylgia[87] (Level A).

Several studies have investigated the benefit of manipulation of the carpal bones in conditions such as carpal tunnel syndrome. In a comparative trial, Davis et al.[88] found comparable outcomes to medical care when manipulation was combined with ultrasound and wrist supports. In two case reports, Valente and Gibson[89] and Russell[90] advocated manipulation to the neck, wrist, and elbow in the treatment of two 40+-year-old females with conditions of CTS and cubital tunnel syndrome, respectively. Hafner et al.[91] reported comparable outcomes of medical and chiropractic intervention of manipulation of the wrist. Despite the purported benefits, Ernst[92] acknowledged that no hard evidence exists to support "chiropractic" manipulation for the care of CTS (Level C).

Manipulation to the cervical spine is associated with immediate hypoalgesia to the elbow,[93,94] which does not decline during repeated use.[95] There is Level B evidence of short-term gain using these procedures.

Summary

- Significant evidence exists to support early controlled active movement for healing of fractures and ligamentous injuries of the elbow–wrist–hand.
- Mobilization with movement may yield effective outcomes if implemented in patients with lateral epicondylitis.
- Evidence exists to the benefit of cervical mobilization for reduction of elbow pain in lateral epicondylitis.
- Some evidence exists to support the use of manipulation of the wrist for both elbow and wrist pain.

Chapter Questions

1. Describe the overlap in contribution of potential concordant pain between the elbow, wrist, and hand.

2. Briefly outline the biomechanical characteristics of the elbow. Identify how the degrees of freedom are passively assessed. Repeat this process for the wrist and hand.

3. Identify the benefits and disadvantages of using a single scale for the elbow, wrist, and hand.

4. Suggest the potential manual therapy treatments used in conditions associated with stiffness, laxity, and pain for the elbow, wrist, and hand.

Patient Cases

Case 9.1: Cyrus Flint (52-year-old male)

Diagnosis: Lateral elbow pain.

Observation: He demonstrates large forearms and heavy musculature.

Mechanism: He notes pain after a weekend of woodworking. His mechanism was associated with heavy gripping and twisting.

Concordant Sign: Resisted wrist extension.

Nature of the Condition: He indicates the problem is a nuisance but it is painful during normal activities only. He is able to modulate the pain with ibuprofen.

Behavior of the Symptoms: The pain is isolated to the lateral elbow of the patient with some referral of symptoms to the thumb.

Pertinent Patient History: He has a long-term history of osteoarthritis. He was diagnosed with prostate cancer in 1987.

Patient Goals: Pain is his primary concern.

Baseline: At rest, 3/10 NAS for pain; when worst, 5/10 pain.

Examination Findings: Active resisted extension of the wrist is the most painful movement. There is some discomfort during elbow extension with a varus force. A PA of the humeral head is also concordant.

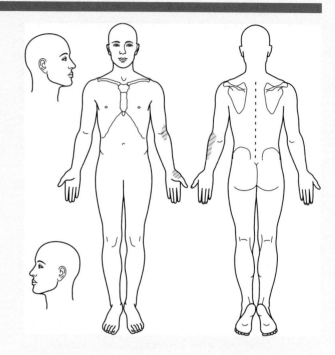

1. Based on these findings, what else would you like to examine?
2. Is this patient a good candidate for manual therapy?
3. What is the expected prognosis of this patient?
4. What treatments do you feel presented in this book may be beneficial for this patient?

Case 9.2: Carol Downing (41-year-old female)

Diagnosis: Status post-colles fracture.

Observation: She exhibits swelling and thickness around her wrist. The left wrist is poorly defined.

Mechanism: She has been casted for the last 8 weeks. She just had the cast removed 2 days ago.

Concordant Sign: Wrist extension and flexion are equally painful.

Nature of the Condition: At present, she does not feel confident in her strength or mobility to actively use the wrist.

Behavior of the Symptoms: The discomfort she feels involves a sharp pain during movements followed by a dull ache during rest.

Pertinent Patient History: She had a hysterectomy at age 32.

Patient Goals: She is interested in increasing the mobility and strength of her wrist.

Baseline: Her pain at rest is 2/10 and increases to 6/10 during movement.

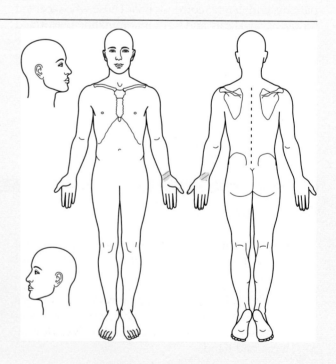

Examination Findings: Active and passive physiological movements are equally limited and painful in flexion and extension. Her thumb exhibits no pain with movements. Her accessory mobility is significantly limited.

1. Based on these findings, what else would you like to examine?
2. Is this patient a good candidate for manual therapy?
3. What is the expected prognosis of this patient?
4. What treatments do you feel presented in this book may be beneficial for this patient?

PEARSON
myhealthprofessionskit

Use this address to access the Companion Website created for this textbook. Simply select "Physical Therapy" from the choice of disciplines. Find this book and log in using your username and password to access video clips and the anatomy and arthrological information.

References

1. Bystrom S, Hall C, Welander T, Kilbom A. Clinical disorders and pressure–pain threshold of the forearm and hand among automobile assembly line workers. *J Hand Surg.* 1995;20B:782–790.
2. Ono Y, Nakamura R, Shimaoka M, Hiruta S, Hattori Y, Ichihara G. Epicondylitis among cooks in nursery schools. *Occup Environ Med.* 1998;55:172–179.
3. Walker-Bone KE, Palmer KT, Reading I, Cooper C. Criteria for assessing pain and nonarticular soft-tissue rheumatic disorders of the neck and upper limb. *Semin Arthritis Rheum.* 2003;33(3):168–184.
4. Katz JN, Larson MG, Sabra A, et al. The carpal tunnel syndrome: Diagnostic utility of the history and physical examination findings. *Ann Intern Med.* 1999;112:321–327.
5. Atroshi I, Breidenbach W, McCabe S. Assessment of the carpal tunnel outcome instrument in patients with nerve-compression symptoms. *J Hand Surg.* 1997;22:222–227.
6. Gunnarsson L, Amilon A, Hllestrand P, Leissner P, Philipson L. The diagnosis of carpal tunnel syndrome: Sensitivity and specificity of some clinical and electrophysiological tests. *J Hand Surg.* 1997;22:34–27.
7. O'Gradiagh D, Merry P. A diagnostic algorithm for carpal tunnel syndrome based on Bayes's theorem. *Rheumatology.* 2000;39:1040–1041.
8. Bessette L, Keller RB, Lew RA, Simmons BP, Fossel AH, Mooney N, Katz JN. Prognostic value of a hand symptom diagram in surgery for carpal tunnel syndrome. *J Rheumatol.* 1997;24(4):726–734.
9. Priganc V, Henry S. The relationship among five common carpal tunnel syndrome tests and the severity of carpal tunnel syndrome. *J Hand Ther.* 2003;16:225–236.
10. Dugas J, Andrews J. in Altchek D, Andrews J. *The athlete's elbow.* Philadelphia; Lippincott Williams and Wilkins: 2001.
11. Daniels J, Zook E, Lynch J. Hand and wrist injuries. Part 1: Non-emergent evaluation. *Am Family Phys.* 2004;69:1941–1948.
12. Haque M, Adams J, Borenstein D, Wiesel S. *Hand and wrist pain.* 2nd ed. Danvers, MA ; Lexis Publishing: 2000.
13. Kapandji I. *The physiology of the joint: The elbow flexion and extension.* 2nd ed. Vol 1. London; Livingstone: 1970.
14. Chaparro A, Rogers M, Fernandez J, Bohan M, Choi SD, Stumpfhauser L. Range of motion of the wrist: implications for designing computer input devices for the elderly. *Disabil Rehabil.* 2000;22(13–14):633–637.
15. Ebara S, Yonenobu K, Fujinara K, Yamashita K, Ono K. Myelopathic hand characterized by muscle wasting: A different type of myelopathic hand in patients with cervical spondylosis. *Spine.* 1988;13:785–791.
16. Colebatch J, Gandevia S. The distribution of muscular weakness in upper motor neuron lesions affecting the arm. *Brain.* 1989;112:749–763.
17. Mehta JA, Bain GI. Posterolateral rotatory instability of the elbow. *J Am Acad Orthop Surg.* 2004;12(6):405–415.
18. Higgs PE, Young VL. Cumulative trauma disorders. *Clin Plast Surg.* 1996;23(3):421–433.
19. Sanders M. *Management of cumulative trauma disorders.* Boston; Butterworth-Heinemann: 1997.
20. Kim DH, Kam AC, Chandika P, Tiel RL, Kline DG. Surgical management and outcome in patients with radial nerve lesions. *J Neurosurg.* 2001;95(4):573–583.
21. Kiuru MJ, Haapamaki VV, Koivikko MP, Koskinen SK. Wrist injuries; diagnosis with multidetector CT. *Emerg Radiol.* 2004;10(4):182–185.
22. Pao VS, Chang J. Scaphoid nonunion: diagnosis and treatment. *Plast Reconstr Surg.* 2003;112(6):1666–1676.
23. Macdermid JC, Wessel J. Clinical diagnosis of carpal tunnel syndrome: A systematic review. *J Hand Ther.* 2004;17(2):309–319.
24. Gupta K, Benstead T. Symptoms experienced by patient with carpal tunnel syndrome. *J Canadian Neuro Sci.* 1997;24(4):338–342.

25. Viera A. Management of Carpal Tunnel Syndrome. *Am Fam Physic.* 2003;68(2);265–273.

26. Lehtinen I, Kirjavainen T, Hurme M, Lauerma H, Martikainen K, Rauhala E. Sleep-related disorder in carpal tunnel syndrome. *Acta Neuro Scand.* 1996;93:360–365.

27. Bongers P, Kremer A, ter Laak J. Are psychosocial factors, risk factors for symptoms and signs of the shoulder, elbow or wrist/hand? A review of the epidemiological literature. *Am J Ind Med.* 2002;41:315–342.

28. Henderson M, Kidd BL, Pearson RM, White PD. Chronic upper limb pain: An exploration of the biopsychosocial model. *J Rheumatol.* 2005;32(1):118–122.

29. Bergqvist U, Wolgast E, Nilsson B, Voss M. Musculoskeletal disorders among visual display terminal workers: Individual, ergonomic, and work organizational factors. *Ergonomics.* 1995;38(4):763–776.

30. Bernard B, Sauter S, Fine L, Petersen M, Hales T. Job task and psychosocial risk factors for work-related musculoskeletal disorders among newspaper employees. *Scand J Work Environ Health.* 1994;20(6):417–426.

31. Engstrom T, Hanse JJ, Kadefors R. Musculoskeletal symptoms due to technical preconditions in long cycle time work in an automobile assembly plant: A study of prevalence and relation to psychosocial factors and physical exposure. *Appl Ergon.* 1999;30(5):443–453.

32. Lagerstrom M, Wenemark M, Hagberg M, Hjelm EW. Occupational and individual factors related to musculoskeletal symptoms in five body regions among Swedish nursing personnel. *Int Arch Occup Environ Health.* 1995;68(1):27–35.

33. LaStayo PC, Wheeler DL. Reliability of passive wrist flexion and extension goniometric measurements: A multicenter study. *Phys Ther.* 1994;74(2):162–174.

34. Horger MM. The reliability of goniometric measurements of active and passive wrist motions. *Am J Occup Ther.* 1990;44(4):342–348.

35. Mayerson NH, Milano RA. Goniometric measurement reliability in physical medicine. *Arch Phys Med Rehabil.* 1984;65(2):92–94.

36. Adams BD, Grosland NM, Murphy DM, McCullough M. Impact of impaired wrist motion on hand and upper-extremity performance. *J Hand Surg [Am].* 2003;28(6):898–903.

37. Morrey BF, Chao EY. Passive motion of the elbow joint. *J Bone Joint Surg Am.* 1976;58(4):501–508.

38. Youm Y, Dryer RF, Thambyrajah K, Flatt AE, Sprague BL. Biomechanical analyses of forearm pronation–supination and elbow flexion–extension. *J Biomech.* 1979;12(4):245–255.

39. Morrey BF, Askew LJ, Chao EY. A biomechanical study of normal functional elbow motion. *J Bone Joint Surg Am.* 1981;63(6):872–877.

40. Wagner C. Determination of the rotary flexibility of the elbow joint. *Eur J Appl Physiol Occup Physiol.* 1977;37(1):47–59.

41. Sarrafian S, Melamed J, Goshgarian G. Study of wrist motion in flexion and extension. *Clin Orthop.* 1977;126:153–159.

42. McGee D. *Orthopedic physical assessment.* 4th ed. Philadelphia: Saunders. 2002.

43. Garcia-Elias M, An KN, Berglund L, Linscheid RL, Cooney WP, Chao EY. Extensor mechanism of the fingers: I. A quantitative geometric study. *J Hand Surgery.* 1991;16A:1130–1136.

44. Li ZM, Kuxhaus L, Fisk JA, Christophel TH. Coupling between wrist flexion–extension and radial–ulnar deviation. *Clin Biomech.* 2005;20(2):177–183.

45. Palmer AK, Skahen JR, Werner FW, Glisson RR. The extensor retinaculum of the wrist: An anatomical and biomechanical study. *J Hand Surg [Br].* 1985;10(1):11–16.

46. Brumfield RH, Champoux JA. A biomechanical study of normal functional wrist motion. *Clin Orthop Relat Res.* 1984;187:23–25.

47. Von Lanz T, Wachsmuth W. *Praktische anatomie.* Berlin; Springer-Verlag: 1959.

48. An N-K, Morrey B. Biomechanics of the elbow. In Morrey B. *The elbow and its disorders.* 3rd ed. Philadelphia; Saunders: 1993.

49. Sucher B. Palpatory diagnosis and manipulative management of carpal tunnel syndrome. *J Am Osteopathic Assoc.* 1994;94:647–663.

50. Rosenberg D, Conolley J, Dellon AL. Thenar eminence quantitative sensory testing in the diagnosis of proximal median nerve compression. *J Hand Ther.* 2001;14(4):258–265.

51. Fairbank SR, Corelett RJ. The role of the extensor digitorum communis muscle in lateral epicondylitis. *J Hand Surg [Br].* 2002;27(5):405–409.

52. Szabo RM, Slater RR Jr, Farver TB, Stanton DB, Sharman WK. The value of diagnostic testing in carpal tunnel syndrome. *J Hand Surg [Am].* 1999;24(4):704–714.

53. Morrey B. The posttraumatic stiff elbow. *Clin Orthop.* 2005;431:26–35.

54. Kim S, Shin S. Arthroscopic treatment for limitation of motion of the elbow. *Clin Orthop.* 2000;375:1401–1448.

55. Chinchalker S, Szekeres M. Rehabilitation of elbow trauma. *Hand Clinic.* 2004;20:363–374.

56. Akalin E, El O, Peker O, et al. Treatment of carpal tunnel syndrome with nerve and tendon gliding exercises. *Arch Phys Med Rehab.* 2002;81(2):108–113.

57. Chiu T, Wright A. To compare the effects of different rates of application of a cervical mobilization technique on sympathetic outflow to the upper limb in normal subjects. *Man Ther.* 1996;1:198–203.

58. Vicenzino B, Collins D, Wright A. An investigation of the interrelationship between manipulative therapy-induced hypoalgesia and sympathoexcitation. *J Manipulative Physiol Ther.* 1998;21:448–453.

59. Sterling M, Jull G, Wright A. Cervical mobilization: Concurrent effects on pain, sympathetic nervous system activity and motor activity. *Man Ther.* 2001;6:72–81.

60. Wright A. Pain-relieving effects of cervical manual therapy. In. Grant R (ed). *Physical therapy of the cervical and thoracic spine.* 3rd ed. New York; Churchill Livingston: 2002.

61. Lovick T. Interactions between descending pathways from the dorsal and ventrolateral periaqueductal gray matter in the rat. In: Depaulis A, Bandler R (eds). *The midbrain periaqueductal gray matter.* New York; Plenum Press: 1991.

62. Vicenzino B, Paungmali A, Buratowski S, Wright A. Specific manipulative therapy treatment for chronic lateral epicondylalgia produces uniquely characteristic hypoalgesia. *Man Ther.* 2001;6:205–212.

63. Simon R, Vicenzino B, Wright A. The influence of an anteroposterior accessory glide of the glenohumeral joint on measures of peripheral sympathetic nervous system function in the upper limb. *Man Ther.* 1997;2(1):18–23.

64. Vincenzion B. Lateral epicondylalgia: a musculoskeletal physiotherapy perspective. *Man Ther.* 2003;8:66–79.

65. Paungmali A, O'Leary S, Souvlis T, Vincenzino B. Naloxone fails to antagonize initial hypoalgesic effect of a manual therapy treatment for lateral epicondylalgia. *J Manipulative Physol Ther.* 2004;27:180–185.

66. Abbott J. Mobilization with movement applied to the elbow affects shoulder range of movement in subjects with lateral epicondylagia. *Man Ther.* 2001;6:170–177.

67. Abbott J, Patla C, Jensen P. The initial effects of an elbow mobilization with movement technique on grip strength in subjects with lateral epicondylagia. *Man Ther.* 2001;6:163–169.

68. Backstrom K. Mobilization with movement as an adjunct intervention in a patient with complicated de Quervain's tenosynovitis: a case report. *J Orthop Sports Phys Ther.* 2002;32:86–97.

69. Maitland GD. *Peripheral manipulation* 3rd ed. London; Butterworth-Heinemann: 1986.

70. Kaufman RL. Conservative chiropractic care of lateral epicondylitis. *J Manipulative Physiol Ther.* 2000;23(9):619–622.

71. Kaufman RL, Bird J. Manipulative management of post-Colles' fracture weakness and diminished active range of motion. *J Manipulative Physiol Ther.* 1999;22(2):105–107.

72. Lin C, Ju M, Huang H. Gender and age effects on elbow joint stiffness in healthy subjects. *Arch Phys Med Rehabil.* 2005;86;82–85.

73. Cook A, Szabo R, Birkholz S, King E. Early mobilization following carpal tunnel release. A prospective randomized study. *J Hand Surg (Br).* 1995;20:228–230.

74. Kay S, Haensel N, Stiller K. The effect of passive mobilization following fractures involving the distal radius: a randomized study. *Aust J Physiother.* 2000;46:93–101.

75. Coyle J, Robertson V. Comparison of two passive mobilizing techniques following Colles' fracture: A multi-element design. *Man Ther.* 1998;3(1):34–41.

76. Cyriax J, Cyriax P. *Cyriax's illustrated manual of orthopaedic medicine.* Boston: Butterworth-Heineman; 1993.

77. Trudel D, Duley J, Zastrow I, Kerr EW, Davidson R, MacDermid JC. Rehabilitation for patients with lateral epicondylitis: A systematic review. *J Hand Ther.* 2004;17(2):243–266.

78. Coppieters MW, Bartholomeeusen KE, Stappaerts KH. Incorporating nerve-gliding techniques in the conservative treatment of cubital tunnel syndrome. *J Manipulative Physiol Ther.* 2004;27(9):560–568.

79. Tal-Akabi A, Rushton A. An investigation to compare the effectiveness of carpal bone mobilization and neurodynamic mobilization as methods of treatment for carpal tunnel syndrome. *Man Ther.* 2000;5:214–222.

80. Heebner ML, Roddey TS. The effects of neural mobilization in addition to standard care in persons with carpal tunnel syndrome from a community hospital. *J Hand Ther.* 2008;21:229–240.

81. Randall T, Portney L, Harris B. Effects of joint mobilization on joint stiffness and active motion of the metacarpal–phalangeal joint. *J Orthop Sports Phys Ther.* 1985;6:30–36.

82. Burke J, Buchberger DJ, Carey-Loghmani MT, Dougherty PE, Greco DS, Dishman JD. A pilot study comparing two manual therapy interventions for carpal tunnel syndrome. *J Manipulative Physiol Ther.* 2007;30(1):50–61.

83. Bisset L, Paungmali A, Vicenzino B, Beller E. A systematic review and meta-analysis of clinical trials on physical interventions for lateral epicondylalgia. *Br J Sports Med.* 2005;39(7):411–422.

84. Herd C, Meserve B. A Systematic review of the effectiveness of manipulative therapy in treating lateral epicondylalgia. *J Man Manip Ther.* 2008;16:225–237.

85. Ishikawa J, Cooney W, Niebur G, Kai-Nan A, Minami A, Kaneda K. The effects of wrist distraction on carpal kinematics. *J Hand Surg.* 1999;24A:113–120.

86. Struijs PA, Kerkhoffs GM, Assendleft WJ, Van Dijk CN. Conservative treatment of lateral epicondylitis. *AM J Sports Med.* 2004;32:462–469.

87. Nagrale A, Herd C, Ganvir S, Ramteke G. Cyriax physiotherapy versus phonophoresis with supervised exercise in subjects with lateral epicondylalgia: A randomized clinical trial. *J Man Manip The*r. 2009;17: 171–178.

88. Davis P, Hulbert J, Kassak K, Meyer J. Comparative efficacy of conservative medical and chiropractic treatments for carpal tunnel syndrome: A randomized controlled trial. *J Manipulative Physiol Ther.* 1998;21:317–326.

89. Valente R, Gibson H. Chiropractic manipulation in carpal tunnel syndrome. *J Manipulative Physiol Ther.* 1994;17:246–249.

90. Russell B. A suspected case of ulnar tunnel syndrome relieved by chiropractic extremity adjustment methods. *J Manipulative Physiol Ther.* 2003;26:602–627.

91. Hafner E, Kendall J, Kendall P. Comparative efficacy of conservative medical and chiropractic treatments for carpal tunnel syndrome: A randomized clinical trial. *J Manipulative Physiol Ther.* 1999;22(5):348–349.

92. Ernst E. Chiropractic manipulation for non-spinal pain: A systematic review. *N Z Med J.* 2003;116(1179):539.

93. Fernández-Carnero J, Fernández-de-las-Peñas C, Cleland JA. Immediate hypoalgesic and motor effects after a single cervical spine manipulation in subjects with lateral epicondylalgia. *J Manipulative Physiol Ther.* 2008;31(9):675–681.

94. Vicenzino B, Paungmali A, Buratowski S, Wright A. Specific manipulative therapy treatment for chronic lateral epicondylalgia produces uniquely characteristic hypoalgesia. *Man Ther.* 2001;6:205–212.

95. Paungmali A, O'Leary S, Souvlis T, Vicenzino B. Hypoalgesic and sympathoexcitatory effects of mobilization with movement for lateral epicondylalgia. *Phys Ther.* 2003;83:374–383.

Manual Therapy of the Lumbar Spine

Chad E. Cook

Objectives

- Understand the basic aspects of lumbar spine biomechanics and anatomy.
- Identify the role of physical and psychosocial factors and low back pain.
- Demonstrate the active physiological, passive physiological, passive accessory components for low back pain.
- Identify common lumbar spine special tests and their respective diagnostic values.
- Identify the pertinent treatment methods for lumbar spine impairment classifications.

Clinical Examination

Differential Diagnosis

Differential diagnosis of low back disorders into subcategories should result in more effective treatment.[1-4] Subcategorization into diagnostic classifications is also beneficial for improvements in research, building consistency in terminology, development of pertinent treatment algorithms, and optimization of surgical selection. McCarthy and colleagues[5] outlined three categorization processes during the initial diagnostic triage: (1) identification of nerve root–related problems, (2) identification of disorders that represent serious pathology, and (3) identification of patients who fall under the classification heading of nonspecific low back pain. This process allows the clinician to differentiate those subjects appropriate for care and categorizes further patients into homogenized groups for optimal treatment.

Step One: Identification of Nerve Root–Related Problems. Assessment of nerve root–related problems requires the *inability* to rule out low back–related leg pain by using a straight leg raise or slump test, and ruling in using specific tests such as those associated with hard neurological findings (e.g., reflex loss, sensation changes, and muscle strength loss).

Step Two: Red Flag Assessment. A concurrent second step involves the differentiation of patients that are appropriate for conservative care such as manual therapy. Within this step, it is imperative to isolate **sinister disorders** and red flags as well as other factors that may retard outcome or foster progression of chronicity. The majority of low back impairments are generally benign, self-limiting disorders,[6-9] nonetheless, in approximately 5% or less of cases, patients may present with a serious, specific disease process that requires emergency intervention.[6] Lurie[6] outlined three major categories of serious, specific disease processes that may not recover well during conventional care. The three major categories include: (1) nonmechanical spine disorders, (2) visceral disease, and (3) miscellaneous. Table 10.1 outlines the selected disorders under each specific category and the estimated prevalence of the dysfunction.

Patient history is more useful than a clinical examination in detecting malignancy, which is rare, accounting for less than 1% of low back pain.[6] Jarvik and Deyo[7] reported that the most diagnostic combination of red flags used to identify malignancy were age >50, history of cancer, unexplained weight loss, and failure of conservative care. The cluster of these variables demonstrated a sensitivity of 100% and a specificity of 60%. Infective spondylitis is another nonmechanical condition and is associated with a fever (sensitivity of 98%), although this finding is not specific to this disorder (specificity of 50%).[6] Ankylosing spondylitis is often associated (specificity of 82%) with early or slow onset, age <40, long-term discomfort (>3 months), morning stiffness, and improvement of discomfort

■ TABLE 10.1 Serious, Specific Low Back Diseases[6]

Category	Specific Disorders	Examples of Disorders
1) Nonmechanical Spine Disorders (±1%)	Neoplasia	Metastases, lymphoid tumor, spinal cord tumor
	Infection	Infective spondylitis, epidural abscess, endocarditis, herpes zoster, Lyme disease
	Seronegative spondyloarthritides	Ankylosing spondylitis, psoriatic arthritis, reactive arthritis, Reiter's syndrome, inflammatory bowel disease
2) Visceral Disease (1–2%)	Pelvic	Prostaitis, endometriosis, pelvic inflammatory disease
	Renal	Nephrolithiasis, pyelonephritis, renal papillary necrosis
	Aortic aneurysm	Aortic aneurysm
	Gastrointestinal	Pancreatitis, cholecystitis, peptic ulcer disease
3) Miscellaneous	Paget's disease	Paget's disease
	Parathyroid disease	Parathyroid disease
	Hemoglobinopathies	Hemoglobinopathies

with exercise, although a combination of these factors results in low sensitivity (23%).[8] Lurie[6] suggests including historical factors such as family history, thoracic stiffness, thoracic pain, and heel pain to further improve the specificity. The detection of cauda equina problems are most accurately identified by urinary retention (sensitivity of 90%, specificity of 95%).[9–11] In addition, red flags are potentially significant physiological risk factors for developing chronic low back pain if not appropriately assessed. These physical factors include evidence of radicular symptoms into the lower extremity, peripheralization of symptoms during treatment or movements, and narrowing of the intervertebral space upon radiological examination. Others have warned that no hard evidence exists that allows identification of the presence of specific physical factors that may lead to negative outcomes.[12–16]

Step Three: Diagnostic Classification. The third and final phase of diagnostic classification involves categorizing patients into homogenized groups (such as nonspecific low back pain) for better treatment. Low back classification models categorize homogeneous conditions by using one of three classification index strategies: (1) status index, (2) prognostic index, and (3) the patient response-based model. Status index models such as those created by Bernard and Kirkaldy-Willis[17] and Moffroid et al.[18] involve the use of physical impairment classifications (diagnoses) designed to discriminate among faulty pathological tissue. Groups are subdivided into homogenous categories based on suspected pain generators. Prognostic index models such as pain-related fear, coping behavior, and so on, are primarily used to predict the future outcome of the patient and to target prospectively those with potentially poor progression.[19] Prognostic index models are typically obtained from statistical analysis of preexisting data and may involve subclassifications based on like-type outcomes. Prognostic index models are retrospective in nature but have been suggested for use prospectively.[20]

Patient response-based models provide clinicians with potential exercise and treatment selections based on the patient's response to movements during an examination. Classification using the patient response-based method addresses symptom elicitation (using pain provocation or reduction methods) with various movements for diagnostic assessment. This classification model (provocation, reproduction, and reduction) assesses the response of singular or repeated movements and/or positions on the patient's concordant complaint of pain or abnormality of movement. Treatment techniques are often similar to the direction and form of the assessment method. The particular treatment technique is based on the movement method that reproduces the patient's pain in a way designed to yield a result that either reduces pain or increases range of motion. The direction, amplitude, forces, and speed of the treatment depends on the patient response during and after the application. This method consists of within-treatment and between-treatment patient response parameters of provocation, reproduction, and reduction that have shown to predict good overall outcomes.[20–23] Within the literature, this process of classification has further been subdivided into two primary forms: (1) diagnostic classification based on signs and symptoms, and (2) classification based on expectations of treatment outcomes.

Diagnostic classification based on signs and symptoms is the hallmark of most low back classification systems. Physicians have developed many classification techniques that place diagnostic labels on signs and symptoms (and imaging findings) to implicate the "guilty structure." The usefulness of these diagnostic labels seldom guide rehabilitation clinicians' decisions related to the prognosis or treatment of patients with low back pain.[19] Numerous International Classification of Diseases, 9th revision (ICD-9) codes outline specific back impairments, each with subtle differences in characteristics. In many cases, diagnostic equipment that is frequently used to classify low back pain is not discriminatory enough to specify a disorder. Lastly, some physicians do not agree on the occurrence of certain impairments, which may lead to over- or underreporting of the prevalence. These "labels" offer little or no confirmation of the nature, severity, irritability, or stage of the back impairment.

The patient response-based classification is a mechanism commonly referred to throughout this textbook. This classification occurs after results from assessment are analyzed.[19] An example, such as the Mechanical Diagnosis and Treatment (MDT) method (also known as the *McKenzie method*), allows for modification of classification based on follow-up findings.[20] Each classification is dependent upon each patient response to the assessment methods and the corresponding change in treatment approach. This approach does not rely on specific paradigms because each patient may exhibit unique symptoms, which do not lend to one dogmatic approach. However, these methods also have weaknesses as well as strengths. The MDT classification does not recognize spine instability or categories consisting of sinister pathologies such as tumors or fractures.[19]

A recent classification system by Peterson et al.[24,25] involves the merger of diagnostic and patient response indices into a single diagnostic classification. The purpose of this system is to identify clinically homogenous subgroups of patients with nonspecific low back pain that are outlined specifically with the symptomatic causal structures.[24] The process involves three steps in classifying a patient's condition, much of which is based on the MDT classification system. However, the system is designed to strengthen some of the areas in which the MDT classification system initially failed to discern, such as subclassification for the categories of zygopophyseal joint syndrome, sacroiliac joint syndrome, myofascial pain, adverse neural tension, and abnormal pain syndromes.[25]

A common low back impairment classification system is the *Quebec Task Force* (QTF) classification model. This model consists of 12 categories of impairments, often based on location of symptoms, imaging results, and chronicity of pain. One challenge to this model is that rehabilitation clinicians often do not have access to imaging and occasionally the imaging results are flawed. In addition, the intertester reliability between the QTF is unknown.[19] All categories are not mutually exclusive, lending to the chance of classification into more than one group.[19] The QTF model does not associate treatment with diagnosis.[26] Lastly, like the treatment response-based classification, not all impairment categories are represented (i.e., spine instability, fracture).

One reason the task of classification is difficult is that there is sparse evidence to support the relationship between specific physical factors and the ability to predict the severity of a lumbar pathology.[27,28] Similarly, there is little evidence to support that specific physical factors are accurate predictors of disability.[29,30] Essentially, low back recovery is poorly related to the severity of impairment, the type of treatment received, and/or the surgical procedure.

At present, no single diagnostic classification system has demonstrated superiority over another.[24,25] There are numerous pain generators of the lumbar spine, many that are clinically difficult to isolate secondary to convergence.[31] Sources can include the bone, which is innervated by the sympathetic trunk, gray rami communicantes, and the plexuses of the anterior and posterior longitudinal ligament. Additionally, muscles, thoraco-lumbar fascia (which contains nociceptive nerve endings), dura mater (which is innervated by an extensive plexus of the lumbar sinuvertebral nerve complex), the epidural plexus, ligaments, zygopophyseal joints that are innervated by the medial branches of the lumbar dorsal rami, and frequently, the intervertebral discs all share common nerve attachments.[32–34]

Spitzer reports that most incidences of low back pain do not have a readily demonstrable and identifiable pathological basis.[28] Often the selected pathological process is generally not the established cause of the pain[35] or may not occur in isolation. Despite these challenges, selected authors have suggested prevalence of "at-fault" structures that may be the pain generators of low back impairment. Bogduk[35] reported the most common site is typically discogenic (39%), followed by the zygopophyseal joints (15%), the sacroiliac joint (13%), and undefined (33%). Laslett reported estimates of 15–40% of low back pain originating in the zygopophyseal joints.[36]

Summary

- Even with clinical and diagnostic tests, the cause of most low back impairments is unknown.
- The lumbar intervertebral disc is the primary pain generator in the lumbar spine, accounting for the majority of impairments.
- A lumbar spine classification system may yield homogeneous outcomes for research, treatment, and assessment.
- The treatment response-based classification system may offer the most clinician-friendly classification model and typically does not suffer from many of the validity challenges of other classification models.
- At present, no classification system has been proven more valid than another has, but for manual therapy clinicians, the treatment response-based classification may allow adaptability to each individual patient.

Clinical Examination

Observation

For individuals with **postural syndromes,** observation and the symptoms associated with long-term positioning is a prime assessment tool. O'Sullivan[37] has used observations to determine positional preferences of spine instability patients. His classifications were based on position intolerance and theoretical instabilities on these positions. Additionally, Cook, Brismee, and Sizer[38] reported that certain postural intolerances were characteristic to patients with clinical lumbar spine instability. Granata and Wilson have associated the maintenance of selected trunk postures with the propensity for spine instability.[39]

A decreased **willingness to move** is also an observational method worth addressing and has been related to poor treatment outcomes.[40,41] Avoidance of certain movements because of fear of reinjury or increased pain is common in patients with chronic low back impairment.[42] This reluctance may be associated with fear of movement-related pain that may lead to a cascade of further problems. **Catastrophizing behavior,** a symptom frequently associated with decreased willingness to move, is also common in those with poor low back–related outcomes.[42]

Although not conclusively definitive, physiometric findings may assist the clinician in categorizing patient presentations. Physiometric findings are poorly reliable and are not always associated with patient outcomes, but when combined with other indicators are useful in patient assessment. Abnormal side-to-side weight-bearing asymmetry has been recognized in

patients with low back pain versus controls.[43] Other non-empirical-based findings such as flattened posture, excessive lordosis, or generalized poor posture may be associated with selected pathologies.

Riddle and Rothstein[44] found that detection of a lateral shift (Figure 10.1 ■) demonstrated poor inter-rater reliability during an examination. Kilpikoski et al.[45] also found poor reliability for visual detection of lateral shift but did agree on the directional preference of each centralizing patient. The directional preference

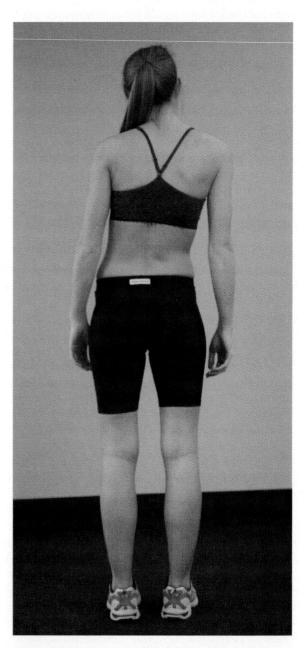

■ **Figure 10.1** Example with a right lateral shift. Shift detection is determined by analyzing the position of the trunk over the pelvis. In this example, the patient's trunk is shifted right over the pelvis.

corresponds to a movement or position that decreases pain symptoms, a movement that may include any active range of motion in the sagittal or coronal plane. Clare, Adams, and Maher[46] found moderate reliability (0.48–0.64) in the detection of a lateral shift and proposed the use of a photograph to dissect the sagittal plane to improve results. Tenhula et al.[47] suggested that response to a shift correction demonstrated useful clinical information during an examination confirming the presence of a lateral shift in patients with low back pain. The authors advocated the use of repeated side glides for analysis of centralization or peripheralization of symptoms, a finding supported by Young,[48] in association with repeated movement testing. Centralization of symptoms is associated with positive outcomes and a reduced tendency for disability.[29]

Patients may exhibit a lateral shift toward or away from his or her report of pain. If the shift is toward the pain the shift is described as an ipsilateral shift and may be associated with a central disc herniation. If the shift is away from the report of pain, the shift is described as a contralateral shift and may be associated with a posterolateral disc herniation.

Patient History

Vroomen et al.[49] found that consistency in history taking varied among clinicians and was strongest in the areas of muscle strength and sensory losses, intermediate for reflex changes, and poor in the areas of a specific spine examination. Most significantly, the authors suggested that the clinicians should concentrate further on history taking to extract useful components for clarification. This suggestion is supported by other studies that found that gender differences,[50] occupations that require vigorous activity, occupations that expose the individual to vibration, the report of an unpleasant work environment,[50–53] prior history of back problems,[54] and a sedentary lifestyle,[52,54] corresponded to certain classifications of low back pain. A standardized approach to the subjective evaluation provides a useful format for the clinician and reduces the potential of errors of omission.

Young et al.[55] reported the link between patient history and physical examination factors in order to associate common subjective complaints with specific impairments. Their findings suggested that pain while rising from sitting was positively associated with both sacroiliac pain and discogenic pain, but negatively associated zygopophyseal pain. O'Sullivan et al.[56] reported correlations between complaint of back pain and time spent sitting. Relief during immediate sitting is strongly suggestive of spinal stenosis,[12] demonstrating a sensitivity of 0.46 and a specificity of 0.93.

Difficulty with toileting and the Valsalva maneuver during sitting is not specific to a particular disorder but is recognized as a common complaint during low back pain.[8] Wide-based gait or abnormalities of gait are commonly associated with stenosis; however, these symptoms are not specific to stenosis and may involve any low back–related pathology.[6]

Deyo and friends[11] suggests that when attempting to ascertain information that may be helpful to determine outcome based on history, the most useful items are failed previous treatments, substance abuse history, and disability compensation. Additionally, reviewing for the presence of depression may be helpful in determining whether this potential covariate will reduce the chance of successful recovery. Since no single scale exists that succinctly identifies all of these psychosocial characteristics, a careful and judicious history may be the only mechanisms for evaluation.

Area of the Symptoms Although radicular and referred pain are caused by many structures, isolation of origination of pain will help identify the "guilty" structure or movement impairment. Discounting myelopathy, essentially two primary types of referred pain can arise from the lumbar spine: (1) somatic referred pain, which is caused by noxious stimulation of structures or tissue intrinsic to the lumbar spine and (2) radicular pain that is caused by irritation of the lumbar or sacral nerve roots that pass through the lumbar vertebral canal or foramina.[57] Viscera can also refer pain to the lumbar region but is much less common. Secondary to convergence, somatic referred pain may arise from nearly any source of local lumbar or lumbosacral pain.[58] Clinically, the characteristics of somatic referred pain are often described as deeply perceived, diffuse, and hard to localize.[58] Causal structures may include ligaments, the surrounding musculature, zygopophyseal joints, and/or the intervertebral discs, each of which can refer pain to the lower extremities.[57,58]

Pain originating from the zygopophyseal joints can refer to the greater trochanter, posterior lateral thigh, buttock, groin, and below the knee,[59,60] and pain originating from the dura may cause back or leg symptoms. Smyth and Wright[61] found that dural-pain is typically isolated with traction stimulus and Kuslich et al.[62] found that dural-pain may be referred to the back, buttock, and the upper and lower leg. Typically, zygopophyseal, disc, and dural-pain have variable pain patterns but it is common to see symptoms below the knee for all three conditions.[57] Robinson[57] reported that common somatic referred pain descriptors are characterized by predictable identifiers. Pain is typically in the back or lower extremities, characterized as deep, achy, diffuse, poorly localized, dull, and cramp-like.

Radicular pain indicates that the origin of the pain generator is in the nerve root and may be associated with chemical or mechanical trauma. Radicular pain may display "hard" nerve findings that may include motor losses, sensory deficits, or pain in a dermatome distribution,[63] although these findings are specific and not sensitive. As with somatic referred pain, radicular symptoms may correspond to the level of dysfunction. L4 will radiate to the hip and anterolateral aspect of thigh (never to foot). L5 will radiate to the posterior side of the leg into the great toe, S1 to the posterior leg, distal–lateral to the foot and little toe, and S2 to the posterior side of the thigh, down to the bend of the knee, but never into the foot. McCullough and Waddell[64] and Smyth and Wright[61] differentiated L5 and S1 by the location of the symptoms; L5 is located at the dorsum of the foot, and S1 is located at the lateral aspect of the foot. However, L5–S1 pain does not always cause pain that refers to the foot or toe.

In general, radicular pain is characterized by the identifiers of intense, radiating, severe, sharp, darting, and lancinating, and is well localized, in comparison to somatic referred pain.[57] Caution should be used in diagnosing based on complaint of radiculopathy since description of the pain yields low diagnostic value.[65] To summarize, the area of the symptoms for low back may be associated with numerous structures including ligaments, dura, vertebrae, musculature, zygopophyseal, and intervertebral discs. Anterior thigh pain can be L2–3 dermatome or somatic pain from multiple structures. Groin pain can be somatic pain from local structures, somatic pain from the back, or L1–2 dermatomes. Posterior thigh pain can be somatic referred pain from many structures, S1–2 dermatomes, and L5–S1 disc or joint structures. Lastly, foot pain can be L5–S1 radiculopathy, somatic referred pain from disc (more rare), sacroiliac (less rare), dura (rare), or zygopophyseal (less rare).[57]

Summary

- The patient history may be the most important process of the low back examination, especially when differentiating red flags.
- Most of the pain patterns encountered during an examination vary between and within structures.
- The clinician should target the patient's concordant sign during each examination.
- A measurable baseline is imperative for comparative analysis before, during, and after each intervention and treatment technique.

Physical Examination

Active Physiological Movements

Centralization Phenomenon The **centralization phenomenon,** a hallmark of many low back classification programs, was initially recognized by McKenzie in the 1950s and first extensively documented in the 1980s.[66] Centralization is liberally defined as a movement, mobilization, or manipulation technique targeted to pain radiating or referring from the spine, which when applied abolishes or reduces the pain distally to proximally in a controlled predictable pattern.[67] This procedure has been well documented as a predictor of patient care outcomes, specifically suggesting that noncentralizers (those in which peripheral pain does not centralize with movements, mobilization, or manipulation) have poorer outcomes than those who do.[26,29] Others have used the centralization phenomenon to subclassify patients for research study.[68–71] Werneke and Hart[29] found patients' failure to centralize (noncentralizers) were at greater odds for higher pain intensity, failure to return to work, and interference with daily outcomes, and had a higher likelihood of further healthcare costs. Additionally, centralizing behavior is 95% sensitive and 52% specific for the presence of disc syndrome.[68] Without question, the evidence suggesting the inclusion of the centralization phenomenon in a spinal evaluation is quite compelling.

Available Range of Motion While useful in detecting asymmetries in available range of spinal motion, there is little evidence to support the singular use of "total available range of motion" as a predictor for low back impairment. Poor range of spinal motion is a common finding among asymptomatic spines, as is "normal" total range of motion in symptomatic spines. Parks and colleagues found a very poor correlation between total range of motion and functional assessment scores[72] and Haswell[73] reported poor to moderate clinician agreement for reproduction of active physiological movements within an examination session.

The Use of Repeated Movements Young et al.[55] suggested that repeated movements are essential in detection of discogenic pain. Repeated motions are useful to determine the irritability of a patient and the directional preference of their movements. If a patient's condition is easily exacerbated with minimal repeated motions, then further care should advance cautiously. The term "directional preference" reflects the preference of repeated movement in one direction that will improve pain and the limitation of range, whereas movement in the opposite direction causes signs and symptoms to worsen.[74]

The Use of Sustained Movements or Postures
Sustained movements or postures also are essential to detect the pain behavior of the patient. Patients may exhibit preferences in directions of sustained holds or may demonstrate reduction of pain once a segment is stretched or tension is released. In some occasions, repeated movements may be too painful to examine in a patient, thus the use of sustained movements or postures may provide an alternative examination mechanism.

Active Physiological Flexion

The purpose of active physiological flexion is to examine the influence of the movement on the patient's concordant sign and to determine the effect of repeated or sustained movements and whether this response centralizes the patient's concordant pain.

1. The patient is first positioned in a neutral standing position and baseline pain and radicular/referred symptoms are requested.

2. The patient is instructed to flex forward to his or her first point of pain and the pain is queried to determine if concordant (Figure 10.2 ■).

3. The patient is then instructed to progress past the first point of pain; symptoms are again queried.

4. The patient is then instructed to perform repeated movements past and/or near the end range of the motion.

5. While performing the movement, the patient is instructed to report whether his or her symptoms are worsening, improving, or staying the same, and/or centralizing, peripheralizing, or neither. It is imperative that the clinician also identify whether range of motion increases or decreases during movement.

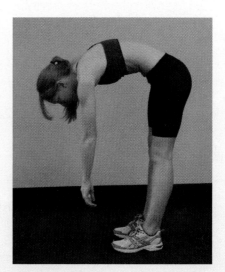

■ **Figure 10.2**   Flexion of the Lumbar Spine

6. If repeated flexion to end range was pain-free, gently "take up the slack" and apply firm pressure to engage the end-feel.

7. At the end-feel position, if pain-free, apply small repeated oscillations to rule out this motion (Figure 10.3 ■).

8. If pain was present during flexion, the overpressure is unnecessary.

(Continued)

If the repeated or sustained movements and overpressure are pain-free, the movement can be identified as nonprovocative. Maitland[75] stated that a joint (or movement) could not be classified as normal unless the range is pain-free during movement and passively with the inclusion of an overpressure. He suggested placing firm pressure at the end of the available range, then applying small oscillatory movements at that end range. Only one study has investigated this phenomenon in rehabilitation assessment. Peterson and Hayes[76] reported that abnormal pathological end-feels are associated with more pain than normal end-feels during passive physiological motion testing at the knee or shoulder. They suggested that the presence of this finding may indicate dysfunction and thus should be assessed during the clinical examination.

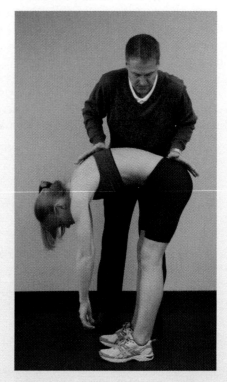

■ **Figure 10.3**　Flexion with Overpressure

Active Extension-Repeated Movements

The purpose of active physiological extension is to examine the influence of the movement on the patient's concordant sign and to determine the effect of repeated or sustained movements and whether this response centralizes the patient's concordant pain.

① The patient is first positioned in a neutral standing position.

② The hands of the patient are placed on each side of his or her hips and baseline pain and radicular/referred symptoms are reported.

③ The patient is instructed to extend backward to his or her first point of pain and the pain is queried to determine if concordant (Figure 10.4 ■).

④ The patient is then instructed to progress past the first point of pain; symptoms are again queried.

⑤ The patient is then instructed to perform repeated movements past and/or near the end range of the motion.

⑥ While performing the movement, the patient is instructed to report whether his or her symptoms are worsening, improving, or staying the same, and/or centralizing, peripheralizing, or neither. It is imperative that the clinician also identify whether range of motion increases or decreases during movement.

⑦ If end-range repeated extension was pain-free, gently "take up the slack" and apply firm pressure to engage the end-feel.

⑧ At the end-feel position, if pain-free, apply small repeated oscillations to rule out this motion (Figure 10.5 ■).

⑨ If pain occurs during extension at any time during the range, the overpressure is unnecessary.

In the event that a patient does not demonstrate centralization with standing repeated movements, it may be relevant to assess the movements in a prone or supine position. Patients who demonstrate a high degree of irritability may require off-loading of the spine in order to centralize with repeated movements or sustained postures. The clinician may adopt this examination position if he or she suspects a high degree of irritability and an increased likelihood of centralization with prone or supine movements.

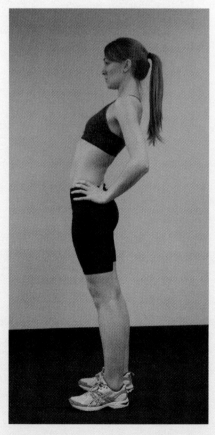

■ Figure 10.4 Repeated Extension of the Lumbar Spine

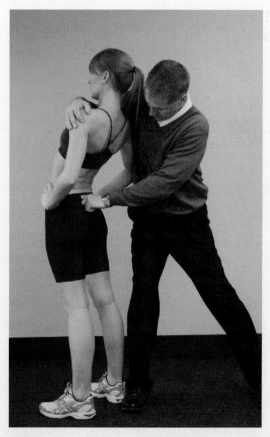

■ Figure 10.5 Extension with Overpressure

Active Side Flexion with Repeated Motions

Past studies have suggested that asymmetry between left and right side bending is a good predictor of disability[77] and is associated with severity of low back pain symptoms.[78] Causes of range-of-motion loss may include posterolateral disc irritation on one side versus the other, nerve root irritation with traction, and/or disc degenerative height changes that influence the axis of motion.

1. The patient is first positioned in a neutral standing position.

2. The hands of the patient are placed on each side of his or her hips and baseline pain and radicular/referred symptoms are queried.

3. The patient is instructed to bend to the right side to his or her first point of pain; the pain is queried to determine if concordant (Figure 10.6 ■).

4. The patient is then instructed to progress past the first point of pain and to perform repeated movements past and/or near the end range of the motion.

5. While performing the movement, the patient is instructed to report whether his or her symptoms are worsening, improving, or staying the same, and/or centralizing, peripheralizing, or neither. It is imperative that the clinician also identify whether range of motion increases or decreases during movement.

6. If end-range repeated side flexion was pain-free, gently "take up the slack" and apply firm pressure to engage the end-feel.

7. At the end-feel position, if pain-free, apply small repeated oscillations to rule out this motion (Figure 10.7 ■).

8. If pain is encountered at any point of the range of side flexion, the overpressure is unnecessary.

9. The movement is repeated on the opposite side.

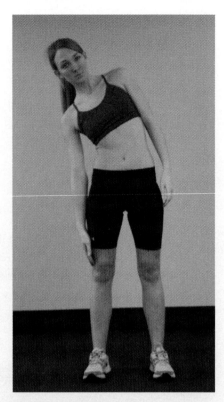

■ **Figure 10.6**   Repeated Side Flexion of the Lumbar Spine

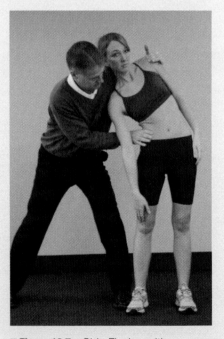

■ **Figure 10.7**   Side Flexion with Overpressure

Active Rotation (Sitting), No Repeated Motions

Very little axial transverse plane rotation of the lumbar spine exists in normal subjects. Previous studies suggest that normal rotation range of motion varies from a high of 3 degrees at L3–4 to a low of .5 degrees at L5–S1.

1. To test rotation, the patient is instructed to cross (tightly) his or her arms on the chest while sitting on the treatment table.

2. The clinician uses his or her knee to block the knees of the patient to reduce compensation at the pelvis (Figure 10.8 ■).

3. Further instructions and emphasis on proper posture will ensure the lumbar spine is isolated.

4. The patient is instructed to rotate as far as possible to the right side and pain is again queried. If painful, it is imperative to determine if the pain is concordant.

5. If pain-free, gently "take up the slack" and apply firm pressure to engage the end-feel.

6. At the end-feel position, if pain-free, apply small repeated oscillations to rule out this motion (Figure 10.9 ■).

7. If pain occurs at any time during the movement, the overpressure is unnecessary.

8. Repeat on the opposite side.

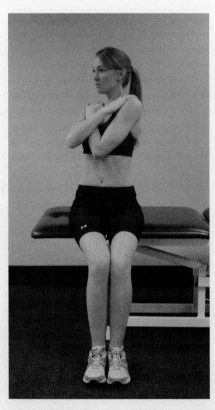

■ **Figure 10.8** Active Rotation to the Right

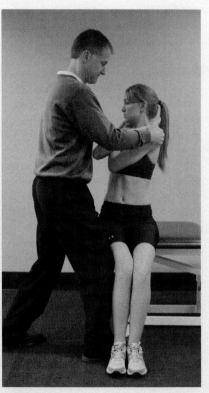

■ **Figure 10.9** Rotation to the Right with Overpressure

Combined Active Physiological Movements

Combining physiological movements allows movement to occur in a number of planes and may improve the ability to implicate a specific structure. Sizer and colleagues[79] advocate the significance of sagittal- versus rotational-based motions in detection of discogenic symptoms. Pain, reproduced during sagittal repeated motions, is typically indicative of a dysfunction of discogenic origin, whereas pain during rotation may indicate facet joint pathology. Nonetheless, further work is needed to support this claim.

Combined movements or "quadrant" movements may be useful in ruling out origination of pain from the lumbar spine. The motions are considered very provocative (sensitive) but do not have the capacity to define the origin or specific structure at fault. A negative finding during the combined tests may be more useful than a positive finding.

1. To test the quadrant position of flexion, the patient is first positioned in a neutral standing position.

2. The patient is instructed to reach downward with both hands toward the right ankle (Figure 10.10 ■) and the patient is queried for reproduction of symptoms.

3. Then, the patient is instructed to reach down with both hands toward the right ankle.

4. Again, the patient is queried for reproduction of symptoms.

5. For the extension quadrant, the patient is instructed to extend, rotate, and side-flex toward the left side (Figure 10.11 ■) and symptoms are assessed.

6. Then, the patient is instructed to extend, rotate, and side-flex toward the right side.

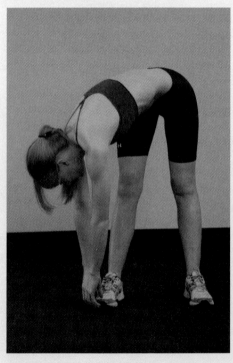

■ **Figure 10.10** Combined Flexion, Side Flexion, and Rotation

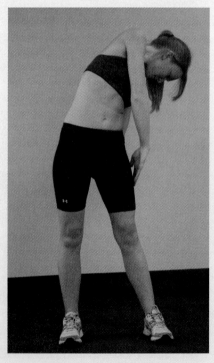

■ **Figure 10.11** Combined Extension, Side Flexion, and Rotation

Summary

- Active range of motion is necessary to elicit the concordant sign of the patient.

- Repeated motions will dictate whether the patient is a centralizer versus a peripheralizer and will contribute to predicting the likelihood of a positive long-term outcome.

- Detection of range-of-motion totals and comparing this to a presumed normal is less beneficial for the clinician than asymmetrical findings during bilateral movements.

Passive Movements

Passive Physiological Movements The primary benefit of passive physiological assessment is to determine if the response associated with passive movements is the same as the earlier investigated active movements. Passive physiological coupling assessment of the spine does not provide useful information since there is no specific "normal" coupling pattern.[80]

Strender et al.[81] demonstrated good reliability among experienced manual therapists for detection of passive physiological movements in a sidelying position. Others[82] have found relatively poor percent agreement between two manual therapists using a similar method of assessment. Most authors have debated the clinical utility, reliability, and validity of passive physiological findings, suggesting that passive physiological assessment of segmental motion may be too discrete, too minute, and thus too unreliable to yield beneficial information.[83–85] Indeed, useful findings are likely very specific but lack sensitivity and potentially usefulness in clinical practice.

Essentially, the most useful benefit to passive physiological assessment may be the comparison of active to passive movement. More passive range of motion may suggest a decreased willingness to volitionally move or pain that manifests during a weight-bearing posture. Although the usefulness of passive physiological assessment is debated, some clinicians would argue that their palpation capabilities provide helpful information for treatment selection.

Physiological Flexion and Extension

Physiological flexion and extension may provide the clinician with an understanding of the available sagittal movements of the lumbar spine.

1. To test flexion and extension, the patient is asked to lay on his or her side with the hips bent to 45 degrees and the knees to 60 degrees.

2. The clinician places the knees of the patient against his or her anterior–superior iliac spine to further stabilize the patient's lower extremities. This also allows the clinician to move the patient into flexion and extension using his or her trunk to support the lower extremities. Assessment of flexion and extension may require the clinician to lift up the knees of the patient (into slight side flexion) in order to reduce the drag on the plinth.

3. During the movements of flexion and extension, the clinician palpates the interspinous spaces of the patient's low back (a technique known as the "piano" grip) (Figure 10.12 ■) for an assessment of quality and quantity of movement at various spinal levels (Figure 10.13 ■).

(Continued)

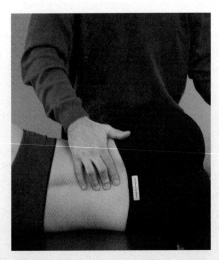

■ **Figure 10.12** The Piano Grip for Interspinous Space Palpation

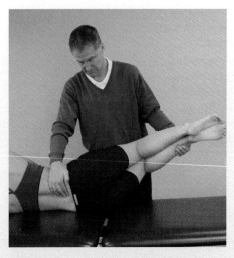

■ **Figure 10.13** Passive Physiological Flexion and Extension

Physiological Side Bending

During passive physiological side flexion, the clinician is concerned with determining the level of motion for each selected spinal segment in comparison to adjacent segments.

1. To perform the assessment, the patient is asked to lay on his or her side with the hips bent to 45 degrees and the knees to 60 degrees.

2. The clinician then grabs both the ankles of the patient to enable a lift as one lever arm; if the patient is large, the clinician can substitute by using one leg.

3. The clinician palpates the interspinous spaces using a piano grip (Figure 10.12).

4. The clinician gently lifts the legs feeling for separation and movement between the spinous processes (with caudal lifting at the legs, expect movement distal to proximal) (Figure 10.14 ■).

5. The method is repeated for the opposite side.

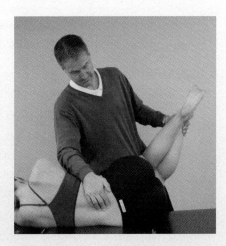

■ **Figure 10.14** Passive Physiological Side Flexion

Physiological Rotations

Physiological rotations involve isolated rotation of a single passive segment of the lumbar spine.

1. Patient is asked to lay on his or her side and is positioned at 45 degrees of hip flexion and approximately 60 degrees of knee flexion.

2. The clinician uses his or her forearm to take up the slack in the hip and his or her first and second finger to loop underneath the spinous process of L5 (or the targeted caudal segment).

3. Using a force of his or her forearm placed on the side of the rib cage and by gently applying a force on L4 (or the targeted cephalic segment) toward the treatment table with his or her thumb, the clinician applies a distraction moment at the L4–L5 facet (Figure 10.15 ■). The force is in a diagonal direction to emphasize the distraction of the facets. Excessive movement, pain, or gapping should be noted, since ideally, rotation is minimal.

4. The clinician should then progress cephalically and perform the same procedure for L5–S1, L3–L4, L2–L3, and L1–L2.

5. Testing the opposite side may also be useful.

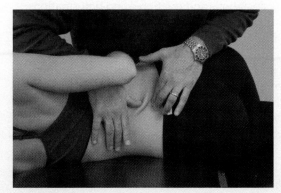

■ **Figure 10.15** Physiological Rotation, Passive Assessment

Summary

- Passive physiological range-of-motion assessment is marred by poor interclinician agreement.
- Perhaps the most useful information collected during passive physiological assessment is the comparison between active physiological motions.
- Assessment of concordant pain should still be the objective of passive physiological assessment.

Passive Accessories Passive accessory assessment is designed to address the relationship of pain intensity with the pathological movement or the level of stiffness, information that must be confirmable from patient to therapist.[86] Most authors use the terms "joint stiffness" and "motion detection" interchangeably by hypothesizing that stiffness is the detection of motion available within the examined joint,[87–92] although this concept is not always synonymously agreed upon by all clinicians.[92] The behavior and location of movement stiffness may dictate the level of pathology and theoretically may qualify a determinable level of motion loss.

Physiological accessory motions may include many of the traditional principles of arthrokinematic motion, including a central or unilateral posterior–anterior (PA), anterior–posterior (AP), arthrokinematic glide, and joint compression. The PA accessory motion is a commonly used therapeutic assessment tool for the low back and is a fundamental assessment tool in clinical judgment of both pain provocation and motion assessment.[93,94]

While detecting spinal accessory stiffness alone has not been shown to be consistently reliable,[92–95] several authors have suggested that palpating for pain accompanying stiffness or movement dysfunction is both reliable and valid.[86,87,96] Phillips and Twomey[96] examined 32 subjects with a format of both verbal and nonverbal responses accompanied with passive intervertebral and passive accessory intervertebral movements. In both a prospective and retrospective study, they too found that the manual clinicians displayed a higher level of sensitivity with verbal versus nonverbal manual diagnosis.

Dickey et al.[97] reported a strong relationship between reported pain and the measured amount of vertebral accessory motion during physiological movement. They reported that both intervertebral motions (translations and rotations) and deformations (compression and distraction movements) have a high degree of interaction with pain (as one increases so does the other). Jull and colleagues[87] used passive articular intervertebral movements (PAIVMs) to identify proven symptomatic zygopophyseal levels with very high levels of sensitivity. A similar study found reliability of motion detection to vary widely (kappa .00–.23) compared to verbal response (kappa .22–.65).[56] Others[98] found similar findings but to a lesser degree. Pain during these studies was reported during active physiological movements (flexion, extension, right to left side bending, and vice versa) but does suggest the importance of intersegmental motion assessment and accessory joint play.

The PA assessment has been used as a component of a clinical prediction rule for manipulation of the spine in two studies.[99,100] Both studies indicated that detectable PA stiffness in combination with other factors found during the examination was related to a higher likelihood that the patient would benefit with manipulation. This suggests that detection of stiffness by the clinician, when used in concert with other findings, may be beneficial for treatment outcomes. Fritz and colleagues[101] has correlated the treatment outcome with the assessment of posterior–anterior stiffness in a clinical population. The authors found that patients who displayed hypomobility during the clinician's assessment in the examination were more likely to improve with manipulation and patients who displayed hypermobility were more likely to improve with stabilization. Conversely, Hicks et al.[102] has identified that the presence of hypermobility (along with other variables) found during the examination (using a PA) is a predictor of success for patients undergoing a stabilization approach.

One study has indicated there is no relationship between the changes of stiffness of the overall perceived improvement by the patient.[103] They also found that changes in stiffness were not necessarily related to treatment applied.

Central Posterior–Anterior

Maitland suggested that assessment using a central posterior–anterior (CPA) is most beneficial when patients report midline or bilateral symptoms.[75] The CPA involves a three-point movement targeted to the spinous process of the patient. Under force application, all lumbar segments translate and rotate in a three-point fashion, although the segment that receives the direct force application moves greater than the surrounding segments.[104]

1. The technique is applied using a pisiform contact to the spinous process of the lumbar spine (Figure 10.16 ■). The force should be very light at first, followed by progressing intensities.

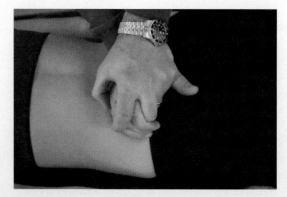

■ **Figure 10.16** Central Posterior–Anterior Intervertebral Assessment

② The clinician starts proximal and moves distal on the patient's spine asking for the reproduction of the concordant sign of the patient.

③ A segment can only be cleared if a significant amount of PA force is applied with no complaint of pain by the patient. A painful segment should elicit the concordant sign during the PA, and may reproduce radicular or referred symptoms at first.

④ Repeated movement or sustained holds help determine the appropriateness of the technique; diminished findings with repeated movements may be an indicator that the technique is useful.

Unilateral Posterior–Anterior

A unilateral posterior–anterior (UPA) also involves a three-point movement targeted to the facet, lamina, or transverse process of the targeted segment.[104]

① Using a thumb pad to thumb nail contact (Figure 10.17 ■) the clinician applies a gentle force perpendicular to the targeted transverse process of the lumbar spine (right or left). The force should be about 4 kg or thumb nail blanching at first. By placing the PA force laterally on the transverse process, more rotation is elicited.

② The UPAs are preformed proximal with a proximal to distal progression.

③ The clinician should ask for the reproduction of the concordant sign of the patient.

④ Repeated movement or sustained holds help determine the appropriateness of the technique and a segment can only be cleared if a significant amount of PA force is applied.

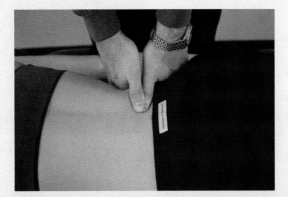

■ **Figure 10.17** Unilateral Posterior–Anterior
Intervertebral Assessment

L5–S1 Differentiation

The proximity of the L5–S1 facet to the sacroiliac joint may cause confusion for clinicians during differential assessment of the facet and sacroiliac joint. Both areas refer pain that covers similar anatomical regions and the L5–S1 facet is very close to the sacroiliac joint, lying midway between the L5 spinous process and the deep-set sacroiliac joint. In most patients, the joints are less than 1 inch from one another. A theoretical triangle exists between the L5–S1 facet and the sacroiliac joint (Figure 10.18 ■). The tip of the triangle is at the L5 spinous process and the sides of the triangle are present at the sacroiliac joint. Midway in the upper sides of the triangle are the L5–S1 facets.

Correct palpation can effectively target each segment and allow the clinician to perform a UPA pain provocation maneuver.

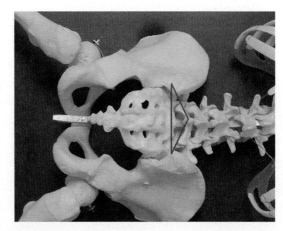

■ **Figure 10.18** The Triangle of L5–S1 and the Sacroiliac Joint

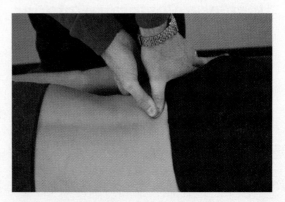

■ **Figure 10.19** UPA Force to L5–S1 Facet

1. The clinician palpates the sacral base by first identifying the superior border of the posterior–superior iliac spine (PSIS).

2. The fifth lumbar vertebra is then palpated as the first prominent spinous process superior to the sacral base.

3. The clinician applies a UPA force midway between the spinous process of L5 and the PSIS (sacroiliac joint). This force should identify the L5–S1 facet (Figure 10.19 ■).

4. The clinician then applies a UPA force at an angle medial to the PSIS of the same side (Figure 10.20 ■). This force should identify the sacroiliac joint and/or structures surrounding or overlaying the joint.

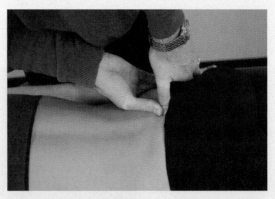

■ **Figure 10.20** UPA Force (at angle) to Sacroiliac Joint

Concordant pain should identify which of the two regions (or both) should be focused on during treatment.

Transverse Glide

The transverse glide is a combined translation and rotation assessment method. In most cases, the transverse glide is identified by the patient as a greater provocateur than a UPA or CPA. This assessment method should be used with caution since it may lead to soreness and easier reproduction of symptoms.

1. Using a thumb pad, the clinician hooks the targeted spinous process, removing the slack associated with soft tissue.

2. If the pain of the patient is reported on the left, the clinician should move to the right side of the patient (Figure 10.21 ■) and push the spinous process to the left. By placing the lateral force on the spinous process, rotation is elicited.

3. The transverse glides are initiated proximal with a proximal to distal progression.

4. The clinician should ask for the reproduction of the concordant sign of the patient.

5. The pathological segment should elicit the concordant sign of the patient during the mobilization, and may reproduce radicular or referred symptoms.

6. Repeated movement or sustained holds help determine the appropriateness of the technique.

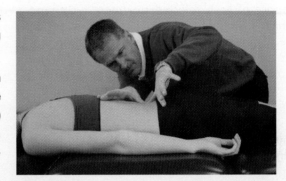

■ **Figure 10.21** Transverse Glide of the Lumbar Spine

Summary

- Passive accessory assessment may yield useful information in the detection of lumbar pathology.
- Passive accessory assessment is useful in isolating the dysfunctional segment.
- Passive accessory assessment may be unreliable when assessment of "Stiffness-only" is the goal.
- Passive accessory assessment is beneficial when pain provocation is the purpose of the segmental examination.

Clinical Special Tests

Palpation Generally, palpation of the lumbar spine is not useful in implicating selected tissue because of a condition called convergence. Convergence occurs when a number of structures that are innervated by the same systems send afferent messages to the brain, and the brain is unable to ascertain where and what structure the afferent messages were from. In addition, the location of the structure targeted by the clinician may not be the actual structure targeted. Billis et al.[105] reported poor reproducibility among clinicians for identifying the L5 spinous process. Clinicians and manual therapists demonstrated more reproducibility than students did, but all subjects were seemingly inaccurate. French et al.[106] reported similar findings for palpatory mechanisms used prior to the administration of chiropractic techniques. Subsequently, palpation-based treatments in the absence of patient report of concordant pain may yield variable findings among clinicians.

Manual Muscle Testing The use of manual muscle testing of the lumbar musculature is controversial. The construct of a manual muscle test for lumbar impairment assumes the resisted weakness implicates a weakness and subsequent impairment. However, because the lumbar spine's musculature is complex, the global musculature (prime movers) may exhibit no strength losses while the local musculature may be both weak and may demonstrate motor control problems. Local musculature weakness (multifidi and transverses abdominus) and motor loss commonly demonstrates subtle quantifiable clinical features[107] with inconsistent findings during manual muscle testing. In essence, gross manual muscle testing of the trunk may yield variable information for subjects with low back pain. Finite muscle testing using a stabilizer or blood pressure cuff or measures of endurance may yield information that is more useful.

Treatment Techniques

Targeted Outcome

The purpose of each selected treatment technique should have a singular focus toward improving the outcome of the patient. Treatment should directly influence the concordant sign of the patient; therefore, active, positional, and passive techniques should directly stimulate the concordant sign during the application of the technique. Treatment techniques that initially cause an increase in symptoms or peripheralizing pain (temporary) may eventually be appropriate techniques. It may take time before symptoms resolve and the clinician needs to assess the findings with either repeated movements or a static hold. These techniques are only considered inappropriate to use if the patient exhibits worsening of symptoms, particularly peripheralization during continued application and at the end of treatment.

Understanding of the "when" to use a specific technique was outlined in the examination section. The patient's response to repeated movements and/or sustained stretches are indicators of whether a specific treatment choice is appropriate or not. The selections can provide one of three potential positive outcomes: (1) reduction of pain, (2) normalization of range, and (3) centralization or abolishment of symptoms. The

obtainment of any of these three outcomes will validate the treatment method used in the previous treatment. A treatment selection that provides no change in the patient, or results in negative consequences, is either an inappropriate treatment selection or is designed to provide benefits in due time (e.g., lumbar stabilization exercises). The nexus of the patient response-based method requires that the clinician identify the effectiveness of the specific manual therapy approach within and between each patient session.[23]

Treatment-Based Classification

Delitto and colleagues have advocated the use of a treatment-based classification (TBC) model.[70] They based their classification partly on the response of a patient to treatment, constructed from key history and examination findings. Similar to the MDT classification, the TBC places patients into homogenous groups purportedly to allow more specific treatment intervention, yet unlike the MDT classification, the TBC provided a classification for groups unrepresented such as instability.

The focus of the TBC model is less on diagnosis and more on improvement of treatment,[108] and has been reduced to four specific classifications that involve categorization based on key history and clinical findings (Figure 10.22 ■). These categories include (1) specific exercise, (2) mobilization, (3) immobilization, and (4) traction.[109] The specific exercise category involves patients who may demonstrate postural preferences, may exhibit centralization behavior with selected movements, or may demonstrate reduction of pain during active and passive techniques. The mobilization group

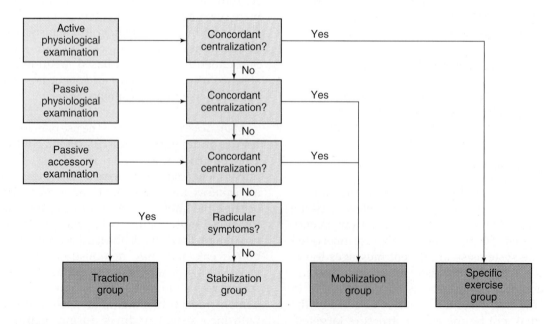

■ **Figure 10.22** Algorithm for the Treatment-Based Classification

generally demonstrates local, unilateral low back pain, or sacroiliac joint–related pain. The immobilization group may exhibit frequent bouts of similar back pain and could be associated with instability. Lastly, the traction group exhibits signs and symptoms of nerve root compression, no improvement with lumbar movements, and a potential lateral shift that is unimproved with lateral translations. Although this model has demonstrated poor reliability,[110] there is evidence of construct validity.[108]

The benefit of using the TBC classification is that the examination distills out which categories of the TBC in which the patient falls. For example, if a patient exhibits centralization behavior, they would fall into the specific exercise group. If a patient exhibits substantiated findings of radiculopathy, they fall into the traction group. If a patient exhibits centralization during active movements and improves with mobilization, they could qualify in both categories. Findings of worsening with both active and passive movements, and no findings of radiculopathy, suggest the patient should fall within the immobilization group. Each category is not considered mutually exclusive.

Specific Exercise Classification   Within the TBC model, and as defined by this book, the specific exercise classification involves specific directionally based exercises. The hallmark of this approach is associated with the centralization phenomenon. As mentioned, the centralization phenomenon is a useful tool in identifying the presence of a discogenic pain[68] and whether the patient will exhibit a positive outcome versus a concordant group that does not demonstrate centralization behavior.[29] Centralization is defined as "a situation in which pain arising from the spine and felt laterally from the midline or distally is reduced and transferred to a more central or near midline position when certain movements are performed."[66,67] Examination techniques that lead to centralization behavior during the examination are carried over to treatment. In some cases, it may take several treatment visits to ascertain the result of repeated motions and to determine if the patient is a centralizer.

This book adopts a very liberal definition for the term "centralization." Active or passive techniques that centralize, reduce, or *abolish* symptoms during application are considered possible techniques of

Active Treatment Techniques — Repeated Motions

Treatment involving repeated motions should directly relate to the findings of the examination. If the patient exhibited decreases of pain or centralization of symptoms during a movement such as repeated extension, the repeated extension is advocated. The same process occurs if the patient demonstrates improvement with another direction of movement such as forward flexion or left or right side flexion. Repeated movements in prone are advocated if the patient is irritable and does not demonstrate centralization in a loaded position. Repeated movements such as extension are performed in standing (Figure 10.23 ■) or prone.

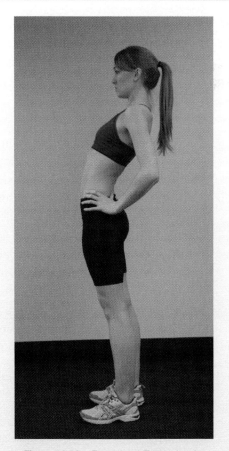

■ **Figure 10.23**   Repeated Extension in Standing

Active Physiological Sustained Postural Holds

Treatment involving a postural hold is also extracted from the examination. In some cases, the postural hold may serve as prepositioning for a mobilization procedure (Figures 10.24 ■ and 10.25 ■).

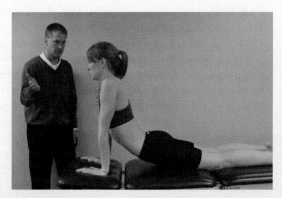

■ **Figure 10.24**   Static Hold for Low Back Extension in Prone

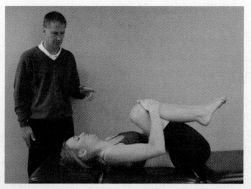

■ **Figure 10.25**   Static Hold for Low Back Flexion in Supine

Treatment Techniques–Side Glides

Side glides are a positional- or movement-based technique designed to correct a positional shift. Typically, patients exhibit a lateral shift described by analyzing the position of the thoracic trunk over the pelvis. In Figure 10.26 ■, the patient exhibits a left lateral shift as the thoracic spine is shifted over the pelvis. Correcting the shift would require a pull of the patient's pelvis in the direction as the shift and push the thoracic spine in the opposite direction of the shift, or a technique described as a "right"-side glide. This technique is appropriate to use if the symptoms centralize upon completion of a bout of therapy.

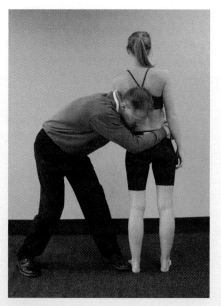

■ **Figure 10.26**   Side Glide for Lateral Shift Correction

1   The patient stands with shifted side facing the clinician.

2   After instructing the patient regarding the procedure at hand, the clinician places one shoulder compressed to the trunk of the patient while wrapping his or her arms around the pelvis of the patient.

③ Using sequential movements, the clinician glides the thoracic spine in the opposite direction as he or she pulls the pelvis.

④ Treatment is based on a positive response during repeated trials for the patient. If the patient exhibits centralization during the side glide, several bouts of the process are repeated. If the patient peripheralizes during repeated movements during the procedure the patient may be a candidate for traction under the TBC criteria.

Combined Movements: Passive Accessory Mobilization in Prepositions

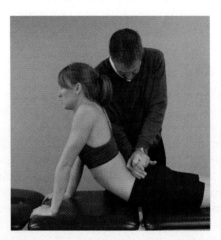

■ **Figure 10.27**   Passive Accessory CPA during Prone Press-Ups

This book adopts a liberal definition of the specific exercise classification of the TBC.[108] The use of passive procedures to enhance the movement in a specific direction is plausible if this movement positively influences the concordant sign of the patient. For example, with the exception of an isolated L5–S1 dysfunction, if a patient benefits from repeated end-range extension the patient may benefit from repeated passive accessory mobilization to the spine at a preposition of end-range extension because both actions create a similar three-point movement of the spine.[111] Subsequently, prepositions that target the concordant movements of side flexion, extension, or nerve tension may be useful prior to the application of a CPA or UPA technique (Figure 10.27 ■–10.29 ■). Each technique is only performed if the effects of the procedure are similar to what occurs during the specific concordant active physiological movement.

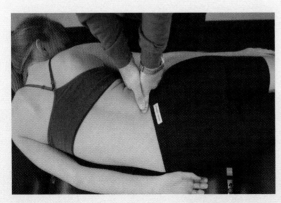

■ **Figure 10.28**   Passive Accessory UPA during Right Side Flexion

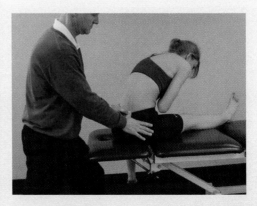

■ **Figure 10.29**   UPA during Sitting with Straight Leg Raise

choice. Unlike the definitions supported by other authors, a centralization response may occur from a number of structures, which are nondiscogenic that originate from radiculopathic or somatic referred pain.

Mobilization Classification   Patients that fall within the mobilization classification may benefit from mobilization or manipulation. This text advocates that there is a high likelihood that a considerable amount of overlap exists between the specific exercise and mobilization classifications. Use of the patient response-based method allows the selection of mobilization procedures based on the positive response during the examination. Consequently, an examination method may also be used as a treatment approach.

Generalized Techniques

Mobilization Procedures from the Examination Mobilization methods selected based on the response of the patient's examination may also be plausible treatment options. Generally, the methods are selected based on the desired response of the patient once the techniques were applied during the examination. Chiradejnant et al.[112] reported that the direction of the technique may make little difference in the outcome of the patient. In their study, randomly selected spine mobilization techniques performed at the *targeted* level demonstrated no difference when compared to therapist-selected techniques. Nevertheless, evidence does suggest that the technique does result in the best outcome when applied directly to the desired concordant segment.[109]

Others[99] have advocated the use of treatment decision rules such as clinical prediction rules (CPR) for determining if patients are appropriate for manipu-

lation early within the care cycle. One CPR consists of (1) < 16 days of symptoms, (2) hip internal rotation of at least 35 degrees, (3) lumbar segmental hypomobility tested with a spring test (a version of a central posterior–anterior mobilization), (4) no symptoms distal to the knee, and 5) a score of < 19 on the work subscale of the Fear-Avoidance Beliefs Questionnaire as the five mechanisms of the rule. Four of five of these findings increased the post-test odds of a short-term positive response from manipulation by 25-fold and demonstrated better outcomes than nonspecific stabilization exercises.[92] This CPR has been investigated by two other independent trials[113,114] and has not demonstrated as strong of efficacy. Although there may be a number of reasons why subsequent studies have not supported the rule (different spectrum of patients, different treatment techniques, and differences in amount of applications of the treatment), the key point to consider is that each patient is individual and may need modification in their intervention program outside a blanketed manipulation method.

The manipulation procedure that was performed to the experimental group is a technique commonly associated with sacroiliac joint manipulation. To perform the procedure, the patient lies in a supine position and is requested to lace both hands behind the neck. The clinician places his or her arm through the arms of the patient's and grasps the arm of the patient closest to the table (Figure 10.30 ■). An alternative method involves the clinician reaching posteriorly and grasping the scapula of the patient. The clinician side-bends the patient away and rotates/flexes the patient toward him or her, while applying pressure to the distal anterior–superior iliac spine (ASIS). The clinician continues to apply rotation toward him- or herself until the

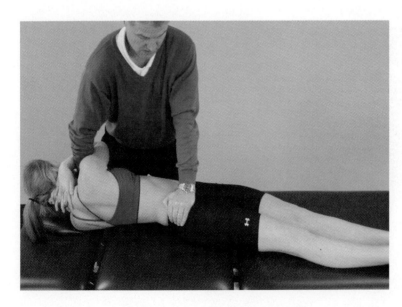

■ **Figure 10.30** Grade V of Ileum on Sacrum

Sidelying Rotational Mobilization

A common mobilization procedure used to gap the zygopophyseal joints superiorly from the table or "close" the segment inferiorly on the table is a sidelying rotational mobilization.

1. The patient should be in a sidelying position and depending on the intent of the procedure, the patient will lie with the painful side up (if the desire is to "open" a facet) or lie with the painful side down (if the clinician plans to "close" the segment). The decision on which side to place the patient is based on the examination results.

2. The patient's lower leg is straightened and the upper leg is slightly flexed (the knee of the upper leg should not be in contact with the table).

3. The clinician grasps the upper arm and gently flexes and rotates the patient cephalically. The clinician only rotates to the point they feel movement at the segment superior to his or her targeted joint.

4. Once found, the clinician places the hand of the patient underneath the side of his or her head.

5. The clinician places his or her ASIS just cephalic to the patient's ASIS. His or her forearm then pulls the patient's pelvis snuggly to the clinician's thigh and hip.

6. The clinician then places his/her forearm posteriorly on the rib cage (interlocked through the arm of the patient).

7. Using a hand position that is similar to passive physiological rotation testing, the clinician stabilizes the targeted segments for great emphasis for the mobilization.

8. The clinician pulls upward on the lateral aspect of the spinous process of the caudal segment by pulling up away from the table.

9. Conversely, the clinician uses his or her thumb to push downward toward the table on the lateral aspect of the cephalic spinous process (Figure 10.31 ■).

10. The patient is rotated slightly to further stabilize or "lock" the position.

11. For additional isolation, the clinician loads the patient through his or her body and can shift the emphasis of the procedure toward the upper, middle, and lower segments by weight shifting cephalically to caudally (cephalic shift emphasizes upper segments, the caudal shift lowers segments).

12. Mobilization is performed based on the patient response. The technique is applied as a gentle oscillation by loading the patient and by pushing down toward the table with the cephalic hand and pulling upward away from the table with the caudal hand (Figure 10.32 ■).

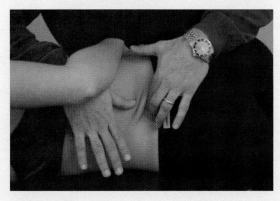

■ **Figure 10.31**   Hand Position for the Mobilization

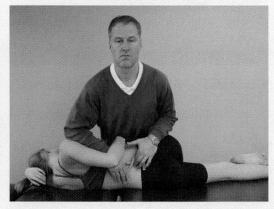

■ **Figure 10.32**   Opening Procedure Causing Gapping of Superior Zygopophyseal Joints

ASIS begins to rise from the table. Once resistance is encountered from the ASIS, the clinician applies a curvilinear AP force through the ASIS of the patient.

Targeted-Specific Techniques Targeted specific techniques are designed to provide a more specific treatment to a targeted segment.

Sidelying Rotational Manipulation (Opening Technique)

The rotational manipulation is useful for patients with chronic stiffness of the lower back or who demonstrate an opening disorder (pain during forward flexion or pain during side flexion away). The technique may be indicated if UPAs or transverse glides do not provide enough vigor to relieve (completely) the patient's symptoms. Additional patient candidates include those that report difficulty moving into rotation or another direction due to a limitation or block. The same placement principles used in the sidelying mobilization procedure are used in the patient set-up for the manipulation (Figure 10.33 ■).

1. The thrust is performed by taking up the slack and prepositioning the patient at the limit. Since the limit is a combined movement of side flexion and rotation, the technique is not performed at end-range rotation.

2. The final procedure involves a quick thrust performed by loading downward (toward the table) on the patient (Figure 10.34 ■). A common mistake involves the clinician pulling and pushing too vigorously with the fingers. The technique should involve loading through the body of the patient more so than forceful hand movements.

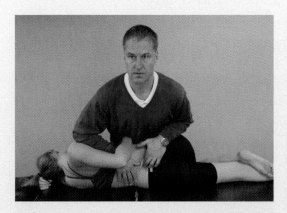

■ **Figure 10.33** Preposition prior to Manipulative Thrust

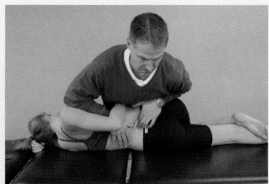

■ **Figure 10.34** Thrust Procedure

Adjustment for Upper Segments

An adjustment of upper segments involves the same set-up as previously suggested, with one added step. The single added step involves shifting the patient and the clinician's hold cephalically to further engage the upper segments (Figure 10.35 ■). To the patient, the targeted segment will feel more "locked," thus it is important to query the patient after the adjustment. Sometimes it takes several attempts to isolate the most secure locked position.

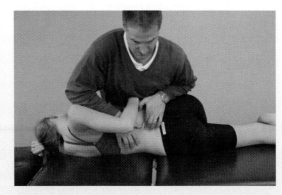

■ **Figure 10.35** Adjustment for the Upper Segments in a Rotational Manipulation

Adjustment for Lower Segments

An adjustment for the lower segments involves the same set-up as previously, with one added step. The single added step involves shifting the patient and the clinician's hold caudally to further engage the lower segments (Figure 10.36 ■). To the patient, the targeted segment will feel more "locked," thus it is important to query the patient after the adjustment. Sometimes it takes several attempts to isolate the most secure locked position.

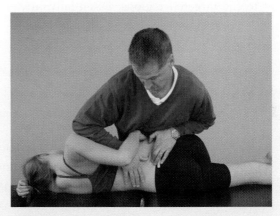

■ **Figure 10.36** Adjustment for the Lower Segments in a Rotational Manipulation

Closing Technique

For patients with closing dysfunctions (e.g., extension and side flexion to one side) one can perform a closing manipulation.

① The patient lays in a sidelying position with the painful side upward.

② The patient's lower leg is slightly flexed and the clinician grasps the upper arm and gently rotates the trunk of the patient cephalically.

(Continued)

③ The patient's spine is placed in slight extension.

④ The clinician uses his or her thumb to push downward toward the table on the lateral aspect of the cephalic spinous process at the cephalic segment.

⑤ Using his or her forearm, the clinician locks the top side buttock and pushes cephalically to further close the joint (Figure 10.37 ■).

⑥ The thrust involves a quick push into further extension and side flexion with the forearm of the clinician (by pushing on the top side buttock).

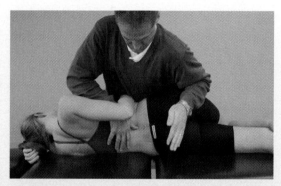

■ **Figure 10.37** Closing Manipulation of the Low Back

Traction Group Many clinicians use motorized traction to treat lumbar disc–related problems. This book advocates the use of manual traction to more appropriately isolate the force and direction of treatment to the targeted regions. Essentially, any activity that decompresses the intervertebral foramen is considered a plausible traction–related technique since there is little evidence to support a "reduction" of the disc with traction.

Hooklying Traction

For patients with irritability, lumbar traction may provide enough relief to advance to techniques that are more vigorous. Although the benefit of traction (or distraction) for the disc is disputed, the benefit of gentle traction techniques for pain relief is substantiated.

① The patient assumes a hooklying position in supine.

② The clinician hooks the proximal aspect of the patient's lower leg (below the knees) with their hands and gently pulls caudally (Figure 10.38 ■). The intent of the treatment is to reduce symptoms, thus the amount of force during the pull is dependent on symptom report from the patient.

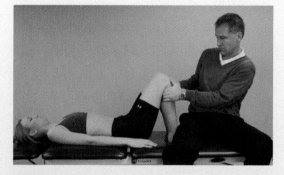

■ **Figure 10.38** Hooklying Lumbar Traction

Sidelying Traction

1. The patient assumes a sidelying position with the painful disc up. There are three steps to this traction technique.

2. First, the clinician promotes on opening side-bending (side-bending away from the painful side), either though a caudal pressure placed on the patient's iliac crest, or through prepositioning.

3. Second, the thorax of the patient should be rotated posteriorly to further concentrate the traction force through the lower back.

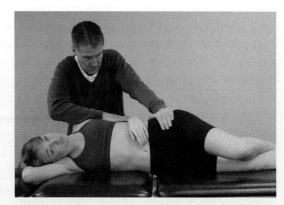

■ **Figure 10.39** Sidelying Traction Technique: Incorporation of Anterior Rotation

4. Third, the clinician then applies a posterior to anterior force to the posterior iliac crest (while maintaining the side flexion force) (Figure 10.39 ■). The intent of the treatment is to reduce and centralize symptoms.

Leg Pull Procedure

Another traction technique involves a single distraction of the lumbar spine with the hip in slight internal rotation. The slight internal rotation force increases the amount of distraction on the lumbar spine and decreases separation at the hip. The procedure also allows the lumbar spine to side flexion away and open the symptomatic side.

1. The patient assumes a supine position.

2. The clinician lifts the patient's leg approximately 1.5–2 feet from the table and pulls the leg while monitoring the symptoms of the patient (Figure 10.40 ■).

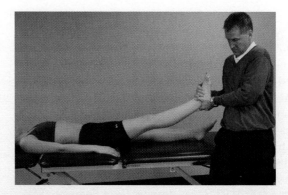

■ **Figure 10.40** Leg Pull Traction

Summary

- The clinician must first identify the concordant sign of the patient and treatment should be directed toward this finding.
- The TBC is a classification method that allows categorizing of patient treatment approaches.
- The four divisions of the TBC include a stabilization group, mobilization group, specific exercise group, and traction group.
- For unknown reasons, conditions with the same diagnosis may lead to dissimilar outcomes.

Treatment Outcomes

The Evidence

Treatment Based on Classification This book advocates a patient response-based treatment, homogenized into a classification model. At present, only a few studies have investigated this form of analysis but have yielded positive results. One study established criterion validity,[108] whereas another found better outcomes when compared against a control group that received exercises based on standardized suggested guidelines.[115] Cook and colleagues[20] reported the outcomes of exercise programs based on the patient response-based method of classification and limited study selection to those that compared the classified approach to a pragmatic or true control. Only five studies were included, four of which demonstrated evidence of improvement over pragmatic controls.

Clinical Prediction Rules In a recent systematic review of decision rules for back pain, May and Rosedale[116] evaluated the validity of CPRs advocated for the prescription of specific treatments. Of the 16 studies identified, only five were related to validation of the rules and seven were related to spine manipulation. Based on the author's analyses, all derivation-based studies were scored as "high quality," whereas none of the validation-based studies demonstrates good quality. Since this publication, one additional validation study has been published as well.[114]

The most cited CPR was derived from Flynn et al.[99] The study identified five variables: (1) score of less than 19 on the Fear-Avoidance Belief Questionnaire, (2) no symptoms distal to the knee, (3) symptom duration of less than 16 days, (4) at least one hip with more than 35 degrees of internal rotation, and (5) hypomobility of the lumbar spine during a posterior–anterior assessment. The study was validated by Childs et al.[100] on a similar patient population and found that those who

met the clinical prediction rule and received spinal manipulative therapy were more likely to improve in pain and disability than those who met the rule and receive general low back exercises.

Others have investigated the same rule in a different population, using different treatment parameters and inclusion criteria. Hancock et al.[113] used the same criteria but intervened using mostly mobilization techniques. In their study, there was no difference in pain or disability between those who met the CPR criteria and whether they received mobilization/manipulation or not. In a slightly different design that included only two of five CPR criteria (in addition to age > 35), Hallegraeff et al.[114] found improvements in disability at $2^1/_2$ weeks, but not pain or range of motion. It is important to note that the authors also provided four additional sessions of manipulation rather than the two sessions of the original authors. At present, the use of a CPR with the parameters outlined by Flynn et al.[99] may provide good outcomes for pain and disability, but evidence suggests changes associated with disability are likely greater (Level C).

Thrust and Nonthrust Techniques For the purpose of this chapter, manual therapy will be divided into two separate categories of treatment: spinal manipulative therapy and mobilization (nonthrust manipulation). Within the lumbar spine, the primary difference between the two forms of treatment is the velocity and range of the techniques being performed and the use of a thrust for manipulation.[117] A thrust technique focuses on the prepositioning of the segment to end range and the use of a high-velocity, low-amplitude thrust at that end range,[118] whereas a nonthrust technique employs oscillation anywhere in range.[119,120] Thrust techniques are often accompanied by an audible pop or cavitation,[121,122] whereas with mobilization, no such audible is expected.

A number of studies have examined the effects of thrust and nonthrust techniques on the lumbar spine. Correspondingly, several systematic reviews of randomized controlled trials addressing these interventions for lumbopelvic pain have been written in recent years. In summary, the evidence outlined provided within the studies does not appear to be definitive in conclusion. Notable findings include the prevailing methodological weaknesses of most studies[117,123] and weaknesses associated with failure to cluster patients into groups who respond best to various forms of interventions.[124] Mior[123] have also raised a concern whether or not clinician training, skill level, and specific thrust techniques selected may also alter the outcomes of the interventions, although recent research has demonstrated that experience and training may not influence the outcome of intervention[125,126] and that the selection and dosage of a particular technique may not be of primary importance.[109,127] As a whole, the quality of the studies that have examined thrust and nonthrust techniques limits the usefulness of findings in treatment planning.[128]

Nonthrust Techniques Most studies that have examined the effectiveness of nonthrust techniques have also included thrust techniques in the interventional design. When directly compared with a thrust procedure, nonthrust techniques have been found to produce less short-term pain relief,[119] although in combination, greater short-term pain relief has been demonstrated when compared with placebo, or care from a general practitioner.[119] Long term, there is Level B evidence that a combined approach of thrust and nonthrust techniques are more effective than modalities and home exercises,[119] although inferior to back exercise, following surgery for disc herniation.[119,129]

Thrust Techniques A number of reviews have examined the effectiveness of thrust techniques to the lumbar spine.[119,123,130,131] For acute lumbopelvic pain, six total randomized controlled trials indicate that there is moderate evidence that thrust techniques have enhanced short-term results compared with nonthrust manipulation and detuned diathermy. Conversely, there is limited evidence that thrust techniques produce better short-term results compared with a combo treatment of diathermy, exercise, and/or ergonomic instruction.[113] There is moderate evidence that thrust techniques with exercise were similar in effect to nonsteroidal anti-inflammatory drugs (NSAIDs) with exercise for short- and long-term pain relief (Level B). There is moderate evidence that a combination of thrust/nonthrust is more effective than physical therapy and a home exercise program for disability reduction and overall patient improvement in the long term. There is also moderate evidence that thrust/nonthrust produces superior results to general medical practice care or placebo in the short term. There is limited evidence that for short-term improvement in pain and disability, thrust/nonthrust is superior to physical therapy, back exercise, placebo, no treatment, a combination of traction, exercise, use of a corset, and transcutaneous electrical nerve stimulation (Level A).

Sufficient evidence exists that thrust techniques are more effective than a sham procedure, placebo, or other treatments that are either ineffective or harmful, but there is insufficient evident at the writing of this book to suggest that thrust is superior to other treatments that demonstrate clinical effectiveness. These other treatments include conventional physical therapy, exercise, analgesics, and back school. When reviewing the data analysis, it is clear that thrust manipulation demonstrated greater improvements than most other treatments in the majority of the studies but when the data is pooled these differences do not constitute statistically or clinically significant levels.[131]

Although thrust is suggested as more effective on patients with acute symptoms, results suggest that nearly the same amount of evidence to support a treatment of thrust manipulation exists for chronic low back pain sufferers as acute low back sufferers.[132] However, when manipulation is added to extension exercises, no additional benefit occurs[133] (Level B).

Traction and Decompression There is conflicting evidence on the benefit of traction for the lumbar spine.[134,135] When the subject pool includes those with sciatica and those without sciatica in any stage of healing, the evidence strongly suggests that traction as a single treatment is not more effective than other treatments, sham, or placebo. When subjects are further subclassified to those with sciatica, the evidence is not as strong because it is conflicting, but still suggests that traction as a single treatment is not particularly effective.

A recent clinical prediction rule using mechanical lumbar traction was created to identify patients who might benefit from traction.[136] The study found that (1) noninvolvement of manual work, (2) low-level fear-avoidance beliefs (<20.5), (3) no neurological deficit, and (4) age above 30 years responds well to mechanical traction. The presence of all four variables (positive likelihood ratio = 9.36) increased the probability of response rate with mechanical lumbar traction from 19.4 to 69.2%. Ironically, the population who benefited may not meet the typical population one would use traction upon.

Summary

- Few clinical trials have examined the benefit of mobilization and manipulation of the lumbar spine.
- There are no studies that have investigated a direct comparison between mobilization and manipulation.
- Clinical prediction rules for thrust and nonthrust manipulation of the lumbar spine have yielded mixed results.
- Most positive results for thrust and nonthrust manipulation have occurred in small, poorly designed studies.
- Future studies are needed to examine the benefit of mobilization and manipulation of the lumbar spine.

Chapter Questions

1. Which movement-based phenomenon has been shown to relate to positive outcomes?

2. How does the physiological anatomy of the facet joint limit rotation?

3. Which physiological motion allows more degrees of movement in the lumbar spine: flexion-extension, rotation, or side flexion?

4. Why do tests that require manual assessment of minute movements have poor reliability?

5. At present, is the literature definitive in its exploration of the benefits of manual therapy for the lumbar spine?

6. Which method of assessment (pain provocation or movement assessment) has the highest degree of reliability?

7. What procedure is suggested initially for patients who exhibit centralization behavior of the lumbar spine?

Patient Cases

Case 10.1: Lonnie Wright (44-year-old male)

Diagnosis: Lumbar radiculopathy
Observation: He exhibits a flat low back with a slight shift to the right.
Mechanism: He notes his pain began after lifting a couch at home.

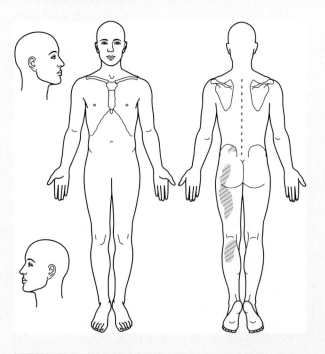

Concordant Sign: His worst pain occurs after long-term sitting. He reports left-sided leg pain to the calf.
Nature of the Condition: He indicates that the condition has greatly affected his work as a plumber. He also notes that it takes several hours for his condition to decrease once it is irritated.
Behavior of the Symptoms: The low back hurts nearly all the time but the leg pain appears worse after bouts of sitting or bending over.
Pertinent Patient History: He reports a history of chronic low back pain.
Patient Goals: He is interested in reducing the leg pain primarily. He indicates he can live with the back pain.
Baseline: The leg pain is 5/10, whereas the back pain is 3/10.
Examination Findings: Extension (active and passive) worsens back pain but improves leg pain. Flexion lessens back pain but worsens leg pain. UPA to the left side of L5–S1 reduces leg pain. Leg pull traction reduces leg pain from 5/10 to 3/10.

1. Based on these findings, what else would you like to examine?
2. Is this patient a good candidate for manual therapy?
3. What is the expected prognosis of this patient?
4. What treatments do you feel presented in this book may be beneficial for this patient?

Case 10.2: Monique Jackson (76-year-old female)

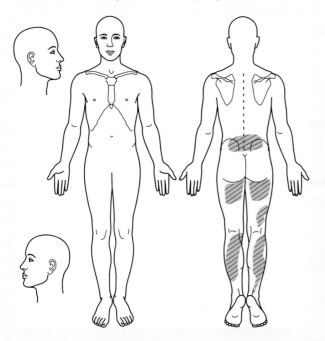

Diagnosis: Low back strain
Observation: Ms. Jackson has excessive lordosis and walks with a very wide based gait.
Mechanism: Insidious onset of pain that has lasted for over 20 years.

Concordant Sign: Pain in legs is worse during extension.
Nature of the Condition: She has declined in her functional activities mainly because of her bilateral leg pain. She notes that the symptoms are unpredictable to her and that there is nothing she does that will dictate the symptoms.
Behavior of the Symptoms: Unpredictable.
Pertinent Patient History: A number of health problems including diabetes, obesity, and a bout of cancer 11 years ago.
Patient Goals: She is concerned that her current problem is the start of an eventual decline of her well-being.
Baseline: The pain in her legs is 4/10, whereas the pain in her back is 2/10.
Examination Findings: Her legs are worsened with extension and improved with sitting and flexion. PAs are not helpful nor is traction.

1. Based on these findings, what else would you like to examine?
2. Is this patient a good candidate for manual therapy?
3. What is the expected prognosis of this patient?
4. What treatments do you feel presented in this book may be beneficial for this patient?

Case 10.3: Larry Flintstone (25-year-old male)

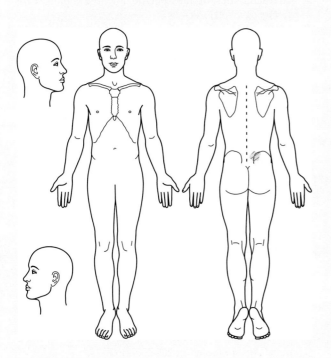

Diagnosis: Lumbar strain
Observation: Larry is an overweight young man with no apparent shift.
Mechanism: He notes a bout of low back pain only after working in a long-term flexed position. The pain occurred during return to extension from flexion.
Concordant Sign: Passive or active extension or side flexion to the right.
Nature of the Condition: He indicates he can tolerate the position well. It feels better after "working it out." He functions as a grocer and is able to tolerate the job demands well.
Behavior of the Symptoms: The pain is localized to the right side of the low back with no reports of leg pain.
Pertinent Patient History: Nothing significant.
Patient Goals: He is interested in getting rid of his current low back pain.
Baseline: His baseline pain is 2/10 and it is 7/10 when he moves into extension.
Examination Findings: Extension and side flexion to the right are painful and concordant. A UPA to

the right L5–S1 facet reproduces concordant symptoms.

1. Based on these findings, what else would you like to examine?

2. Is this patient a good candidate for manual therapy?
3. What is the expected prognosis of this patient?
4. What treatments do you feel presented in this book may be beneficial for this patient?

PEARSON
myhealthprofessionskit™

Use this address to access the Companion Website created for this textbook. Simply select "Physical Therapy" from the choice of disciplines. Find this book and log in using your username and password to access video clips and the anatomy and arthrological information.

References

1. Borkan JM, Koes B, Reis S, Cherkin DC. A report from the second international forum for primary care research on low back pain: Re-examining priorities. *Spine*. 1998;23:1992–1996.
2. Bouter LM, van Tulder MW, Koes BW. Methodologic issues in low back pain research in primary care. *Spine*. 1998;23:2014–2020.
3. Leboeuf-Yde C, Lauritsen JM, Lauritsen T. Why has the search for causes of low back pain largely been non-conclusive? *Spine*. 1997;22:877–881.
4. Spitzer WO. Scientific approach to the assessment and management of activity related spinal disorders. A monograph form clinicians. Report of the Quebec Task Force on Spinal Disorders. *Spine*. 1987;Suppl. S1–59.
5. McCarthy C, Arnall F, Strimpakos N, Freemont A, Oldham J. The biopsychosocial classification of nonspecific low back pain: A systematic review. *Physical Therapy Reviews*. 2004;9:17–30.
6. Lurie JD. What diagnostic tests are useful for low back pain? *Best Pract Res Clin Rheumatol*. 2005;19(4):557–575.
7. Deyo R, Phillips W. Low back pain. A primary care challenge. *Spine*. 1996;21(24):2826–2832.
8. Deyo RA. Nonsurgical care of low back pain. *Neurosurg Clin N Am*. 1991;2(4):851–862.
9. Hart LG, Deyo RA, Cherkin DC. Physician office visits for low back pain: Frequency, clinical evaluation, and treatment patterns from a U.S. national survey. *Spine*. 1995;20(1):11–19.
10. Jarvik JG, Deyo RA. Imaging of lumbar intervertebral disk degeneration and aging, excluding disk herniations. *Radiol Clin North Am*. 2000;38(6):1255–1266.
11. Deyo RA, Rainville J, Kent DL. What can the history and physical examination tell us about low back pain? *JAMA*. 1992;268(6):760–765.
12. McIntosh G, Frank J, Hogg-Johnson S. Prognostic factors for time receiving workers' compensation benefits in a cohort of patient with low back pain. *Spine*. 2000;26:758–765.
13. Hadijistavropoulos H, Craig K. Acute and chronic low back pain: Cognitive, affective, and behavioral dimensions. *J Consult Clin Psychol*. 1994;62:341–349.
14. Hunter S, Shaha S, Flint D, Tracy D. Predicting return to work: A long-term follow-up study of railroad workers after low back injuries. *Spine*. 1998;23:2319–2328.
15. Frymoyer J. Predicting disability from low back pain. *Clin Orthop*. 1992;(279):101–109.
16. Schultz iZ, Crook J, Berkowkitz J, Meloche GR, Milner R, Zuberbier OA. *Biophysical multivariate predictive model of occupational low back disability*. New York; Springer: 2005.
17. Bernard T, Kirkaldy-Willis W. Recognizing specific characteristics of nonspecific low back pain. *Clin Orthop*. 1987;217:266–280.
18. Moffroid M, Haugh L, Henry S, Short B. Distinguishable groups of musculoskeletal low back pain patients and asymptomatic control subjects based on physical measures of the NIOSH Low Back Atlas. *Spine*. 1994;19:1350–1358.
19. Riddle DL. Classification and low back pain: A review of the literature and critical analysis of selected systems. *Phys Ther*. 1998;78:708–737.
20. Cook C, Hegedus E, Ramey K. Physical therapy exercise intervention based on classification using the patient response method: A systematic review of the literature. *J Manual Manip Ther*. 2005;13:158–168.
21. Aina A, May S, Clare H. The centralization phenomenon of spinal symptoms: A systematic review. *Man Ther*. 2004;9:134–143.
22. Tuttle N. Do changes within a manual therapy treatment session predict between-session changes for patients with cervical spine pain? *Aust J Physiother*. 2005;51:43–48.
23. Hahne AJ, Keating JL, Wilson SC. Do within-session changes in pain intensity and range of motion predict between-session changes in patients with low back pain? *Aust J Physiother*. 2004;50(1):17–23.
24. Peterson T, Laslett M, Thorsen H, Manniche C, Ekdahl C, Jacobsen S. Diagnostic classification of non-specific low

back pain: A new system integrating patho-anatomic and clinical categories. *Physiother Theory Pract.* 2003;19:213–237.

25. Peterson T, Laslett M, Thorsen H, Manniche C, Ekdahl C, Jacobsen S. Inter-tester reliability of a new diagnostic classification system for patients with non-specific low back pain. *Aust J Physiother.* 2004;50:85–94.

26. Werneke M, Hart D. Categorizing patients with occupational low back pain by use of the Quebec Task Force Classification system versus pain pattern classification procedures: discriminant and predictive validity. *Phys Ther.* 2004;84(3):243–254.

27. Bigos SJ, Davis GE. Scientific application of sports medicine principles for acute low back problems. The Agency for Health Care Policy and Research Low Back Guideline Panel (AHCPR, Guideline #14). *J Orthop Sports Phys Ther.* 1996;24(4):192–207.

28. Spitzer W. Diagnosis of the problem (the problem of diagnosis). *Spine.* 1987;12(suppl):S16–S21.

29. Werneke M, Hart D. Centralization phenomenon as a prognostic factor for chronic low back pain. *Spine.* 2001;25:758–764.

30. Frymoyer J. Predicting disability from low back pain. *Clin Orthop.* 1993;279:101–109.

31. Bogduk N, Macintosh JE, Pearcy MJ. A universal model of the lumbar back muscles in the upright position. *Spine.* 1992;17(8):897–913.

32. Bogduk N. The sources of low back pain. In: Jayson M (ed). *The lumbar spine and back pain.* 4th ed. Edinburgh; Churchill Livingstone: 1992.

33. Bogduk N. Lumbar dorsal ramus syndrome. *Med J Aust.* 1980;2:537–541.

34. Bogduk N, Macintosh JE. The applied anatomy of the thoracolumbar fascia. *Spine.* 1984;9(2):164–170.

35. Bogduk N. The anatomical basis for spinal pain syndromes. *J Manipulative Physiol Ther.* 1995;18(9):603–605.

36. Laslett M. Breakout session. American Academy of Orthopedic Manual Physical Therapists. Reno, Nevada. 2003.

37. O'Sullivan P. Lumbar segmental instability: Clinical presentation and specific stabilizing exercise management. *Man Ther.* 2000;5(1):2–12.

38. Cook C, Brismee JM, Sizer P. Subjective and objective descriptors of clinical lumbar spine instability: A Delphi study. *Man Ther.* 2006;11(1):11–21.

39. Granata KP, Wilson SE. Trunk posture and spinal stability. *Clin Biomech.* 2001;16:650–659.

40. Tubach F, Leclerc A, Landre M, Pietri-Taleb F. Risk factors for sick leave due to low back pain: A prospective study. *J Occup Environ Med.* 2002;44:451–458.

41. Fritz J, George S. Identifying psychosocial variables in patients with acute work-related low back pain: The importance of fear-avoidance beliefs. *Phys Ther.* 2002;82: 973–983.

42. Roelofs J, Peters ML, Fassaert T, Vlaeyen JW. The role of fear of movement and injury in selective attentional processing in patients with chronic low back pain: A dot-probe evaluation. *J Pain.* 2005;6(5):294–300.

43. Childs JD, Piva SR, Erhard RE, Hicks G. Side-to-side weight-bearing asymmetry in subjects with low back pain. *Man Ther.* 2003;8(3):166–169.

44. Riddle D, Rothstein J. Intertester reliability of McKenzie's classifications of the syndrome types present in patients with low back pain. *Spine.* 1993;18(10):1333–1344.

45. Kilpikoski S, Airaksinen O, Kankaanpaa M, Leminen P, Videman T, Alen M. Interexaminer reliability of low back pain assessment using the McKenzie method. *Spine.* 2002;27(8):207–214.

46. Clare HA, Adams R, Maher CG. Reliability of detection of lumbar lateral shift. *J Manipulative Physiol Ther.* 2003;26(8):476–480.

47. Tenhula JA, Rose SJ, Delitto A, et al. Association between direction of lateral lumbar shift, movement tests, and side of symptoms in patients with low back pain syndrome. *Phys Ther.* 1990;70(8):480–486.

48. Young S. Personal communication. March 17, 2005.

49. Vroomen PC, de Krom MC, Wilmink JT, Kester AD, Knottnerus JA. Diagnostic value of history and physical examination in patients suspected of lumbosacral nerve root compression. *J Neurol Neurosurg Psychiatry.* 2002;72(5):630–634.

50. Boos N, Rieder R, Schade V, Spratt KF, Semmer N, Aebi M. 1995 Volvo Award in clinical sciences: The diagnostic accuracy of magnetic resonance imaging, work perception, and psychosocial factors in identifying symptomatic disc herniations. *Spine.* 1995;20(24):2613–2625.

51. Elfering A, Semmer NK, Schade V, Grund S, Boos N. Supportive colleague, unsupportive supervisor: the role of provider-specific constellations of social support at work in the development of low back pain. *J Occup Health Psychol.* 2002;7(2):130–140.

52. Luoma K, Riihimaki H, Luukkonen R, Raininko R, Viikari-Juntura E, Lamminen A. Low back pain in relation to lumbar disc degeneration. *Spine.* 2000;25(4): 487–492.

53. Luoma K, Riihimaki H, Raininko R, Luukkonen R, Lamminen A, Viikari-Juntura E. Lumbar disc degeneration in relation to occupation. *Scand J Work Environ Health.* 1998;24(5):358–366.

54. Hasenbring M, Marienfeld G, Kuhlendahl D, Soyka D. Risk factors of chronicity in lumbar disc patients: A prospective investigation of biologic, psychologic, and social predictors of therapy outcome. *Spine.* 1994;19: 2759–2765.

55. Young S, April C, Laslett M. Correlation of clinical examination characteristics with three sources of chronic low back pain. *Spine J.* 2003;3(6):460–465.

56. O'Sullivan PB, Mitchell T, Bulich P, Waller R, Holte J. The relationship between posture and back muscle endurance in industrial workers with flexion-related low back pain. *Man Ther.* 2006;11(4):264–271.

57. Robinson J. Lower extremity pain of lumbar spine origin: Differentiating somatic referred and radicular pain. *J Man Manip Ther.* 2003;11:223–234.

58. Bogduk N. *Clinical anatomy of the lumbar spine and sacrum.* 3rd ed. New York; Churchill Livingstone: 1997.

59. Marks R. Distribution of pain provoked from lumbar facet joints and related structures during diagnostic spinal infiltration. *Pain.* 1989;39:37–40.

60. Mooney V, Robertson J. The facet syndrome. *Clin Orthop.* 1976;115:149–156.

61. Smyth MJ, Wright V. Sciatica and the intervertebral disc: An experimental study. *J Bone Jnt Surg.* 1959;40A: 1401–1418.

62. Kuslich S, Ulstrom CL, Michael CJ. The tissue origin of low back pain and sciatica: A report of pain response to tissue stimulation during operations on the lumbar spine using local anesthesia. *Ortho Clin North Am.* 1991;22:181–187.

63. Norlen G. On the value of the neurological symptoms in sciatica for the localization of a lumbar disc herniation. *Acta Chir Scadinav Supp.* 1944;95:1–96.

64. McCullough JA, Waddell G. Variation of the lumbosacral myotomes with bony segmental anomalies. *J Bone Joint Surg.* 1980;62:475–480.

65. Lauder T, Dillingham TR, Andary M. Effect of history and exam in predicting electrodiagnostic outcome among patients with suspected lumbosacral radiculopathy. *Am J Phys Med Rehabil.* 2000;79:60–68.

66. McKenzie R. *The lumbar spine: Mechanical diagnosis and therapy.* Waikanae, New Zealand; Spinal Publications: 1981.

67. Aina A, May S, Clare H. The centralization phenomenon of spinal symptoms: A systematic review. *Man Ther.* 2004;9:134–143.

68. Donelson R, Aprill C, Medcalf R, Grant W. A prospective study of centralization of lumbar and referred pain. A predictor of symptomatic discs and annular competence. *Spine.* 1997;22:1115–1122.

69. Erhard R, Delitto A, Cibulka M. Relative effectiveness of an extension program and a combined program of manipulation and flexion and extension exercises in patients with acute low back syndrome. *Phys Ther.* 1994;74:1093–1100.

70. Delitto A, Erhard R. Bowling R. A treatment-based classification approach to low back syndrome: Identifying and staging patients for conservative treatment. *Phys Ther.* 1995;75:470–489.

71. Long A, Donelson R, Fung T. Does it matter which exercise?: A randomized control trial of exercise for low back pain. *Spine.* 2004;29:2593–2602.

72. Parks KA, Crichton KS, Goldford RJ, McGill SM. A comparison of lumbar range of motion and functional ability scores in patients with low back pain: Assessment for range of motion validity. *Spine.* 2003;28(4):380–384.

73. Haswell K. Interexaminer reliability of symptom-provoking active sidebend, rotation, and combined movement assessments of patients with low back pain. *J Man Manip Ther.* 2004;12:11–20.

74. Donelson R, Silva G, Murphy K. Centralization phenomenon: Its usefulness in evaluating and treating referred pain. *Spine.* 1990;15:211–213.

75. Maitland GD. *Maitland's vertebral manipulation.* 6th ed. London; Butterworth-Heinemann: 2001.

76. Peterson C, Hayes K. Construct validity of Cyriax's selective tension examination: Association of end-feels with pain at the knee and shoulder. *J Orthop Sports Phys Ther.* 2000;30(9):512–521.

77. Waddell G, Somerville D, Henderson I, Newton M. Objective clinical evaluation of physical impairment in chronic low back pain. *Spine.* 1992;17(6):617–628.

78. Wong TK, Lee RY. Effects of low back pain on the relationship between the movements of the lumbar spine and hip. *Hum Mov Sci.* 2004;23(1):21–34.

79. Sizer P, Phelps V, Dedrick G, Matthijs O. Differential diagnosis and management of root related pain. *Pain Prac* 2002;2:98–121.

80. Cook C. Lumbar Coupling biomechanics: A literature review. *J Man Manip Ther.* 2003;11(3):137–145.

81. Strender L, Sjoblom A, Ludwig R, Taube A, Sundell K. Interexaminer reliability in physical examination of patients with low back pain. *Spine.* 1997;22(7):814–820.

82. Love R, Brodeur R. Inter- and intra-examiner reliability of motion palpation for the thoracolumbar spine. *J Manipulative Physio Ther.* 1987;19:261–266.

83. Lee M, Latimer J, Maher C. Manipulation: Investigation of a proposed mechanism. *Clin Biomech.* 1993;8: 302–306.

84. Maher C, Adams R. Reliability of pain and stiffness assessments in clinical manual lumbar spine examinations. *Phys Ther.* 1994;74(9):801–811.

85. Maher C, Latimer J. Pain or resistance: The manual therapists' dilemma. *Aust J Physiother.* 1992;38(4):257–260.

86. Jull G, Treleaven J, Versace G. Manual examination: Is pain provocation a major cue for spinal dysfunction? *Aust J Physiother.* 1994;40:159–165.

87. Jull G, Bogduk N, Marsland A. The accuracy of manual diagnosis for cervical zygopophyseal joint pain syndromes. *Med J Aust.* 1988;148(5):233–236.

88. Boline P, Haas M, Meyer J, Kassak K, Nelson C, Keating J. Interexaminer reliability of eight evaluative dimensions of lumbar segmental abnormality: Part II. *J Manipulative Physiol Ther* 1992;16(6):363–373.

89. Bjornsdottir SV, Kumar S. Posteroanterior spinal mobilization: State of the art review and discussion. *Disabil Rehabil.* 1997;19(2):39–46.

90. Hestoek L, Leboeuf-Yde C. Are chiropractic tests for the lumbo-pelvic spine reliable and valid?: A systematic critical literature review. *J Manipulative Physiol Ther.* 2000;23:258–275.

91. Macfadyen N, Maher CG, Adams R. Number of sampling movements and manual stiffness judgments. *J Manipulative Physiol Ther.* 1998;21(9):604–610.

92. Maher C, Simmonds M, Adams R. Therapists' conceptualization and characterization of the clinical concept of spinal stiffness. *Phys Ther.* 1998;78:289–300.

93. Anson E, Cook C, Comacho C, Gwilliam B, Karakostas T. The use of education in the improvement in finding R1 in the lumbar spine. *J Man Manip Ther.* 2003;11(4): 204–212.

94. Cook C, Turney L, Miles A, Ramirez L, Karakostas T. Predictive factors in poor inter-rater reliability among physical therapists. *J Man Manip Ther.* 2002;10(4): 200–205.

95. van Trijffel E, Anderegg Q, Bossuyt P, Lucas C. Interexaminer reliability of passive assessment of intervertebral motion in the cervical and lumbar spine: A systematic review. *Man Ther.* 2005 (e-pub).

96. Phillips DR, Twomey LT. A comparison of manual diagnosis with a diagnosis established by a uni-level lumbar spinal block procedure. *Man Ther.* 2000;1(2):82–87.

97. Dickey JP, Pierrynowski MT, Bednar DA, Yang SX. Relationship between pain and vertebral motion in chronic low-back pain subjects. *Clin Biomech.* 2002;17(5):345–352.

98. Hicks G, Fritz J, Delitto A, Mishock J. Interrater reliability of clinical examination measures for identification of lumbar segmental instability. *Arch Phys Med Rehabil.* 2003;84(12):1858–1864.

99. Flynn T, Fritz J, Whitman J, Wainner R, Magel J, Rendeiro D, Butler B, Garber M, Allison S. A clinical prediction rule for classifying patients with low back pain who demonstrate short-term improvement with spinal manipulation. *Spine.* 2002;27(24):2835–2843.

100. Childs JD, Fritz JM, Flynn TW, et al. A clinical prediction rule to identify patients with low back pain most likely to benefit from spinal manipulation: A validation study. *Ann Intern Med.* 2004;141(12):920–928.

101. Frtiz JM, Whitman J, Childs J. Lumbar spine segmental mobility assessment: An examination of validity for determining intervention strategies in patient with low back pain. *Arch Phys Med Rehabil.* 2005;86:1745–1752.

102. Hicks G, Fritz JM, Delitto A, McGill S. Preliminary development of a clinical prediction rule for determining which patients with low back pain will respond to a stabilization exercise program. *Arch Phys Med Rehabil.* 2005;86:1753–1762.

103. Ferreira ML, Ferreira PH, Latimer J, Herbert RD, Maher C, Refshauge K. Relationship between spinal stiffness and outcome in patients with chronic low back pain. *Man Ther.* 2009;14:61–67.

104. Lee R, Evans J. An in vivo study of the intervertebral movements produced by posteroanterior mobilization. *Clin Biomech.* 1997;12:400–408.

105. Billis EV, Foster NE, Wright CC. Reproducibility and repeatability: errors of three groups of physiotherapists in locating spinal levels by palpation. *Man Ther.* 2003;8(4):223–232.

106. French SD, Green S, Forbes A. Reliability of chiropractic methods commonly used to detect manipulable lesions in patients with chronic low-back pain. *J Manipulative Physiol Ther.* 2000;23(4):231–238.

107. Niere K, Torney SK. Clinicians' perceptions of minor cervical instability. *Man Ther.* 2004;9(3):144–150.

108. George S, Delitto A. Clinical examination variables discriminate among treatment-based classification groups: A study of construct validity in patients with acute low back pain. *Phys Ther.* 2005;85(4):306–314.

109. Chiradejnant A, Latimer J, Maher C, Stepkovitch N. Does the choice of spinal level treated during posteroanterior (PA) mobilization affect treatment outcome? *Physiotherapy Theory Practice.* 2002;18:165–174.

110. Heiss DG, Fitch DS, Fritz JM, Sanchez W, Roberts K, Buford J. The interrater reliability among physical therapists newly trained in a classification system for acute low back pain. *J Orthop Sports Phys Ther.* 2004;34(8):430–439.

111. Rebain R, Baxter GD, McDonough S. A systematic review of the passive straight leg raising test as a diagnostic aid for low back pain (1989 to 2000). *Spine.* 2002;27(17):E388–395.

112. Chiradejnant A, Maher C, Latimer J, Stepkovitch N. Efficacy of therapist selected versus randomly selected mobilization techniques for the treatment of low back pain: A randomized controlled trial. *Aust J Physiotherapy.* 2003;49:233–241.

113. Hancock M, Maher CG, Latimer J, Herbert RD, McAuley JH. Independent evaluation of clinical prediction rule for spinal manipulative therapy: A randomized controlled trial. *Eur Spine J.* 2008;17:936–943.

114. Hallegraeff JM, de Greef M, Winters JC, Lucas C. Manipulative therapy and clinical prediction criteria in treatment of acute nonspecific low back pain. *Percept Mot Skills.* 2009;108:196–208.

115. Fritz JM, Delitto A, Erhard RE. Comparison of classification-based physical therapy with therapy based on clinical practice guidelines for patients with acute low back pain: A randomized clinical trial. *Spine.* 2003;28(13):1363–1371.

116. May S, Rosedale R. Prescriptive clinical prediction rules in back pain research: A systematic review. *J Man Manip Ther.* 2009;17:36–45.

117. Assendelft WJ, Morton SC, Yu EI, Suttorp MJ, Shekelle PG. Spinal manipulative therapy for low back pain. A meta-analysis of effectiveness relative to other therapies. *Ann Intern Med.* 2003;138(11):871–881.

118. Shirley D. Manual therapy and tissue stiffness. In: Boyling JD, Jull GA (eds). *Grieve's modern manual therapy: The vertebral column.* London; Churchill Livingstone: 2004.

119. Bronfort G, Haas M, Evans RL, Bouter LM. Efficacy of spinal manipulation and mobilization for low back pain and neck pain: A systematic review and best evidence synthesis. *Spine J.* 2004;4(3):335–356.

120. Maitland GD, Hengeveld E, Banks K, English K. *Maitland's vertebral manipulation.* London; Butterworth-Heinemann: 2001.

121. Flynn TW, Childs JD, Fritz JM. The audible pop from high-velocity thrust manipulation and outcome in individuals with low back pain. *J Manipulative Physiol Ther.* 2006;29(1):40–45.

122. Lewit K. The contribution of clinical observation to neurobiological mechanisms in manipulative therapy. In: Korr IM (ed). *The neurobiological mechanisms in manipulative therapy.* New York; Plenum Press: 1978.

123. Mior S. Manipulation and mobilization in the treatment of chronic pain. *Clin J Pain.* 2001;17(4 suppl):S70–76.

124. Schiotz E, Cyriax J. *Manipulation Past and Present.* London, UK: Heinemann, 1975.

125. Whitman JM, Fritz JM, Childs JD. The influence of experience and specialty certifications on clinical outcomes for patients with low back pain treated within a standardized physical therapy management program. *J Orthop Sports Phys Ther.* 2004;34(11):662–672.

126. Cohen E, Triano JJ, McGregor M, Papakyriakou M. Biomechanical performance of spinal manipulation therapy by newly trained vs. practicing providers: Does experience transfer to unfamiliar procedures? *J Manipulative Physiol Ther.* 1995;18(6)347–352.

127. De Coninck SLH. *Orthopaedic medicine Cyriax: Updated value in daily practice, part II: Treatment by deep transverse massage, mobilization, manipulation and traction.* Minneapolis, MN: OPTP; 2003.

128. Furlan AD, Clarke J, Esmail R, Sinclair S, Irvin E, Bombardier C. A critical review of reviews on the treatment of chronic low back pain. *Spine.* 2001;26(7):E155–162.

129. Timm KE. A randomized-control study of active and passive treatments for chronic low back pain following L5 laminectomy. *J Orthop Sport Phys Ther.* 1994;20(6):276–286.

130. van Tulder MW, Koes BW, Bouter LM. Conservative treatment of acute and chronic nonspecific low back pain: A systematic review of randomized controlled trials of the most common interventions. *Spine.* 1997;22(18):2128–2156.

131. Assendelft WJJ, Morton SC, Yu EI, Suttorp MJ, Shekelle PG. Spinal manipulative therapy for low back pain. *Cochrane Database Syst Rev.* 2007:CD000447.

132. Lawrence DJ, Meeker W, Branson R, et al. Chiropractic management of low back pain and low back-related leg complaints: A literature synthesis. *J Manipulative Physiol Ther.* 2008;31(9):659–674.

133. Rasmussen J, Laetgaard J, Lindecrona AL, Qvistgaard E, Bliddal H. Manipulation does not add to the effect of extension exercises in chronic low back pain: A randomized controlled, double blind study. *Joint Bone Spine.* 2008;75:708–713.

134. Clarke J, van Tulder M, Blomberg S, de Vet H, van der Heijden G, Bronfort G. Traction for low back pain with or without sciatica: An updated systematic review within the framework of the Cochrane collaboration. *Spine (Phila Pa 1976).* 2006;31(14):1591–1599.

135. Harte AA, Baxter GD, Gracey JH. The efficacy of traction for back pain: A systematic review of randomized controlled trials. *Arch Phys Med Rehabil.* 2003;84(10): 1542–1553.

136. Cai C, Pua YH, Lim KC. A clinical prediction rule for classifying patients with low back pain who demonstrate short-term improvement with mechanical lumbar traction. *Eur Spine J.* 2009;18(4):554–561.

Manual Therapy of the Sacroiliac Joint and Pelvis

Chad E. Cook

Objectives

- Understand the biomechanics and gross movements of the sacroiliac joint.
- Understand the biomechanics of the pubic symphysis and sacroiliac joint.
- Outline an evidence-based examination process.
- Differentiate low back problems from sacroiliac joint problems.
- Identify manual therapy treatment methods that restore normal sacroiliac and pelvis function.

Clinical Examination

Differential Diagnosis

There are two apparent causes of sacroiliac joint (SIJ)/pelvis pain: mechanical and nonmechanical. Huijbregts[1] outlines several non-mechanical pathologies that affect the SIJ, including infections, inflammatory, metabolic, and iatrogenic conditions. These nonmechanical pathologies are not the focus of this book, but deserve mention. Relatively uncommon conditions that affect the SIJ such as ankylosing spondylitis, psoriatic arthritis, Reiter's syndrome, systemic lupus erythematosus, Sjoegren's syndrome, gout, Paget's disease, tuberculosis, and various bacterial infections are best addressed by a traditional medical physician. Generally, these disorders demonstrate nonmechanically based patterns and fail to respond to conservative care; however, worth noting is that all are difficult to diagnosis using traditional manual therapy evaluative methods.

Early osteopathic literature promoted clinical assessment methods that relied heavily on palpatory and observable phenomena.[2,3] Many of these procedures were adopted by manual therapists of multiple professions, specifically physical therapists, with little questioning regarding their diagnostic or clinical value. Many of these methods are still used in clinical practice despite having been shown to have questionable reliability and diagnostic validity.[4–8] Examples of early emphases during assessment include objective assessment of "free movement," observation of displacement during sitting or standing, measurement of leg length change during supine to sit position, and symptomatic identifiers such as buttock pain and groin pain.[2]

The current, most universally accepted criterion standard for implication of a sacroiliac problem is a videofluoroscopic-guided anesthetic block injection into the SIJ.[9,10] Worth noting is that this criterion standard has been recently questioned[11] for its benefit and is certainly not a perfect "gold standard." Laslett et al.[12] described an alternate method where fluoroscopic-guided arthrographs were used to provoke concordant symptoms, followed by instillation of a small volume of anesthetic for abolishment of symptoms. This method should result in an 80% reduction in pain for the test to be considered positive. Nonetheless, despite the rigor associated with these diagnostic clarification methods there are some limitations associated with false positive rates,[10] and leaking outside the SIJ.[13]

The *European Guidelines on the Diagnosis and Treatment of Pelvic Girdle Pain*[14] suggested that the use of SIJ injections as a diagnostic tool is inappropriate in a number of conditions that could still qualify as SIJ or pelvic pain. For example, pain in the long dorsal ligament or pubic symphysis would not yield a positive test with double injections but is still considered a form of pelvic disorder. Additionally, most SIJ injection methods are compared against clinical "reference standards" and vice versa. Some studies have been compared against questionable clinical tests and may yield inappropriate information.

Others have suggested the utility of a clinical diagnosis as the criterion standard for determining SIJ pain. Cibulka and Koldehoff[5] suggested the use of a clinical diagnosis based on regional pain classification, the response of direct treatment techniques, and the restoration of pelvic symmetry as a diagnostic method. This suggestion may yield questionable benefit specifically when diagnosing based on response to treatment. Since the SIJ and low back are highly integrated, the likelihood of applying a specific treatment that fails to address other regional anatomic sites is minute. In fact, a recent paper investigating palpatory assessment of selected SIJ movement tests found asymmetries in patients with low back pain as well as pelvis pain.[15] Additionally, restoration of pelvic symmetry is based on the theory that asymmetry is quantifiable, a theory that has yet to be enumerated within the literature. Such fine, precision-based assessments are highly at risk for bias, and certainly unproven for reliability.

There is some debate that both clinical examination findings and injections yield separate and beneficial findings. Maigne et al.,[16] Laslett,[17] and Berthelot et al.[11] argue that pathological changes to soft tissue around the SIJ may serve as a pain generator and would not be identified during an interarticular injection. Laslett[17] suggests the use of both a movement-based assessment that has demonstrated validity, such as the McKenzie assessment for directional preference, and the inclusion of an intra-articular block, performed together, are necessary for diagnosis of SIJ pain. One of the hallmarks of the McKenzie approach is the theory that patients who demonstrate centralization behavior (centralizers) have problems that originate from the low back,[18] and noncentralizers are generally "other" disorders. There is strong evidence that centralization is associated with a lumbar disc dysfunction,[19] thus the use of this assessment method is suggested during sacroiliac pelvic disorder assessment to rule out the lumbar spine.

In a past clinical case control study, this hypothesis has shown to exhibit validity. In 2003, Laslett et al.[12] divided a population of chronic back patients into centralizers and noncentralizers. The centralizers were proposed low back dysfunction patients, purportedly associated with disc dysfunction, and were removed from the study. The noncentralizers were then examined with a battery of sacroiliac tests including an intra-articular block to distill further the findings. A large portion of these patients did present with positive findings and were considered to have SIJ pain.

Lastly, recent evidence has suggested that SIJ pain is best classified into homogenous entities. Albert and colleagues[20] reported that there are five classifications of pregnancy-related pelvic joint pain and provide prevalence rates for each classification. These authors identified pelvic girdle syndrome, symphysiolysis, one-sided sacroiliac pain, double-sided sacroiliac pain, and miscellaneous categories for pregnancy-related pain. Of the five, pelvic girdle syndrome displayed an incidence of 6%, symphysiolysis 2.3%, one-sided sacroiliac pain 5.5%, double-sided sacroiliac pain 6.3%, and miscellaneous categories 1.6%.

One notable concept of the Albert et al.[20,21] studies was the suggestion that not all SIJ pain representations are the same. In a 2000 study, findings when various SIJ tests were administered on subjects in disparate classifications demonstrated differences in sensitivity and specificity.[21] This suggests that some of the variability associated with special clinical tests may be associated with the variability of the diagnosis as well as the variability of testing and test methods selected. Subsequently, an understanding that various forms of SIJ pain are necessary and should inform the examiner that a very open-minded approach is necessary before condemning the likelihood of SIJ pain based on the absence of selected findings.

Summary

- There are two apparent causes of SIJ/pelvis pain: mechanical and nonmechanical. Mechanical causes are associated with instability and displacement. Nonmechanical causes are associated with infections and disease processes.

- Historic osteopathic methods of SIJ assessment lean heavily on palpation and observation, two methods that have not demonstrated reliability or validity.

- The current gold standard for diagnosis of SIJ pain is a videofluoroscopic-guided anesthetic block injection into the SIJ, although not all researchers agree with this selection.

- Some researchers have suggested the use of a clinical diagnosis for the "reference standard," mainly because many diagnostic methods compare the finding against clinical standards.

- There may be different "kinds" of pelvic disorders, thus many special clinical tests may present with different levels of sensitivity and specificity based on the "flavor" of the disorder.

Observation

The role of posture and its influence on pelvic pain is well studied. Selected postures can alter SIJ motion and place tension on the stabilizing ligaments, yet abnormalities of anatomy[22] and posture[23] are not reliable predictors of cause of pain. Snijders et al.[24] reported that slumped sitting postures created a counternutation moment and tension upon the iliolumbar ligament and long dorsal ligament. It is proposed that the selected stress placed on these innervated ligaments may be a source of low back pain.[24]

Sturesson et al.[25] reported that the straddle position (stride standing) leads to primarily sagittal rotation and movement of the ilia on the sacrum. Others have reported that stabilization of the pelvis is enhanced during soft-seated sitting since this motion complements the action of the oblique abdominal muscles and the contribution of these muscles for stability of the SIJ.[26]

It is worth noting that one significant problem associated with using observation is the potential overfocus on movement "feel," postural position, or visual assessment.[27] Potter and Rothstein[28] examined intertester reliability among clinicians at determining appropriate pelvic symmetry. The percent agreement among clinicians was very poor, suggesting this tool has little transferability from clinician to clinician. Others[29,30] have demonstrated that asymmetric findings were not associated with low back pain or sacroiliac pain. Levangie[30] found that leg length discrepancy, anterior superior iliac spine (ASIS) and posterior superior iliac spine (PSIS) bilateral comparisons, and iliac crest height determination presented diagnostic information that was actually more detrimental for determining a diagnosis of SIJ pain than beneficial. Clearly, little evidence exists that asymmetry is an identifier of a pelvic dysfunction and even less evidence exists that clinicians can reliably see or feel palpation or visual based, structural observation. Subsequently, this book does not advocate observational methods that involve determination of asymmetry.

One critical finding to consider is the prevalence of SIJ/pelvic impairment in pregnant or post-pregnant females. Nearly 50% of pregnant or recently pregnant females experienced some iteration of pelvic pain.[31–33] With pre-examination odds this high, the likelihood of pelvic involvement in nonspecific low back pain is notable.

Summary

- Various positions or postures do not appear to be effective for diagnosis of SIJ-related pain.
- Clearly, little evidence exists that asymmetry is an identifier of a pelvic dysfunction and even less evidence exists that clinicians can reliably see or feel palpation or visual-based structural observation.

Patient History

The most important aspect of the subjective history is the identification of nonmechanical symptoms or risk factors associated with infections and inflammatory, metabolic, and iatrogenic conditions. Peloso and Braun[34] indicate that many of the symptoms associated with ankylosing spondylitis, psoriatic arthritis, Reiter's syndrome (reactive arthritis), arthritis associated with inflammatory bowel disease, and undifferentiated spondyloarthropathies present with similar "symptoms" to those of mechanical SIJ/pelvis pain. For example,

these disorders commonly demonstrate pain with prolonged activity, tenderness over the SIJ or buttocks, potential involvement in the knees and hips, and restrictions in activities of daily living. However, selected symptoms are dissimilar to SIJ/pelvic pain, including involvement of the shoulders; restrictions in motion, specifically spine flexion, extension, and side flexion; pain at the thoraco-lumbar junction; and improvement with moderate activity. Additionally, medical and laboratory work-up may find markers in the blood or tissue that identify these selected nonmechanical disorders. Medical screening is warranted in any situation where symptoms are contradictory to clinical reasoning.

Numerous authors have reported common subjective or patient history–based complaints that they have associated with sacroiliac pain.[10] Lateral buttock pain is the predominant symptom of patients with a sacroiliac joint pain.[35] Nonetheless, the pain may also radiate down the posterior thigh, into the groin, into the anterior thigh, or transfer as distal as the foot or toes.[1] Slipman et al.[36] reported that the onset of pain occurs from a traumatic event such as a fall, or positional movements that generate force upon the SIJ such as torsion, heavy lifting, prolonged lifting, rising from a stooped position, or during a motor vehicle accident when the foot is depressed on the brake. Others have associated SIJ pain with long-term positioning such as crossing the legs or assuming a slumped position.

Pain Maps

Pain maps have been developed to outline the area of sensory change. Fortin et al.[37,38] suggested that SIJ-related pain results in an area approximately 3 centimeters wide and 10 centimeters long, just inferior to the PSIS. These findings were determined after injecting asymptomatic individuals in the SIJ and determining areas of hyperesthesia using light touch. Others have reported the same finding, identifying that pain isolated to the PSIS region, is sensitive for SIJ pain.[39]

Slipman et al.[40] reported contradictory findings in symptomatic subjects, pointing out that many patients reported symptoms into the lower lumbar, groin, thigh, ankle, and lower leg, in patterns dissimilar to Fortin et al.[37,38] Dreyfuss et al.[29] suggested the use of a pain map yields limited value for discriminating SIJ origin. Using intra-articular injections for patients with and without SIJ disorders, the authors compared pain patterns of several patients, and no specific pattern emerged for SIJ pain versus a dysfunction of another origin.[29] Broadhurst et al.[39] reported the absence of pain in the lumbar region was associated with SIJ dysfunction, and identified the presence of pain in the groin as significant. Groin pain was not considered a useful clinical tool in Dreyfuss et al.'s report.[29]

The *European Guidelines on the Diagnosis and Treatment of Pelvic Girdle Pain*[14] advocate that pain location should be considered but only in conjunction with other findings. These authors identified groin pain, pain below L5, pain in the region of the PSIS, and absence of pain in the lumbar spine as plausible, albeit not discriminatory, findings, with some evidence-based support. Young et al.[41] reported that most of the patients with injection-confirmed SIJ had pain lateral and below L5, whereas discogenic patients presented with midline pain. Slipman et al.[36] theorized that variability in pain referral patterns exist because the joint's innervation is highly variable, pain may be referred from internal and external structures, and pain referral may be dependent on the distinct location of the SIJ injury. At best, location of pain offers limited assistance in isolating SIJ/pelvis pain. See Figure 11.1 ■.

Summary

- An effective history should include the dissemination of nonmechanical disorders of the pelvis.
- There is mixed evidence of the usefulness of pain maps in identifying SIJ disorders. It does appear that in most cases, SIJ pain tends to be unilateral, can refer to the lower extremity (as far as the foot), and does have significant overlap with referred patterns of the lumbar spine.
- SIJ pain is commonly lateral and caudal to L5 when compared with discogenic lumbar pain, but not in all cases.
- The variation in pain distribution may be reflective of the largeness of the joint and the different sensory groups that supply aspects of the joint.

Physical Examination

The sacroiliac joint's morphology is extremely complex, which adds to the difficulty in appropriately examining and treating the region.[42,43] The complexity is further augmented by the paucity of clinical findings that are distinctly associated with SIJ pain.[29] Additionally, since the actual SIJ motion is so small and potentially subclinical, many manual examination methods are simply not useful. In essence, clinicians often operate in a large degree of uncertainty to whether the condition is SIJ-associative or not. Since injections are not routinely performed as part of manual therapy practice or diagnostic intervention, the likelihood of absolute identification of pain of sacroiliac origin based on traditional diagnostic principles is low.

Active Physiological Movements

Some authors have reported a relationship of active physiological movements with SIJ pain. Rost et al.[31] reported that most patients in a subclassification of pelvic pain that occurred during pregnancy reported pain during weight-bearing activities such as walking. Schwarzer et al.[44] reported that no planar active physiological movements are associated with SIJ pain, a finding also supported by Maigne et al.[16] Dreyfuss et al.[29] reported no significant active physiological movements such as movement toward lying down and movement toward a sitting posture that were associated with SIJ pain. Their study did report that standing was associated with a 3.9 likelihood

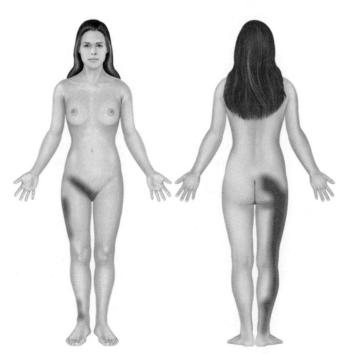

■ **Figure 11.1** Commonly Reported Pain Distribution for the Sacroiliac Joint

ratio versus nonstanding. Young et al.[41] reported that patients with confirmed SIJ pain (through fluoroscopically guided double injections) reported pain during rising from sitting. In their study, patients who experienced pain during sit to stand were 28 times more likely to have SIJ pain when concurrently positive with three of five special clinical tests. However, these findings in isolation are not significant enough to implicate SIJ related pain. In Young's study, patients with discogenic pain also reported pain during rising from sitting, which suggests that the inclusion of a single active physiological examination finding provides little diagnostic value for the clinician.

Lastly, some clinicians continue to focus on and espouse the merits of palpatory assessment during active physiological movements.[5,45,46] For this book, these methods are not supported. This does not suggest that the palpatory methods used by other clinicians are not effective in the hands of selected practitioners and when combined with numerous other examination processes. However, there is a preponderance of evidence that for the lay clinician, the reliability and diagnostic value of movement assessment techniques of the SIJ are fairly low.

Young et al.[41] reported that repeated movements are essential in detection of discogenic pain symptoms. Long et al.[18] and Laslett et al.[12] advocate that patients who centralize are most likely lumbar impairments and should be treated with directional preference exercises. Young et al.[41] does report that during the prepositioning of an innominate to allow specific anterior or posterior rotation, in some cases the patients will report a reduction of pain; however, this process does not occur during normal lumbar physiological assessment. The benefit of this finding is that it allows a discriminatory examination process in which low back impairments are separated from SIJ impairments. Patients who fail to centralize are classified as nonradiographic instability or sacroiliac impairment and require additional testing. Intentionally, for this textbook, the active physiological component of the SIJ examination is identical to the lumbar component.

"SIJ pain has no special distribution of features and is similar to symptoms arising from other lumbosacral structures. There are no provoking or relieving movements or positions that are unique or especially common to SIJ pain."[47] Subsequently, SIJ examination in absence of a lumbar spine screen may yield biased findings. This suggests that it is imperative to "rule out" the presence of lumbar spine pain prior to SIJ examination, but to also recognize that the two conditions can occur concomitantly.

The reader is directed toward the lumbar spine examination, including active physiological movements with overpressures, and passive accessory movements outlined in Chapter 10. Any isolated pain provoking, reducing, or centralization-based movement performed in lumbar flexion, side flexion, extension, or rotation likely implicates the lumbar spine.

In cases where no centralization or abolition of pain results from active physiological movements of the lumbar spine, further active physiological movements are used to distill out a directional preference with repeated forces on the SIJ. Young[48] described two techniques to initiate anterior and posterior rotation of a single innominate: sit to stand and the lunge. In addition, a step and bend technique can be used to increase posterior rotation of the innominate on one side.

Sit to Stand

Sit to stand has been implicated as a movement that is provocative in patients with SIJ pain. To date, only one study has investigated the diagnostic accuracy of the movement to implicate pelvic girdle pain and the findings were poor.[49]

Lunge for Anterior Rotation

A lunge has been investigated in one diagnostic accuracy study and demonstrated a small increase in post-test probability in the patient population.[49]

1 To test this motion, the patient assumes a lunge position, the painful extremity functioning as the trail leg.

2 The patient lunges forward until force is encountered on the posterior trail leg (Figure 11.2 ■).

3 The patient repeats the anterior lunge maneuver to determine if pain is reduced with repeated movements.

4 Resting symptoms are reassessed upon completion.

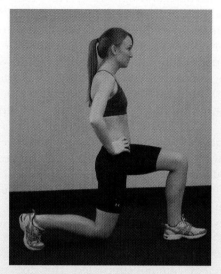

■ **Figure 11.2**   Anterior Rotation Lunge

Step and Bend for Posterior Rotation

1 The patient places the painful side extremity up on a 2- to 3-foot platform (right side in Figure 11.3 ■).

2 The patient then leans forward placing a backward or posterior torque on the innominate.

3 The patient repeats the posterior rotation technique to determine if pain is reduced with repeated movements.

4 Resting symptoms are reassessed upon completion.

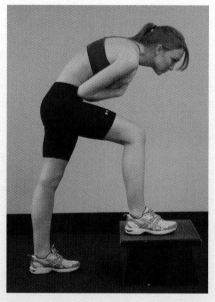

■ **Figure 11.3**   Posterior Rotation Step and Bend

Summary

- SIJ pain has no special distribution of features and is similar to symptoms arising from other lumbosacral structures.
- Patients with SIJ often report pain during unilateral weight bearing, sit to stand, and standing versus not standing.
- There is a preponderance of evidence that for the lay clinician, the reliability and diagnostic value of movement assessment techniques of the SIJ are poor.
- There is considerable evidence that patients who demonstrate centralization during a traditional lumbar examination do not have SIJ disorders.

Passive Physiological Movements

Cibulka and colleagues[4] reported that passive rotation asymmetry of the hip was positively associated with sacroiliac pain, a finding that has been demonstrated *in vitro* by others.[50] Additionally, there is evidence that suggests that a relationship between free hip range of motion and the sacroiliac joint exists, although the direction of that relationship is uncertain. For example, Pollard and Ward[51] reported an improvement in hip range of motion after manipulation of the sacroiliac joint. In the Cibulka et al. study,[4] patients were classified as having sacroiliac pain only using regional pain classification, the response of the direct treatment technique, and after restoration of pelvic symmetry.

Others have advocated the use of physiological end-range provocation movements of the innominates performed in sidelying.[52,53] Theoretically, these movements create torque on the intra- and extra-articular structures and could reproduce pain. Because of the complexity associated with both intra- and extra-articular structures, the ability to determine the required "direction" of the dysfunction based on feel, single movement provocation, or observation is evasive. For example, if anterior rotation of the right innominate on the sacrum is painful during end-range movement, several structures could be at fault. Extra-articular structures such as the long dorsal ligament may be irritated or internal structures such as the capsule may be impinged. This dilemma is the most significant challenge associated with an examination because adequate carryover to treatment is difficult to hypothesize. This necessitates the use of repeated end-range movements to outline whether the examination movement may be helpful as a treatment procedure.

Passive Physiological Posterior Rotation (Nutation)

Physiological rotation is necessary to determine the direction of treatment for the impairment. Unfortunately, none of the palpation-based tests has demonstrated reliability and validity to the point where these are useful to determine treatment direction. Subsequently, pain provocation and the response to repeated movements will serve to dictate the type of innominate impairment and the direction needed for treatment such as manipulation. One study has investigated passive nutation and found poor diagnostic accuracy for identifying SIJ pain.[49] Posterior rotation of the innominate on the sacrum provides a similar movement to sacral **nutation.**

1. The patient assumes a sidelying position, the painful side is placed upward away from the table, and resting symptoms are assessed.

2. The painful-sided leg is flexed beyond 90 degrees to engage the pelvis and to promote passive physiological flexion.

3. The clinician then situates his or her body into the popliteal fold of the painful-sided leg to "snug up" the position. The plinth-sided leg remains in an extended position.

4. The clinician then places his or her hands on the ischial tuberosity and the ASIS to promote further physiological rotation (Figure 11.4 ■).

5. The patient's pelvis is passively moved to the first sign of concordant pain.

(Continued)

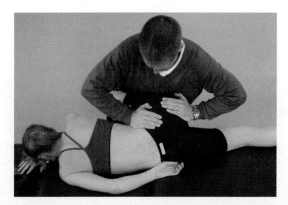

■ **Figure 11.4**   Passive Physiological Posterior Rotation: Nutation

⑥ The clinician then moves the patient beyond the first point of pain toward end range and the patient's symptoms are assessed for concordance.

⑦ The clinician then applies repeated motions at the end range to determine if the patient's concordant pain abolishes or increases. It is imperative to determine a pattern during this step since this step will determine the direction selected for treatment.

⑧ If concordant pain is bilateral, the process is repeated on the opposite side.

Passive Physiological Anterior Rotation (Counternutation)

One study has investigated passive counternutation and found poor diagnostic accuracy for identifying SIJ pain.[49] Passive **counternutation** assessment is similar in concept to nutation but requires selected changes in the pattern.

① The patient assumes a sidelying position, the painful side up. Resting symptoms are assessed.

② The painful-sided leg is extended and the plinth side leg is flexed to 90 degrees: the motion is the mirror image of passive physiological nutation in which the lower leg is wrapped around the waist of the clinician (not viewable in Figure 11.5 ■).

③ The clinician cradles the top leg with the caudal side hand and encourages further movement into hip extension. The cranial side forearm is placed on the PSIS and promotes anterior rotation of the innominate.

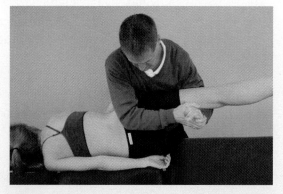

■ **Figure 11.5**   Passive Physiological Anterior Rotation: Counternutation

④ The patient's pelvis is passively moved to the first sign of concordant pain. The clinician then moves the patient beyond the first point of pain toward end range and the patient's symptoms are reassessed for concordance.

⑤ The clinician then applies repeated motions at the end range to determine if the patient's concordant pain abolishes or increases. Again, it is imperative to determine a pattern during this step since this step will determine the direction selected for treatment.

⑥ If concordant pain is bilateral, the process is repeated on the opposite side.

Passive Accessory Movements

Essentially, there are no studies that have assessed the merit of passive accessory movements of the SIJ. Traditionally, many clinicians have suggested that conventional PAs and APs may be beneficial in identifying "movement-related pain" and could be helpful in isolating the side of the lesion. In order to provide additional information, repeated passive accessory movements should cause a change in the concordant pain of the patient. In this manner, passive accessory movements may provide additional benefit or confirmatory information. When used in the context of "feel" for movement, in lieu of pain provocation, a passive accessory approach has diminished value because the range of motion and actual movements of the SIJ are so small.

As investigated with passive physiological movements, end-range repeated movements might be helpful to determine if the examination movements are plausible treatment techniques. The passive accessory movements should be applied to the painful side of the SIJ/pelvis for maximum discriminatory value. A passive accessory movement may be beneficial if repeated passive physiological movements cause a reduction of pain during the examination process; otherwise, the value is highly redundant to passive physiological movements.

Unilateral and Bilateral Anterior–Posterior Movements of the Innominate

Both the unilateral and bilateral anterior–posterior (AP) of the innominate promotes posterior rotation of the innominate with respect to the sacrum. Although both techniques should be examined, determination of which technique to use is based on the most complete reproduction of symptoms.

① The patient assumes a supine position and resting symptoms are assessed.

② For a unilateral AP (Figure 11.6 ■), the clinician applies a light posterior pressure at the ASIS to promote posterior rotation of the innominate. The AP should be applied just to the first report of pain. For a bilateral AP, the same process occurs with the contact points of both ASIS (Figure 11.7 ■).

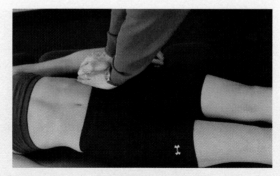

■ **Figure 11.6** Unilateral AP of the ASIS

(Continued)

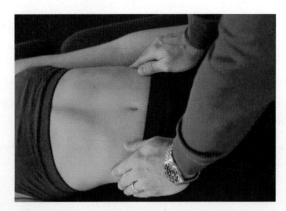

■ **Figure 11.7** Bilateral AP of the ASIS

③ The clinician then applies the force beyond the first point of pain and reassesses the patient's concordant sign.

④ The clinician then applies 5–30 seconds of repeated end-range oscillations to determine the behavior of the concordant pain. Because the SIJ is a strong and irregular joint, a significant load may be required to produce symptoms.[34] A positive sign that would implicate this method as an appropriate treatment choice is reduction of pain with continuous oscillations.

⑤ If a unilateral AP is performed, the clinician can repeat on the opposite side.

Unilateral and Bilateral Posterior–Anterior Movements of the Innominate

Both the unilateral and bilateral posterior–anterior (PA) of the innominate promotes anterior rotation of the innominate on the sacrum. Both techniques should be examined and determination of which technique to use is based on the most complete reproduction of symptoms.

① The patient assumes a supine position and resting symptoms are assessed.

② For a unilateral PA (UPA), the clinician applies a light posterior pressure at the PSIS with a thumb pad to thumb nail contact to promote anterior rotation of the innominate (Figure 11.8 ■). The UPA should be applied just to the first report of

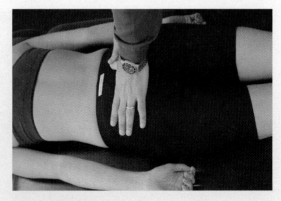

■ **Figure 11.8** Unilateral PA of the PSIS

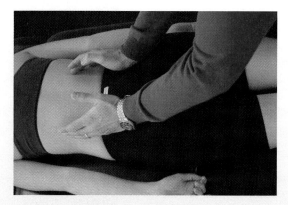

■ **Figure 11.9** Bilateral PA of the PSIS

pain. For a bilateral PA, the same process occurs with the contact points of both PSIS using the pisiforms of both hands (Figure 11.9 ■).

③ The clinician then applies the force beyond the first point of pain and reassesses the patient's concordant sign.

④ The clinician then applies 5–30 seconds of repeated end-range oscillations to determine the behavior of the concordant pain. Because the SIJ is a strong and irregular joint, a significant load may be required to produce symptoms.[27] A positive sign that would implicate this method

Summary

- Passive rotation asymmetry of the hip is positively associated with sacroiliac dysfunction, a finding that has been demonstrated *in vitro* by several investigators.

- Because palpation, observation, and single movement examination methods do not provide the examiner with credible criteria for assessment, the use of repeated end-range movements are advocated as a diagnostic and treatment method.

- There are no studies that assess the merit of passive accessory-based movements. When used in the context of "feel" for movement, in lieu of pain provocation, a passive accessory approach has diminished value because the range of motion and actual movements of the SIJ are so small.

Special Clinical Tests

Palpatory Mechanisms A wealth of literature is dedicated to the examination of the diagnostic value associated with special clinical tests and diagnostic tests. Most investigators agree that the minute amount of displacement associated with an SIJ pain make radiographic imaging inefficient.[54,55] Generally, traditional x-rays and CT scans are not beneficial in detecting mechanical SIJ dysfunction.[56,57] In contrast, for pubic symphysis disorders, the Chamberlain x-ray is a valid method.[58] Because of the limited value in these traditional diagnostic tests for the SIJ, the videofluoroscopically guided intra-articular diagnostic block is the recognized criterion standard,[29,59,60] but only for intra-articular disorders.[14]

Numerous "signs" of sacroiliac pain are advocated by various clinicians including regional abnormalities in length tension relationships, leg length changes, static and dynamic osseous landmarks, provocation movements, and selected postures.[29] Despite the variety of suggested examination methods, few conclusive tests are accepted universally for their diagnostic value in isolating SIJ pain.

Some authors suggest there is no evidence to support the use of mobility testing for dysfunction of the sacroiliac joints.[27,61] However, deep palpation to the pubic symphysis is associated with osteitis pubis or instability of the pubic symphysis,[21,62] and Vleeming et al.[63] suggests that painful palpation over the long dorsal ligament may implicate irritation of that ligament.

Levangie[30] reported poor diagnostic values of selected palpation-based assessment of symmetry for the pelvis. In her study, Levangie did not isolate SIJ patients through diagnostic block; therefore the findings were associated with patients with long-term nonspecific low back pain that may have included SIJ impairment.

The diagnostic value of each of the findings is very poor, suggesting that palpation-based methods are not helpful in identifying SIJ pain. If used in combination with other measures, the values may have utility, but alone these findings offer conflicting or very poor diagnostic value. The reader is recommended to consult the sister textbook[64] to this textbook to review the diagnostic values of each test. In summary, the palpatory tests included in (Figures 11.10– 11.12 ■) have very low diagnostic value, very poor reliability, and may have little to no value in clinical practice for *diagnosing* SIJ pain or dysfunction.

Movement-Based Testing Several movement-based assessments exist and have been studied for reliability and diagnostic accuracy. Four of the movement-based assessments, the Gillet test, the long sit test, the standing flexion test, and the sitting flexion test (Figures 11.13–11.16 ■), involve measurement of asymmetry during selected movement procedures. Comprehensively, these tests demonstrate poor reliability and very little diagnostic value.[65,66] Levangie[30] used a mechanical device to improve the reliability of the movement-based assessments to avoid

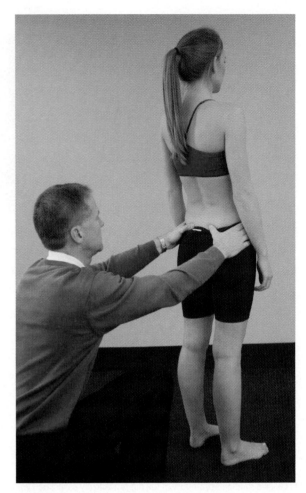

■ **Figure 11.11** PSIS Symmetry in Standing

the problems associated with poor consistency and support this limited utility of these measures. The reader is recommended to consult the sister textbook[64] to this textbook to review the diagnostic values of each test. It is arguable whether the movement-based assessment provides any diagnostic value for detecting SIJ-related pain.

Provocation-Based Testing Restrictive use of isolated pain provocation tests has questionable utility.[11,16,43,60] In construct, some have promoted the use of pain provocation tests only when clustered together with other tests.[12,27,66,67] When compared to palpation and movement-based assessment, pain provocation tests yield higher reliability and diagnostic value scores for diagnosing SIJ pain (when clustered). Specifically, reliability is better, often producing interclinician agreement values that qualify as "fair" to "good."[65]

For this text, a cluster of pain provocation tests are used to implicate the SIJ as the origin of pain. The tests are not designed to identify a dysfunction nor do the

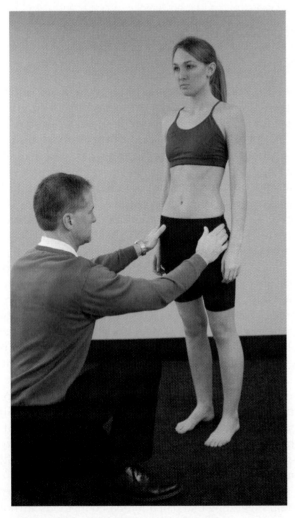

■ **Figure 11.10** ASIS Symmetry in Standing

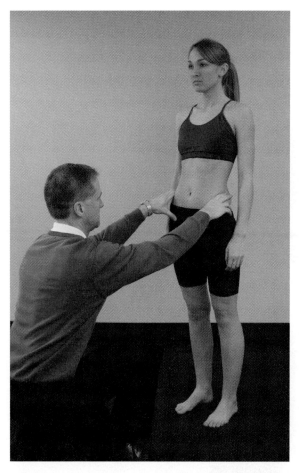

■ **Figure 11.12**   Iliac Crest Height during Standing

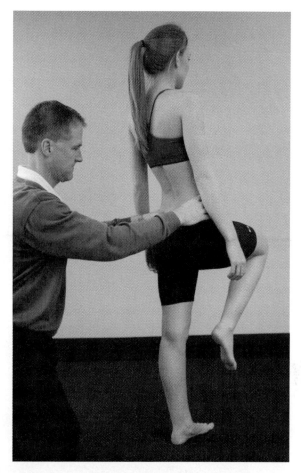

■ **Figure 11.13**   The Gillet Test

tests solely implicate the SIJ and rule out the lumbar spine. The four tests advocated by this book are the Thigh Thrust, Compression Test, the Distraction Test, and the Sacral Thrust. Each is described below. If a person cannot assume a prone position, one may choose to use the thigh thrust, Patrick test, (Figure 11.17 ■), compression, distraction, and the Gaenslen's test (Figure 11.18 ■).

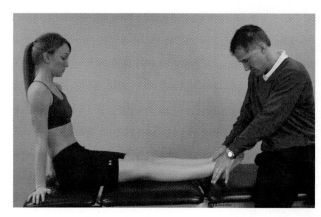

■ **Figure 11.14**   The Long Sit Test

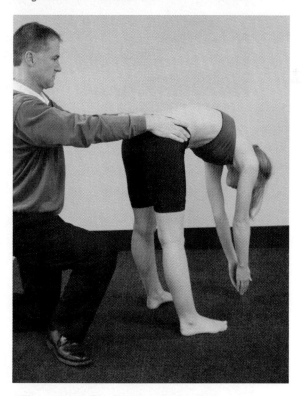

■ **Figure 11.15**   The Standing Flexion Test

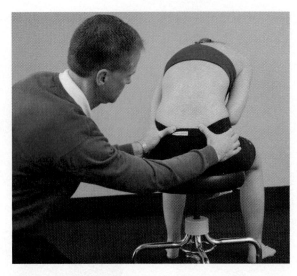

■ **Figure 11.16**   The Sitting Flexion Test

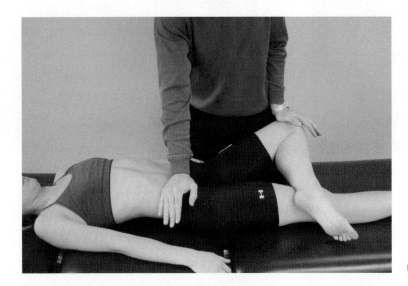

■ **Figure 11.17**   Patrick's Test

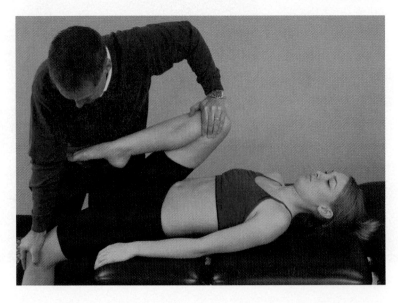

■ **Figure 11.18**   Gaenslen's Test

Thigh Thrust

The Thigh Thrust is a useful clinical test that has been included as part of a cluster of SIJ tests in recent studies. The Thigh Thrust is also known as the Ostgaard test, the 4P test, and the Sacrotuberous stress test, and involves a downward force of the thigh that causes a posterior translation of the innominate on the sacrum. Concordant pain reproduction is considered a positive test.

1. The patient is positioned in supine and resting symptoms are assessed. The clinician stands on the opposite side of the painful side of the patient.

2. The painful-sided knee is flexed to 90 degrees.

3. The clinician places his or her hand under the sacrum to form a stable "bridge" for the sacrum.

4. A downward pressure is applied through the femur (at the knee) to force a posterior translation of the innominate on the sacrum (Figure 11.19 ■). The force is held for at least 30 seconds and if no pain occurs, a slight bounce at the end of the 30 seconds to further provoke the joint is used.

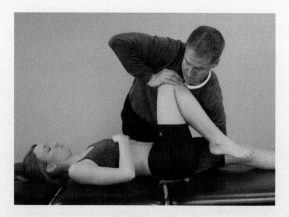

5. The patient's symptoms are assessed to determine if they are concordant. A positive test is concordant pain that is posterior to the hip or near the SIJ.

■ Figure 11.19   The Thigh Thrust

Sacral Spring Test

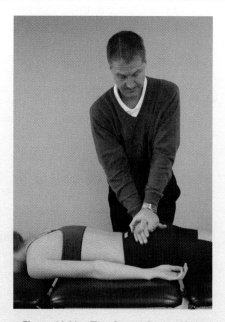

The Sacral Spring Test is one of the four pain provocation tests advocated by Laslett and colleagues.[47] The test theoretically provides an anterior shearing force of the sacrum on both of the ilia.

1. The patient assumes a prone position after assessment of resting symptoms.

2. The clinician palpates the second or third spinous process of the sacrum then applies a series of five to seven downward thrusts on the sacrum at S3 (Figure 11.20 ■). By targeting the midpoint of the sacrum, the clinician is less likely to force the lumbar spine into hyperextension. A positive test is a reproduction of the concordant sign during downward pressure.

■ Figure 11.20   The Sacral Spring Test

Sacroiliac Compression Test

1. The patient assumes a sidelying position with his or her painful side up, superior to the plinth (left side in Figure 11.21 ■).

2. After assessment of resting symptoms, the clinician then cups the iliac crest of the painful side and applies a downward force through the ilium for up to 30 seconds. As with the other SIJ tests, considerable vigor is required to reproduce the symptoms; in some cases repeated force is necessary. A positive test is reproduction of the concordant sign of the patient.

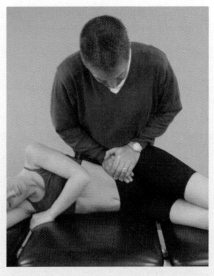

■ **Figure 11.21** The SI Compression Test

SI Distraction Test

The SI Distraction Test is similar in concept to the Compression Test but utilizes an opposite direction of force.

1. After resting symptoms are assessed the patient assumes a supine position.

2. The medial aspect of both anterior–superior iliac spines is palpated by the clinician. The clinician crosses his or her arms, creating an X at the forearms and a force is applied in a lateral–posterior direction (Figure 11.22 ■). For comfort, it is often required that the clinician relocate his or her hands on the ASIS several times.

3. The clinician applies a vigorous static force for 30 seconds in an attempt to reproduce the concordant sign of the patient. A positive test is reproduction of the concordant sign of the patient.

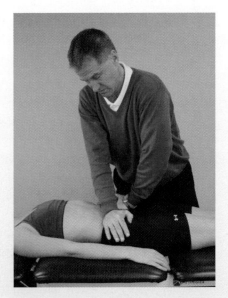

■ **Figure 11.22** The Sacroiliac Distraction Test

Combining Tests (Clusters)

Several studies have purported the benefit of combining selected SIJ tests to improve the reliability and diagnostic value. Kokmeyer et al.[67] showed improvement when three of five tests were positive, suggesting the findings were more discriminate than using only one test. Others have advocated the benefit of palpation or movement-based tests, although it is possible that the methods used to determine these results were methodologically flawed.[68] Laslett and colleagues[12] and Young[48] used the discriminatory criteria of both centralization assessment and diagnostic blocks to determine patients with sacroiliac pain. Using a combination of three of five tests, the positive likelihood ratio improved to 4.16. Laslett et al.[12] suggested that this cluster of tests is necessary versus one single test to rule out the potential for single tester error. Furthermore, Laslett and colleagues[47] have outlined that finding two of four positive tests when testing the thigh thrust, distraction, compression, and sacral thrust, in the absence of centralization of the spine, is indicative of a positive SIJ dysfunction. The authors advocate testing the thigh thrust and distraction first and that any combination of two positive findings is indicative of SIJ dysfunction. In an independent study, van der Wurff and associates found similar diagnostic accuracy using three of five tests[69] (Table 11.1 ■).

■ **TABLE 11.1** Diagnostic Value of Selected Combined SIJ Special Clinical Tests

Author	Reliability	Sensitivity	Specificity	+LR	-LR
Distraction, Thigh Thrust, Gaenslen's Test, Compression, and Sacral Thrust					
Laslett et al.[12] (3 of 5)	NT	91	78	4.16	0.11
Thigh Thrust, Distraction, Sacral Thrust, and Compression Tests					
Laslett et al.[47] (2 of 4)	NR	88	78	4.00	0.16
Thigh Thrust, Distraction, Sacral Thrust, and Compression Tests					
Van der Wurff et al.[69] (3 of 5)	NR	85	79	4.02	0.19

NR, not reported; NT, not tested.

Manual Muscle Testing   Rost et al.[31] suggested that resisted sidelying abduction (Figure 11.23 ■) is symptomatic with patients experiencing hypermobility of the sacroiliac and pubic symphysis. In contrast, assessment of loss of hip adduction strength (secondary to pain) may be useful in implicating postpartum pelvic pain syndrome. Additionally, the nature of the Active Straight Leg Raise (not pictured), which involves pain during active hip flexion, may also implicate pelvic instability.

Summary

- The most useful palpation-based special tests appear to be direct palpation of the pubic symphysis and long dorsal ligament.
- Manual muscle testing appears to yield useful information, specifically resisted hip adduction and possibly resisted hip flexion.
- No observation or palpation for location-based tests appears to demonstrate acceptable reliability or validity.
- A cluster of two of four special clinical tests has demonstrated fair to moderate validity for adjusting post test probability of injection-confirmed SIJ pain. These tests include the sacral spring, the compression and distraction tests, and the thigh thrust.

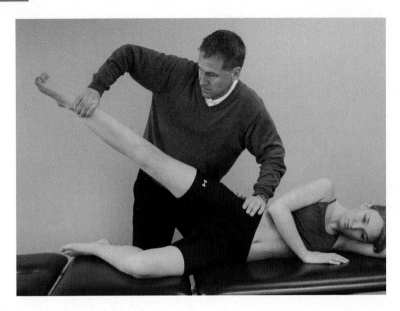

■ **Figure 11.23**   The Resisted Abduction Test

Diagnosis and Treatment Decision Making

Indeed, isolation of the presence of a sacroiliac or pelvic impairment is a challenge. Further assessment of the homogenous category of SIJ impairment is all the more difficult. Nevertheless, the critical use of appropriate examination findings will improve the likelihood that one will not miss an SIJ/pelvic problem.

Palpation-based examination methods have long been a hallmark of diagnosing SIJ pain. Unfortunately, there is little reliability or validity to these methods and they may serve only to bias the clinician to an incorrect diagnosis. In fact, numerous guru-based educators have suggested multitudes of various SIJ directional faults such as up-slips, down-slips, inflares, outflares, superior shears, and inferior shears. Unfortunately, there is no biomechanical literature that supports the absolute existence of these phenomena, nor are there diagnostic methods to support a positional diagnosis. Subsequently, most evidence-based studies have outlined dysfunction primarily associated with SIJ inflammatory disorders, such as anterior rotation of the innominate on the sacrum, posterior rotation of the innominate on the sacrum, and superior shear of the pubis with respect to the opposite side. Typically, superior shear of the pubis is associated with ipsilateral anterior rotation of the innominate on the sacrum.[58] Bilateral conditions of said disorders are plausible as well. By limiting our examination to these findings, the likelihood of correctly identifying the disorder is substantially improved. Because determining the correct side and the direction of the dysfunction is crucial for manual therapy and surgical treatment,[30,58] considerable effort should be dedicated to this exploration.

By using evidence-based information, the chance of appropriately identifying the presence of an SIJ dysfunction is improved (although still challenging). The steps include (1) ruling out the presence of a disc-related lumbar spine impairment or an impairment that responds well to lumbar spine-related treatments and (2) using evidence-based special tests to appropriately identify the presence of SIJ-related disorders.

Use of the criteria developed by George and Delitto[70] allows the clinician to segregate treatment responses of the lumbar spine into four primary categories (see Chapter 10). Treatment directed at traction, specific exercise, and mobilization groups are methods used for a lumbar spine disorder. Failure to improve in any of the lumbar-directed responses may be suggestive of clinical instability or SIJ pain (Figure 11.24). Using centralization and other aspects of lumbar spine treatment to rule out back disorders versus other disorders is a method designed to carefully discriminate and improve the likelihood of a correct diagnosis. By using the centralization phenomenon and 10% pretest prevalence, the likelihood of correctly identifying an SIJ pain increases from 10 to 40%. Including other discriminatory factors such as gender, pregnancy, the pain during palpation of the long dorsal ligament, and incident of injury would provide even further conclusive information.

As stated, Laslett et al.[47] suggest the use of two of four positive tests to outline SIJ-related pain (Figure 11.25 ■). A combination of two positive thigh thrust, distraction, compression, or sacral thrust

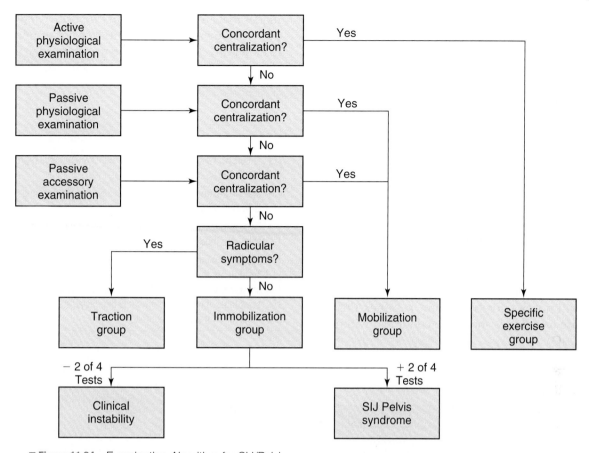

■ **Figure 11.24**   Examination Algorithm for SIJ/Pelvis

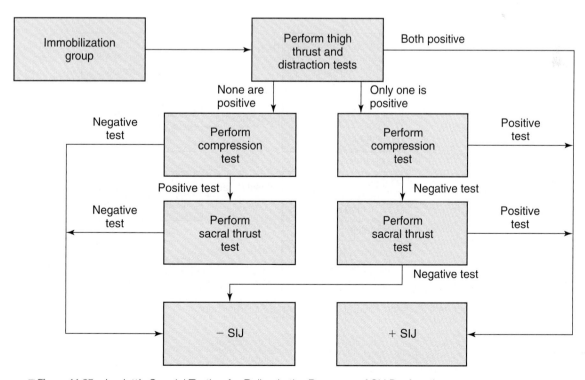

■ **Figure 11.25**   Laslett's Special Testing for Ruling in the Presence of SIJ Dysfunction

tests, in the absence of centralization of the spine, is suggestive of SIJ pain. This finding is a modification from the original three of five tests suggested also by Laslett et al.[12] Ruling "out" the lumbar spine and a positive two of four tests for SIJ is associated with a four times likelihood that SIJ pain is truly present.

The last aspect of the evidence-based model involves treatment decision making (Figure 11.26 ■). Although the findings of ruling out lumbar spine and two of four positive tests increase the probability of accurately diagnosing SIJ pain, the tests do not outline what form of treatment is appropriate for the patient. To determine whether a patient benefits from a manual therapy–oriented approach, a series of manual techniques are used to assess patient response. Either the patient will positively respond to techniques that are counternutation or nutation based, or they will not positively respond to either. Positive response techniques should be continued with tech-

niques that are associated with the positive movement pattern. However, if a patient does not respond well to either direction of movement, stabilization is likely the suggested treatment approach and should be implemented.

Summary

- Theoretical position-based impairments are not well represented within the literature.

- One way to improve the diagnostic accuracy of detecting SIJ pain is by ruling out the lumbar spine.

- Two of four positive SIJ tests after having ruled out the lumbar spine are moderately indicative of SIJ pain.

- Appropriate treatment is associated with desired patient response. Treatments that are associated with nutation or counternutation are appropriately administered if they reduce patient complaint of symptoms. If neither treatment is beneficial, stabilization may be the desired treatment approach.

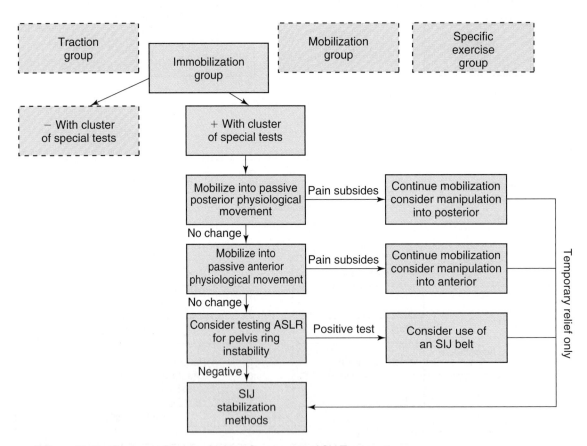

■ **Figure 11.26** Treatment Decision-Making Component of SIJ Treatment

Treatment Techniques

There may be no other region of the body that so much effort has been dedicated toward examination and diagnosis yet so little study has been performed regarding treatment. At present, there are no studies that comprehensively and prospectively analyze the effectiveness of active stretching, muscle energy, manipulation, or mobilization for SIJ/pelvic treatment.[71] Numerous anecdotal findings suggest various forms of physical therapy and chiropractic treatment yield modest benefits for reduction of pain.[72] The *European Guidelines on the Diagnosis and Treatment of Pelvic Girdle Pain*[14] reports they cannot recommend the use of any of these methods because no single randomized clinical or pragmatic trial has been performed.

There may be several reasons for this finding. First, conclusive diagnosis of SIJ pain requires diagnostic blocks and is an expensive and a time-consuming step, thus homogenizing groups in certain SIJ/pelvis groups is difficult. Second, few clinicians agree on the appropriate treatment for SIJ. Third, the understanding that instability is a common cause of SIJ/pelvis pain is a relatively contemporary finding.

As with other anatomical regions, the SIJ and pelvis may exhibit different forms of impairment. It is unfair to assume that all SIJ pain will exhibit the same set of symptoms, involve the same anatomical tissue, and will demonstrate a similar form of outcome. The joint is very large and has different regions with different referred pain patterns. The size of the joint requires a variety of types of treatment; treatment needs modification for the older population.[73]

In 2002, Albert et al.[20] introduced five subgroups of posterior pelvic pain syndrome (PPPP), including SIJ pelvic girdle syndrome (pain in the SIJ and pubic symphysis), symphysiolysis, one-sided SIJ syndrome, double-side SIJ syndrome, and mixed. Albert believes that although this finding is based on clinical examination and was from a population of 2,269 pregnant patients, the plausibility exists that nonpregnant patients may suffer from similar dysfunctions.[74] Anatomically and biomechanically, these disparate problems could represent clinically in very dissimilar ways.

Active Physiological Movements

Self-correction methods of SIJ pain allow the patient to "self-treat" in the absence of an attending clinician. Although there are numerous methods of self-treatment, those methods that are targeted toward the complimentary rotational displacements are the easiest for the patient to understand and perform in isolation.

Standing Rotation

If the patient responded well to repeated counter-nutation of the innominate in sidelying, a standing rotation technique may be applicable as a home program.

1 The patient's leg (on the symptomatic side) is placed on a box or some other structure approximately 2–3 feet high.

2 The patient then leans forward over the leg to encourage posterior pelvic rotation (on the right side in Figure 11.27 ■).

3 Repeated oscillations are used to "mobilize" the innominate.

4 The patient can repeat the procedure throughout the day.

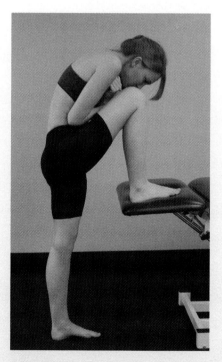

■ **Figure 11.27**   Standing Rotation

External Rotation with Trunk Flexion

If the patient responded well to repeated counter-nutation of the innominate in sidelying, external rotation with trunk flexion may also be applicable.

1. To perform this as a home program, the patient sits with the leg on the symptomatic side crossed at the knee. This movement promotes external rotation of the hip and corresponding posterior innominate movement of the pelvis.

2. The patient then leans forward to further the posterior rotation of the pelvis (Figure 11.28 ■).

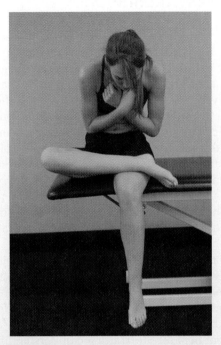

■ **Figure 11.28** External Rotation with Flexion

The Standing Extension Stretch

If the patient responded well to repeated nutation of the innominate in sidelying, a standing extension stretch may be useful.

1. The patient places the knee or foot of the symptomatic leg posterior to the hip (right side in Figure 11.29 ■).

2. The patient extends backward by "sagging" the pelvis to promote anterior rotation of the innominate.

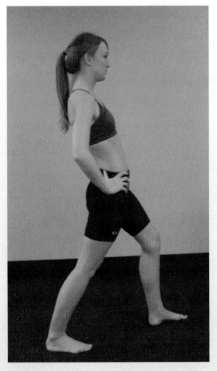

■ **Figure 11.29** Standing Extension Stretch

Passive Physiological Movements

Passive physiological movements are designed to identify a directional movement that may be pain reducing for the patient.

Posterior Rotation of the Innominate on the Sacrum

This technique is selected if repeated physiological rotations led to pain relief or abolishment of symptoms during the clinical examination.

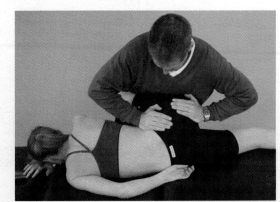

■ **Figure 11.30** Physiological Posterior Rotation of the Innominate

1. The patient assumes a sidelying position, the painful side up and resting symptoms are assessed.

2. The painful-sided leg is flexed beyond 90 degrees to engage the pelvis and to promote passive physiological flexion.

3. The clinician then situates his or her body into the popliteal fold of the painful-sided leg to "snug up" the position. The plinth-sided leg remains in an extended position (Figure 11.30 ■).

4. The clinician then places his or her hands on the ischial tuberosity and the ASIS to promote physiological rotation.

5. The patient's pelvis is passively moved to the first sign of concordant pain, then the method is repeated at or near end range while respecting the patient's concordant sign.

Anterior Rotation of the Innominate on the Sacrum

This technique is selected if repeated physiological rotations led to pain relief or abolishment of symptoms during the clinical examination.

1. The patient assumes a sidelying position, the painful side up, and resting symptoms are assessed.

2. The painful-sided leg is extended and the plinth-sided leg is flexed to 90 degrees. The motion is the mirror image of passive physiological nutation.

3. The clinician cradles the leg with the caudal side hand and encourages further movement into hip extension.

④ The cranial-sided hand is placed on the PSIS and promotes anterior rotation of the innominate (Figure 11.31 ■).

⑤ The clinician then places his or her hand on the ischial tuberosity and forearm on the ASIS to further promote physiological rotation.

⑥ The patient's pelvis is passively moved to the first sign of concordant pain, then the method is repeated at or near end range while respecting the patient's concordant sign.

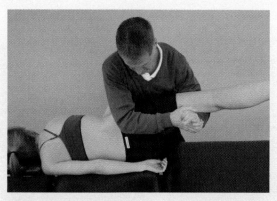

■ **Figure 11.31** Physiological Anterior Rotation of the Innominate

Passive Physiological Anterior Rotation in Prone

This technique is selected if repeated physiological anterior rotation of the innominate led to pain relief during the passive physiological examination, yet end-range movements were poorly tolerated in the sidelying position.

① The patient assumes a prone position and resting symptoms should be assessed.

② The clinician stands to the same side as the leg where concordant symptoms are identified.

③ The clinician places the cephalic hand on the PSIS while the caudal hand lifts the knee and thigh (Figure 11.32 ■).

④ Using a sequential motion, the clinician then applies a downward glide to the PSIS (promoting anterior rotation of the innominate) at the same time he or she performs passive hip extension. The amount of force applied to the PSIS can be modulated. The treatment should elicit the concordant sign of the patient.

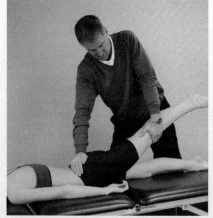

■ **Figure 11.32** Passive Physiological Anterior Rotation in Prone

Passive Accessory Movements (PAIVMS)

There are numerous methods of passive accessory techniques, many of which are redundant to the passive physiological procedures. Selection of a technique should distill out of the examination. For example, the use of a unilateral AP to the right ASIS should only be selected if pain reduces while performing repeated movements during the initial examination.

Unilateral Gapping During Rotation

One method designed to encourage posterior glide is the unilateral gap. By placing the lumbar spine in a coupled position (meaning concurrent rotation and side flexion) the ligamentous and capsular system of the lumbar spine is in apposition and will demonstrate decreased movements. By using this set-up, translation on the innominate should provide more isolated forces to the pelvis versus the low back.

1. The patient lies in a sidelying position and the painful side is placed up.

2. The clinician then rotates skyward to L5 to couple the ligaments and facets.

3. The cephalic hand is placed flush against L5 to provide a block to the lumbar spine and the caudal hand is placed on the ASIS to provide a force anteriorly to posteriorly (Figure 11.33 ■). Repeated movements should result in abolishing or diminishing symptoms.

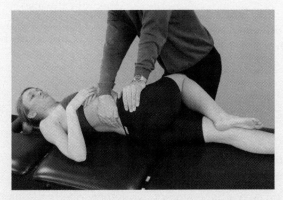

■ **Figure 11.33**   Unilateral Gapping of SIJ in Sidelying

Posterior Shear of Innominate on Sacrum

The posterior shear mobilization/manipulation of the innominate is very similar to the Thigh Thrust Test. The technique should only be used if posterior glide techniques such as an AP yield beneficial results during the examination.

1. The patient is positioned in supine for the procedure and resting symptoms are assessed.

2. The clinician stands on the opposite side of the painful side of the patient. The painful-sided knee (right side in Figure 11.34 ■) is flexed to 90 degrees.

3. The clinician places his or her hand under the sacrum to form a stable "bridge" for the sacrum. A downward pressure is applied through the femur to force a posterior translation of the pelvis. Repeated movements may be necessary and/or a thrust can be used for a manipulative procedure.

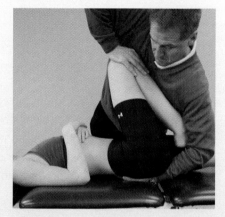

■ **Figure 11.34** Posterior Shear of Innominate on Sacrum

Manually Assisted Movements

Muscle energy techniques are commonly used as treatment techniques of the SIJ/pelvis. Since bombardment of neurophysiological input is the goal of the treatment, three techniques will be discussed that theoretically also correct an anteriorly rotated innominate, a posteriorly rotated innominate, and a displaced pubic symphysis.

Adduction Isometric of the Pubic Symphysis

Mens et al.[58] point out that instability of the pelvis results in superior migration of the impaired (painful)-sided pubis during weight bearing. One method to relocate this migration is the adduction isometric treatment, commonly referred to as the "shot gun." In reality, this method is as likely as powerful for its neurophysiological effects as its biomechanical effects.

1. The patient assumes a hooklying supine position and resting symptoms are queried.

2. The clinician provides a series of resisted bilateral hip abduction bouts in which the patient is requested to push out against the clinician-applied resistance for several bouts of 6-second holds.

3. Slowly, the clinician allows further hip abduction in the hooklying position until the knees are wide enough apart to allow the clinician to place his or her forearm, lengthwise, between the knees.

(Continued)

④ After the last abduction isometric bout, the clinician requests a strong and quick adduction isometric contraction against the forearm resistance (Figure 11.35 ■). Often, the patient experiences some discomfort and an audible with this activity. Since the core of the problem is generally instability, the patient may benefit from the application of a SIJ belt directly after this procedure.

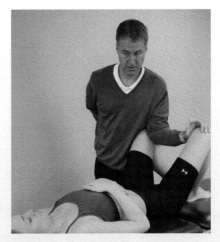

■ **Figure 11.35** Correction of Displacement of Pubic Symphysis

Muscle Energy Technique to Initiate Posterior Rotation

If the patient displays pain during physiological posterior rotation of the innominate in sidelying that is improved with repeated movements into posterior rotation, he or she may be a good candidate for a muscle energy technique. The technique is effective, because the patient controls the amount of force applied through the SIJ.

① The patient assumes a hooklying supine position and resting symptoms are queried.

② The leg on the painful side is flexed at the knee and hip and raised into as much hip flexion as the patient can tolerate.

③ The opposite extremity is positioned in relative extension or neutral position.

④ Using his or her body, the clinician then leans into the flexed leg (left leg in Figure 11.36 ■) to provide a stable barrier for resistance.

■ **Figure 11.36** Muscle Energy Technique to Initiate Posterior Rotation

⑤ The opposite arm is extended and placed on the knee of the patient as a counterforce.

⑥ The patient is instructed to push downward with the knee and hip against the resistance of the clinician while simultaneously flexing the opposite hip against the hand resistance. A series of three to five bouts of 5-second holds are beneficial.

⑦ Upon completion, the concordant movement of the patient is reassessed.

Muscle Energy Technique to Initiate Anterior Rotation

If the patient displays pain during physiological anterior rotation of the innominate in sidelying that is improved with repeated movements into anterior rotation, he or she may be a good candidate for a muscle energy technique.

1. The patient assumes a hooklying supine position and resting symptoms are queried.

2. The leg on the painful side is extended off the table and the opposite leg is flexed at the hip and the knee. The position is the opposite of that in Figure 11.36. It is best for the clinician to stand to the opposite side of the leg on the painful pelvis.

3. Using his or her body weight, the clinician then leans into the flexed leg (nonpainful side) to provide a stable barrier for resistance. The opposite arm is extended and placed on the knee of the patient.

4. The patient is instructed to lightly push downward (in hip extension) against the resistance of the clinician while simultaneously flexing the leg on the painful side (right leg in Figure 11.37 ■) against the hand resistance. A series of three to five bouts of 5-second holds are beneficial.

5. Upon completion, the concordant movement of the patient is reassessed.

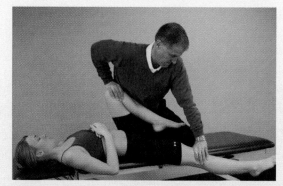

■ **Figure 11.37** Muscle Energy Technique to Initiate Anterior Rotation

Manipulation

Manipulation maneuvers are designed to bombard the region with neurophysiological inputs, and provide correction of displacement and pain relief upon application.[25] Previously, using a purported SIJ technique, Flynn et al.[76] outlined that an audible was not necessary for a positive treatment outcome.[77] Using an innovative audiographic method to record cavitation sounds, Beffa and Mathews[78] indicated that the audible associated with a manipulation isn't always at the targeted segment of the adjustment.

Roentgen stereophotogrammetric analysis suggests that manipulation does not alter the position of the SIJ.[79] However, improvements in clinically identified asymmetry do occur after manipulation, a finding also reported by Tullberg et al.[79] who hypothesized this response as associative soft-tissue changes. Considerable evidence exists that manipulation does have the capacity to affect soft tissue around the SIJ, since the H-reflex is decreased after manipulation[80] and may alter the feed-forward mechanism in the deep transverse abdominus.[81]

The following techniques are described with the underlying assumption that repeated passive physiological or accessory movements did not provide pain relief. However, even if repeated movements provide pain relief, manipulation can be a treatment of choice. The manipulative procedures would be performed in the same direction that pain decreased with passive accessory movements versus the opposite direction, as described in the following examples.

Sidelying Manipulation into Anterior Rotation

The sidelying manipulation into anterior rotation is a technique that may be beneficial if the patient had decreased symptoms during anterior rotation of the innominate.

1. The patient assumes a sidelying position and resting symptoms are queried.

2. The painful-sided leg is extended and the plinth-sided leg is flexed to 90 degrees. The motion is the mirror image of passive physiological counternutation.

3. The clinician cradles the leg with the caudal side hand and encourages further movement into hip extension (Figure 11.38 ■). The cranial side forearm is placed on the PSIS and promotes anterior rotation of the innominate and a quick but firm thrust is applied at end range. Rarely does an audible occur.

4. The patient's concordant sign should be reassessed directly after the treatment.

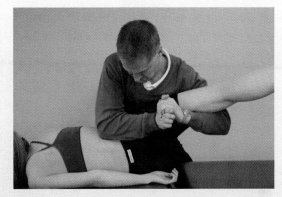

■ **Figure 11.38** Sidelying, Manipulation into Anterior Rotation

Sidelying Manipulation into Posterior Rotation

The sidelying manipulation into posterior rotation is a technique that may be beneficial if the patient had decreased symptoms during posterior rotation of the innominate.

1. The patient is placed in a sidelying position, the painful side up.

2. The painful-sided leg is flexed beyond 90 degrees to engage the pelvis and to promote passive physiological flexion.

3. The clinician then situates his or her body into the popliteal fold of the painful-sided leg to "snug up" the position, whereas the plinth-sided leg remains in an extended position (Figure 11.39 ■).

4. The clinician then places his or her hands on the ischial tuberosity and the ASIS to promote further physiological rotation.

5. The patient's pelvis is passively moved to end range. A quick but firm thrust is applied at end range; rarely does an audible occur.

6. The patient's concordant sign should be reassessed directly after the treatment.

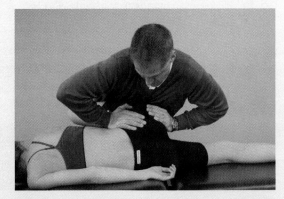

■ **Figure 11.39** Sidelying, Manipulation into Posterior Rotation

Anterior to Posterior Innominate Thrust

The anterior to posterior innominate thrust (Chicago Roll) is well described in previous studies.[82] There is some question whether the procedure actually manipulates the SIJ or the fifth facet of the lumbar spine. Nonetheless, a patient who demonstrates pain with repeated anterior rotation of the innominate may be a good candidate for this procedure. The technique is described in further detail in Chapter 10.

1. The patient assumes a supine position after a baseline assessment of symptoms.

2. The patient interlocks his or her fingers behind the neck and the elbows are pulled together.

3. The clinician side-flexes the patient's body away and rotates the patient's body toward them (in opposition) (Figure 11.40 ■).

4. The patient is rolled until end range and the clinician then applies a quick thrust at end range to the patient's ASIS.

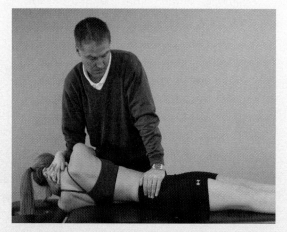

■ **Figure 11.40** The Anterior to Posterior Innominate Thrust

Posterior to Anterior PSIS Thrust

The anterior PSIS thrust may be beneficial in patients that report decreased pain with repeated passive physiological anterior rotation.

1. The patient assumes a prone position.

2. The clinician stands to the same side as the leg where concordant symptoms are identified.

3. The clinician places the cephalic hand on the PSIS while the caudal hand lifts the knee and thigh (Figure 11.41 ■).

4. Using a sequential motion, the clinician then applies a downward glide to the PSIS (promoting anterior rotation of the innominate) at the same time he or she performs passive hip extension. At end range, the clinician provides a quick thrust.

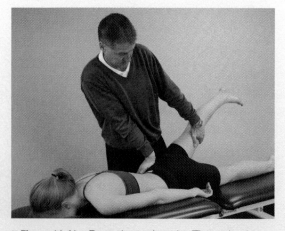

■ **Figure 11.41** Posterior to Anterior Thrust (patient prone, thrust to PSIS)

Cyriax Grade V SIJ Manipulation

Cyriax[83] described a procedure in which the lower limb of the painful-sided pelvis is distracted quickly, thus causing a manipulative force throughout the pelvis. Because a patient who exhibits pubic symphysis dysfunction often displays superior displacement of one pubis on the other, this method may demonstrate benefit. Thus, this technique is appropriate for a patient who has a positive Chamberlain x-ray, or has pain with repeated anterior rotation of the innominate.

1. The patient assumes a supine position after assessment of baseline symptoms.

2. The clinician elevates the extended leg approximately 30 degrees and internally rotates the hip to tension the hip joint. Distraction is applied on the lower extremity to remove any slack.

3. The lower leg is gently oscillated (up and down) to relax the patient. Once the patient has relaxed and has allowed the full weight of the leg to fall into the clinician's hands a quick longitudinal thrust is applied in an upward and distal direction (Figure 11.42 ■).

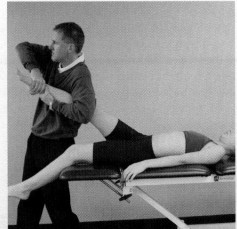

■ **Figure 11.42**   Long Leg Lever Thrust (Cyriax Grade V)

Summary

- Many of the documented SIJ disorders are associated with pain during pregnancy.
- More research is needed on this area of SIJ classification.
- A cornucopia of manual therapy methods exists for pelvic treatment; the benefits of these methods are still unknown, but are supported by anecdotal evidence.

Treatment Outcomes

The Evidence

Anecdotally, manual therapy has provided promising findings during clinical practice and has been advocated as an intervention as efficacious.[84] What is ironic is the absolute disconnect between the global passion clinicians have regarding SIJ examination and the very few trials associated with manual therapy treatment of the SIJ (Level C). In a study by Galm et al.[85] manual therapy led to more rapid improvements in a two-sample comparison of patients classified as SIJ pain with documented concurrent herniated disc. Manual therapy was the only treatment difference between the two groups. Prone position mobilization and manipulation procedures were selected because these methods were considered safe for a patient with disc impairment.[86] Shearar et al.[87] found pre- to post-test improvements in pain and disability in patients with clinically determined SIJ dysfunction, improvements that were present at 3 weeks follow-up. Additionally, Lukban et al.[88] suggested, "Manual physical therapy may be a useful therapeutic modality for patients diagnosed with high-tone pelvic floor dysfunction, and sacroiliac dysfunction." Intervention seemed to be most useful in patients with primary complaints of urinary frequency, suprapubic pain, and dyspareunia.

On the other hand, several laboratory-based studies do exist. Biomechanically, it does *not* appear that an SIJ thrust completely and solely targets the SIJ only.[78] There also appears to be no change in joint position before and after manipulation (even after confirmation of a clinical change by the attending physiotherapist).[32,79] This suggests that biomechanical changes to the SIJ are less pronounced than what many clinicians may assume.

Neurophysiologically, a number of changes have been reported. Suter et al.[89] reported that quadriceps inhibition occurred after manipulation to the SIJ in side-lying. Others have reported reductions in the H-reflex after manipulation,[80] changes in hormone levels directly post-treatment,[90] reduction of lower extremity symptoms,[80] and improvement of pain[75,87,91] after SIJ manipulation, despite the likelihood that the manipulation does not substantially change the position of the innominate on the sacrum.[79] Pain is also decreased in patients with related hip and SIJ symptoms.[91]

Manual therapy to the SIJ functions to improve feed-forward mechanism of the transverse abdominus[92] and may assist in reducing soft-tissue tension.[93] Furthermore, there is a significant decrease in reflex excitability even after cutaneous stimulation.[80,94] Fast thrusts have greater neurophysiological effects[94] and a thrust only works if muscle or joint capsule is engaged vigorously.[80] The thrust must be performed on symptomatic subjects[51] and variable results may likely be a reflection of complex innervation pattern (rami from L5–S3) and large joint, although one study has reported the cervical spine manipulation also creates changes to the SIJ.[51] All of these studies identify the short-term effects of manipulation and none has analyzed the benefits comparatively versus other treatment methods.

Summary

- No randomized or pragmatic trials have investigated the benefit of muscle energy, stretching, mobilization, or manipulation for confirmed SIJ-related pain.
- There are a number of neurophysiological changes associated with SIJ manual therapy but there does not appear to be evidence to support biomechanical changes.

Patient Cases

Case 11.1: Lindsey Knowles (24-year-old female)

Diagnosis: Sciatica

Observation: Endomorphic body compensation. Body mass index = 32.

Mechanism: She notes subtle pain that began during pregnancy and worsened during post-pregnancy.

Concordant Sign: Her worst pain occurs during lifting her baby and during long-term walking.

Nature of the Condition: She indicates she often requires long-term sitting breaks to decrease the back and leg pain. It has decreased her activity after the pregnancy.

Behavior of the Symptoms: The back and leg pain occur simultaneously.

Pertinent Patient History: No prior history of low back pain or pelvic pain. This is her first pregnancy.

Patient Goals: She is interested in increasing her activity.

Baseline: The leg pain is 2/10, whereas the posterior pelvic pain is 5/10.

Examination Findings: No active or passive movements reproduce her symptoms. She does have three of four positive test findings with the thigh thrust, compression, and sacral thrusts.

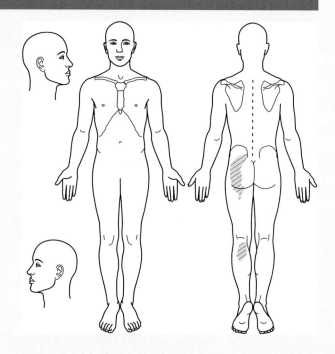

1. Based on these findings, what else would you like to examine?
2. Is this patient a good candidate for manual therapy?
3. What is the expected prognosis of this patient?
4. What treatments do you feel presented in this book may be beneficial for this patient?

Case 11.2: Carol Harstburger (26-year-old female)

Diagnosis: Low back strain

Observation: Carol is a very thin female that is obviously a runner.

Mechanism: Insidious onset of pain that has occurred over the last 3 months.

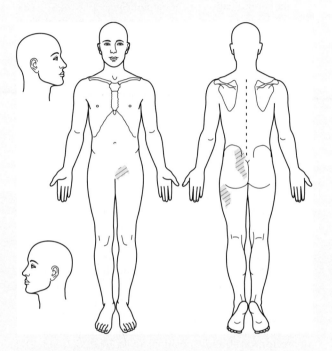

Concordant Sign: Running.

Nature of the Condition: She notes that 2 miles into a run she begins to feel posterior pelvic pain. The pain worsens with extension or left leg standing and prevents her from running.

Behavior of the Symptoms: Worsens during running.

Pertinent Patient History: She notes a significant weight loss of over 30 pounds in the past 2 years. This has been concurrent with her increase in mileage.

Patient Goals: She wants to be able to run without pain.

Baseline: Baseline her pain is 1/10 but increases to 4/10 during running.

Examination Findings: Nothing reproduces her symptoms. Only the sacral thrust is painful.

1. Based on these findings, what else would you like to examine?
2. Is this patient a good candidate for manual therapy?
3. What is the expected prognosis of this patient?
4. What treatments do you feel presented in this book may be beneficial for this patient?

Chapter Questions

1. Describe why the majority of sacroiliac pain involves the tendency of the joint to succumb toward hypermobility.

2. Describe the biomechanical relationship between the pelvis joints and the lumbar spine. Indicate the difficulties in separating the two areas during an examination.

3. Outline the five suggested classification groups for pelvic girdle pain.

4. Describe the use of clusters for special clinical tests of the sacroiliac spine.

5. Outline an effective treatment mechanism for SIJ pain.

References

1. Huijbregts P. Sacroiliac joint dysfunction: Evidence-based diagnosis. *Orthopaedic Division Review.* 2004;8: 18–44.

2. Johnson W. Sacroiliac strain. *J Am Osteopathic Association.* 1964;63:1015–1029.

3. Stoddard A. Conditions of the sacroiliac joint and their treatment. *Physiother.* 1958;44:97–101.

4. Cibulka MT, Sinacore D, Cromer G, Delitto A. Unilateral hip rotation range of motion asymmetry in patients with sacroiliac joint regional pain. *Spine.* 1998;23: 1009–1015.

5. Cibulka MT, Koldehoff R. Clinical usefulness of a cluster of sacroiliac joint tests in patients with and without low back pain. *J Orthop Sports Phys Ther.* 1999;29(2): 83–89.

6. Vincent-Smith B, Gibbons P. Inter-examiner and intra-examiner reliability of the standing flexion test. *Man Ther.* 1999;4(2):87–93.

7. Tong HC, Heyman OG, Lado DA, Isser MM. Interexaminer reliability of three methods of combining test results to determine side of sacral restriction, sacral base position, and innominate bone position. *J Am Osteopath Assoc.* 2006;106(8):464–468.

8. Robinson HS, Brox JI, Robinson R, Bjelland E, Solem S, Telje T. The reliability of selected motion- and pain provocation tests for the sacroiliac joint. *Man Ther.* 2007;12(1):72–79.

9. Saal JS. General principles of diagnostic testing as related to painful lumbar spine disorders: A critical appraisal of current diagnostic techniques. *Spine.* 2002;27(22):2538–2545.

10. Freburger JK, Riddle D. Using published evidence to guide the examination of the sacroiliac joint region. *Phys Ther.* 2001;81:1135–1143.

11. Berthelot JM, Labat JJ, LeGoff B, Gouin F, Maugars Y. Provocative sacroiliac joint maneuvers and sacroiliac joint block are unreliable for diagnosing sacroiliac joint pain. *Joint Bone Spine.* 2006;73(1):17–23.

12. Laslett M, Young SB, Aprill CN, McDonald B. Diagnosing painful sacroiliac joints: A validity study of a McKenzie evaluation and sacroiliac provocation tests. *Aust J Physiotherapy.* 2003;49:89–97.

13. Hogan QH, Abram SE. Neural blockade for diagnosis and prognosis: A review. *Anesthesiology.* 1997;86(1): 216–241.

14. Vleeming A, Albert H, Ostgaard H, Stuge B, Sturesson B. European Guideline on the Diagnosis and Treatment of Pelvic Girdle Pain. *Eur Spine J.* 2008;17(6):794–819.

15. Arab AM, Abdollahi I, Joghataei MT, Golafshani Z, Kazemnejad A. Inter- and intra-examiner reliability of single and composites of selected motion palpation and pain provocation tests for sacroiliac joint. *Man Ther.* 2009;14(2):213–221.

16. Maigne JY, Aivaliklis A, Pfefer F. Results of sacroiliac joint double block and value of sacroiliac pain provocation tests in 54 patients with low back pain. *Spine.* 1996;21(16):1889–1892.

17. Laslett M. The value of the physical examination in diagnosis of painful sacroiliac joint pathologies. *Spine.* 1998;23(8):962–964.

18. Long A, Donelson R, Fung T. Does it matter which exercise?: A randomized control trial of exercise for low back pain. *Spine.* 2004;29(23):2593–2602.

19. Werneke M, Hart D, Cook D. A descriptive study of the centralization phenomenon. *Spine.* 1999;24:676–683.

20. Albert H, Godskesen M, Westergaard J. Evaluation of clinical tests used in classification procedures in pregnancy-related pelvic joint pain. *Eur Spine J.* 2000;9(2): 161–166.

21. Albert HB, Godskesen M, Westergaard JG. Incidence of four syndromes of pregnancy-related pelvic joint pain. *Spine.* 2002;27(24):2831–2834.

22. Jensen M, Brant-Zawadzki M, Obuchowski N, Modic M, Malka S, Ross J. Magnetic resonance imaging of the lumbar spine in people without back pain. *New England J Med.* 1994;331:69–73.

23. Dieck GS, Kelsey JL, Goel VK, Panjabi MM, Walter SD, Laprade MH. An epidemiologic study of the relationship between postural asymmetry in the teen years and subsequent back and neck pain. *Spine.* 1985;10(10): 872–877.

24. Snijders C, Hermans P, Niesing R, Spoor C, Stoekart R. The influence of slouching and lumbar support on iliolumbar ligaments, intervertebral discs, and sacroiliac joints. *Clin Biomech.* 2004;19:323–329.

25. Sturesson B, Uden A, Vleeming A. A radiostereometric analysis of the movements of the sacroiliac joints in the reciprocal straddle position. *Spine.* 2000;25(2):214–217.

26. Snijders C, Bakker M, Vleeming A, Stoeckart R, Stam H. Oblique abdominal muscle activity in standing and in sitting on hard and soft seats. *Clin Biomech.* 1995;10:73–78.

27. Laslett M. Keynote address. Annual conference of the *American Academy of Orthopaedic Manual Physical Therapists.* Reno, NV. 2003.

28. Potter NA, Rothstein JM. Intertester reliability for selected clinical tests of the sacroiliac joint. *Phys Ther.* 1985;65(11):1671–1675.

29. Dreyfuss P, Michaelsen M, Pauza K, McLarty J, Bogduk N. The value of medical history and physical examination in diagnosing sacroiliac joint pain. *Spine.* 1996;21(22):2594–2602.

30. Levangie P. The association between static pelvic asymmetry and low back pain. *Spine.* 1999;24(12):1234–1242.

31. Rost CC, Jacqueline J, Kaiser A, Verhagen AP, Koes BW. Pelvic pain during pregnancy: a descriptive study of signs and symptoms of 870 patients in primary care. *Spine.* 2004;29(22):2567–2572.

32. Sturesson B, Uden G, Uden A. Pain pattern in pregnancy and "catching" of the leg in pregnant women with posterior pelvic pain. *Spine.* 1997;22(16):1880–1883.

33. Berg G, Hammar M, Moller-Jensen J. Low back pain during pregnancy. *Obstet Gynecol.* 1998;1:71–75.

34. Peloso PM, Braun J. Expanding the armamentarium for the spondyloarthropathies. *Arthritis Res Ther.* 2004;6 Suppl 2:S36–43.

35. Chan KF. Musculoskeletal pain clinic in Singapore—sacroiliac joint somatic dysfunction as cause of buttock pain. *Ann Acad Med Singapore.* 1998;27(1):112–115.

36. Slipman C, Patel P, Whyte W. Diagnosing and managing sacroiliac pain. *J Musculoskeletal Med.* 2001;18:325–332.

37. Fortin JD, Aprill CN, Ponthieux B, Pier J. Sacroiliac joint: pain referral maps upon applying a new injection/arthrography technique. Part II: Clinical evaluation. *Spine.* 1994;19(13):1483–1489.

38. Fortin JD, Dwyer AP, West S, Pier J. Sacroiliac joint: pain referral maps upon applying a new injection/arthrography technique. Part I: Asymptomatic volunteers. *Spine.* 1994;19(13):1475–1482.

39. Broadhurst NA, Simmons DN, Bond MJ. Piriformis syndrome: Correlation of muscle morphology with symptoms and signs. *Arch Phys Med Rehabil.* 2004;85(12):2036–2039.

40. Slipman C, Jackson H, Lipetz J. Sacroiliac joint pain referral zones. *Arch Phys Med Rehab.* 2000;81:334–338.

41. Young S, Aprill C, Laslett M. Correlation of clinical examination characteristics with three sources of chronic low back pain. *Spine J.* 2003;3(6):460–465.

42. Harrison DE, Harrison DD, Troyanovich SJ. The sacroiliac joint: A review of anatomy and biomechanics with clinical implications. *J Manipulative Physiol Ther.* 1997;20(9):607–617.

43. Walker JM. The sacroiliac joint: A critical review. *Phys Ther.* 1992;72(12):903–916.

44. Schwarzer A, Aprill CN, Bogduk N. The sacroiliac joint in chronic low back pain. *Spine.* 1995;20:31–37.

45. Lee D. The pelvic girdle. In *An approach to the examination and treatment of the lumbo–pelvic–hip region.* 2nd ed. Edinburgh; Churchill Livingstone: 1999.

46. Cibulka MT, Aslin K. How to use evidence-based practice to distinguish between three different patients with low back pain. J Orthop Sports *Phys Ther.* 2001;31(12):678–688.

47. Laslett M, Aprill C, McDonald B, Young S. Diagnosis of sacroiliac joint pain: Validity of individual provocation tests and composites of tests. *Man Ther.* 2005;10:207–218.

48. Young S. Personal communication. March 17, 2005.

49. Cook C, Massa L, Harm-Ernandes I, et al. Interrater reliability and diagnostic accuracy of pelvic girdle pain classification. *J Manipulative Physiol Ther.* 2007;30(4):252–258.

50. Smidt G, Wei S, McQuade K, Barakatt E, Sun T, Stanford W. Sacroiliac motion for extreme hip positions: A fresh cadaver study. Spine 1997;15:2073–2082.

51. Pollard H, Ward G. The effect of upper cervical or sacroiliac manipulation on hip flexion range of motion. *J Manipulative Physiol Ther.* 1998;21(9):611–616.

52. Wang M, Dumas GA. Mechanical behavior of the female sacroiliac joint and influence of the anterior and posterior sacroiliac ligaments under sagittal loads. *Clin Biomech.* 1998;13(4–5):293–299.

53. Winkle D. Diagnosis and treatment of the spine. In *Nonoperative orthopaedic medicine and manual therapy.* Denver, CO; Aspen Publishing: 1996.

54. Vleeming A, Stoeckart R, Volkers C, Snijders C. Relation between form and function in the sacroiliac joint. Part 1: Clinical anatomic aspects. *Spine.* 1990;15:130–132.

55. Pool-Goudzwaard A, van Dijke G, Mulder P, Spoor C, Snijders C, Stoeckart R. The iliolumbar ligament: Its influence on stability of the sacroiliac joint. *Clin Biomech.* 2003;18:99–105.

56. Moore M. Diagnosis and surgical treatment of chronic painful sacroiliac dysfunction. In: Vleeming A, Mooney V, Dorman T, Snijders C. *Second interdisciplinary world congress on low back pain.* San Diego, CA, 9–11 November, 1995.

57. Ribeiro S, Prato-Schmidt A, van der Wurff P. sacroiliac dysfunction. *Acta Orthop Bras.* 2003;11:118–125.

58. Mens J, Vleeming A, Snijders C, Stam H, Ginai A. The active straight leg raising test and mobility of the pelvic joints. *Eur Spine J.* 1999;8:468–473.

59. Broadhurst NA, Bond MJ. Pain provocation tests for the assessment of sacroiliac joint dysfunction. *J Spinal Disord.* 1998;11(4):341–345.

60. van der Wurff P, Meyne W, Hagmeijer RH. Clinical tests of the sacroiliac joint. *Man Ther.* 2000;5(2):89–96.

61. Laslett M, Williams M. The reliability of selected pain provocation tests for sacroiliac joint pathology. *Spine.* 1994;19(11):1243–1249.

62. Williams P, Thomas D, Downes E. Osteitis pubis and instability of the pubic symphysis. When nonoperative measures fail. *Am J Sports Med.* 2000;28:350–355.

63. Vleeming A, Pool-Goudzwaard AL, Hammudoghlu D, Stoeckart R, Snijders CJ, Mens JM. The function of the long dorsal sacroiliac ligament: Its implication for understanding low back pain. *Spine.* 1996;21(5):556–562.

64. Cook C, Hegedus E. *Orthopedic physical examination tests: An evidence-based approach.* Upper Saddle River, NJ; Prentice Hall: 2008.

65. Robinson HS, Brox J, Robinson R, Bjelland E, Solem S, Telje T. The reliability of selected motion and pain provocation tests for the sacroiliac joint. *Man Ther.* 2007;12:72–79.

66. van der Wurff P. Clinical diagnostic tests for the sacroiliac joint: motion and palpation tests. *Aust J Physiother.* 2006;52:308.

67. Kokmeyer DJ, van der Wurff P, Aufdemkampe G, Fickenscher TC. The reliability of multitest regimens with sacroiliac pain provocation tests. *J Manipulative Physiol Ther.* 2002;25(1):42–48.

68. Fritz JM. How to use evidence-based practice to distinguish between three different patients with low back pain. *J Orthop Sports Phys Ther.* 2001;31(12):689–695.

69. van der Wurff P, Buijs E, Groen G. A multitest regimen of pain provocation tests as an aid to reduce unnecessary minimally invasive sacroiliac joint procedures. *Arch Phys Med Rehabil.* 2006;89:10–14.

70. George S, Delitto A. Clinical examination variables discriminate among treatment-based classification groups: A study of construct validity in patients with acute low back pain. *Phys Ther.* 2005;85(4):306–314.

71. Dreyfuss P, Dreyer SJ, Cole A, Mayo K. Sacroiliac joint pain. *J Am Acad Orthop Surg.* 2004;12:255–265.

72. Bogduk N. Management of chronic low back pain. *Med J Aust*. 2004;180(2):79–83.

73. Dar G, Khamis S, Peleg S, et al. Sacroiliac joint fusion and the implications for manual therapy diagnosis and treatment. *Man Ther*. 2008;13(2):155–158.

74. Albert H, Godskesen M, Westergaard J. Prognosis in four syndromes of pregnancy-related pelvic pain. *Acta Obstet Gynecol Scand*. 2001;80(6):505–510.

75. Michaelsen M. Manipulation under joint anesthesia/analgesia: A proposed interdisciplinary treatment approach for recalcitrant spinal axis pain of synovial joint region. *J Manipulative Physiol Ther*. 2000;23:127–129.

76. Flynn T, Fritz J, Whitman J, Wainner R, Magel J, Rendeiro D, Butler B, Garber M, Allison S. A clinical prediction rule for classifying patients with low back pain who demonstrate short-term improvement with spinal manipulation. *Spine*. 2002;27:2835–2843.

77. Flynn T, Fritz J, Wainner R, Whitman J. The audible pop is not necessary for successful spinal high-velocity thrust manipulation in individuals with low back pain. *Arch Phys Med Rehabil*. 2003;84:1057–1067.

78. Beffa R, Mathews R. Does the adjustment cavitate the targeted joint?: An investigation into the location of cavitation sounds. *J Manipulative Physiol Ther*. 2004;27:e2.

79. Tullberg T, Blomberg S, Branth B, Johnsson R. Manipulation does not alter the position of the sacroiliac joint: A roentgen stereophotogrammetric analysis. *Spine*. 1988;23:1124–1128.

80. Murphy B, Dawson N, Slack J. Sacroiliac joint manipulation decreases the H-reflex. *Electromyogr Clin Neurophysiol*. 1995;35:87–94.

81. Marshall P, Murphy B. The effect of sacroiliac joint manipulation on feed-forward activation times of the deep abdominal musculature. *J Manipulative Physiol Ther*. 2006;29(3):196–202.

82. Childs JD, Fritz JM, Flynn TW, Irrgang JJ, Johnson KK, Majkowski GR, Delitto A. A clinical prediction rule to identify patients with low back pain most likely to benefit from spinal manipulation: A validation study. *Ann Intern Med*. 2004;141(12):920–928.

83. Cyriax JH. *Textbook of orthopaedic medicine*. 11th ed. London; Baillière Tindall: 1984.

84. Grgić V. The sacroiliac joint dysfunction: Clinical manifestations, diagnostics and manual therapy. *Lijec Vjesn*. 2005;127(1–2):30–35.

85. Galm R, Frohling M, Rittmeister M, Schmitt E. Sacroiliac joint dysfunction in patients with imaging-proven lumbar disc herniation. *Eur Spine J*. 1998;7(6):450–453.

86. Lee K, Carlini W, McCormick G, Albers G. Neurologic complications following chiropractic manipulation: A survey of California neurologists. *Neurology*. 1995;45:1213–1215.

87. Shearar KA, Colloca CJ, White HL. A randomized clinical trial of manual versus mechanical force manipulation in the treatment of sacroiliac joint syndrome. *J Manipulative Physiol Ther*. 2005;28(7):493–501.

88. Lukban J, Whitmore K, Kellogg-Spadt S, Bologna R, Lesher A, Fletcher E. The effect of manual physical therapy in patients diagnosed with interstitial cystitis, high-tone pelvic floor dysfunction, and sacroiliac dysfunction. *Urology*. 2001;57(6 Suppl (1)):121–122.

89. Suter E, McMorland G, Herzog W, Bray R. Decrease in quadriceps inhibition after sacroiliac joint manipulation in patients with anterior knee pain. *J Manipulative Physiol Ther*. 1999;22:149–153.

90. Kokjohn K, Schmid D, Triano JJ, Brennan P. The effect of spinal manipulation on pain and prostaglandin levels in women with primary dysmenorrhea. *J Manipulative Physiol Ther*. 1992;15:279–285.

91. Fickel TE. 'Snapping hip' and sacroiliac sprain: Example of a cause–effect relationship. *J Manipulative Physiol Ther*. 1989;12(5):390–392.

92. Marshall P, Murphy B. The effect of sacroiliac joint manipulation on feed-forward activation times of the deep abdominal musculature. *J Manipulative Physiol Ther*. 2006;29(3):196–202.

93. Fisk JW. A controlled trial of manipulation in a selected group of patients with low back pain favouring one side. *N Z Med J*. 1979;90(645):288–291.

94. Herzog W, Conway PJ, Zhang YT, Gál J, Guimaraes AC. Reflex responses associated with manipulative treatments on the thoracic spine: A pilot study. *J Manipulative Physiol Ther*. 1995;18(4):233–236.

Manual Therapy of the Hip

Chad Cook and Christopher Fiander

Chapter

12

Objectives

- Identify the pertinent anatomy and biomechanics of the hip.
- Demonstrate an appropriate and responsive hip examination sequence.
- Identify plausible mobilization and manual therapy treatment techniques for the hip.
- Discuss the influence of mobilization and manual therapy on recovery for hip patients in randomized trials.

Clinical Examination

Differential Diagnosis

Effective clinical examination of the hip requires differentiation of causal pain originators from other structures such as the lumbar spine, pelvis, and in some occasions the knee. Often, the location, frequency, and pattern of pain closely represent those of lumbar spine or pelvic origin. Although there is considerable overlap in patterns, most pain-reproducing procedures of the hip demonstrate pain of intra-articular origin and often exhibit symptoms in the groin with occasional radiation to the knee.[1,2] Thigh and buttock pain and pain with referral below the knee is *generally* associated with structures of the low back or pelvis, not the hip.[1] Nonetheless, documented situations in which hip pain caused radiating pain below the knee and pain into the back have occurred.[3]

Brown and colleagues[3] outlined significant signs and symptoms that differentiated low back and hip pain for diagnostic clarity. The authors reported that for a "hip-only" diagnosis (hip pain and no low back pain), limited internal rotation, groin pain, and/or a limp during gait were positive predictors of a "hip-only" origin. The absence of a short leg, decreased range of motion, and a negative femoral nerve stress test (prone knee flexion) were negatively associated with a "hip-only" diagnosis. In other words, common examination methods such as leg length, range-of-motion losses, and the femoral nerve stress test were less likely to implicate

the hip as the causal factor, thus suggesting the origin of pain/dysfunction is from another structure. Examination items such as a lumbar "list," pain during internal rotation, an antalgic limp, and weakness were not discriminatory predictors of hip versus back pain.

Lauder[4] produced one of the most comprehensive discussions of pain patterns associated with various forms of hip dysfunction in 2002. She reported that disorders of the hip frequently mimic lumbar dysfunction from L1 to L3 (Figure 12.1 ■). Additionally, pain from trochanteric bursitis may refer to the buttock and

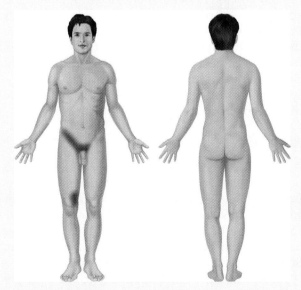

■ **Figure 12.1**   Pain Drawing of Intra-articular Hip Pain

337

slightly anterior to the bursae, occasionally resulting in leg parathesia.[5] Often low back pain and trochanteric bursitis are concurrently reported, although these conditions are typically not directly related.[4]

Observation

Sims[6] recommended a comprehensive lower extremity observational assessment to determine abnormalities of the hip. He suggested that excessive motions at other joints, most notably the foot, could negatively affect the hip. Additionally, visual cues such as decreased stance time or lurching toward the symptomatic hip during the stance phase are signs of an antalgic gait.[7]

Although visual markers such as Q-angle are controversially associated with knee problems, no studies have outlined a relationship with hip pain. Loss of passive extension during standing is indicative of age-related posture and is sometimes associated with osteoarthritis and low back pain. Although obesity is not directly associated with hip bursitis, the relationship has been suggested in a single case study.[8]

Gait

Controlled lateral shift of the center of gravity is one of the six determinants of gait and is a function of the hip musculature, specifically the hip abductors.[9] Another determinant of gait, pelvic rotation, is designed to lengthen the stride of an individual, improving economy by covering greater length with similar energy efforts. This process is designed to reduce the total energy expenditure in human locomotion, and is typically altered only when dysfunction is present. For optimum efficiency, these determinants require full extension, 30 degrees of flexion, at least 10 degrees of external rotation, and approximately 7 degrees of internal rotation, movements that are typical ranges found during joint play.[10] Severe damage to the hip that eliminates these movements can reduce the efficiency of gait up to 47%.[11] Subsequently, clinical gait analysis may identify selected hip pathology, specifically when reports of problems with endurance during propulsion are prominent.

Alignment

As stated in Chapter 11, alignment of the hip and pelvis provides very little differential diagnostic value. Levangie[11] found that leg length discrepancy, anterior superior iliac spine (ASIS) and posterior superior iliac spine (PSIS) bilateral comparisons, and iliac crest height determination presented *diagnostic* information that was actually more detrimental than beneficial.

Measuring leg length is used to conclude if predisposing biomechanical disadvantages may result in increased pain. Various leg length measurements that use a tape measure have demonstrated acceptable reliability when radiographic methods are used as the criterion standard.[12] A common measurement method includes a measure from the inferior border of the greater trochanter to the inferior aspect of the medial malleolus. However, variable correlations to actual impairment or biomechanical dysfunctions exist and the clinician should be wary of a direct cause and effect relationship.[13–15]

Patient History

Behavior of Pain

Groin pain is typically associated with intra-articular hip conditions such as capsulitis, chondritis, and osteoarthritis. In all three of these conditions, referral of pain to the anterior medial knee and lateral knee are commonly reported.[3] Lateral, pinpoint hip pain is generally associated with trochanteric bursitis.[4] Generally, pain worsens upon weight bearing or inactivity for intra-articular pain, and worsens with compression or stretching in extra-articular conditions such as trochanteric bursitis.

Summary

- Many of the pain distribution patterns exhibited by hip conditions are similar to those of the pelvis and lumbar spine.
- The most common pain distribution pattern of the hip is lateral hip pain and/or groin pain.
- A lurching gait and gluteus medius stance is indicative of either pain or osteoarthritis of the hip.
- Little evidence exists to support the use of alignment to identify selected hip dysfunction.

Physical Examination

Active Movements

A relationship between hip range of motion, specifically internal rotation and low back dysfunction, has been suggested in the literature.[16] Flynn and colleagues[17] reported that the clinical prediction rule for identifying patients whom benefit from manipulation was partially based on hip internal rotation findings. Sjoile[18] reported that low back pain in adolescents was related to a decrease in hip mobility in flexion and internal rotation. Others[19] have reported a relationship between hip internal rotation and low back pain in professional golfers. Conversely, McConnell[20] proposes that limited hip extension and external rotation negatively influence the functional mobility of the lumbar spine.

Active Physiological Movements   There are two methods of active physiological testing. One method involves assessment of the planar movement of the hip to ascertain the influence of active movement on selected directions. The second involves **functional testing** to determine which functional activities most closely reproduce the concordant sign of the patient. Both methods are beneficial to explore during a general examination.

Supine Hip Flexion

Hip flexion requires the contractile capability of the anterior hip musculature and causes concurrent tension on the posterior structures of the hip.[21] Injuries to the hamstrings or posterior hip structures are often reported as pain during movements of end-range hip flexion.[21] Others have reported that the loss of a complete hip flexion arc is commonly associated with patients diagnosed with hip pathology.[22]

1. The patient assumes a supine position after assessment of resting symptoms.

2. The patient is instructed to raise his or her hip into flexion to the first point of pain and is then instructed to move beyond the first point of pain toward end range (right hip in Figure 12.2 ■).

3. Upon completion, pain is reassessed for the concordant sign.

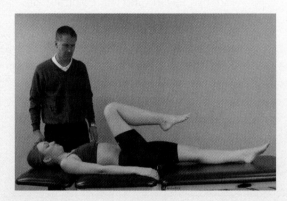

■ **Figure 12.2** Supine Hip Flexion

Sidelying Hip Abduction

Active sidelying abduction may be painful in conditions such as a gluteus medius tear, trochanteric bursitis, or abductor tendinopathy.[23] Weaknesses during active range of motion are found concurrently with **Trendelenburg's sign** and during gait deviations that demonstrate a limp. Commonly, patients attempt to compensate for hip weakness by substituting the hip flexors during a request for hip abduction movements.

1. The patient assumes a sidelying position after assessment of resting symptoms.

2. The patient is instructed to raise his or her non-plinth-sided lower extremity to the first point of pain (in abduction) (Figure 12.3 ■). The patient is instructed to move beyond the first point of pain toward end range.

3. Upon completion, pain is reassessed for the concordant sign.

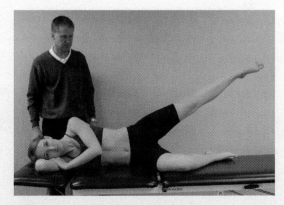

■ **Figure 12.3** Sidelying Hip Abduction

Sidelying Hip Adduction

Pain with hip adduction may be associated with adductor tendonitis, pelvic instability, a sports hernia, or a pubic rami fracture.

1. The patient assumes a sidelying position after assessment of resting symptoms.

2. The patient is instructed to raise his or her plinth-sided lower extremity into hip adduction (right side in Figure 12.4 ■) to the first point of pain and then instructed to move beyond the first point of pain toward end range.

3. Upon completion, pain is reassessed for the concordant sign.

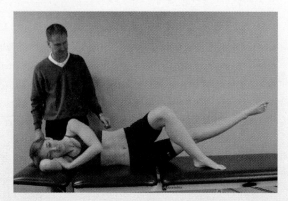

■ **Figure 12.4**   Sidelying Hip Adduction

Prone Hip Extension

Perry et al.[24] suggest that the prone extension position more accurately isolates hip extension musculature and advocate this position for testing of extensor muscles. Findings have shown that hip extension loss is related to increased risk for falls, low back pain, and capsular range-of-motion losses in the hip. Hip extension loss is purported to be a cause of altered lumbopelvic rhythm and lower quarter dysfunction.[25]

1. The patient assumes a prone position after assessment of resting symptoms.

2. The patient is instructed to raise his or her lower extremity into hip extension to the first point of pain (Figure 12.5 ■). The patient is instructed to move beyond the first point of pain toward end range.

3. Upon completion, pain is reassessed for the concordant sign.

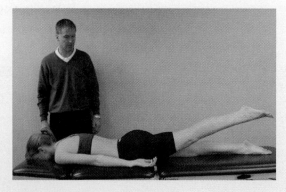

■ **Figure 12.5**   Prone Hip Extension

Sitting Internal Rotation

Hip internal rotation measures are considered sensitive tools for assessing intra-articular symptoms.[26,27] Two studies have reported an association between diminished internal range of motion and a failure to improve with manipulation to the low back.[26,27] Pain during active internal rotation may result from placing tension on the active external rotators such as the piriformis.[28]

1. The patient assumes a sitting position after assessment of resting symptoms.

2. The patient is instructed to rotate his or her lower extremity internally to the first point of pain; then the patient is instructed to move beyond the first point of pain toward end range.

3. Upon completion, pain is reassessed for the concordant sign.

Sitting External Rotation

Sitting external rotation requires the contraction of the external rotators such as the piriformis. Although rarely linked to dysfunction, limited sitting external rotation motion may be caused by extracapsular tightness and may implicate extra-articular structures more so than intra-articular. Although it would seem that active external rotation would elicit pain in some conditions such as a gluteus medius tear, no studies have confirmed or supported this assumption.

1. The patient assumes a sitting position after assessment of resting symptoms.

2. The patient is instructed to rotate his or her lower extremity externally to the first point of pain. The patient is then instructed to move beyond the first point of pain toward end range.

3. Upon completion, pain is reassessed for the concordant sign.

Functional Tests

Functional tests are commonly called **quick tests**[29] and are designed to provide a glimpse of pain provocation with various activities. Additionally, functional tests may be helpful in serving as the concordant movement for examination and re-examination of the patient.

Deep Squat

A deep squat may be effective in determining the contribution of posterior extra-articular hip structures such as the gluteus maximus, or if pain is reproduced anteriorly, may be associated with acetabular impingement syndrome or a tight posterior capsule of the hip. In patients with an antalgic gait, the load and shift requirements of a deep squat may also reproduce intra-articular pain.

1. The patient assumes a standing position after assessment of resting symptoms.

2. The patient is instructed to squat to the first point of pain, and if the movement is painful, the clinician should determine if the movement is concordant (Figure 12.6 ■).

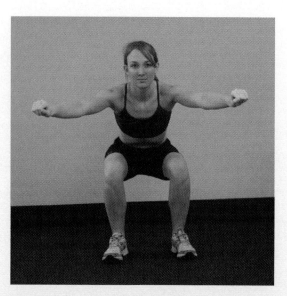

■ **Figure 12.6** Deep Bilateral Squat

Trendelenburg's Stance

Trendelenburg's stance is often used to evaluate weakness or pain in the hip abductors.[1] Weakness of the hip abductors has been linked to knee problems, iliotibial band syndrome, and gait and running abnormalities.[30] Patients with pain or weakness will demonstrate a dropping of the contralateral pelvis during unilateral stance.[1] This movement differs from a lumbar list, a visual finding that is frequently observed in patients with a lumbar dysfunction.

1. The patient assumes a standing position after assessment of resting symptoms.

2. The patient is instructed to stand on one leg (left side in Figure 12.7 ■), while bending the knee of the opposite leg.

3. The clinician should evaluate for opposite-sided (to the weight-bearing leg) pelvic drop and, if present, concordant symptoms on the weight-bearing leg (left side in Figure 12.7).

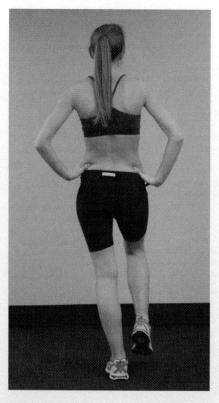

■ **Figure 12.7** Trendelenburg's Stance

Unilateral Step-Up

Arokoski et al.[31] found differences in the ability of symptomatic and asymptomatic patients in climbing stairs. The unilateral step-up also leads to compression forces three to six times the body weight of the individual; therefore, in the presence of intra-articular pain, this procedure may be very sensitive.[32]

1 The patient is instructed to stand with one leg on a 6- to 12-inch step. The lower extremity that is on the step should continue to weight-bear through the bent knee (Figure 12.8 ■).

2 Resting symptoms are assessed then the patient is instructed to straighten the leg on the step, thus lifting the opposite lower extremity from the ground and eliminating weight bearing.

3 The clinician should evaluate the weight-bearing hip for concordant symptoms.

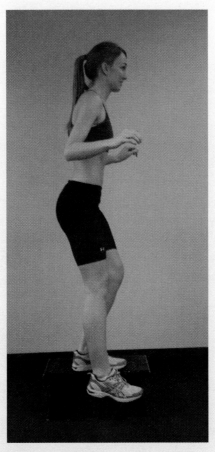

■ **Figure 12.8** Unilateral Step-Up

Axial Rotation Axial rotation incorporates reciprocal internal and external rotation actively in weight bearing, therefore combining increased compressive force with motions that are sensitive to intra-articular involvement and possible degenerative changes in the hip.[26,27,30]

Additionally, Gombotto et al.[33] and others[34] suggest a correlation between lumbar dysfunction and pain and restrictions in hip rotation, including individuals participating in rotational sports. Because axial rotation incorporates lumbopelvic motion, it may assist in screening the lumbar spine and/or implicate a hip-related impairment that is contributing to lumbar dysfunction and pain.

The patient is instructed to stand with his or her feet facing in the sagittal plane and the arms by his or her side. The patient then turns from side-to-side allowing both the trunk and pelvis to move. The patient is encouraged to keep both feet from pronating or supinating off the floor while the axial rotation occurs in an effort to prevent excessive compensatory movement within the lower leg. The clinician makes note of pain provocation or restriction and determines if this occurs ipsilaterally or contralaterally to hypothesize as to the impaired range of motion. For example, in an individual with right hip intra-articular pathology, pain elicited during right axial rotation would suggest internal rotation as the impaired motion, whereas right hip pain during left axial rotation would suggest external rotation as the impaired motion.

Summary

- Pain during active range of motion of the hip is indicative of selected dysfunctions and may prove useful during collection of data.
- Functional testing of the hip can serve as a baseline measure or may reproduce pain during combined movements.

Passive Movements

Passive Physiological Movements Passive physiological movements are necessary to identify potential noncontractile structures that are pain generators.

Flexion

There are numerous types of dysfunctions associated with hip flexion. Lauder[4] reported that often ischial bursitis is reproduced with movements such as passive hip flexion along with resisted hip extension. Cyriax[35] described the "sign of the buttock" as pain during hip flexion that is similar in range to pain during a straight leg raise. A positive "sign of the buttock" may be indicative of a serious pathology in the pelvis, hip, or lumbar spine. Greenwood et al.[36] have reported the benefit of the "sign of the buttock" during differentiation of hip and low back pain. Flexion is occasionally painful in patients with femoroacetabular impingement.

1. The patient is positioned in supine.

2. After assessment of resting symptoms, the clinician passively lifts the hip into flexion to the first point of reported pain; pain is queried to determine if concordant.

3. The clinician passively moves the leg toward end range; pain is again queried accordingly (Figure 12.9 ■). If no pain is present, the clinician applies an overpressure to rule out the specific passive movement of the joint.

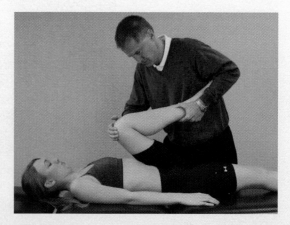

■ **Figure 12.9** Passive Hip Flexion

4. Upon completion, resting symptoms are again assessed.

Abduction

Passive abduction may be restricted in patients with demonstrable osteoarthritis of the hip. Additionally, some evidence exists that lateral hip labrum tears may produce pain during passive contact of the femoral head to the lesion site of the hip.[37]

1 To test abduction, the patient is placed in a supine position.

2 After assessment of resting symptoms, the clinician passively glides the hip into abduction to the first point of reported pain. One hand blocks the pelvis just cephalic to the hip joint to prevent excessive lumbar motion (Figure 12.10 ■). The clinician queries to determine if the pain is concordant, then the clinician passively moves the leg toward end range; pain is again queried accordingly.

3 If no pain is present, the clinician applies an overpressure to rule out the specific passive movement of the joint. Upon completion, resting symptoms are again assessed.

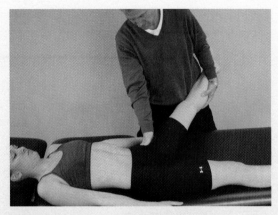

■ **Figure 12.10**   Passive Hip Abduction

Adduction

Passive hip adduction, iliotibial band stretching, and other stretch-related maneuvers may reproduce symptoms in patients who experience trochanteric bursitis.[4] Rarely does passive hip adduction reproduce symptoms in patients with hip osteoarthritis.

1 The patient is placed in a supine position.

2 After assessment of resting symptoms, the clinician passively pulls the opposite hip into adduction to the first point of reported pain. One hand blocks the opposite knee of the patient to prevent excessive lumbar side flexion (Figure 12.11 ■).

3 The clinician queries to determine if the pain is concordant.

4 The clinician then passively moves the leg toward end range; pain is again queried accordingly.

5 If no pain is present, the clinician applies an overpressure to rule out that specific passive movement of the joint.

6 Upon completion, resting symptoms are again assessed.

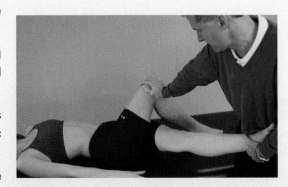

■ **Figure 12.11**   Passive Hip Adduction

Internal Rotation

As with hip flexion, internal rotation has been linked with numerous hip-related patholo-gies.[38,39] Loss of internal rotation is a direct predictor of whether or not a patient with hip pain receives a total hip replacement in the future.[40] This finding is consistent with patients diagnosed with hip osteoarthritis and is strongly associated with hip pain and loss of joint space on an x-ray.[41] Internal rotation is also a criterion of osteoarthritis using the criteria developed by Altman and colleagues.[42] Lastly, patients with piriformis syndrome may complain of reproduction of symptoms with end-range passive internal rotation while the hip maintains an extended position.[43]

1. The patient assumes a supine position and the clinician assesses resting symptoms.

2. The clinician passively cradles the lower leg below the knee and slowly internally rotates the hip to the first point of reported pain. The other hand squeezes the femur and provides a rotational movement in order to reduce the stress placed upon the knee (Figure 12.12 ■).

3. The clinician queries to determine if the pain is concordant.

4. The clinician passively moves the leg toward end range; pain is again queried accordingly.

5. If no pain is present, the clinician applies an overpressure to rule out the targeted passive movement of the joint.

6. Upon completion, resting symptoms are again assessed.

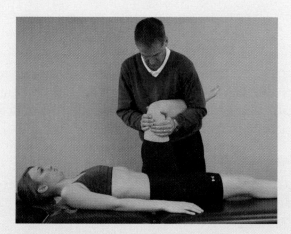

■ **Figure 12.12** Passive Internal Rotation

External Rotation

Arokoski and associates[31] suggested a relationship between hip osteoarthritis and loss of passive external rotation. Additionally, external rotation is occasionally painful when the passive end-range force is applied to internal rotator musculature.

1. The patient assumes a supine position and the clinician assesses resting symptoms.

2. The clinician passively cradles the lower leg below the knee and slowly externally rotates the hip to the first point of reported pain. The other hand squeezes the femur and provides a rotational movement in order to reduce the stress placed upon the knee (Figure 12.13 ■).

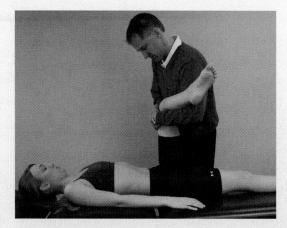

3. The clinician queries to determine if the pain is concordant. The clinician then passively moves the leg toward end range; pain is again queried accordingly.

4. If no pain is present, the clinician applies an overpressure to rule out that specific passive movement of the joint.

5. Upon completion, resting symptoms are again assessed.

■ **Figure 12.13**   Passive External Rotation

Hip Extension

As with active hip extension loss, passive hip extension restrictions are associated with capsular restrictions and long-term pain. Passive hip extension may place tension on the anterior aspect of the hip capsule and labrum, thus reproducing symptoms in that select population.

1. The patient is placed in a prone position.

2. The clinician passively lifts the hip into extension to the first point of reported pain. One hand blocks just cephalically to the hip joint to reduce the amount of lumbar extension that occurs with this procedure (Figure 12.14 ■).

3. The clinician queries to determine if the pain is concordant.

4. Then the clinician passively moves the leg toward end range; pain is again queried accordingly.

(Continued)

⑤ If no pain is present, the clinician applies an overpressure to rule out that specific passive movement of the joint.

⑥ Upon completion, resting symptoms are again assessed.

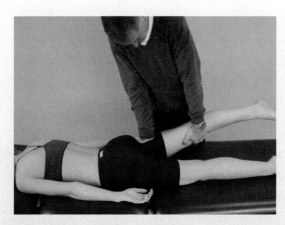

■ **Figure 12.14**   Passive Hip Extension

Passive Accessory Movements Kaltenborn[44] proposed that the close-packed position of the hip joint is extension, internal rotation, and slight abduction. Sims[6] suggested that accessory movement, or available joint play and mobility, in the proposed close-packed position is highly limited. In contrast, Williams[45] argues that no accessory motion exists even within the open-packed position.

Anterior–Posterior Glide

An anterior–posterior glide of the hip may identify pain associated with cartilage compression and will most likely consist of very small movements.

① The technique is performed after placing the patient in a sidelying position.

② The clinician assesses resting symptoms then applies a passive glide of the hip joint using the thumb to lock anterior to the greater trochanter and the heel of the hand to apply the force to the thumb contact point (Figure 12.15 ■).

③ The clinician passively moves toward a posterior direction. Any reproduction of pain that is concordant implicates this assessment method as a possible treatment technique.

④ Upon completion, resting symptoms are again assessed.

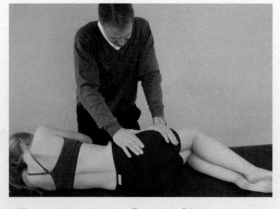

■ **Figure 12.15**   Anterior–Posterior Glide

Posterior–Anterior Glide

A posterior–anterior glide of the hip may identify pain associated with cartilage compression and represents very small movements.

① The technique is performed after placing the patient in a sidelying position.

② The clinician assesses resting symptoms then applies passive glide of the hip joint using the thumb to lock posterior to the greater trochanter and the heel of the hand to apply the force to the thumb contact point (Figure 12.16 ■). The clinician passively glides toward an anterior direction. Any reproduction of pain that is concordant implicates this assessment method as a possible treatment technique.

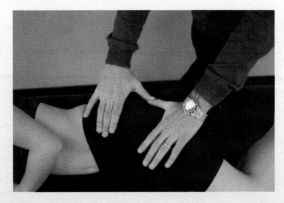

■ **Figure 12.16** Posterior–Anterior Glide

③ Upon completion, resting symptoms are again assessed.

Sidelying Distraction

In cases where the patient's pain is significant, a relaxing, nonaggressive technique such as the sidelying distraction maneuver may be useful.

① The technique is performed after placing the patient in a sidelying position.

② The clinician assesses resting symptoms then applies an inferior passive glide of the hip by using the web space of his or her hand (Figure 12.17 ■). The contact point of the hip includes the surrounding tissue of the greater trochanter.

③ The clinician passively glides the extremity toward a caudal direction. If the patient's upper leg is placed anterior to the tableside leg, the amount of distraction available is greater. Any reproduction of pain that is concordant implicates this assessment method as a possible treatment technique.

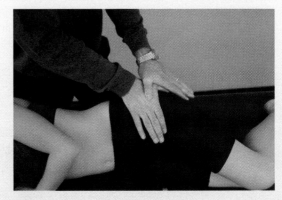

■ **Figure 12.17** Sidelying Distraction

④ Upon completion, resting symptoms are again assessed.

Indirect Distraction

The indirect distraction method involves displacement of the knee and ankle as well as the hip. The technique has been shown to generate up to 200–600 Newtons of distraction force[10] and is useful for a more substantial distraction of the hip than the technique pictured in Figure 12.17. However, because more than one joint is distracted, indirect traction requires greater intensity during application than direct traction.

1. The technique is performed in a supine position after assessment of resting symptoms.

2. The clinician queries the patient for a history of knee or ankle dysfunction that would contraindicate the use of this method. If none, the clinician cradles the ankle of the patient into both of his or her hands (Figure 12.18 ■).

3. The clinician then takes up the slack to preposition the hip into targeted motion. Generally, resting position of the hip includes a moderate degree of flexion and abduction with slight external rotation.[10] The clinician then provides an inferior force by leaning backward while holding the ankle.

4. Upon completion, resting symptoms are again assessed.

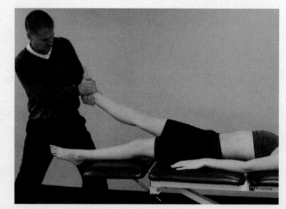

■ **Figure 12.18** Indirect Distraction

Direct Distraction

The accessory movements involved with a direct distraction maneuver are similar to those of the indirect method. This procedure, however, allows the majority of force to transfer through the hip joint and does not involve distraction at the knee or ankle.

1. The technique is performed in a supine position after assessment of resting symptoms.

2. The clinician places the lower extremity over his or her shoulder and places his or hands (ulnar border) near the hip joint for an appropriate contact.

3. Using the shoulder as a fulcrum, the clinician pulls inferiorly with the hands at the hip and pushes cephalically with the shoulder for an inferior distraction (Figure 12.19 ■).

4. The clinician passively glides the joint toward the projected end range; pain is again queried accordingly.

5. Upon completion, resting symptoms are again assessed.

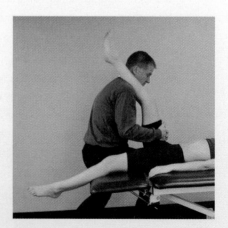

■ **Figure 12.19** Direct Distraction

Combined Movements

Maitland[29] advocated the use of combined movements, specifically if all other hip accessory and physiological movements are pain free. Most combined movements are performed passively for improved efficiency and control. For the hip, combined movements typically include flexion and internal or external rotation, external rotation and abduction, or internal rotation and adduction. When a combined movement is initiated, the peri-articular tissue such as the capsule and ligaments are taut and engaged more effectively than during lax positions. Adding compression and/or distraction further engages the tissue, thus sensitizing the examination method.

Internal Rotation and Adduction

Internal rotation and adduction may increase the tension placed upon the capsule and ligaments and may provide greater stress during a mobilization or stretching method. The movements will also compress the labrum and component of the capsule at end range. Often, this technique is concordant in patients with hip osteoarthritis and/or synovitis.

① The technique is performed in a supine position after assessment of resting symptoms.

② At 90 degrees of flexion, the clinician passively moves the hip into full internal rotation concurrently while applying an adduction force (Figure 12.20 ■).

③ Symptoms are evaluated to determine if the movement produces a concordant response.

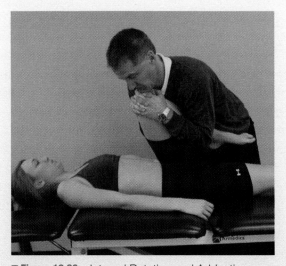

■ **Figure 12.20**   Internal Rotation and Adduction

External Rotation, Flexion, and Abduction

DeAngelis and Busconi[1] suggest that the hip capsule is most lax in external rotation, flexion, and abduction, and report that the patient will often hold his or her hip into this combined movement when an inflammatory process is present.

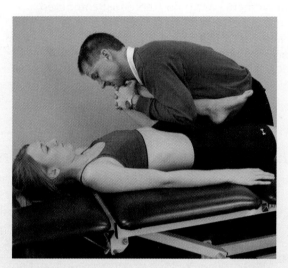

■ **Figure 12.21**   External Rotation, Flexion, and Abduction

1. The technique is performed in a supine position after assessment of resting symptoms.

2. The hip is moved to 90 degrees of flexion; the clinician passively moves the hip into full external rotation concurrently while applying an abduction force (Figure 12.21 ■).

3. Symptoms are evaluated to determine if the movement produces a concordant response.

Extension Quadrants/Combined Movements

The North American Institute of Manual Therapy[46] advocates assessing combined motions in extension, when planar active and passive physiological movements are non-provocative. Testing combined movements in extension is clinically significant given the association of restrictions in hip extension to lumbar and lower quarter dysfunction.[25] If concordant symptoms are reproduced in either extension quadrant, these combined motions may also aid the clinician in treatment selection as one can rationalize using the prone military crawl position or the prone end-range internal rotation position if symptoms are found in the extension/external rotation/abduction or extension/internal rotation/adduction positions, respectively.

1. The patient is prone with the knee flexed and stabilization is offered at the sacrum.

2. The hip is externally rotated as it is brought into extension.

3. The clinician applies an anterior force to the sacrum to stabilize the lumbar spine (Figures 12.22 ■ and 12.23 ■).

④ External rotation continues to be increased as the extended hip is brought into abduction.

⑤ Symptoms are monitored throughout the motion for reproduction of the concordant sign.

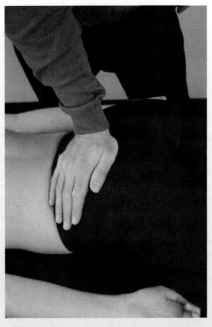

■ **Figure 12.22**   Use of Hand to Stabilize the Sacrum

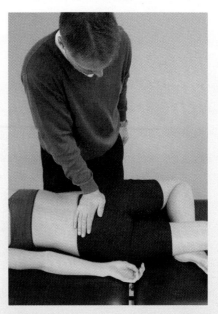

■ **Figure 12.23**   The Military Crawl Position: Sacrum Stabilized by Clinician

Summary

- Of the passive hip movements, the movements most often related to dysfunction include internal rotation, flexion, and occasionally external rotation.
- It is questionable whether passive accessory movements such as the anterior to posterior and posterior to anterior glides create movement within the hip joint.
- Traction techniques generate the greatest amount of displacement at the hip.
- Combined movements may be effective in targeting capsular and ligamentous tissue by prepositioning in tightened positions.

Special Clinical Tests

Unlike other body regions, few hip special clinical tests have been diagnostically validated. Less publication interest has been demonstrated on this topic, possibly since the findings are not as controversial as other body regions (i.e., sacroiliac joint, low back). Consequently, many of the special clinical tests lack testing and demonstrate unknown diagnostic value.

Palpation

No studies were found that measured the reliability or validity of palpation of the hip. Selected authors[46–49] purport the benefit of palpation of the hip, primarily for ruling in or out trochanteric bursitis, hip flexor muscle pain, and ischial tuberosity bursitis.

Muscle Testing

There are mixed findings regarding the benefit of muscle testing. Generally, the reliability of manual muscle testing at the hip is good for hip extensor strength testing.[24] Hip abduction yields variable results since the angle that the hip is placed in may bias the results of the muscle assessment.[43] The use of an external tool such as a dynamometer may improve muscle testing.

Summary

- The special clinical tests of the hip have been less investigated for diagnostic accuracy as compared to many other regions of the body.
- There are mixed benefits to manual muscle testing of the hip, although the authors of this chapter advocate the use of it to gain a comprehensive view of the patient's condition.

Treatment Techniques

Generally, manual therapy treatments associated with the hip involve some mechanism of stretching to improve planes of movement that were concordant during the examination. Techniques designed to improve range of motion includes stretching, manually assisted stretching, and mobilization.

Stretching

Stretching is a form of manual therapy that can be applied passively or through active-assistance of the patient.

Hip Extension Stretch

1. The patient assumes the prone position.

2. Using one hand the clinician blocks the hip joint just cephalic to the gluteal crease. The other hand applies a passive stretch into extension while stabilizing with the blocking hand (Figure 12.24 ■). The position is held for approximately 10–15 seconds.

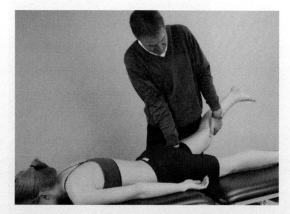

■ **Figure 12.24**   Passive Hip Extension Stretch

Hip Extensor Stretch

1. The patient is positioned in supine.

2. The patient is asked to bring the involved leg into a position of knee and hip flexion.

3. The clinician takes the hip further into flexion to provide a stretch on the posterior structures of the hip. The stretch is amplified by placing a downward pressure through the femur to target the posterior capsule of the hip (Figure 12.25 ■). If the patient complains of pain or "pinching" at the anterior of the hip, the stretch should be ceased.

4. Once a stretch position is achieved, the stretch is sustained for 10–15 seconds.

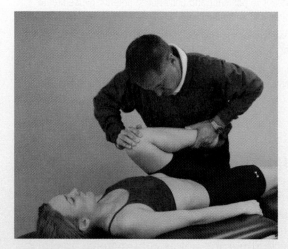

■ **Figure 12.25**   Hip Flexor Stretch

Internal Rotation Stretch

1. The patient assumes a supine position.
2. The clinician passively cradles the lower leg below the knee and slowly internally rotates the hip toward end range. The other hand squeezes the femur and provides a rotational movement in order to reduce the stress placed upon the knee (Figure 12.26 ■).
3. The position is held for approximately 10–15 seconds.

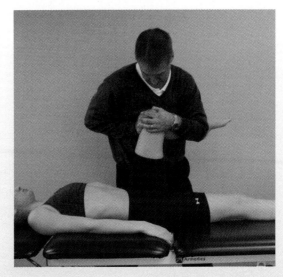

■ **Figure 12.26**   Passive Internal Rotation Stretch

External Rotation Stretch

1. The patient assumes a supine position.
2. The clinician assesses resting symptoms.
3. The clinician passively cradles the lower leg below the knee and slowly externally rotates the hip toward end range. The other hand squeezes the femur and provides a rotational movement in order to reduce the stress placed upon the knee (Figure 12.27 ■).
4. The position is held for approximately 10–15 seconds.

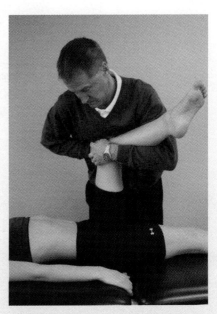

■ **Figure 12.27**   Passive External Rotation Stretch

Muscle Energy Methods

Active assist stretching through use of muscle energy techniques is also a method that is effective for range-of-motion gains.

Extension Muscle Energy

1. The patient is placed in prone.

2. Using one hand the clinician blocks the hip joint just cephalic to the gluteal crease. The other hand applies a passive stretch into extension while blocking the anterior leg with the thigh of the clinician (Figure 12.28 ■). If the hip mobility is too poor to allow the clinician to block with his or her leg, a towel can serve as a substitute block.

3. The patient is instructed to push lightly into hip flexion against the counterforce of the clinician.

4. The position is held for approximately 6 seconds.

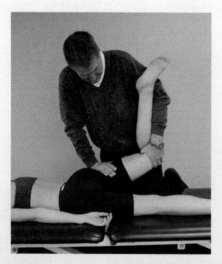

■ **Figure 12.28**   Muscle Energy Stretch to Gain Hip Extension

Hip Internal and External Rotation, Muscle Energy

1. The patient assumes a supine position.

2. The clinician passively cradles the lower leg below the knee and slowly internally rotates the hip toward end range. The other hand squeezes the femur and provides a rotational movement in order to reduce the stress placed upon the knee.

(Continued)

③ The patient is instructed to turn his or her hip lightly into external rotation.

④ The position is held for approximately 6 seconds.

⑤ For external rotation, the clinician passively cradles the lower leg below the knee and slowly externally rotates the hip toward end range. The other hand squeezes the femur and provides a rotational movement in order to reduce the stress placed upon the knee.

⑥ The patient is instructed to turn his or her hip into internal rotation (Figure 12.29 ■).

⑦ The position is held for approximately 6 seconds.

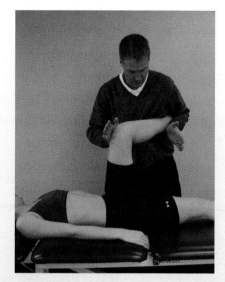

■ **Figure 12.29** Muscle Energy Stretch to Gain Internal Rotation

Mobilization with Traction

Prepositioning in the close-packed position of extension, abduction, and internal rotation reduces the values associated with traction when compared against similar forces placed during a loose-packed position (external rotation, slight flexion, and abduction).

Indirect Traction Treatment

① An indirect traction method requires the assumption of a supine position.

② The clinician queries the patient for a history of knee or ankle dysfunction that would contraindicate the use of this method. If none, the clinician cradles the ankle of the patient into both of his or her hands. The clinician then takes up the slack to preposition the hip into targeted motion. Generally, the resting position of the hip includes a moderate degree of flexion and abduction with slight external rotation.[10]

③ The clinician then provides an inferior force by leaning backward while holding the ankle (Figure 12.30 ■).

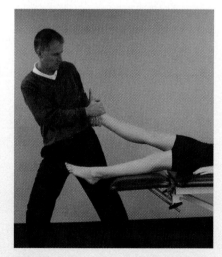

■ **Figure 12.30** Indirect Caudal Glide

(Continued)

④ Upon completion, resting symptoms are again assessed.

On some occasions, the use of a belt may increase the amount of force applied during the indirect traction technique. When the belt is placed in a figure-eight fashion, it will cinch up to the lower extremity during traction and will create a very stable contact with the ankle (Figure 12.31 ■).

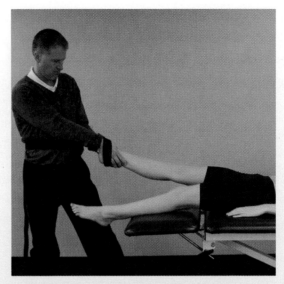

■ **Figure 12.31**   Indirect Caudal Glide with Belt

Direct Traction

A direct traction technique (also performed in supine) differs slightly from an indirect technique.

① The clinician places the lower extremity over his or her shoulder.

② The clinician places his or hands (ulnar border) near the hip joint for an appropriate contact. Using the shoulder as a fulcrum, the clinician pulls inferiorly with the hands at the hip and pushes cephalically with the shoulder for an inferior distraction (Figure 12.32 ■).

③ The clinician passively glides the joint toward the projected end range. Pain is again queried accordingly.

④ Upon completion, resting symptoms are again assessed.

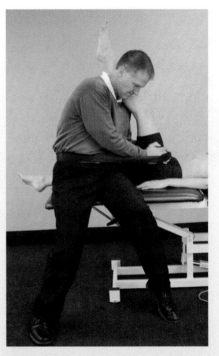

■ **Figure 12.32**   Direct Caudal Glide with Belt

Sims[6] outlines the benefit of selected accessory glides during planar mobilization. He suggests these methods are effective for pain relief and range-of-motion gains. It is arguable whether significant movement actually occurs during the treatment application; however, some evidence does exist for the use of a posterior to anterior technique. Yerys and associates[50] reported that mobilization methods such as a posterior to anterior mobilization (PA) provided a significant improvement in hip extension strength.

Anterior to Posterior Glide

1. The patient assumes a sidelying position.

2. The clinician applies a passive glide of the hip joint using the thumb to lock anterior to the greater trochanter and the heel of the hand to apply the force to the thumb contact point (Figure 12.33 ▪).

3. The clinician passively moves toward a posterior direction. The clinician applies a series of 30-second bouts.

4. Upon completion, resting symptoms are again assessed.

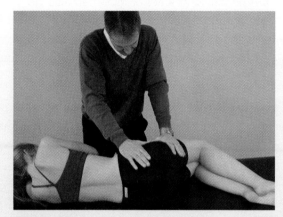

▪ **Figure 12.33**   Anterior–Posterior Glide

Posterior to Anterior Glide

1. The patient assumes a sidelying position.

2. The clinician applies a passive glide of the hip joint using the thumb to lock posterior to the greater trochanter and the heel of the hand to apply the force to the thumb contact point (Figure 12.34 ▪).

3. The clinician passively glides toward an anterior direction. The clinician applies a series of 30-second bouts.

4. Upon completion, resting symptoms are again assessed.

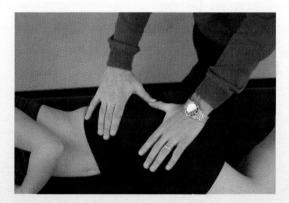

▪ **Figure 12.34**   Posterior–Anterior Glide

Modification of the Posterior to Anterior Glide

A posterior to anterior glide can also be performed in prepositioning of the military crawl position. This method allows greater vigor during a mobilization by prepositioning the patient in a tightened capsular position.

1. The patient assumes a prone position with prepositioning of flexion, abduction, and external rotation of the hip. The position is analogous to a soldier crawling under barbed wire.

2. The clinician applies a passive glide of the hip joint using the thumb to lock posterior to the greater trochanter and the heel of the hand to apply the force to the thumb contact point (Figure 12.35 ■).

3. The clinician passively glides toward an anterior direction. The clinician applies a series of 30-second bouts.

4. Upon completion, resting symptoms are again assessed.

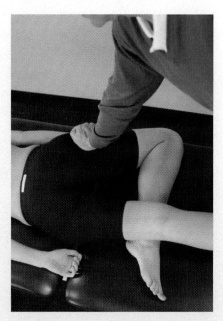

■ **Figure 12.35** Posterior–Anterior Glide, Preposition of Military Crawl

Lateral Glide

The lateral glide is a mobilization method that most likely yields marginal range-of-motion improvement but may be effective in reducing the pain of the patient. The use should be restricted to patients who are pain dominant, who do not tolerate the more aggressive movement-based mobilizations.

1. The patient assumes a supine position.

2. Using a belt and judicious hand placement provides a greater contact point for mobilization anterior and medial to the hip joint. The clinician places his or her shoulder against the knee of the patient to create a counterforce during the mobilization. The mobilization procedure includes a lateral glide of the hip joint at the contact of the medial and anterior hip concurrently with the medial glide of the knee (Figure 12.36 ■). The clinician should perform a series of bouts lasting approximately 30 seconds.

3. Upon completion, resting symptoms are again assessed.

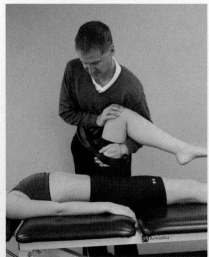

■ **Figure 12.36** Lateral Glide with Belt

Curvilinear Glide

1. The patient assumes a supine position.

2. The hip is prepositioned in flexion, abduction, and external rotation.

3. The clinician places his or her web space of the hand near the lateral crease of the hip joint (just superior to the greater trochanter) (Figure 12.37 ■). The mobilization is targeted medially, anteriorly, and inferiorly. The clinician should perform a series of bouts lastly approximately 30 seconds.

4. Upon completion, resting symptoms are again assessed.

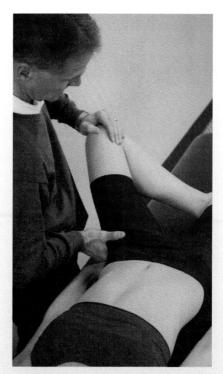

■ Figure 12.37 Posterior–Anterior Glide, Preposition of Curvilinear Glide

Mobilization with Compression

Maitland[29] advocated the use of compression of the hip to stimulate synovial fluid production.[6] As with the majority of procedures presented in this book, concordant findings should drive the decision making when determining whether to use compression.

Passive Internal Rotation with Compression

1. The patient assumes a supine position.

2. The clinician passively cradles the lower leg below the knee and slowly internally rotates the hip toward end range. The other hand squeezes the femur and provides a rotational movement in order to reduce the stress placed upon the knee (Figure 12.38 ■).

3. The clinician performs a series of passive physiological movements into internal rotation. Concurrently, the clinician places a compressive load through the femur into the hip joint of the patient. The technique is performed for a bout of 30 seconds and symptoms are reassessed upon completion of three bouts.

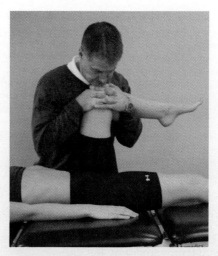

■ Figure 12.38 Passive Internal Rotation with Compression

Compression with an Anterior–Posterior Glide

1 The patient assumes a sidelying position.

2 The clinician placed one palm anterior to the greater trochanter for the anterior–posterior (AP) force. The other hand is placed over the trochanter of the patient and applies a compressive force.

3 The clinician passively moves toward a posterior direction while concurrently providing a compressive force through the trochanter (Figure 12.39 ■). The clinician applies a series of 30-second bouts.

4 Upon completion, resting symptoms are again assessed.

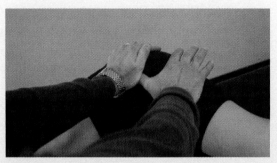

■ **Figure 12.39** Compression with an Anterior Posterior

Passive Hip Flexion with Concurrent Compression

1 The patient assumes a supine position. The procedure is typically targeted for patients with internal rotation restrictions and/or pain.

2 The clinician passively applies a load through the femoral shaft using both hands and his or her chin while concurrently gliding the lower extremity into hip flexion (Figure 12.40 ■). The repeated movements into flexion are targeted at three bouts of 30 seconds each.

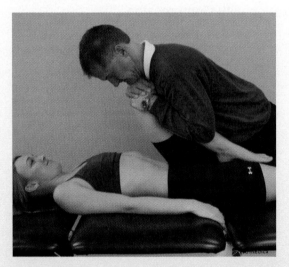

■ **Figure 12.40** Hip Flexion with Compression

Mobilization with Movement

Mobilization with movement typically involves a passive technique performed by the clinician concurrently during an active movement by the patient.

Hip Internal Rotation with a Lateral Glide Mobilization, Mobilization with Movement

1. The technique is performed in supine and is targeted for patients with flexion restrictions/pain.

2. The patient's hip is flexed to 90 degrees and the knee is flexed to mid-range flexion.

3. Using a belt (wrapped around the hip and for support, around the back of the clinician), the clinician applies a lateral glide (Figure 12.41 ■). The patient is instructed to perform active internal rotation during the concurrent hip lateral–inferior glide. The technique is designed to target the posterior capsule. The clinician may emphasize the internal rotation using an active assist movement.

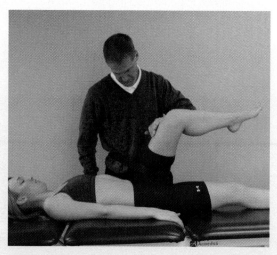

■ **Figure 12.41** Hip Internal Rotation with a Lateral Glide Mobilization, Mobilization with Movement

Hip Flexion with a Lateral-Inferior Glide Mobilization, Mobilization with Movement

1. The patient assumes a supine position.

2. The patient's hip is flexed to 90 degrees and the knee is flexed to end-range flexion.

3. Using a belt (wrapped around the hip and for support, around the back of the clinician), the clinician applies a lateral glide (Figure 12.42 ■). The patient is instructed to perform active flexion during the concurrent hip lateral glide. The clinician may emphasize the flexion using an active assist movement.

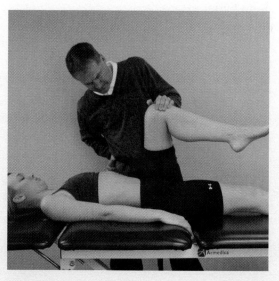

■ **Figure 12.42** Hip Flexion with a Lateral–Inferior Glide Mobilization, Mobilization with Movement

(Continued)

④ To target adduction losses, the hip is prepositioned into adduction and flexion and the same procedure discussed above is performed (Figure 12.43 ■).

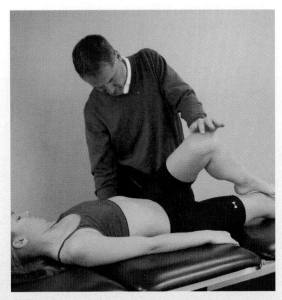

■ **Figure 12.43** Hip Flexion with a Lateral–Inferior Glide Mobilization in Preposition of Adduction, Mobilization with Movement

Hip Extension with Lateral Glide, Mobilization with Movement

This closed kinematic chain technique is designed to target extension.

① The patient stands with the targeted hip prepositioned near the limit of extension.

② Using a belt (wrapped around the hip and for support, around the back of the clinician), the clinician applies a lateral glide. The hands of the clinician push medially on the ilium of the patient to stabilize against the lateral force of the mobilization.

③ The patient is instructed to lunge forward so that the targeted hip moves further into extension during the concurrent hip lateral glide (Figure 12.44 ■).

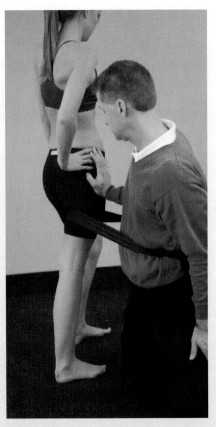

■ **Figure 12.44** Hip Extension with Lateral Glide, Mobilization with Movement

Hip Abduction with a Posterior–Lateral Glide: Mobilization with Movement

This closed kinematic chain technique is designed to target hip abduction.

1. The patient stands with the targeted hip prepositioned near the limit of abduction.

2. Using a belt (wrapped around the hip and for support, around the back of the clinician), the clinician applies a posterior–lateral glide.

3. The hands of the clinician push medially on the ilium of the patient to stabilize against the lateral force of the mobilization.

4. The patient is instructed to lean into further abduction actively during the concurrent hip posterior–lateral glide (Figure 12.45 ■).

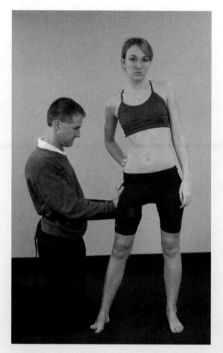

■ **Figure 12.45** Hip Abduction with a Posterior–Lateral Glide, Mobilization with Movement

Manipulation

As with other joints, manipulation can be targeted at the hip joint. Because of the large force required at this joint the most effective manipulation strategies generally include indirect techniques.

Indirect Manipulation

1. The patient assumes a supine position.

2. The clinician queries the patient for a history of knee or ankle dysfunction that would contraindicate the use of this method. If none, the clinician cradles the ankle of the patient into both of his or her hands.

(Continued)

③ The clinician then takes up the slack to preposition the hip into a resting position. Generally, the resting position of the hip includes a moderate degree of flexion and abduction with slight external rotation.[11]

④ The clinician then provides an inferior force by leaning backward while holding the ankle (Figure 12.46 ■).

⑤ At end range, the clinician applies a rapid and quick distraction force to manipulate the hip.

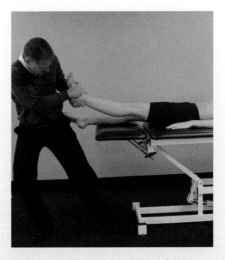

■ **Figure 12.46** Indirect Manipulation

Indirect Manipulation (Cyriax Grade V)

Cyriax[35] described a technique designed to manipulate the SIJ in which the leg is manually thrust into distraction while in a loose-packed position. This method may also manipulate the hip joint as well if the leg is held in slight external rotation.

① The patient assumes a supine position.

② The lower extremity of the patient is prepositioned into flexion, slight external rotation, and slight abduction.

③ Using the arm cephalic to the patient, the clinician cradles the lower leg of the patient and grips the ankle posteriorly.

④ The caudal arm to the patient is flexed at the elbow and the patient's anterior ankle is gripped. A premovement of circumduction allows the patient to relax prior to the manipulation procedure. The manipulation involves a quick distraction into full extension of the knee, thus providing a vacuum-like force through the hip. Patients with ankle, knee, or pelvic disorders are not good candidates for this procedure.

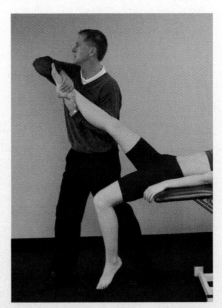

■ **Figure 12.47** Indirect Manipulation (Cyriax Grade V)

Summary

- Treatment techniques for the hip include stretching, mobilization, manipulation, and variations and combinations of these methods.
- Traction may be the most effective technique for joint distraction.
- Manipulation methods generally involve some mechanism of traction indirectly applied to increase the force input.

Treatment Outcomes

The Evidence

Stretching/Muscle Energy/Proprioceptive Neuro-muscular Facilitation (PNF) Stretching Passive stretching, manually assisted stretching, and mobilization have demonstrated equivocal value for range-of-motion gains. Kerrigan and associates[51] suggest that the more vigorous the hip flexor stretching, the more beneficial the gains, despite the age of the individual. Hip flexor stretching has implications to gait and injury prevention, as shown by Rodacki et al.[52] This study found that manual stretching of the hip flexors increased gait speed due to improved pelvic rotation and stride length along with decreased double limb stance time during gait in females (average age, 64.5); and both speed and double limb stance time are suggestive of fall risk in older adults. This finding represents Level C evidence for immediate changes in gait parameters, but has not been studied in patients seeking care specifically for hip dysfunction or for long-term effects.

Manually assistive stretching in the form of muscle energy techniques may be used in patients that demonstrate fear or pain during passive stretching. Medeiros et al.[53] reported similar outcomes when comparing two groups that received isometric contraction and passive stretch procedures.

Mobilization Mobilization with traction has been used in many studies and may result in increased joint distraction. In selected case reports, traction and mobilization methods lead to improvement in internal rotation range of motion,[54] although most studies demonstrated reduction in subjective pain but no changes in range of motion,[21] in one case, as quickly as one visit.[55] Past studies that used radiographic quantification during traction have reported movement up to 10–20 centimeters during distraction.[11,56] Arvidsson[10] identified that an increase in applied force created a direct increase of displacement.

In the most comprehensive study to date, Hoeksma et al.[57] reported statistically significant improvements of hip function and pain in a group that received manual therapy, versus a group that was limited to exercise alone. After 5 weeks, patients in the manual therapy group had significantly better outcomes for pain, stiffness, hip function, and range of motion. Improvements in pain, hip function, and range-of-motion values were still present after 29 weeks. Hoeksma et al.[57] used hip traction and a traction manipulation performed in the limited positions during their clinical trial. There is Level B evidence to support the use of traction and traction manipulation.

In a follow-up analysis, Hoeksma and colleagues[58] attempted to identify subgroups that may be more likely to benefit from manual therapy. The study suggested that subgrouping patients with osteoarthritis based on function, pain, or range of motion does not assist in determining effectiveness of manual therapy. However, those with mild to moderate osteoarthritis on radiographs did respond positively to manual therapy. While no significant change in range of motion is indicated in those with severe findings on radiograph, manual therapy is still more effective than exercise therapy alone for changes in hip function and pain. The authors recognize that subgroups may exist but that the population they studied may have been too homogenous to support the use of subgroupings.

Currier et al.[59] attempted to identify a clinical prediction rule (CPR) for patients with knee OA who may benefit from hip mobilizations. The study includes caudal glides, anterior-to-posterior, and posterior-to-anterior in a flexion, abduction, external rotation position. Five variables were indicative of short-term (48 hours) benefit: hip/groin pain or paresthesia, anterior thigh pain, passive knee flexion less than 122 degrees, passive hip internal rotation less than 17 degrees, and pain with hip distraction. The presence of two variables indicates a positive likelihood ratio of 12.9 with a 97% success rate. This CPR needs to be validated further and provides Level C evidence.

Strain–Counterstrain Lastly, a method known as strain–counterstrain, also known as positional release, is a passive positional technique designed to relieve pain and dysfunction by placing the muscular tissue in a shortened position for a reduction of the tender point.[60] The reliability of assessing the tender points was poor but pain was significantly reduced post-treatment.[61] Another study has demonstrated significantly improved response to a manual muscle test using a dynamometer possibly associated with reducing pain in the targeted segment. Further studies are needed for additional analysis.[60] As such, there is Level C evidence to support the use of strain–counterstrain.

Summary
• There is moderate evidence within the literature that static stretching is beneficial for range-of-motion gains of the hip.
• There is good evidence within the literature that manipulation and traction are beneficial for pain and range of motion at the hip.
• There is limited evidence within the literature to support mobilization of the hip.

Chapter Questions

1. Describe the biomechanics of the hip. Identify which physiological movement demonstrates the greatest potential for mobility.

2. Discuss the capsular pattern theory of the hip. Debate the value of Altman's selection of internal rotation as an osteoarthritis factor.

3. Outline the most common techniques used to increase hip range of motion. Compare the similarities of the techniques.

Patient Cases

Case 12.1: Jeb Lonestar (67-year-old male)

Diagnosis: Hip osteoarthritis.
Observation: He exhibits marked hip restrictions during walking and a painful gait.

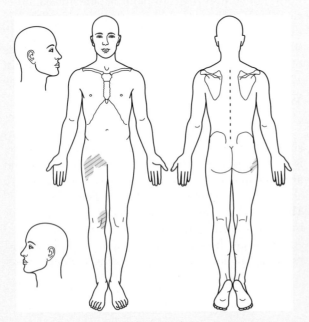

Mechanism: He indicates a very long-term history of hip problems. He reports that he has had pain for over 20 years.
Concordant Sign: Sit to stand.
Nature of the Condition: Notes that he can no longer exercise or walk without immense pain. He does indicate that the condition has also decreased tolerance to long-term sitting.
Behavior of the Symptoms: The pain is localized on the right groin region with a dull ache down the lateral aspect of the right leg.
Pertinent Patient History: He has high blood pressure and has had liver problems in the last 5 years.
Patient Goals: He would like to be more active.
Baseline: At rest, 3/10 NAS for pain; when worst, 4/10 pain.
Examination Findings: Actively and passively, he has pain during internal rotation and flexion. Pain is diminished during hip distraction.

1. Based on these findings, what else would you like to examine?
2. Is this patient a good candidate for manual therapy?
3. What is the expected prognosis of this patient?
4. What treatments do you feel presented in this book may be beneficial for this patient?

Case 12.2: Carlita Montgomery (42-year-old female)

Diagnosis: Femoral acetabular impingement syndrome

Observation: She is overweight.

Mechanism: Symptoms began after exercising in the gym. She started doing loaded squats and now reports pain during long-term sitting or squatting.

Concordant Sign: Loaded squatting.

Nature of the Condition: Primarily, she is concerned that the hip problem will worsen and that it may lead to hip degeneration. The pain only truly hurts while in a squatting or sitting position. The pain resolves quickly once out of that position.

Behavior of the Symptoms: The pain is worse the more active she is.

Pertinent Patient History: No significant history of any medical condition.

Patient Goals: She would like to get back into exercising.

Baseline: Her pain is 1/10 at rest and increases to 6/10 when she squats.

Examination Findings: Pain is present during functional squatting. Pain increases with hip flexion, internal rotation, and adduction. Distraction relieves symptoms but only temporarily.

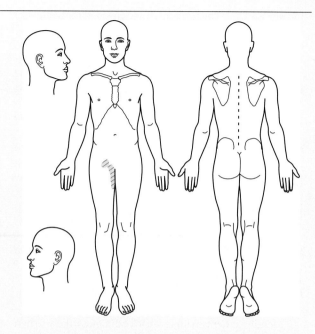

1. Based on these findings, what else would you like to examine?
2. Is this patient a good candidate for manual therapy?
3. What is the expected prognosis of this patient?
4. What treatments do you feel presented in this book may be beneficial for this patient?

PEARSON
myhealthprofessionskit™

Use this address to access the Companion Website created for this textbook. Simply select "Physical Therapy" from the choice of disciplines. Find this book and log in using your username and password to access video clips and the anatomy and arthrological information.

References

1. DeAngelis NA, Busconi BD. Assessment and differential diagnosis of the painful hip. *Clin Orthop Relat Res.* 2003;(406):11–18.
2. Ordeberg G. Characterization of joint pain in human OA. *Novartis Found Symp.* 2004;260:105–115.
3. Brown MD, Gomez-Marin O, Brookfield KF, Li PS. Differential diagnosis of hip disease versus spine disease. *Clin Orthop Relat Res.* 2004;(419):280–284.
4. Lauder T. Musculoskeletal disorder that frequently mimic radiculopathy. *Phys Med Clinics North Am.* 2002; 13:469–485.
5. Collee G, Dijkmans B, Vanderbroucke J, Rozing P, Cats A. A clinical epidemiological study in low back pain: Description of two clinical syndromes. *Br J Rheum.* 1990;29:354–357.
6. Sims K. Assessment and treatment of hip osteoarthritis. *Man Ther.* 1999;4:136–144.
7. Vidigal EC, da Silva OL. Observation hip. *Acta Orthop Scand.* 1981;52(2):191–195.
8. Kandemir U, Bharam S, Philippon M, Fu F. Endoscopic treatment of calcific tendonitis of gluteus medius and minimus. *Arthroscopy.* 2003;19:E1–E4.
9. Waters RL, Mulroy S. The energy expenditure of normal and pathologic gait. *Gait Posture.* 1999;9(3):207–231.

10. Arvidsson I. The hip joint: Forces needed for distraction and appearance of the vacuum phenomenon. *Scand J Rehabil Med*. 1990;22:157–161.

11. Levangie P. The association between static pelvic asymmetry and low back pain. *Spine*. 1999;24(12):1234–1242.

12. Beattie P, Isaacson K, Riddle DL, Rothstein JM. Validity of derived measurements of leg-length differences obtained by use of a tape measure. *Phys Ther*. 1990; 70(3):150–157.

13. Krawiec CJ, Denegar CR, Hertel J, Salvaterra GF, Buckley WE. Static innominate asymmetry and leg length discrepancy in asymptomatic collegiate athletes. *Man Ther*. 2003;8(4):207–213.

14. Friberg O. Clinical symptoms and biomechanics of lumbar spine and hip joint in leg length inequality. *Spine*. 1983;8(6):643–651.

15. Goel A, Loudon J, Nazare A, Rondinelli R, Hassanein K. Joint moments in minor limb length discrepancy: A pilot study. *Am J Orthop*. 1997;26(12):852–856.

16. Childs JD, Fritz JM, Flynn TW, Irrgang JJ, Johnson KK, Majkowski GR, Delitto A. A clinical prediction rule to identify patients with low back pain most likely to benefit from spinal manipulation: A validation study. *Ann Intern Med*. 2004;141(12):920–928.

17. Flynn T, Fritz J, Whitman J, Wainner R, Magel J, Rendeiro D, Butler B, Garber M, Allison S. A clinical prediction rule for classifying patients with low back pain who demonstrate short-term improvement with spinal manipulation. *Spine*. 2002;27(24):2835–2843.

18. Sjolie AN. Low-back pain in adolescents is associated with poor hip mobility and high body mass index. *Scand J Med Sci Sports*. 2004;14(3):168–175.

19. Vad VB, Bhat AL, Basrai D, Gebeh A, Aspergren DD, Andrews JR. Low back pain in professional golfers: The role of associated hip and low back range-of-motion deficits. *Am J Sports Med*. 2004;32(2):494–497.

20. McConnell J. Recalcitrant chronic low back and leg pain—a new theory and different approach to management. *Man Ther*. 2002;7(4):183–192.

21. Lee RY, Munn J. Passive moment about the hip in straight leg raising. *Clin Biomech*. 2000;15(5):330–334.

22. Woods D, Macnicol M. The flexion-adduction test: an early sign of hip disease. *J Pediatr Orthop*. Part B 2000;10:180–185.

23. Kagan A. Rotator cuff tears of the hip. *Clin Orthop Relat Res*. 1999(368):135–140.

24. Perry J, Weiss WB, Burnfield JM, Gronley JK. The supine hip extensor manual muscle test: a reliability and validity study. *Arch Phys Med Rehabil*. 2004;85(8): 1345–1350.

25. Winters MV, Blake CG, Trost JS, Marcello-Brinker TB, Lowe LM, Garber MB, Wainner RS. Passive versus active stretching of hip flexor muscles in subjects with limited hip extension: a randomized clinical trial. *Phys Ther*. 2004;84(9):800–807.

26. Heikkila S, Viitanen JV, Kautiainen H, Kauppi M. Sensitivity to change of mobility tests: Effect of short term intensive physiotherapy and exercise on spinal, hip, and shoulder measurements in spondyloarthropathy. *J Rheumatol*. 2000;27(5):1251–1256.

27. Fritz JM, Whitman JM, Flynn TW, Wainner RS, Childs JD. Factors related to the inability of individuals with low back pain to improve with a spinal manipulation. *Phys Ther*. 2004;84(2):173–190.

28. Huber HM. (abstract). The piriformis syndrome—a possible cause of sciatica. *Schweiz Rundsch Med Prax*. 1990;79(9):235–236.

29. Maitland GD. *Peripheral manipulation* 3rd ed. London; Butterworth-Heinemann: 1986.

30. Fredericson M, Cookingham CL, Chaudhari AM, Dowdell BC, Oestreicher N, Sahrmann SA. Hip abductor weakness in distance runners with iliotibial band syndrome: Hip abductor weakness in distance runners with iliotibial band syndrome. *Clin J Sport Med*. 2000; 10(3):169–175.

31. Arokoski MH, Haara M, Helminen HJ, Arokoski JP. Physical function in men with and without hip osteoarthritis. *Arch Phys Med Rehabil*. 2004;85(4): 574–581.

32. Anderson, MK; Hall, SJ; Martin M. *Sports injury management*. Philadelphia; Lippincott Williams & Wilkins: 2000.

33. Gombotto S, Collins DR, Sahrman SA, Engsberg JR, Van Dillen LR. Gender differences in pattern of hip and lumbopelvic rotation in people with low back pain. *Clin Biomech*. 2006;21:263–271.

34. Scholtes SA, Gombatto SP, Van Dillen LR. Differences in lumbopelvic motion between people with and people without low back pain during two lower limb movement tests. *Clin Biomech*. 2009;24:7–12.

35. Cyriax J. *Textbook of orthopaedic medicine*. 7th ed. Vol. 1. London; Baillierre Tindall: 1978.

36. Greenwood MJ, Erhard RE, Jones DL. Differential diagnosis of the hip vs. lumbar spine: Five case reports. *J Orthop Sports Phys Ther*. 1998;27(4):308–315.

37. Ito K, Leunig M, Ganz R. Histopathologic features of the acetabular labrum in femoroacetabular impingement. *Clin Orthop Relat Res*. 2004;(429):262–271.

38. Warren P. Management of a patient with sacroiliac joint dysfunction: A correlation of hip range of motion asymmetry with sitting and standing postural habits. *J Man Manip Ther*. 2003;11:153–159.

39. Cibulka MT, Threlkeld J. The early clinical diagnosis of osteoarthritis of the hip. *J Orthop Sports Phys Ther*. 2004;34(8):461–467.

40. Birrell F, Croft P, Cooper C, Hosie G, Macfarlane G, Silman A, PCR Hip Study Group. Predicting radiographic hip osteoarthritis from range of movement. *Rheumatology* (Oxford). 2001;40(5):506–512.

41. Reijman M, Hazes JM, Koes BW, Verhagen AP, Bierma-Zeinstra SM. Validity, reliability, and applicability of seven definitions of hip osteoarthritis used in epidemiological studies: A systematic appraisal. *Ann Rheum Dis*. 2004;63(3):226–232.

42. Altman R, Alarcon G, Appelrouth D, et al. The American College of Rheumatology criteria for the classification and reporting of osteoarthritis of the hip. *Arthritis Rheum*. 1991;34(5):505–514.

43. Beatty R. The piriformis muscle syndrome: A single diagnostic maneuver. *Neurosurgery*. 1994;34:512–514.

44. Kaltenborn F. *Manual mobilization of the extremity joints.* 4th ed. Oslo; Olaf Norlis Bokhandel: 1989.

45. Williams P, Bannister L. In: Berry M, Collins P, Dyson M, Dussek J, Ferguson M (eds.) *Gray's anatomy,* 38th ed. Edinburgh; Churchill Livingstone: 1995.

46. NAIOMT. Course notes Level II and III Lower Quadrant. 2008.

47. Caruso F, Toney M. Trochanteric bursitis. A case report of plain film, scintigraphic, and MRI correlation. *Clin Nucl Med.* 1994;19:393–395.

48. Adkins S, Figler R. Hip pain in athletes. *Am Fam Physician.* 2000;61:2109–2118.

49. Jones D, Erhard R. Diagnosis of trochanteric bursitis versus femoral neck stress fracture. *Phys Ther.* 1997;77: 58–67.

50. Yerys S, Makofsky H, Byrd C, Pennachio J, Cinkay J. Effect of mobilization of the anterior hip capsule on gluteus maximus strength. *J Man Manip Ther.* 2002;10: 218–224.

51. Kerrigan DC, Xenopoulos-Oddsson A, Sullivan MJ, Lelas JJ, Riley PO. Effect of a hip flexor-stretching program on gait in the elderly. *Arch Phys Med Rehabil.* 2003;84(1):1–6.

52. Rodacki A, Souza RM, Ugrinowitsch C, Cristopoliski F, Fowler NE. Transient effects of stretching exercises on gait parameters of elderly women. *Man Ther.* 2009; 14:167–172.

53. Medeiros JM, Smidt GL, Burmeister LF, Soderberg GL. The influence of isometric exercise and passive stretch on hip joint motion. *Phys Ther.* 1977;57(5):518–523.

54. Angstrom L, Lindstrom B. (abstract). Treatment effects of traction and mobilization of the hip joint in patients with inflammatory reheumatological diseases and hip osteoarthritis. *Nordisk Fysioterapi.* 2003;7:17–27.

55. Whipple T, Plafcan D, Sebastianelli W. Manipulative treatment of hip pain in a ballet student: A case study. *J Dance Med Science.* 2004;8:53–55.

56. Insulander B. (abstract). Some findings regarding manual traction on hip joints. *Sjukgymnasten.* 1973;4:289–296.

57. Hoeksma HL, Dekker J, Ronday HK, et al. Comparison of manual therapy and exercise therapy in osteoarthritis of the hip: A randomized clinical trial. *Arthritis Rheum.* 2004;51(5):722–729.

58. Hoeksma HL, Dekker J, Ronday HK, Breedveld FC, van den Ende CHM. Manual therapy in osteoarthritis of the hip: Outcome in subgroups of patients. *Rheumatology.* 2005;44:461–464.

59. Currier LL, Froehlich PJ, Carow SD, et al. Development of a clinical prediction rule to identify patients with knee pain and clinical evidence of knee osteoarthritis who demonstrate a favorable short-term response to hip mobilization. *Phys Ther.* 2007;87(9):1106–1119.

60. Wong C, Schauer-Alvarez C. Effect of strain counterstrain on pain and strength in hip musculature. *J Man Manip Ther.* 2004;12:215–223.

61. Wong C, Schauer C. Reliability, validity, and effectiveness of strain counterstrain techniques. *J Man Manip Ther.* 2004;12:107–112.

Manual Therapy
of the Knee

Chad Cook and Robert Fleming

Objectives

- Identify the pertinent structural aspects and biomechanics of the knee.
- Demonstrate an appropriate sequential knee examination.
- Identify plausible mobilization and manual therapy treatment techniques.
- Outline the evidence associated with manual therapy of the knee.

Clinical Examination

Observation

Observation of the appropriate gait parameters and static alignment of the lower extremities are often key components to the clinical examination of the knee. The current literature regarding static alignment focuses on alignment at the foot and ankle and the contribution of this alignment to knee pathology. At present, the literature is inconclusive on the actual contribution.

Selfe[1] reviewed the effect of correction of foot and ankle asymmetries and found that patients experienced an average of 67% reduction in patellofemoral knee pain following the dispensation of foot orthotics. Additionally, rear foot posting produced an immediate and statistically significant medial glide in the patellofemoral joint. Gross and Foxworth[2] reviewed the effect of foot orthoses on the patellofemoral joint and their findings indicate that a significant amount of patients report improvement in their pain; however, there is less clear evidence of how correction of foot and ankle symmetry influences the patellofemoral joint. Hinterwimmer et al.[3] found no difference in patellar kinematics in individuals with lower-extremity asymmetries of genu varum and mild medial compartment osteoarthritis. Livingston and Mandigo[4] reported that the magnitude of right to left rear foot asymmetries was no different between symptomatic and asymptomatic patellofemoral pain groups.

Observational analysis of gait deviations is another component to assessment of the patient with knee pain. In the absence of obvious deviations that occur during significant trauma and swelling, minor gait deviations often are concurrent with knee pain. A gait analysis in patients with patellofemoral pain syndrome (PFPS) found that men and women have similar torque generation at the knee during gait, wider-soled shoes increased knee flexor torque by 30%, and patients with PFPS have a decreased walking velocity and more extended knees during gait than healthy controls. Additional studies[5,6] have demonstrated similar findings. A limitation of many of these studies is that each is laboratory based or had utilized special equipment to measure gait deviations, tools that cannot be carried over to a clinical environment.

Summary

- Posture and foot alignment may suggest knee pain associated with other factors; however, in isolation, asymmetry does not implicate the causal problem.
- A gait analysis is helpful to outcome PFPS and other related knee anomalies, although the actual carryover of the findings to clinical practice are questionable.

Patient History

A key initial goal during patient history should include gathering information to determine whether the condition is mechanical or nonmechanical. With knee disorders, identifying the mechanism of injury and/or onset of pain can aid in determining if the presenting disorder may have involved possible tearing or rupturing of structures or, if the onset of pain is more insidious, a more degenerative or sinister condition may be present. Additionally, the patient history will serve to identify potential movements or activities that are related to the concordant signs. For example, patients with meniscal injuries often report knee pain after twisting their leg while bearing full weight and often will experience a popping or tearing sensation, followed by severe pain. Swelling can take several hours to appear. Ligamentous injuries may occur with a similar mechanism to meniscal tears, and often will be the result of a direct blow to the knee, but swelling often occurs immediately.[7]

Based on criteria of the American College of Rheumatology, osteoarthritis of the knee may be suspected if the following criteria are present: age older than 50, daily knee stiffness for less than 30 minutes, crepitus, bony tenderness, bony enlargement, and no palpable warmth.[7] If four criteria are present, the sensitivity of the characteristics is 84% with a specificity of 89%. If at least three of the criteria are present, the chance of osteoarthritis being present is 62%. Of the five criteria, two of the criteria are considered aspects of patient history (age and stiffness) and two of five criteria increase the probability of osteoarthritis to 4%.[7] With this said, at least one physical exam variable would need to be present to bring probability to acceptable levels. This is in line with the fact that clinical history alone, related to the diagnosis of meniscus or ligamentous tears, can only heighten suspicion and help formulate tentative management strategies and not necessarily differentiate between the two. Combining the physical exam and patient history may be more helpful in determining the pathology associated with these disorders.[7]

Nonmechanical disorders such as septic arthritis will present as an acute onset of knee pain with effusion and warmth; signs and symptoms of infection will be present as well. There will likely be no history of trauma to correlate to the effusion. Patients with this presentation should immediately be referred to a medical physician for appropriate consultation.[7,8]

Because the knee is so necessary during all components of function, a specific functional scale is an excellent adjunct to patient history. The Lower Extremity Function Scale (LEFS) is a region-specific scale that is not limited to use with osteoarthritis. The LEFS is a self-report tool, primarily designed as a performance-based measure.[9] The LEFS is reliable (ICC = 0.95)[10], demonstrates construct validity, and is more sensitive to change than the SF-36.[11] The LEFS can measure multiple joints of the lower extremity[10] and is used conjunctively with measures of pain and physical exertion.

Summary

- The purpose of the subjective examination is to identify the concordant mechanical disorders associated with the knee.

- Based on criteria of the American College of Rheumatology, osteoarthritis of the knee may be suspected if the following criteria are present: age older than 50, daily knee stiffness for less than 30 minutes, crepitus, bony tenderness, bony enlargement, and no palpable warmth.

- Nonmechanical disorders often include acute onset of knee pain with effusion, warmth, and signs and symptoms of infection.

- The Lower Extremity Functional Scale is a valid, self-report, region-specific questionnaire that measures problems associated with activities of daily living.

Physical Examination

Active Physiological Movements

Active movements during a clinical examination are used to identify physical impairments that are relevant to the concordant signs. By determining the behavior of the concordant signs toward selected active movements, the clinician can effectively identify potential active physiological treatment approaches.

Plane-Based Active Range of Motion Assessment of active range of motion of the knee can be assessed in different manners that will help not only in determining objective range of motion of the knee, but also the relativity of the impairment to the concordant signs. Non-weight bearing active range-of-motion movements (AROM) can be performed in sitting or supine positions (Figure 13.1 ■). These positions will influence the stressing of tissues surrounding the knee in different ways.

Functional Active Range-of-Motion Testing AROM performed in a weight-bearing position, while less convenient to attain objective measurements of range of motion, allows for a closer replication of functional positions and movements that are relevant to the concordant signs. For example, pain-reproducing movements for the knee may often include ascending and descending stairs and squatting. Cliborne et al.[12] used a "functional squat test" as one outcome measure following a program of hip mobilization in patients

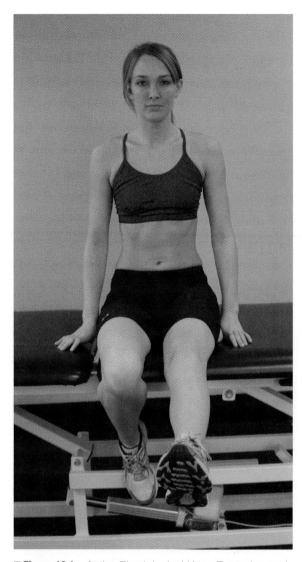

■ Figure 13.1 Active Physiological Knee Extension and Flexion in Sitting Position

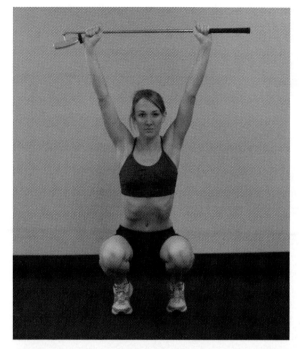

■ Figure 13.2 The Functional Squat Test

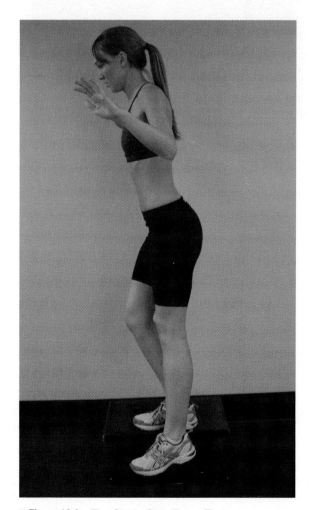

■ Figure 13.3 The Single Step-Down Test

with knee osteoarthritis. The procedure included having the patient stand with his or her feet comfortably apart, then squatting down until either pain limits the range or the heels come off the floor.

A single step-down test is used to measure functional control of the knee during eccentric and concentric knee movements (Figure 13.3 ■). The single step-down test is useful for patients who lack the range of motion to perform the functional squat test.

Hop tests are often used with patients that are post–anterior cruciate ligament (ACL) reconstruction as a means to determine functional activity tolerance and predict dynamic knee stability and possible future injury (Figure 13.4 ■). The Hop test appears to have potential to predict dynamic knee stability, but currently the literature suggests that the predictive capability of these tests is questioned.[13]

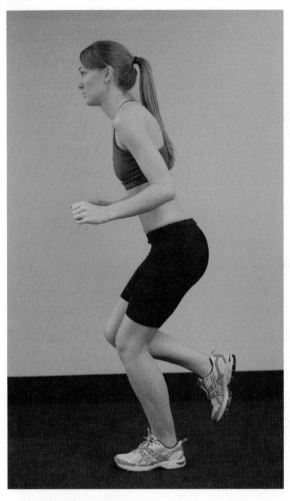

■ **Figure 13.4**   The Hop Test

Summary

- Active range of motion techniques should include functional activities and plane-based movements.
- Functional tests should be geared toward the concordant reproduction of the patient's complaint.

Passive Movements

Passive Physiological Movements   Passive physiological movements of the knee are similar to active physiological movements and are used to confirm the relationship of movement to the concordant signs. Additionally, passive physiological movements of the knee allow for a more complete examination of component movements (i.e., tibial rotation) that are difficult to actively replicate and occur during functional movement. Abnormal "end-feels" of movement such as stiffness or locking have been found to be associated with a patient's concordant sign.[14,15] The clinician should strive to correlate any detection of abnormal movement to the concordant signs.

Passive Physiological Knee Flexion

① The patient assumes a supine position.

② The clinician grasps the patient's leg just proximal to the knee with one hand and just distal on the tibia with the other. The clinician may find it necessary to use a portion of his or her chest to support the leg while applying movement. Additionally, the clinician should strive to maintain the lower extremity/hip in a consistent, neutrally rotated position (this can be modified as needed to correlate to the concordant signs).

③ The clinician gently moves the knee into the flexion (sagittal) plane, stopping at the first point of pain (Figure 13.5 ■).

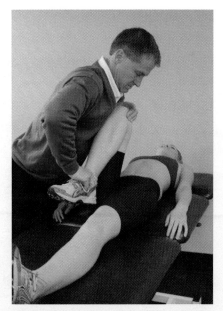

■ **Figure 13.5**   Passive Physiological
Knee Flexion

4 The clinician assesses for symmetry of motion and for reproduction of concordant signs while moving the knee beyond the first point of pain, progressing toward end range as the patient's complaint of pain allows. Repeated movements or sustained holds into knee flexion are then performed to the point of range that allows assessment of the response of the repeated movements on the patient's pain (or like symptoms). As needed, the clinician can apply force (overpressure) to the end of range to assess for pain response.

Knee Flexion with Abduction and Adduction

Combined passive movements are used to examine further available physiological range in an effort to find concordant signs and improve the sensitivity of the examination.

1 To perform this assessment, the clinician follows the procedures in Figure 13.5 and flexes the knee to 10–20 degrees short of end of available range.

2 The clinician firmly grasps the distal femur with one hand while holding the lateral femur against his or her chest. This handling will help ensure that the clinician *does not allow femoral rotation* during this phase of the examination. The clinician's other hand will grasp the distal tibia/ankle.

3 As the clinician flexes the knee, he or she directs the heel toward the direction of the greater trochanter of the hip (producing abduction movement of the tibia) (Figure 13.6 ■). Movement will occur up until pain is reproduced, then gently past this point as tolerated.

(Continued)

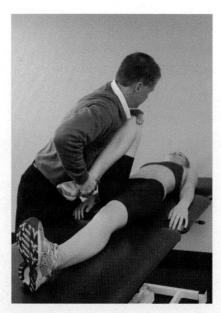

■ **Figure 13.6** Knee Flexion and Abduction

④ If the concordant sign is not reproduced, this movement can then be repeated with the tibia held in various degrees of available tibia internal rotation.

⑤ As needed, the clinician can apply force (overpressure) to the end of range to assess for pain response.

⑥ For knee flexion with adduction, the clinician flexes the knee, he or she directs the heel toward the direction of the groin (producing adduction movement of the tibia) (Figure 13.7 ■). Movement will occur up until pain is reproduced, then gently past this point as tolerated. If the concordant sign is not reproduced, this movement can then be repeated with the tibia held in various degrees of available tibia external rotation. As needed, the clinician can apply force (overpressure) to the end of range to assess for pain response.

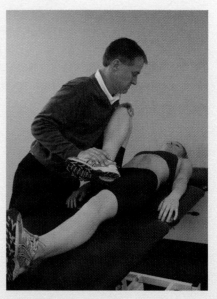

■ **Figure 13.7** Knee Flexion with Adduction

Passive Physiological Extension

The range of motion of full and terminal knee extension is often much less than flexion, thus handling procedures are dramatically different.

1 The patient assumes a supine position and the clinician grasps the lateral ankle with one hand, while the palm of the other hand is placed on the tibial tubercle.

2 Using side-bending of the trunk and a simultaneous force on the above-noted contact areas with the hands, the clinician then produces an extension movement of the knee, stopping at the first point of pain (Figure 13.8 ■).

3 The clinician assesses for symmetry of motion and for reproduction of concordant signs while moving the knee beyond the first point of pain; progressing toward end range as the patient's complaint of concordant pain allows.

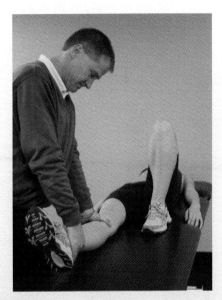

■ **Figure 13.8** Passive Knee Extension

4 Repeated movements into knee extension are then performed to the point of the extension range that pain allows to assess the response of the repeated movements on the patient's pain (or like symptoms). As needed, the clinician can apply force (overpressure) to the end of range to assess for pain response.

Knee Extension with Adduction and Abduction

As noted previously, combined passive movements are used to examine further available physiological range in an effort to find concordant signs and improve the sensitivity of the examination.

1 To perform knee extension with abduction, the clinician follows the procedures in Figure 13.8 and extends the knee to 10–15 degrees short of end of available range.

2 The clinician grasps the tibia/lateral ankle as noted above, but will move the palm contact just lateral to the tibial tubercle.

3 As the clinician extends the knee, using side-bending of the trunk and a simultaneous force on these contact areas with the hands, the clinician then produces an extension–abduction movement of the knee (abduction movement of the tibia) (Figure 13.9 ■). Movement will occur up until pain is reproduced, then gently past this point as tolerated. As needed, the clinician can apply force (overpressure) to the end of range to assess for pain response.

(Continued)

④ To perform an adduction movement with extension, the clinician grasps the lateral ankle as noted above, but will move palm contact just medial to the tibial tubercle and will lean over the leg for proper body alignment.

⑤ As the clinician extends the knee, using side-bending of the trunk and a simultaneous force on these contact areas with the hands, the clinician then produces an extension–adduction movement of the knee (adduction movement of the tibia) (Figure 13.10 ■). Movement will occur up until pain is reproduced, then gently past this point as tolerated. As needed, the clinician can apply force (overpressure) to the end of range to assess for pain response.

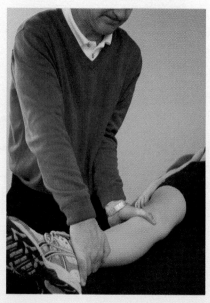

■ **Figure 13.9** Knee Extension with Abduction

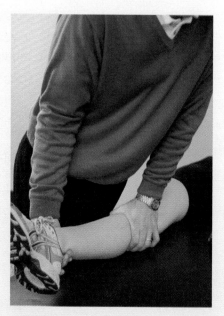

■ **Figure 13.10** Knee Extension with Adduction

Tibial Internal and External Rotation

Approximately 20 degrees of rotation occurs at the tibiofemoral joint. Restrictions are common and may require physiological intervention.

① The patient assumes a supine position.

② The clinician cradles the tibia on his or her forearm and grasps the foot distally at the heel.

③ The ankle of the patient is passively dorsiflexed to create a stable lever during rotation and the knee is flexed to approximately 90 degrees (Figure 13.11 ■).

④ The clinician applies a passive internal rotation to the first point of pain. Repeated movements or sustained holds are applied to determine if the movements reduce pain. The activity is repeated toward end range.

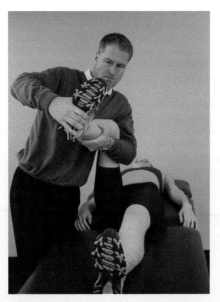

■ **Figure 13.11** Tibial Internal Rotation
at 90 Degrees of Knee Flexion

⑤ The clinician then applies a passive external rotation to the first point of pain. Repeated movements or sustained holds are applied to determine if the movements reduce pain (Figure 13.12 ■). The activity is repeated toward end range.

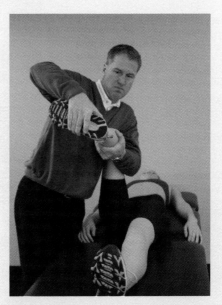

■ **Figure 13.12** Tibial External Rotation
at 90 Degrees of Knee Extension

Summary

- The purpose of passive physiological testing is to reproduce the concordant sign of the patient.
- By incorporating adduction, abduction, and rotations in the plane-based movements of flexion and extension, the clinician may more accurately isolate the disorder of the patient.

Passive Accessory Movements for the Tibiofemoral Joint Assessment of passive accessory movement of the knee is used to evaluate component motion of a joint segment/region, including the relevance to the patient's impairment and concordant signs. As we have repeated throughout this text, assessment of position and/or orientation or movement of the body/joint segments without inclusion of the relevance to the concordant signs will yield less useful clinical information and will limit the clinician's ability to analyze further the patient's response to movements.

The following describes the procedures of passive accessory movement testing of the knee. It is important to note that the assessment of accessory glides necessitates movements in varying ranges of physiological ROM. Careful analysis will allow the clinician to establish the relevance of an impairment of accessory motion to physiological ROM and to the concordant signs that may have been established in the active and/or passive physiological components of the examination.

Posterior–Anterior Mobilization of the Tibiofemoral Joint

1. The patient assumes a supine position with the patient's knees prepositioned at 60–80 degrees of flexion.

2. The clinician will grasp the proximal tibia with both hands, wrapping the fingers around to the posterior tibia.

3. The clinician then gently moves the tibia on the femur in a posterior to anterior direction, stopping at the first point of pain (Figure 13.13 ■). The pain is assessed for the concordant sign. In knee flexion ranges of less than approximately 60 degrees, the clinician will need to ensure he or she moves his or her body from posterior to anterior and slightly caudal to attempt not to passively flex the patient's knee. Additionally, the clinician will need to ensure a consistent position of the hip for all ranges assessed.

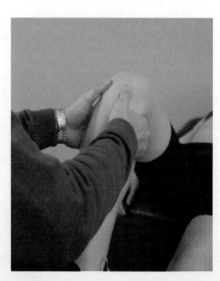

■ **Figure 13.13** Posterior–Anterior Mobilization of the Tibiofemoral Joint

4. The clinician assesses for quality of motion and for reproduction concordant signs while moving the knee beyond the first point of pain, progressing toward end range as the patient's complaint of pain allows. Repeated movements are then performed to the point of range/movement that pain allows, to assess the response of the repeated movements on the patient's pain (or like symptoms).

Anterior–Posterior Mobilization of the Tibiofemoral Joint

1. The patient assumes a supine position and flexes the knee to approximately 60–80 degrees of flexion.

2. The clinician places both thumbs on the tibial tubercle and allows the fingers to rest on the posterolateral aspects of the tibia.

3. Pushing with the thumbs, the clinician then gently moves the tibia on the femur in an anterior to posterior direction, stopping at the first point of pain (Figure 13.14 ■).

4. The clinician assesses for quality of motion and for reproduction of concordant signs while moving the knee beyond the first point of pain, progressing toward end range as the patient's complaint of pain allows. Repeated movements are then performed to the point of range/movement that pain allows, to assess the response of the repeated movements on the patient's pain (or like symptoms).

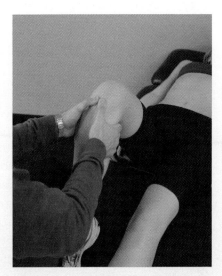

■ **Figure 13.14**   Anterior–Posterior Mobilization of the Tibiofemoral Joint

The movement of the tibia on the femur may isolate the outer horns of the menisci and force movement of the menisci. Movement of the tibia posteriorly on the femur results in anterior movement of the menisci on the femur. Figure 13.15 ■ illustrates this process.

The movement of the tibia anteriorly on the femur in a flexed position may force posterior migration of the meniscus with respect to the tibia. Figure 13.16 ■ illustrates this phenomenon.

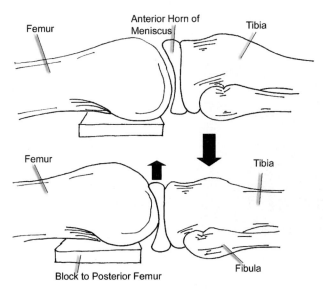

■ **Figure 13.15**   Theoretical Movement of the Anterior Horn of the Meniscus

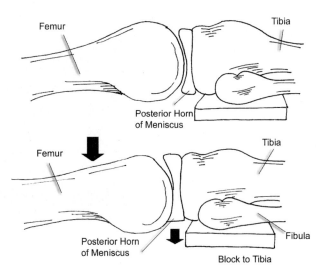

■ **Figure 13.16**   Theoretical Movement of the Posterior Horn of the Meniscus

Medial and Lateral Shear of the Tibiofemoral Joint

1. The patient assumes a supine position.

2. The clinician can place a small bolster behind the femur to allow the knee to rest in approximately 10–20 degrees of flexion or if the knee of the patient is small, the clinician can hold the knee during the assessment.

3. For medial shear, the clinician uses one hand to grasp the medial aspect of the distal femur, in the region of the condyles, while with the other hand the clinician grasps the lateral aspect of the proximal tibia (Figure 13.17 ■). The clinician will stabilize the femur while applying a medially directed movement of the tibia on the femur, stopping at the first point of pain. The procedure can also be tested at 90 degrees of flexion.

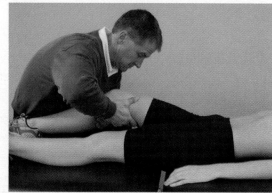

■ **Figure 13.17** Medial Glide of the Tibia on the Femur

4. For lateral shear, the clinician uses one hand to grasp the lateral aspect of the distal femur, in the region of the condyles, while with the other hand the clinician grasps the medial aspect of the proximal tibia (Figure 13.18 ■). The clinician will stabilize the femur while applying a laterally directed movement of the tibia on the femur, stopping at the first point of pain. The procedure can also be tested at 90 degrees of flexion.

5. The clinician will assess for quality of motion and assess for reproduction of concordant signs while moving the knee beyond the first point of pain, progressing toward end range as the patient's complaint of pain allows. Repeated movements are then performed to the point of range/movement that pain allows, to assess the response of the repeated movements on the patient's pain (or similar symptoms).

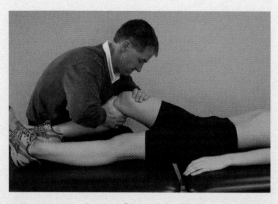

■ **Figure 13.18** Lateral Glide of the Tibia on the Femur

Rotations of the Tibiofemoral Joint

1. The patient assumes a hooklying position (the knee should be flexed to 80–90 degrees) and the clinician stabilizes the patient's foot by sitting on the dorsum of the foot.

2. The clinician grabs the lateral half of the tibia with one hand and stabilizes the femur with the other. The clinician then applies a medially directed and anterior rotation to the lateral half of the tibia (Figure 13.19 ■).

3. For a lateral and anterior rotation, the clinician grabs the medial half of the tibia with one hand and stabilizes the femur with the other. The clinician then applies a lateral and anterior rotation to the lateral half of the tibia (Figure 13.20 ■).

4. For a medial and posterior rotation, the clinician grabs the lateral half of the tibia with one hand and stabilizes the femur with the other. The clinician then applies a medial and posterior rotation to the lateral half of the tibia (Figure 13.21 ■).

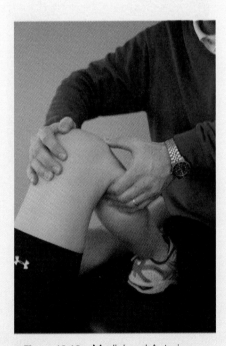

■ **Figure 13.19** Medial and Anterior Rotation of the Tibia on the Femur

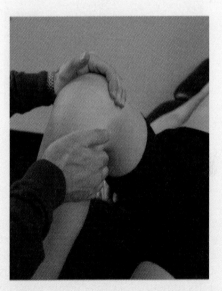

■ **Figure 13.20** Lateral and Anterior Rotation of the Tibia on the Femur

(Continued)

⑤ Lastly, for a lateral and posterior rotation, the clinician grabs the medial half of the tibia with one hand and stabilizes the femur with the other. The clinician then applies a lateral and posterior rotation to the lateral half of the tibia (Figure 13.22 ■).

⑥ For all rotations, movements are repeated or sustained (at the first point of pain and at end range) to determine if concordant and whether the pain abolishes with movements.

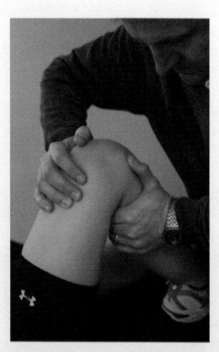

■ **Figure 13.21** Medial and Posterior Rotation of the Tibia on the Femur

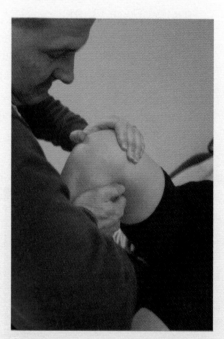

■ **Figure 13.22** Lateral and Posterior Rotation of the Tibia on the Femur

Passive Accessory Movements of the Patello-femoral Joint During movement from flexion to extension, the patella starts in a medially tilted position and then shifts to neutral, lastly shifting to a laterally tilted position while in extension.[16] Additionally, the patella moves distally during progressive extension to flexion, variably moves from anterior to posterior (in many cases the patella just moved posteriorly), and variably moves progressively laterally during knee flexion.[17] Consequently, it is important to assess the numerous ranges of patella mobility.

Cephalad and Caudal Movements of the Patellofemoral Joint

1. The patient assumes a supine position.

2. The clinician places the distal aspect of the patella between his or her thumb and index finger, cupping the hand slightly (Figure 13.23 ■).

3. The clinician then gently glides the patella in cephalad direction, stopping at the first point of pain.

4. The clinician will assess for quality of motion and assess for reproduction of concordant signs while moving the patella beyond the first point of pain, progressing toward end range as the patient's complaint of pain allows. Repeated movements are then performed to the point of range/movement that pain allows, to assess the response of the repeated movements on the patient's pain (or like symptoms).

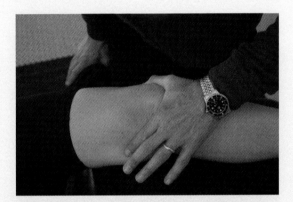

■ **Figure 13.23**   Cephalic Glide of the Patella

5. For caudal movement assessment, the clinician can follow the steps for cephalad movement of the patella, but will move the patella in a caudal direction and contacts the patella at the superior-most region (Figure 13.24 ■).

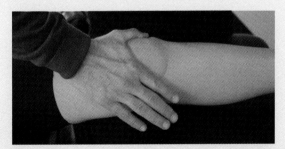

■ **Figure 13.24**   Caudal Glide of the Patella

Medial and Lateral Movements of the Patellofemoral Joint

Medial and lateral movements of the patellofemoral joint are also tested in a supine position with slight knee flexion. It is generally useful to place the knee of the clinician under the knee of the patient, functioning as a bolster.

1. To test lateral movement the clinician will sit on the lateral side of the knee and place the fingers against the medial border of the patella.

2. The clinician will produce a laterally directed movement of the patella (Figure 13.25 ■), stopping at the first point of pain.

3. The clinician will assess for quality of motion and assess for reproduction of concordant signs while moving the patella beyond the first point of pain, progressing toward end range as the patient's complaint of pain allows. Repeated movements are then performed to the point of range/movement that pain allows, to assess the response of the repeated movements on the patient's pain (or like symptoms).

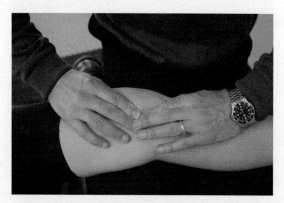

■ **Figure 13.25**   Lateral Glide of the Patella

4. To test medial movement, the clinician will stand on the lateral side of the knee and place the thumbs against the lateral border of the patella (Figure 13.26 ■). The clinician can follow the above steps for lateral movement of the patella but produce movement in a medially directed direction.

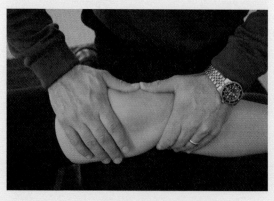

■ **Figure 13.26**   Medial Glide of the Patella

Medial and Lateral Tilt Movements of the Patellofemoral Joint

Based on the anatomy of the posterior facet of the patella, medial and lateral "tilting" or rotation of the patella in the transverse plane is an accessory movement of the patellofemoral joint. Tilting is tested in a supine position with the knee placed in slight flexion.

1 To create a medial tilt, the clinician will place one of his or her thumbs or palm on the medial half of the patella, while the other thumb or thenar eminence blocks the lateral aspect of the patella (to limit the patella from moving laterally).

2 The clinician will produce a medial "tilting" movement of the patella by pushing on the medial half of the patella in an anterior to posterior direction, stopping at the first point of pain (Figure 3.27 ■).

3 The clinician will assess for quality of motion and assess for reproduction of concordant signs while moving the patella beyond the first point of pain, progressing toward end range as the patient's complaint of pain allows. Repeated movements are then performed to the point of range/movement that pain allows, to assess the response of the repeated movements on the patient's pain (or like symptoms).

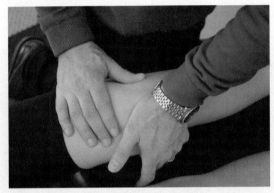

■ Figure 13.27   Medial Tilt of the Patella

To create and test a lateral tilt, the clinician can follow the above steps but with lateral tilting, by producing movement in an anterior to posterior direction on the lateral half of the patella. The clinician should also be sure to block the medial border of the patella (with the thumbs of fingers) to prevent a medial movement of the patella during the lateral tilting movement (Figure 13.28 ■).

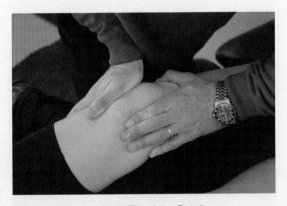

■ Figure 13.28   Lateral Tilt of the Patella

Medial and Lateral Rotation Movements

The medial and lateral rotation described in this section refers to rotation in the frontal plane (i.e., the apex [superior border] of the patella directed medially is medial rotation). Each is tested in a supine position with slight knee flexion.

1. The patient assumes a supine position.

2. To test medial rotation, the clinician sits on the lateral side of the knee and grasps the patella with both hands, placing the apex of the patella in the web space of the caudal hand and the superior aspect of the patella in the web space of the cephalad hand (Figure 13.29 ■).

3. To produce a medially directed rotation the clinician will rotate the apex of the patella medially, stopping at the first point of pain. The clinician may find it helpful when producing these movements to take up tissue slack around the knee. This can be accomplished by placing the hands on the patella and placing the cephalic hand medially (about 2 o'clock position) and the caudal hand just opposite the cephalad hand (about 8 o'clock position). Firmly grasping the soft tissues the clinician moves his or her hands back to the original position. This technique should allow the clinician to feel more localized movement of the patella versus the surrounding soft tissues.

4. The clinician will assess for quality of motion and for reproduction of concordant signs while moving the patella beyond the first point of pain, progressing toward end range as the patient's complaint of pain allows.

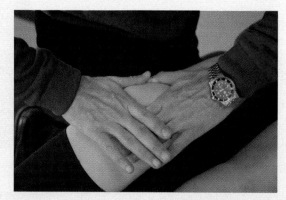

■ **Figure 13.29**   Medial Rotation of the Patella

Lateral rotational movements are tested similarly to the above steps but movement of the inferior aspect of the patella is produced in a lateral direction (Figure 13.30 ■). In all patella assessments, repeated movements are then performed to the point of range/movement that pain allows, to assess the response of the repeated movements on the patient's pain (or like symptoms).

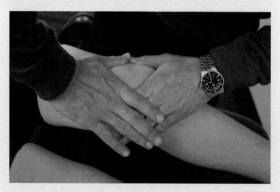

■ **Figure 13.30**   Lateral Rotation of the Patella

Patellar Compression Compression of joint surfaces in examination is purported to aid in determining if a patient's symptoms are from a "joint surface disorder," that is, possible changes to the joint surfaces that may contribute to a patient's symptoms.[18] It is unknown whether pain from compression of a joint surface correlates to tissue changes of the joint surfaces. With this in mind, the reader is encouraged to consider compression as an additional examination technique that may reveal concordant signs. Additionally, compression can be used to aid in ruling out the involvement of a joint region when examination movements are assessed with strong compression without symptom provocation.[18] Common clinical findings that suggest examination with compression include:[18]

1. The standard examination movements do not clearly correlate to the patient's symptoms.
2. The patient complains of pain through the range of movement.
3. There is crepitus of the joint with movement.
4. Heavy work or activity causes minor symptoms ("compressive loads").
5. Lying on the involved joint provokes symptoms.

There are varieties of joint regions that require examination with compression and the patellofemoral joint is one of them. For the patellofemoral joint, cephalad/caudal, medial/lateral, medial/lateral tilt, and medial/lateral rotation movements can be performed with compression. The clinician can perform the previously described examination movements of the patellofemoral joint with compression, then assess for relevance to concordant signs. Compression is achieved by moving the patella toward the femur, gently at first, then producing the previously described movements. As with any other accessory examination technique, the clinician should consider assessing with the knee while positioned in various ranges of physiological range of motion.

Patellar Distraction In essence, the set-up for patellar distraction is the opposite of compression. Gently, the clinician will need to use the pads of the fingers to grasp the lateral and medial posterior facet region of the patella and produce a movement of the patella away from the femur. Assessment then includes producing cephalad/caudal, medial/lateral, medial/lateral tilt, and medial/lateral rotation movements while sustaining distraction. The clinician's goals will remain the same of relating the relevance of provoking movements to concordant signs.

Summary

- The purpose of passive accessory testing is to reproduce the concordant sign of the patient.
- Appropriate isolation of passive accessory testing may require prepositioning of the knee to implicate symptoms.
- Strategies such as compression are effective in isolating painful conditions.
- Combined accessory movements may tighten structures and further implicate causal problems.

Posterior–Anterior Glide of Superior Tibial–Fibular Joint

The superior tibial–fibular joint region should be included in a comprehensive evaluation of the knee. This structure can contribute to pain and dysfunction in the knee region and plays an integral role in the interaction between the foot/ankle and the knee.

1. The patient assumes a sidelying position with the area examined facing upward.

2. The clinician should aim to position the lower extremity in a relatively neutral position of hip adduction (i.e., towel or pillow between knees). The clinician will stand behind the patient and palpate for the posterior margin of the head of the fibula.

(Continued)

③ The clinician will then place the pads of his or her thumbs against the posterior margin of the head of the fibula. Using the thumbs, the clinician produces a posterior to anterior directed movement, stopping at the first point of pain (Figure 13.31 ▪).

④ The clinician will assess for quality of motion and assess for reproduction of concordant signs while moving the fibula beyond the first point of pain, progressing toward end range as the patient's complaint of pain allows.

⑤ Repeated movements are then performed to the point of range/movement that pain allows, to assess the response of the repeated movements on the patient's concordant pain.

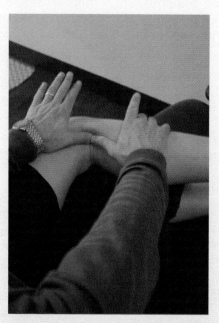

▪ **Figure 13.31**   Posterior–Anterior Glide of the Tibial–Fibular Joint

The above-described movement should then be performed with compression. This is achieved by leaving one thumb on the posterior margin of the fibula and taking the interthenar groove of the other hand and placing it on top of the thumb. Compression is achieved by pushing downward toward the plinth while simultaneously producing the posterior to anterior movement.

Anterior–Posterior Glide of the Tibial–Fibular Joint

1. The patient assumes a sidelying position with the area examined facing upward.

2. The clinician should aim to position the lower extremity in a relatively neutral position of hip adduction (i.e., towel or pillow between knees). The clinician stands in front the patient and palpates for the anterior margin of the head of the fibula.

3. The clinician then places the pads of his or her thumbs against the anterior margin of the head of the fibula (Figure 13.32 ■). Using the thumbs, the clinician produces an anterior to posterior directed movement, stopping at the first point of pain.

4. The clinician will assess for quality of motion and assess for reproduction of concordant signs while moving the fibula beyond the first point of pain, progressing toward end range as the patient's complaint of pain allows.

5. Repeated movements are then performed to the point of range/movement that pain allows, to assess the response of the repeated movements on the patient's concordant pain.

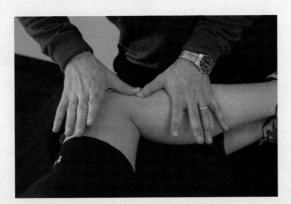

■ **Figure 13.32**   Anterior–Posterior Glide of the Tibial–Fibular Joint

The previously described movements should then be performed with compression. This is achieved by leaving one thumb on the anterior margin of the fibula and taking the interthenar groove of the other hand and placing it on top of the thumb. Compression is achieved by pushing downward toward the plinth while simultaneously producing the anterior to posterior movement.

Cephalad and Caudal of the Tibial–Fibular Joint

1 The patient assumes a sidelying position with the area examined facing upward.

2 The clinician should aim to position the lower extremity in a relatively neutral position of hip adduction (i.e., pillow or towel between knees). The clinician will stand anteriorly to the patient and palpate for the anterior and posterior margins of the head of the fibula.

3 The clinician then grasps the rear foot of the same lower extremity. The clinician will ensure that the rear foot is clear of the table to produce eversion and inversion movements of the rear foot.

4 The clinician will indirectly produce cephalad and caudal movements of the fibula by producing eversion (cephalad fibula) (Figure 13.33 ■) or inversion (caudal fibula) (Figure 13.34 ■) of the rear foot. Simultaneous palpation of the superior fibula occurs during these movements. Movement occurs up to the first point of pain.

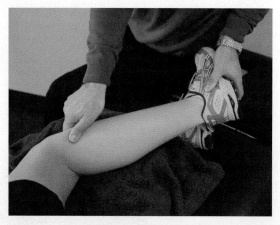

■ **Figure 13.33** Cephalic Glide of the Tibular–Fibular Joint

5 The clinician will assess for quality of motion and assess for reproduction of concordant signs while moving the fibula beyond the first point of pain (by moving the rear foot), progressing toward end range as the patient's complaint of pain allows.

6 Repeated movements are then performed to the point of range/movement that pain allows, to assess the response of the repeated movements on the patient's concordant pain.

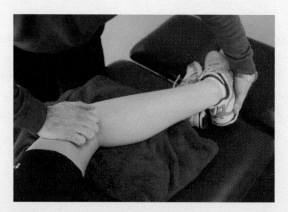

■ **Figure 13.34** Caudal Glide of the Tibular–Fibular Joint

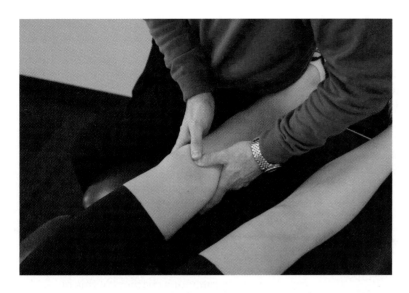

■ **Figure 13.35** Palpation of the Medial Tibial Joint Line in Extension

Special Clinical Tests

Palpation

Palpatory tests for the knee are best divided into two main categories:(1) palpation for the presence of joint line tenderness and (2)palpation for the presence of a fracture. See Table 13.1 ■.

Palpation for Joint Line Tenderness

Palpation for joint line tenderness is a basic maneuver used to implicate meniscal injuries or general effusion of the knee.[19] Since the anterior–medial aspect of the medial meniscus becomes prominent during internal rotation and flexion, it may be advantageous to preposition the knee in this position during the palpation procedure. Extension of the knee may further improve the sensitivity of this palpation procedure (Figure 13.35 ■).

Palpation for Knee Fractures

The **Ottawa Knee Rules** are a prospective set of clinical findings that are designed to assist in determining whether referral for a radiograph is necessary to rule

■ **TABLE 13.1**   Special Clinical Tests for Palpation (Joint Line Tenderness)

Author	Sensitivity	Specificity	LR+	LR−
Barry et al.[20]	86	43	1.5	0.32
Noble & Erat[21]	73	13	0.8	2.1
Fowler & Lubliner[22]	85	30	1.2	0.5
Saengnipanthkul et al.[23]	58	74	2.2	0.6
Kurosaka et al.[24]	55	67	1.6	0.67
Anderson & Lipscomb[25]	77	NR	NA	NA
Akseki et al. medial meniscus[26]	88	44	1.6	0.27
Akseki et al. lateral meniscus[26]	67	80	3.4	0.41
Karachalios et al. medial meniscus[27]	71	87	5.5	0.33
Karachalios et al. lateral meniscus[27]	78	90	7.8	0.24
Eren medial meniscus[28]	86	67	2.6	0.20
Eren lateral meniscus[28]	92	97	30.7	0.08

out a fracture.[29] There are five components to the Ottawa Knee Rules: (1) age > 55, (2) tenderness at the head of the fibula, (3) isolated tenderness of patella during palpation, (4) inability to flex knee to 90 degrees, and (5) inability to bear weight both immediately and in the emergency department. If any of the criteria are positive, the patient should be referred for a radiograph. The Ottawa Knee Rules are recognized as the most valid mechanism to determine whether plain film radiographs are necessary in the event of acute trauma.[7]

Manual Muscle Testing

Manual muscle testing (break test) of knee flexion and/or extension with a hand-held dynamometer has demonstrated good reliability in studies. (1) that have used children as subjects;[30] (2) for subjects' status post–hip fracture,[31] (3) for patients with cerebral palsy,[32] (4) for patients with spinal muscular atrophy[33] and (5) for community-dwelling older adults[34] However, manual muscle testing was considered poor when tested using subjects that were healthy.[35] The inclined squat strength test is considered an alternative to the break test and is considered more functional. The test has demonstrated good reliability using subjects with no known pathology.[36]

Treatment Techniques

Manual therapy treatment of knee disorders should focus on identifying physical impairments that are related to concordant signs. Physical impairments can range from disorders associated with motor control, active, and passive mobility, or passive structure competence of the systems of the knee.

Active or passive mobilization in any direction may be beneficial for the patient with osteoarthritis.[37] Activities such as active quadriceps contractions have been shown to reduce negative biochemical parameters within the knee associated with osteoarthritis.[37] Compression-based mobilizations may be most effective at producing these changes and have been shown to lead to better outcomes than treatments with no compression.[38] As with the previous chapters of this book, the examination methods are often similar to the treatment procedures.

Mobilization Techniques

Mobilization techniques are those performed by the clinician that are strictly passive in nature.

Compression Mobilization of the Tibiofemoral Joint

1. The patient assumes a prone position.

2. The clinician stabilizes the tibia by applying a perpendicular grip to the tibia and fibula with his or her mobilizing arm.

3. The knee is bent toward the concordant region of pain (flexion in Figure 13.36 ■).

4. The clinician applies a compressive load through the tibiofemoral joint by loading the heel of the patient with the nonmobilizing hand.

5. The clinician applies oscillations (a posterior–anterior mobilization in Figure 13.36) during compression for treatment of the patient with the mobilizing hand near the knee.

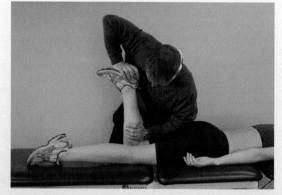

■ **Figure 13.36** Prone Compression Mobilization of the Tibiofemoral Joint

The procedure can also be performed with the patient in a supine position. Rather than using a PA- or AP-based mobilization, the movement incorporated by the clinician may involve oscillatory flexion–extension in small ranges at the concordant position of the knee (Figure 13.37 ■).

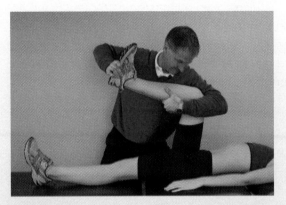

■ **Figure 13.37**   Supine Compression Mobilization of the Tibiofemoral Joint

Compression Mobilization of the Patellofemoral Joint

1 The patient assumes a supine position.

2 The clinician may place his or her knee under the patient's knee to slightly flex the tibiofemoral joint.

3 The clinician applies a load to the patella by placing his or her hand on top of the knee cap. The patient may apply small active oscillatory movements of the tibiofemoral joint during compression by the clinician or the clinician may apply a compression force with patellofemoral mobilization (Figure 13.38 ■).

4 To improve the targeted specificity of the technique, alterations in knee extension or flexion may be added.

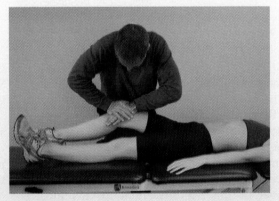

■ **Figure 13.38**   Compression Mobilization of the Patellofemoral Joint

Scoop Mobilization for the Posterior Horn

Because the menisci of the knee are frequently injured or fail to move during knee flexion and extension, the menisci are often targeted for treatment. Anterior–posterior mobilizations of the tibia and femur respectively, should assist in differentiating the anterior and posterior horn of the meniscus. Posterior horn injuries are typically worse during flexion of the knee and during functional activities such as squatting. The scoop mobilization is used to target the posterior horn of the meniscus.

1. The scoop mobilization can be performed in a sitting, prone, or supine, hooklying position (Figure 13.39 ■).

2. The clinician flexes the patient to the first point of pain or toward end-range flexion.

3. The clinician places his or her hands at the joint line posteriorly to the knee of the patient.

4. The clinician then further flexes the knee toward end-range flexion. The mobilization procedure is a curvilinear posterior to anterior pull (which is also upward) that targets the menisci. The technique is most effective near end-range flexion.

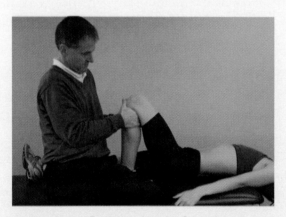

■ **Figure 13.39** Posterior–Anterior Scoop Mobilization in Supine

Tibial Shear at Multiple Ranges The tibial shear mobilization is performed at various ranges throughout the knee. Because the capsule is engaged at greater degrees of flexion, the tibial shear mobilization near full flexion tends to target the capsule more significantly than other stabilizing structures of the knee. A tibial shear in extension may place greater emphasis on the menisci. Concordant pain found during selected angles of passive physiological testing typically identifies the most appropriate position for linear mobilization of the tibia. To improve the targeted specificity of the technique, knee extension or flexion may be altered (Figure 13.40 ■).

Tibial Rotation at Multiple Ranges Occasionally, rotation is more sensitive at reproducing the concordant sign than the tibial shear methods. Subsequently, rotational mobilizations may be effective at various ranges as well. As with the tibial shear methods, concordant pain found during various angles of passive physiological testing typically identifies the most appropriate position for rotational mobilization of the tibia. To improve the targeted specificity of the technique, knee extension or flexion may be altered (Figure 13.41 ■).

Passive Stretching Techniques

Passive stretching techniques typically isolate soft tissue restrictions, but may also be useful in improving joint mobility.

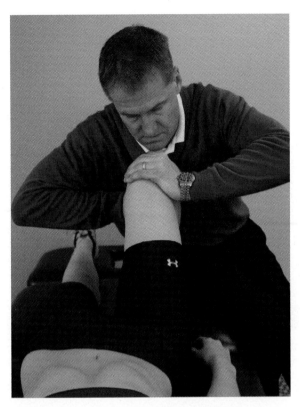

■ **Figure 13.40**   Lateral Tibial Shear at 90 Degrees
of Flexion

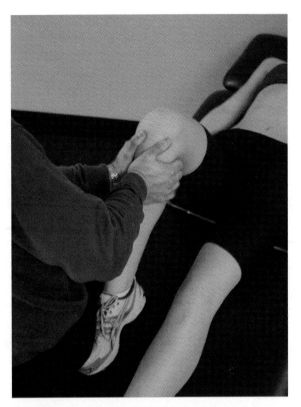

■ **Figure 13.41**   Rotation Mobilization at 90 Degrees
of Flexion

Hamstring Stretches

Several studies have described various hamstring stretching methods. It appears that any form of hamstring stretching (i.e., hold–relax, static hold) tends to provide the same level of improvement in range of motion, albeit with only minimal long-term carryover.[39-41] A hold–relax stretch is a form of muscle energy technique that allows a patient to govern the amount of stretch force provided.

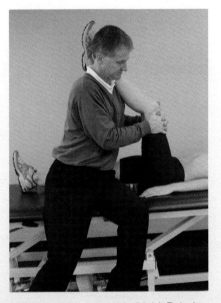

■ **Figure 13.42**   Isometric (Hold–Relax) Hamstring Stretching of the Patient

1. The patient assumes a supine position.

2. The hip is prepositioned into 90 degrees and knee extension is taken to the point of hamstring restriction.

3. The clinician places the heel of the patient on his or her shoulder (Figure 13.42 ■).

4. The patient is instructed to push downward into the shoulder for a hold time of 10–15 seconds; a submaximal contraction is appropriate.

5. The clinician slowly moves the knee into further extension after each isometric contraction of the patient.

Hip Flexor and Knee Extensor Stretch

There is some difficulty in stretching the hip flexors and knee extensors on one's own.

1. The patient is placed in prone position.

2. The knee is flexed and the hip is passively taken into extension. To improve the emphasis of the stretch, it is useful to place a towel or a sandbag under the knee of the patient.

3. The patient is instructed to flex his or her hip against a counterforce of the clinician (Figure 13.43 ■).

4. To isolate the knee extensors, the patient is instructed to extend his or her knee against the counterforce provided by the clinician at the tibia.

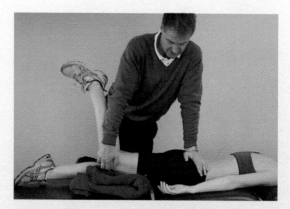

■ **Figure 13.43** Isometric (Hold–Relax) Hip Flexor/Knee Extensor Stretching of the Patient

Mobilization with Movements

Mobilization with movement techniques typically involve passive contributions by the clinician with concurrent active movement performed by the patient.

Internal Rotation of the Tibia during Active-Assist Knee Flexion

1. The patient assumes a supine (hooklying) position.

2. The knee is flexed to 15 degrees from the physiological limit.

3. The clinician supplies a passive internal rotation physiological mobilization and instructs the patient to actively flex his or her knee toward the limit of tibiofemoral flexion (Figure 13.44 ■).

4. Movement into flexion is performed rhythmically, with the clinician moving the knee back toward extension after each procedure.

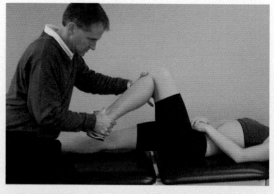

■ **Figure 13.44** Internal Rotation of the Tibia during Active-Assist Knee Flexion, Mobilization with Movement

Internal Rotation of the Tibia during Active-Assist Knee Flexion in Closed Chain

1. The technique is performed in standing position with the affected extremity placed on a chair or a plinth and the knee flexed to 15 degrees from the physiological limit.

2. The clinician supplies a passive internal rotation mobilization force and instructs the patient to flex his or her knee toward the limit of tibiofemoral flexion while bearing weight through the foot (Figure 13.45 ■).

3. Active movement into flexion is performed rhythmically and concurrently with passive internal rotation, with the clinician moving the knee back toward extension after each procedure.

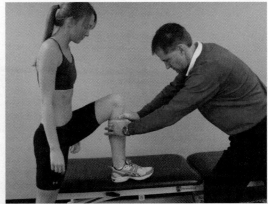

■ **Figure 13.45**   Internal Rotation of the Tibia during Active-Assist Knee Flexion in Closed Chain, Mobilization with Movement

Anterior Glide of the Superior Tibial–Fibular Joint during Active-Assist in Closed Chain

1. The technique is performed in standing position with the affected extremity placed on a chair or a plinth and the knee is flexed to 15 degrees from the limit.

2. The clinician supplies a posterior to anterior glide to the tibiofemoral joint while stabilizing the femur under his or her shoulder (in the armpit).

3. The clinician instructs the patient to flex his or her knee toward the limit of flexion while bearing weight through the foot (Figure 13.46 ■).

4. Movement into flexion is performed rhythmically, with the clinician moving the knee back toward extension after each procedure.

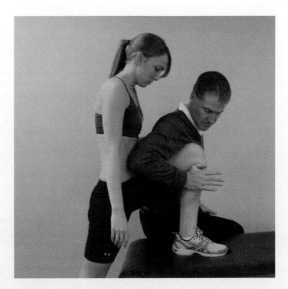

■ **Figure 13.46**   Anterior Glide of the Superior Tibial–Fibular Joint during Active-Assist in Closed Chain, Mobilization with Movement

Prone Scoop Mobilization with Active-Assist Flexion

To enhance flexion at end range, the clinician can apply a scoop mobilization (as discussed previously in supine) while concurrent active flexion to the patient's limit.

1. The technique may best be performed in prone position.

2. The clinician applies a posterior to anterior force at the posterior aspect of the knee while the patient actively moves the knee into flexion (Figure 13.47 ■).

3. By flexing his or her wrist the clinician further isolates the PA force.

4. The clinician's opposite hand is used to guide the knee into flexion.

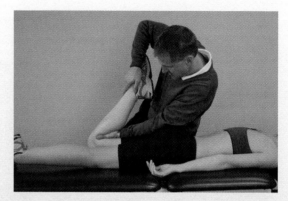

■ **Figure 13.47**   Prone Scoop Mobilization with Active-Assist Flexion, Mobilization with Movement

Knee External Rotation with Active Extension in Closed Chain

1. The patient assumes a supine position with the knee extended toward near limit.

2. The plantar aspect of the foot is compressed against a bolster or a foam wedge.

3. The clinician applies an externally rotated mobilization force while instructing the patient to extend the knee and compress against the foam wedge or bolster (Figure 13.48 ■).

4. The process is repeated several times in an attempt to improve extension.

5. In some cases, the superior tibular–fibular joint can be substituted for the tibiofemoral joint.

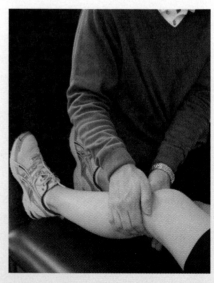

■ **Figure 13.48**   Knee External Rotation with Active Extension in Closed Chain, Mobilization with Movement

Manipulation

Manipulation techniques involve a thrust technique performed at or near the restricted range of the patient.

Manipulation of the Tibiofemoral Joint

Meyer et al.[42] describe a tibiofemoral manipulation in which the tibia is rapidly distracted from the femur. The technique was used concurrently with patellofemoral mobilization and led to a positive consequence in a single case study.

1. The technique is performed in a prone position.

2. The clinician uses a belt to stabilize the femur.

3. The knee is slightly flexed to the targeted range of discomfort.

4. The clinician can preposition the knee in internal or external rotation, depending on the concordant pain of the patient. The manipulation includes a rapid distraction of the tibia on a fixed femur (Figure 13.49 ■).

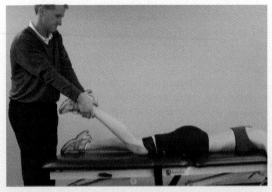

■ **Figure 13.49**   Tibiofemoral Distraction Manipulation of the Knee

Summary

- The majority of manual therapy treatment methods are distilled from the examination process.
- Mobilization with movement may enhance the patient's active use of the extremity toward restricted ranges.
- Adding components such as compression, end-range movements, and distraction may increase the usefulness of manual therapy treatment.

Treatment Outcomes

The Evidence

Mobilization and Manipulation of the Tibiofemoral Joint   There is Level B evidence that nonthrust joint mobilization provides short-term hypoalgesic effects on patients with osteoarthritis[43] and Level C evidence that pain is reduced with nonthrust and thrust manipulation in patients with anterior knee pain[44,45] There is Level A evidence that nonthrust mobilization is beneficial in reducing pain and improving disability scores in patients with osteoarthritis.[46–48] This finding suggests that mobilization should always be part of a treatment protocol for patients with osteoarthritis of the knee.

Noel et al.[38] reported that mobilization with compression, a long axis compression technique of the tibia in a flexed position, led to significantly greater preset range-of-motion goals versus the comparative group, which did not receive mobilization with compression. Mobilizations were performed at end range, were concordantly painful, and were rated as unpleasant by more recipients.

Patellofemoral Mobilization   Assessment of patellar mobility does appear in the literature as a common component to the treatment of patellofemoral pain syndrome. Studies have examined the assessment of static patellar orientation, particularly medial and lateral orientation and mobility assessment. With the exception of one study, these assessments demonstrated poor reliability.[49–52] One study that did demonstrate acceptable levels of reliability included experienced manual therapists and a single subject.[53]

Less evidence exists that manual therapy is beneficial for patients with patellofemoral pain syndrome.[54–56] (Level C). Crossley and colleagues[54,55] reported improvements in knee flexion during stair climbing compared to placebo treatment. Manual therapy mobilization was a component of treatment but was combined with taping, biofeedback, and strengthening exercises. The *Philadelphia Panel Guidelines* found no evidence to support any form of manual or nonmanual treatment of patellofemoral pain syndrome, specifically friction massage, which has demonstrated no benefits in numerous studies.[56]

Static Stretching A number of weaker studies have demonstrated long-term effectiveness of hamstring static stretching, distal or proximal on joint position sense,[57] mobility,[58] static stretching with an external device for range of motion of the knee,[59] and improvement in flexibility of the quadriceps after dedicated stretching.[60] What is unknown is the carryover effect for function for these static stretching procedures, thus the information remains Level C.

Targeted Other Joints for Carryover to the Knee
There is Level C evidence of short-term (transient) benefit from manipulation of the hip[61] and the lumbar spine[62] in reducing pain at the knee. However, there is insufficient evidence to support the routine use of this treatment approach at this time.[63]

Summary

- Outside the use of manual therapy for the treatment of arthritis, few studies have examined the effectiveness of treatment for the knee.
- Little evidence exists to support the use of manual therapy for patellofemoral pain syndrome, although when combined with other treatments, the technique may be beneficial.
- There is some evidence that transient benefit may occur at the knee after manipulation of the hip or low back.
- Some evidence exists that including compression with mobilization increases the return of range of motion quicker than an absence of compression.

Chapter Questions

1. How does the biomechanics of the knee factor into the selection of the manual therapy treatment approach?

2. Describe how the femoral condyle dictates the likelihood of PFPS.

3. Outline the method in which a mobilization to the tibia or femur can isolate the menisci.

4. Describe how compression may positively affect a condition during manual therapy of the knee.

5. Describe three variations of plane-based mobilization that may alter the outcome of the technique.

Patient Cases

Case 13.1: Wally Tiltson (36-year-old male)

Diagnosis: Internal derangement of the knee.
Observation: He exhibits an extension deficit of 10 degrees.
Mechanism: He tore his anterior cruciate ligament over 20 years ago. He did not receive a repair. Since then he has noticed increased stiffness and mobility in his knee.
Concordant Sign: Squatting: the pain is posterior to the knee.

Nature of the Condition: The problem is a nuisance because he indicates he cannot squat or perform functional activities that require squatting. The condition is not irritable, as it only hurts when he is in a squatted position.
Behavior of the Symptoms: The pain is isolated to the posterior knee, although stiffness is felt throughout the knee.
Pertinent Patient History: 20-year history of ACL-deficient knee. Osteoarthritis at other joints.
Patient Goals: He is concerned he has a torn meniscus and his goal is to determine what he can safely do.

Baseline: Leg pain at rest, 2/10 NAS for pain; when worst, 7/10 pain during squatting.

Examination Findings: Range is limited for all movements. Gross joint play is decreased throughout. Full functional squatting is concordant. Shear testing reproduces concordant findings.

1. Based on these findings, what else would you like to examine?
2. Is this patient a good candidate for manual therapy?
3. What is the expected prognosis of this patient?
4. What treatments do you feel presented in this book may be beneficial for this patient?

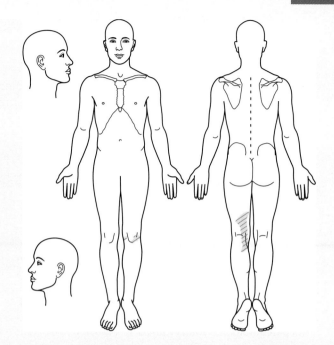

Case 13.2: Rachel Robertson (72-year-old female)

Diagnosis: Osteoarthritis of the knee.
Observation: Enlarged knee with varus deformity.
Mechanism: Multiyear history of osteoarthritis of her knee. There was no major incident that triggered symptoms, although she reports pain initiated while working as a maid.

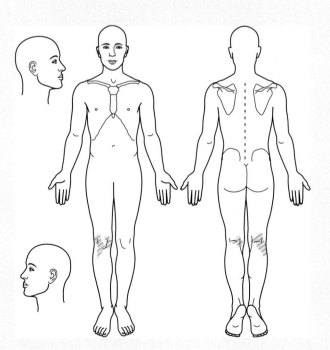

Concordant Sign: She claims her knee catches during walking but cannot isolate the movement.
Nature of the Condition: She reports she can no longer walk for exercise or attend her aquatics class. As such, she has gained approximately 20 pounds in the last 6 months. Her cardiologist has also indicated that she has heart problems that need exercise for maintenance. The condition is irritable.
Behavior of the Symptoms: The pain is present anteriorly along the joint line of the knee. Referred pain goes to the foot of the patient.
Pertinent Patient History: She has a long-term history of low back pain.
Patient Goals: She is interested in decreasing her knee pain so that she can start exercising again.
Baseline: His current symptoms are at 3/10; when worse, 5/10.
Examination Findings: Knee flexion and extension are both painful. Rotation is painful as well.

1. Based on these findings, what else would you like to examine?
2. Is this patient a good candidate for manual therapy?
3. What is the expected prognosis of this patient?
4. What treatments do you feel presented in this book may be beneficial for this patient?

References

1. Selfe J. The patellofemoral joint: A review of primary research. *Crit Rev Phys Rehabil Med*. 2004;16(1):1–30.
2. Gross MT, Foxworth JL. The role of foot orthoses as an intervention for patellofemoral pain. *J Orthop Sports Phys Ther*. 2003;33(11):661–670.
3. Hinterwimmer S, von Eisenhart-Rothe R, Siebert M, Welsch F, Vogl T, Graichen H. Patella kinematics and patellofemoral contact areas in patients with genu varum and mild osteoarthritis. *Clin Biomech*. 2004;19(7):704–710.
4. Livingston LA, Mandigo JL. Bilateral rearfoot asymmetry and anterior knee pain syndrome. *J Orthop Sports Phys Ther*. 2003;33(1):48–55.
5. Otsuki T, Nawata K, Okuno M. Quantitative analysis of gait patterns in patients with osteoarthrosis of the knee before and after total knee arthroplasty: Gait analysis using a pressure measuring system. *J Orthop Sci*. 1999;4(2):99–105.
6. Lafuente R, Belda JM, Sanchez-Lacuesta J, Soler C, Poveda R, Prat J. Quantitative assessment of gait deviation contribution to the objective measurement of disability. *Gait Posture*. 2000;11(3):191–198.
7. Jackson JL, O'Malley PG, Kroenke K. Evaluation of acute knee pain in primary care. *Ann Intern Med*. 2003;139(7):575–588.
8. Chu S, Yang S, Lue K, Hsieh Y. Clinical significance of gelatinases in septic arthritis of native and replaced knees. *Clin Orthop Rel Res*. 2004;427:179–183.
9. Stratford P, Kennedy D, Pagura S, Gollish J. The relationship between self-report and performance-related measures: Questioning the content validity of timed tests. *Arthritis Rheum*. 2003;49:535–540.
10. Watson C, Propps M, Ratner J, Zeigler D, Horton P, Smith SS. Reliability and responsiveness of the Lower Extremity Functional Scale and the anterior knee pain scale in patients with anterior knee pain. *J Orthop Sports Phys Ther*. 2005;35:136–146.
11. Binkley J, Stratford P, Lott S, Riddle D. The Lower Extremity Functional Scale (LEFS): scale development, measurement properties, and clinical application. North American Orthopaedic Rehabilitation Research Network. *Phys Ther*. 1999;79:371–383.
12. Cliborne AV, Wainner RS, Rhon DI, Judd CD, Fee TT. Clinical hip tests and a functional squat test in patients with knee osteoarthritis: Reliability, prevalence of positive test findings, and short-term response to hip mobilization. *J Orthop Sports Phys Ther*. 2004;34(11):676–683.
13. Fitzgerald GK, Lephart SM, Hwang JH, Wainner RS. Hop tests as predictors of dynamic knee stability. *J Orthop Sports Phys Ther*. 2001;31(10):588–597.
14. Hayes W, Petersen C, Falconer J. An examination of Cyriax's passive motion tests with patients having osteoarthritis of the knee including commentary by Twomey LT, with author response. *Phys Ther*. 1994;74:697–708.
15. Petersen C, Hayes K. Construct validity of Cyriax's selective tension examination: Association of end-feels with pain at the knee and shoulder. *J Orthop Sports Phys Ther*. 2000;30:512–527.
16. Ahmed AM, Duncan NA, Tanzer M. In vitro measurement of the tracking pattern of the human patella. *J Biomed Eng*. 1999;121:222–228.
17. Laprade J, Lee R. Real-time measurement of patellofemoral kinematics in asymptomatic subjects. *Knee*. 2005;12:63–72.
18. Maitland G. *Peripheral manipulation*. 3rd ed. London; Butterworth-Heinemann: 1994.
19. Malanga G, Andrus A, Nadler S, McLean J. Physical examination of the knee: A review of the original test description and scientific validity of common orthopedic tests. *Arch Phys Med Rehabil*. 2003;84:592–603.
20. Barry OCD, Smith H, McManus F, MacAuley P. Clinical assessment of suspected meniscal tears. *Ir J Med Sci*. 1983;152:149–151.
21. Noble J, Erat K. In defense of the meniscus: A prospective study of 200 meniscectomy patients. *J Bone Joint Surg*. 1980;62:7–11.
22. Fowler P, Lubliner J. The predictive value of five clinical signs in the evaluation of meniscal pathology. *Arthroscopy*. 1989;5:184–186.
23. Saengnipanthkul S, Sirichativapee W, Kowsuwon W, Rojviroj S. The effects of medial patellar plica on clinical diagnosis of medial meniscal lesion. *J Med Assoc Thai*. 1992;75(12):704–708.
24. Kurosaka M, Yagi M, Yoshiya S, Muratsu H, Mizuno K. Efficacy of the axially loaded pivot shift test for the diagnosis of a meniscal tear. *International Orthop*. 1999;23:271–274.
25. Anderson AF, Lipscomb AB. Preoperative instrumented testing of anterior and posterior knee laxity. *Am J Sports Med*. 1989;17(3):387–392.
26. Akseki D, Ozcan O, Boya H, Pinar H. A new weight-bearing meniscal test and a comparison with McMurray's test and joint line tenderness. *Arthroscopy*. 2004;20(9):951–958.

27. Karachalios T, Hantes M, Zibis AH, Zachos V, Karantanas AH, Malizos KN. Diagnostic accuracy of a new clinical test (the Thessaly test) for early detection of meniscal tears. *J Bone Joint Surg Am.* 2005;87(5):955–962.

28. Eren OT. The accuracy of joint line tenderness by physical examination in the diagnosis of meniscal tears. *Arthroscopy.* 2003;19(8):850–854.

29. Emparanza JI, Aginaga JR; Estudio Multicentro en Urgencias de Osakidetza: Reglas de Ottawa (EMUORO) Group. Validation of the Ottawa Knee Rules. *Ann Emerg Med.* 2001;38(4):364–368.

30. Escolar DM, Henricson EK, Mayhew J, et al. Clinical evaluator reliability for quantitative and manual muscle testing measures of strength in children. *Muscle Nerve.* 2001;24(6):787–793.

31. Roy MA, Doherty TJ. Reliability of hand-held dynamometry in assessment of knee extensor strength after hip fracture. *Am J Phys Med Rehabil.* 2004;83(11): 813–818.

32. Taylor NF, Dodd KJ, Graham HK. Test–retest reliability of hand-held dynamometric strength testing in young people with cerebral palsy. *Arch Phys Med Rehabil.* 2004;85(1):77–80.

33. Merlini L, Mazzone ES, Solari A, Morandi L. Reliability of hand-held dynamometry in spinal muscular atrophy. *Muscle Nerve.* 2002;26:64–70.

34. Ford-Smith CD, Wyman JF, Elswick RK Jr, Fernandez T. Reliability of stationary dynamometer muscle strength testing in community-dwelling older adults. *Arch Phys Med Rehabil.* 2001;82:1128–1132.

35. Agre JC, Magness JL, Hull SZ, et al. Strength testing with a portable dynamometer: Reliability for upper and lower extremities. *Arch Phys Med Rehabil.* 1987; 68(7):454–458.

36. Munich H, Cipriani D, Hall C, Nelson D, Falkel J. The test–retest reliability of an inclined squat strength test protocol. *J Orthop Sports Phys Ther.* 1997;26(4):209–213.

37. Mivaguchi M, Kobayashi A, Kadoya Y, Ohashi H, Yamano Y, Takaoka K. Biochemical change in joint fluid after isometric quadriceps exercise for patients with osteoarthritis of the knee. *Osteoarthritis Cartilage.* 2003;11:252–259.

38. Noel G, Verbruggen LA, Barbaix E, Duquet W. Adding compression to mobilization in a rehabilitation program after knee surgery: A preliminary clinical observational study. *Man Ther.* 2000;5:102–107.

39. Bonner BP, Deivert RG, Gould TE. The relationship between isometric contraction durations during hold–relax stretching and improvement of hamstring flexibility. *J Sports Med Phys Fitness.* 2004;44:258–261.

40. de Weijer VC, Gorniak GC, Shamus E. The effect of static stretch and warm-up exercise on hamstring length over the course of 24 hours. *J Orthop Sports Phys Ther.* 2003;33:727–733.

41. Roberts JM, Wilson K. Effect of stretching duration on active and passive range of motion in the lower extremity. *Br J Sports Med.* 1999;33:259–263.

42. Meyer JJ, Zachman ZJ, Keating JC, Traina AD. Effectiveness of chiropractic management for patellofemoral pain syndrome's symptomatic control phase: A single subject experiment. *J Manipulative Physiol Ther.* 1990;13:539–549.

43. Moss P, Sluka K, Wright A. The initial effects of knee joint mobilization on osteoarthritic hyperalgesia. *Man Ther.* 2007;12:109–118.

44. Gugel MR, Johnston WL. Osteopathic manipulative treatment of a 27-year-old man after anterior cruciate ligament reconstruction. *J Am Osteopath.* 2006;106(6): 346–349.

45. van der Dolden PA, Roberts DL. Six sessions of manual therapy increase knee flexion and improve activity in people with anterior knee pain: A randomised controlled trial. *Aust J Physiother.* 2006;52(4):261–264.

46. Deyle G, Allison S, Matekel R, et al. Physical therapy treatment effectiveness for osteoarthritis of the knee: A randomized comparison of supervised clinical exercise and manual therapy procedures versus a home exercise program. *Phys Ther.* 2005;85:1301–1317.

47. Deyle GD, Henderson NE, Matekel RL, Ryder MG, Garber MB, Allison SC. Effectiveness of manual physical therapy and exercise in osteoarthritis of the knee: A randomized, controlled trial. *Ann Intern Med.* 2000;132(3):173–181.

48. Pollard H, Ward G, Hoskins W, Hardy K. The effect of a manual therapy knee protocol on osteoarthritic knee pain: A randomised controlled trial. *JCCA J Can Chiropr Assoc.* 2008;52:229–242.

49. Manske RC, Davies DJ. A non-surgical approach to examination and treatment of the patellofemoral joint, part 1. Examination of the patellofemoral joint. *Critical Reviews in Physical & Rehabilitation Medicine.* 2003;15(2):141–166.

50. Watson CJ, Leddy HM, Dynjan TD, Parham JL. Reliability of the lateral pull test and tilt test to assess patellar alignment in subjects with symptomatic knees: student raters. *J Orthop Sports Phys Ther.* 2001;31(7): 368–374.

51. Watson CJ, Propps M, Gait W, Redding A, Dobbs D. Reliability of McConnell's classification of patellar orientation in symptomatic and asymptomatic subjects, including commentary by McConnell J and Dye SF with author responses. *J Orthop Sports Phys Ther.* 1999;29(7):379–393.

52. Powers CM, Mortenson S, Nishimoto D, Simon D. Criterion-related validity of a clinical measurement to determine the medial/lateral component of patellar orientation. *J Orthop Sports Phys Ther.* 1999;29(7):372–377.

53. Herrington LC. The inter-tester reliability of a clinical measurement used to determine the medial/lateral orientation of the patella. *Man Ther.* 2002;7(3):163–167.

54. Crossley K, Bennell K, Green S, McConnell J. A systematic review of physical interventions for patellofemoral pain syndrome. *Clin J Sport Med.* 2001;11(2):103–110.

55. Crossley KM, Cowan SM, McConnell J, Bennell KL. Physical therapy improves knee flexion during stair ambulation in patellofemoral pain. *Med Sci Sports Exerc.* 2005;37(2):176–183.

56. Harris GR, Susman JL. Managing musculoskeletal complaints with rehabilitation therapy: Summary of the Philadelphia Panel evidence-based clinical practice guidelines on musculoskeletal rehabilitation interventions. *J Fam Pract.* 2002;51(12):1042–1046.

57. Ghaffarinejad F, Taghizadeh S, Mohammadi F. Effect of static stretching of muscles surrounding the knee on knee joint position sense. *Br J Sports Med*. 2007;41: 684–687.

58. Fasen JM, O'Connor AM, Schwartz SL, et al. A randomized controlled trial of hamstring stretching: comparison of four techniques. *J Strength Cond Res*. 2009; 23:660–667.

59. Bonutti PM, McGrath MS, Ulrich SD, McKenzie SA, Seyler TM, Mont MA. Static progressive stretch for the treatment of knee stiffness. *Knee*. 2008;15:272–276.

60. Peeler J, Anderson JE. Effectiveness of static quadriceps stretching in individuals with patellofemoral joint pain. *Clin J Sports Med*. 2007;17:234–241.

61. Currier LL, Froehlich PJ, Carow SD, et al. Development of a clinical prediction rule to identify patients with knee pain and clinical evidence of knee osteoarthritis who demonstrate a favorable short-term response to hip mobilization. *Phys Ther*. 2007;87(9):1106–1119.

62. Iverson CA, Sutlive TG, Crowell MS. Lumbopelvic manipulation for the treatment of patients with patellofemoral pain syndrome: Development of a clinical prediction rule. *J Orthop Sports Phys Ther*. 2008;38(6): 297–309.

63. Brantingham JW, Globe G, Pollard H, Hicks M, Korporaal C, Hoskins W. Manipulative therapy for lower extremity conditions: expansion of literature review. *J Manipulative Physiol Ther*. 2009;32:53–71.

Manual Therapy of the Foot and Ankle

Ken Learman and Chad Cook

Objectives

- Outline the pertinent clinically relevant anatomy of the foot and ankle.
- Understand the clinical examination of the foot and ankle.
- Outline an effective treatment program for various foot and ankle impairments.
- Identify the outcomes associated with orthopedic manual therapy to the foot and ankle.

Clinical Examination

Differential or Contributory Diagnoses

Consequential foot and ankle disorders are common with conditions such as diabetes. These disorders may exist as stand-alone dysfunctions or primary pathologies. Peripheral vascular disease, a common comorbidity in patients with diabetes, may lead to skin breakdown, pain, burning symptoms, and secondary musculoskeletal disorders of the foot and ankle.[1]

Neurological conditions may mimic foot and ankle dysfunction and require careful differentiation. Individuals with a history of alcoholism, diabetes, and vitamin deficiency are more likely to report radiculopathic-mimicking symptoms than those without these comorbidities.[2] A comprehensive lumbar examination may be required if the patient reports radiating or burning pain at the ankle.[2,3] Discomfort that exhibits radicular-like symptoms may be associated with a nerve root entrapment or radicular pain from the lumbar spine.[2,3] Conditions such as tarsal tunnel syndrome often result in pain patterns that are nonspecific.[2] In many cases, patients with tarsal tunnel syndrome report increased pain at night, often awakening the patient.[2]

Ottawa Ankle Rules

The Ottawa ankle rules were developed in 1992 to reduce the necessity of radiographic imagery after the occurrence of an ankle sprain. Prior to the onset of these rules, nearly every ankle sprained was x-rayed even though less than 15% of ankle sprains result in a fracture.[4,5] The rules dictate the need for an ankle radiograph if a patient demonstrates (1) bone tenderness at the posterior edge or tip of the lateral malleolus and/or (2) bone tenderness at the posterior edge or tip of the medial malleolus, and/or (3) inability to bear weight both immediately and in emergency room. The rules also dictate the need for a foot radiograph if a patient demonstrates (1) bone tenderness at the base of the fifth metatarsal bone, and/or (2) bone tenderness at the navicular, and/or (3) inability to bear weight both immediately and in the emergency room. A summary of several studies has demonstrated that the negative presence of these factors is excellent at ruling out the presence of a fracture ($-LR = 0.07$; $CI = 0.03-0.18$).[5]

Summary

- A myriad of nonmechanical disorders exist for the foot. These disorders consist of neurological, referred pains, and vascular disorders.
- The *Ottawa ankle rules* are specific measurements designed to identify patients with a fracture after an ankle sprain.

Observation

Primarily, observational methods in detecting foot and ankle disorders are focused on three criteria. The first criterion involves inspection of the foot and ankle during standing. Abnormal alignment of the forefoot and hindfoot that is associated with a concordant pain (pain during stance) may require specific intervention such as orthotics or stabilization. The status of the longitudinal arch may provide the clinician with an understanding of the support mechanisms of the foot and the biomechanical consequences associated with important findings. For example, failure of the longitudinal arch may result in a phenomenon known as "too many toes." This phenomenon when viewed posteriorly appears to demonstrate too many digits (Figure 14.1 ■) when in reality the fallen arch increases the amount of pronation during static stance.

The second criterion includes a gait evaluation. Patients should be asked to walk toward and then away from the examiner, walking forward and backward. If no abnormality is revealed by basic gait, then the subject could be asked to walk on toes both toward and away from the examiner followed by walking on heels in maximum dorsiflexion toward and away. If this is not provocative of symptoms and compensation, the subject could be asked to hop on toes and hop on heels to attempt to stimulate the concordant sign.[6]

The third criterion involves a skin and nail inspection. Trophic changes may be indicative of peripheral vascular disease. Pigmentation may be associated with venous insufficiency. Significant callus formation may be a consequence of abnormal gait or increased pressure during weight bearing. Toenail disorders may be a result of psoriasis, poor blood flow, and/or infection.[2]

Summary

- Observational strategies during the examination of the ankle foot complex (AFC) include biomechanical assessment of hindfoot and forefoot alignment.

- Often, a gait evaluation will identify a concordant abnormality in the ankle foot complex (AFC).

- Inspection of the skin and toenails may assist in identifying disorders such as vascular problems, psoriasis, and infections.

Patient History

Important history items collected during a subjective examination include the presence of comorbidities, any relevant past history of ankle disorders, a history of surgery, and occupational and avocation demands.[2] Ascertaining the mechanism of injury may assist in determining the likelihood of the presence of a fracture. High-impact injuries or profound ankle sprains should automatically initiate the assessment of the Ottawa ankle rules discussed earlier.[7]

The behavior of the symptoms may help outline the cause of the disorder. Locking disorders that exhibit an intermittent pattern may be indicative of osteochondritis dissecans (OD) of the talar dome.[7] Pain associated with OD should be queried to differentiate from anterior impingement at the joint line. Anterior impingement is consistently triggered during dorsiflexion at end range while OD may occur intermittently and during different planes of movement.

Lateral ankle pain associated with a sprain is the most common form of ankle injury and usually results from an inversion sprain.[8] Often, individuals report a previous injury that was similar in context. Some may report a "pop" during the injury, which may represent a tear in the surrounding ligamentous structure.[8] A pop is also associated with Achilles tendon tears and should be differentiated using the appropriate physical examination methods.

Conditions such as plantar fasciitis are more common in middle-aged individuals and usually begin with a gradual onset of symptoms. Pain is typically isolated to the plantar aspect of the heel and is worsened during gait without shoe wear that stabilizes the

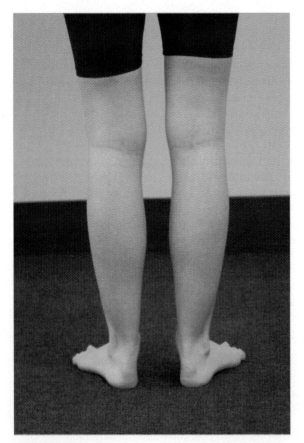

■ **Figure 14.1** Observation of Abnormal Ankle Biomechanics during Stance: Too Many Toes

foot. Plantar fasciitis differs from midfoot arthritis in etiology, but exhibits very similar characteristics. Patients will also complain of pain without supportive shoe wear, but will generally complain of pain in the arch or forefoot region, specifically at the Lisfranc joint.

Disability associated with AFC impairment is occasionally underreported. It has been stated that at least one-third of the time required for recovery is associated with the failure of appropriate measurement for ankle patients.[9] One reason may be associated with the relatively small loss of range of motion noted in acute ankle sprains. Small losses of range of motion can lead to significant reports of disability and adding activity limitation measures to the assessment may improve prediction of duration of disability and return to activity.[9]

Summary

- One essential element of the patient history during the examination of an AFC is the mechanism of injury.

- One of the reasons patients fail to recover is the inability to measure properly the disability associated with an AFC.

Physical Examination

Active Physiological Movements

The focus of the active physiological examination is the reproduction of the concordant sign during activities.[7] Eliciting the concordant sign may require variations of physical activities, responses, or functional activities. By examining the activity performed during the concordant complaint the clinician may improve the likelihood of isolating the disorder.

A common method of elicitation of the concordant sign is the use of functional movements. Some of the movements such as stance and gait were discussed in the observation section of this chapter. Others, such as hopping, running, occupational-related activities, and additional static positions may further distill the underlying elements of the concordant pain. Because the quantities of functional movements that affect the ankle are of large quantity, it is impossible to represent these movements pictorially. However, functional activities such as single leg hopping, step-ups (Figure 14.2 ■), and talar rotation during unilateral stance (Figure 14.3 ■) may be useful in eliciting the concordant sign. Lark et al.[10] reported that older adults required necessary range of motion at the ankle, specifically controlled dorsiflexion, in order to ambulate using stairs. A step-down is a modification that may be useful to determine the availability of functional range of motion.

The peroneus longus assists in propulsion of the foot during push-off. One method of assessing the ability of

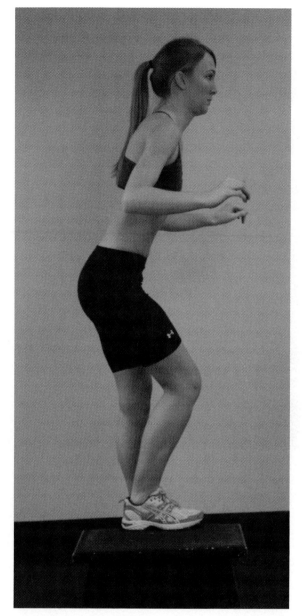

■ Figure 14.2   Step-Ups

the peroneus longus to stabilize during this process is the bilateral peroneus longus test. This test involves the simultaneous action of plantarflexion and eversion during weight bearing. Weakness or injury to the peroneus longus will result in the concordant reproduction of pain or inability to perform upon demand.

Summary

- The focus of the active physiological examination is the reproduction of the concordant sign during activities.

- Functional movements are best performed to outline the problems associated with the AFC.

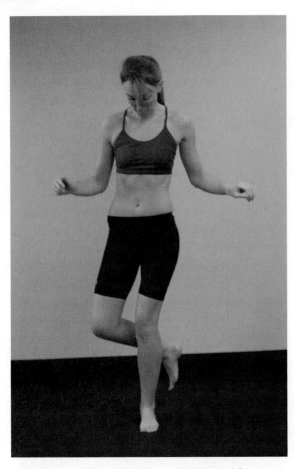

■ **Figure 14.3** Talar Rotation during Unilateral Stance

Passive Movements

Passive Physiological Movements Although passive movements of the foot and ankle involve axes of movements that are multiplanar, it is easiest to define the movements by plane of motion. These planes include plantarflexion, dorsiflexion, abduction, adduction, and the combined planar movements of inversion and eversion.

Plane-Based Movements Plane-based movements are those that are aligned with sagittal, coronal, and transverse movements.

Plantarflexion

1. The patient is placed in prone position with the knee flexed.
2. Resting pain is assessed.
3. The examiner places the posterior hand on the postero-plantar calcaneus and the anterior hand on the dorsal forefoot.
4. The foot and ankle are then passively plantarflexed to the first point of concordant pain (if present). Repeated movements or sustained holds are applied to determine if the symptoms increase or decrease.
5. The foot and ankle is then passively moved toward end range, allowing the same process of assessment for repeated movements and sustained holds. Differentiation of whole foot (Figure 14.4 ■) and midfoot (Figure 14.5 ■) can be made with hand placement changes.

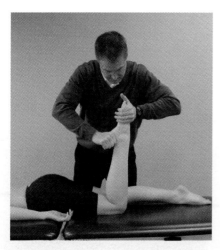

■ **Figure 14.4**   Plantarflexion of the Whole Foot

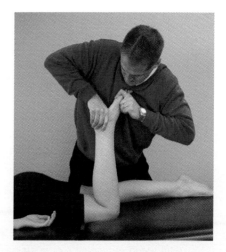

■ **Figure 14.5**   Plantarflexion of the Midfoot

⑥ The clinician stabilizes the hindfoot and passively applies a plantarflexion force on the midfoot.

⑦ Pain and range behavior is reassessed.

⑧ The forefoot can be differentiated from the midfoot by stabilizing the midfoot and forcing the forefoot into plantarflexion (Figure 14.6 ■).

⑨ Pain and range behavior is reassessed.

⑩ A comparison of the patient's reaction to pain with the various positions implicates which anatomical region is the likely source of the pain.

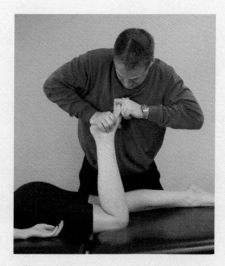

■ **Figure 14.6**   Forefoot Plantarflexion

Dorsiflexion

1. The patient is placed in prone position with the knee flexed.

2. Resting pain is assessed.

3. The examiner places the posterior hand on the postero-dorsal calcaneus (over the calcaneal tendon) and the other hand on the palmar surface of the foot.

4. The foot and ankle are then passively dorsiflexed to the first point of concordant pain (if present) (Figure 14.7 ■). Repeated movements or sustained holds are applied to determine if the symptoms increase or decrease.

5. The foot and ankle is then passively moved toward end range, allowing the same process of assessment for repeated movements and sustained holds.

6. Differentiation of hindfoot from the midfoot is made by stabilizing the hindfoot and promoting dorsiflexion of the midfoot (Figure 14.8 ■). Pain and range behavior is reassessed.

7. Differentiation of the forefoot from the midfoot is made by stabilizing the midfoot and applying a dorsiflexion force to the forefoot (Figure 14.9 ■). Pain and range behavior is reassessed.

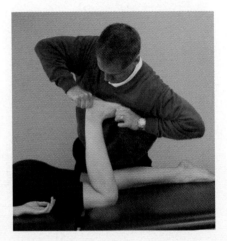

■ **Figure 14.7** Dorsiflexion of the Whole Foot

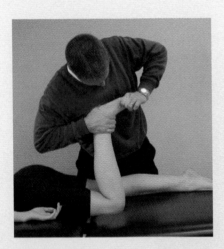

■ **Figure 14.8** Dorsiflexion of the Midfoot from the Hindfoot

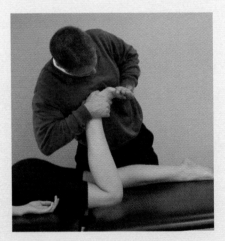

■ **Figure 14.9** Dorsiflexion of the Forefoot

Abduction

1️⃣ The patient is placed in prone position with the knee flexed.

2️⃣ Resting pain is assessed.

3️⃣ The examiner places the posterior hand on the postero-lateral calcaneus and the anterior hand on the medial forefoot.

4️⃣ The foot and ankle are then passively abducted (Figure 14.10 ■) to the first point of concordant pain (if present). Repeated movements or sustained holds are applied to determine if the symptoms increase or decrease.

5️⃣ The foot and ankle is then passively moved toward end range, allowing the same process of assessment for repeated movements and sustained holds.

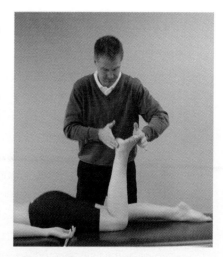

■ **Figure 14.10**   Abduction of the Whole Foot

6️⃣ Differentiation of hind, mid, and forefoot can be made with hand-placement changes. The midfoot is differentiated by stabilizing the hindfoot and promoting abduction at the transversetarsal joint (Figure 14.11 ■). Pain and range behavior is reassessed.

7️⃣ The forefoot and midfoot can be differentiated by stabilizing the midfoot and abducting the forefoot (Figure 14.12 ■). Pain and range behavior is reassessed.

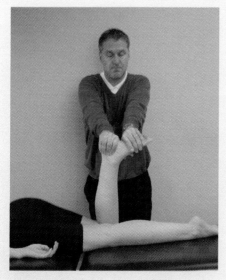

■ **Figure 14.11**   Abduction of the Midfoot in Relation to the Hindfoot

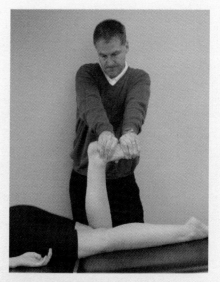

■ **Figure 14.12**   Adduction of the Forefoot Relative to the Midfoot

Adduction

① The patient is placed in prone with the knee flexed.

② Resting pain is assessed.

③ The examiner places the posterior hand on the postero-medial calcaneus and the anterior hand on the lateral forefoot.

④ The foot and ankle are then passively adducted to the first point of concordant pain (if present). Repeated movements or sustained holds are applied to determine if the symptoms increase or decrease.

⑤ The foot and ankle is then passively moved toward end range (the right leg is tested in Figure 14.13 ■), allowing the same process of assessment for repeated movements and sustained holds.

⑥ Differentiation of hind, mid, and forefoot can be made with hand-placement changes. Differentiation of the midfoot relative to the hindfoot is accomplished by stabilizing the hindfoot and promoting adduction at the transverse joint (Figure 14.14 ■). Pain and range behavior is established.

⑦ Differentiation of the forefoot from the midfoot is accomplished by stabilizing the midfoot and promoting adduction at the Lisfranc joint (Figure 14.15 ■). Pain and range behavior is reassessed.

⑧ A comparison of the patient's reaction to pain with the various positions implicates which anatomical region is the likely source of the pain.

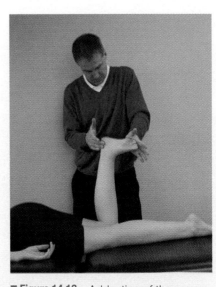

■ **Figure 14.13** Adduction of the Whole Foot

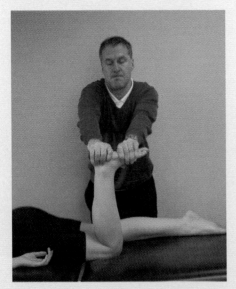

■ **Figure 14.14** Adduction of the Midfoot Relative to the Hindfoot

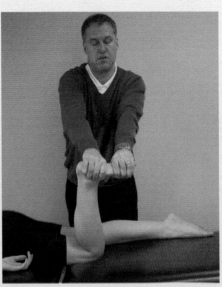

■ **Figure 14.15** Abduction of the Forefoot on the Midfoot

Abduction

1. The patient is placed in prone position with the knee flexed.

2. Resting pain is assessed.

3. The examiner places the posterior hand on the postero-lateral calcaneus and the anterior hand on the medial forefoot.

4. The foot and ankle are then passively abducted (Figure 14.10 ■) to the first point of concordant pain (if present). Repeated movements or sustained holds are applied to determine if the symptoms increase or decrease.

5. The foot and ankle is then passively moved toward end range, allowing the same process of assessment for repeated movements and sustained holds.

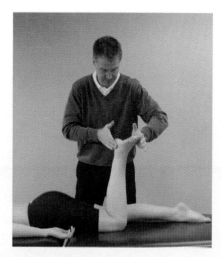

■ **Figure 14.10** Abduction of the Whole Foot

6. Differentiation of hind, mid, and forefoot can be made with hand-placement changes. The midfoot is differentiated by stabilizing the hindfoot and promoting abduction at the transversetarsal joint (Figure 14.11 ■). Pain and range behavior is reassessed.

7. The forefoot and midfoot can be differentiated by stabilizing the midfoot and abducting the forefoot (Figure 14.12 ■). Pain and range behavior is reassessed.

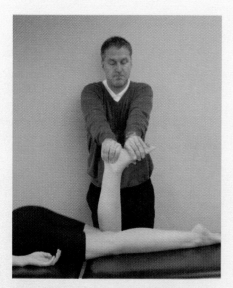

■ **Figure 14.11** Abduction of the Midfoot in Relation to the Hindfoot

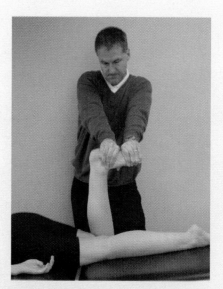

■ **Figure 14.12** Adduction of the Forefoot Relative to the Midfoot

Adduction

1. The patient is placed in prone with the knee flexed.

2. Resting pain is assessed.

3. The examiner places the posterior hand on the postero-medial calcaneus and the anterior hand on the lateral forefoot.

4. The foot and ankle are then passively adducted to the first point of concordant pain (if present). Repeated movements or sustained holds are applied to determine if the symptoms increase or decrease.

5. The foot and ankle is then passively moved toward end range (the right leg is tested in Figure 14.13 ■), allowing the same process of assessment for repeated movements and sustained holds.

6. Differentiation of hind, mid, and forefoot can be made with hand-placement changes. Differentiation of the midfoot relative to the hindfoot is accomplished by stabilizing the hindfoot and promoting adduction at the transverse joint (Figure 14.14 ■). Pain and range behavior is established.

7. Differentiation of the forefoot from the midfoot is accomplished by stabilizing the midfoot and promoting adduction at the Lisfranc joint (Figure 14.15 ■). Pain and range behavior is reassessed.

8. A comparison of the patient's reaction to pain with the various positions implicates which anatomical region is the likely source of the pain.

■ **Figure 14.13** Adduction of the Whole Foot

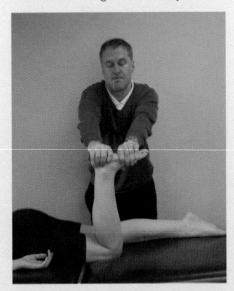

■ **Figure 14.14** Adduction of the Midfoot Relative to the Hindfoot

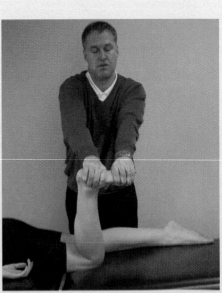

■ **Figure 14.15** Abduction of the Forefoot on the Midfoot

Combined Passive Physiological Movements Combined passive physiological movements are useful in detection of articular or capsular structures. Inversion and eversion are considered combined movements.

Inversion

1 The patient is placed in prone position with the knee flexed.

2 Resting pain is assessed.

3 The examiner places the posterior hand on the calcaneus (fingers medially and thumb laterally) and the anterior hand on the forefoot (fingers medially and thumb laterally).

4 The foot and ankle are then passively inverted (Figure 14.16 ■) as the clinician pushes the foot away from his or her body in a curvilinear fashion. This movement occurs to the first point of pain and the process is repeated at end range as well. Behavior with repeated movements or sustained holds is recorded.

5 Differentiation of hind, mid, and forefoot can be made with hand-placement changes. The midfoot is differentiated from the hindfoot by blocking the hindfoot and promoting an inversion movement at the midfoot (Figure 14.17 ■). Pain and range behavior is assessed.

6 The forefoot can be differentiated by stabilizing the midfoot and promoting inversion at the forefoot. Pain and range behavior is reassessed.

7 A comparison of the patient's reaction to pain with the various positions implicates which anatomical region is the likely source of the pain.

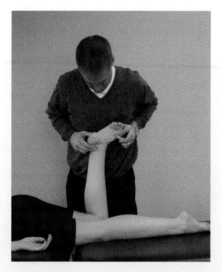

■ **Figure 14.16**   Inversion of the Whole Foot

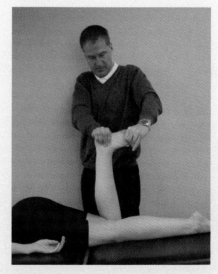

■ **Figure 14.17**   Inversion of the Midfoot with Respect to the Hindfoot

Eversion

1. The patient is placed in prone with the knee flexed.

2. Resting pain is assessed.

3. The examiner places the posterior hand on the calcaneus (fingers medially and thumb laterally) and the anterior hand on the forefoot (fingers medially and thumb laterally).

4. The foot and ankle are then passively inverted (Figure 14.18 ■) as the clinician pushes the foot away from his or her body in a curvilinear fashion. This movement occurs to the first point of pain and the process is repeated at end range as well. Behavior with repeated movements or sustained holds is recorded.

5. Differentiation of hind, mid, and forefoot can be made with hand-placement changes. The midfoot is differentiated from the hindfoot by blocking the hindfoot and promoting an eversion movement at the midfoot (Figure 14.19 ■). Pain and range behavior is assessed.

6. The forefoot can be differentiated by stabilizing the midfoot and promoting eversion at the forefoot. Pain and range behavior is reassessed.

7. A comparison of the patient's reaction to pain with the various positions implicates which anatomical region is the likely source of the pain.

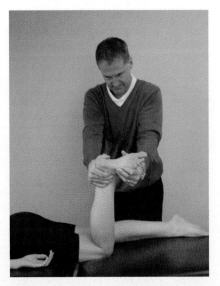

■ **Figure 14.18** Eversion of the Whole Foot

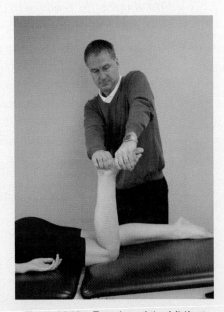

■ **Figure 14.19** Eversion of the Midfoot with Respect to the Hindfoot

Summary

- The purpose of passive physiological movements is to reproduce the concordant sign.
- Passive physiological movement further localizes AFC movements that contribute to concordant patient complaints.
- Passive physiological movements may be single-plane or combined to engage the articular or surrounding structures.

Passive Accessory Movements The arthrokinematics at the multiple joints of the ankle foot complex are wrought with multiplanar movements, complicated rolling and gliding behaviors, and variable facet architecture. By addressing the pain provocation response the clinician is able to determine the concordant response and can cross the boundaries of complexities among the numerous joints.

Antero–Posterior Glide of the Inferior Tibial Fibular Joint

1. The patient assumes a sidelying position with the medial border of the foot placed on the plinth, the clinician is standing in front of the patient facing the foot.

2. Resting symptom level is assessed.

3. The clinician places one thumb on the anterior border of the distal fibula (the anterior border is oblique so care must be taken to stay on the bone), whereas the other hand stabilizes the tibia.

4. The clinician performs a joint play movement by mobilizing the distal fibula directly posteriorly (Figure 14.20 ■) until the patient first reports concordant discomfort. The movement is repeated or sustained to assess the response of the movement.

5. The movement is then performed near end range. The movement is also repeated or sustained to assess the response of the movement on the concordant sign.

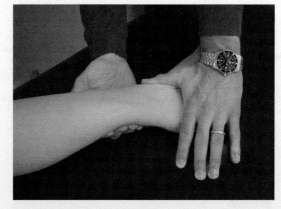

■ **Figure 14.20**   Anterior–Posterior Glide of the Inferior Tibial Fibular Joint

Postero–Anterior Glide of the Inferior Tibial Fibular Joint

1. The patient assumes a sidelying position with the medial border of the foot placed on a plinth, the clinician is standing behind the patient facing the heel.

2. Resting symptom level is assessed.

3. The clinician places one thumb on the posterior shelf of the distal fibula, whereas the other hand stabilizes the tibia.

4. The clinician performs a joint play movement by mobilizing the distal fibula directly anteriorly (Figure 14.21 ■) until the patient first reports concordant discomfort. The movement is repeated or sustained to assess the response of the movement.

5. The movement is then performed near end range. The movement is also repeated or sustained to assess the response of the movement on the concordant sign.

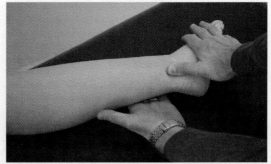

■ **Figure 14.21**   Posterior–Anterior Glide of the Inferior Tibial Fibular Joint

Caudal Glide of the Inferior Tibial Fibular Joint

1. The patient assumes a sidelying position with the medial border of the foot placed on a plinth.

2. The clinician stands cephalically to the foot of the patient.

3. The clinician performs a caudal glide of the fibula by inverting the hindfoot until the patient reports concordant discomfort (Figure 14.22 ■). The movement is sustained or repeated to assess the outcome of the technique.

4. The movement is then performed at end range to elicit a concordant sign. If concordant, repeated or sustained movements are performed.

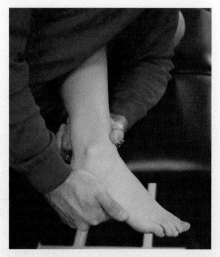

■ **Figure 14.22** Caudal Glide of the Inferior Tibial Femoral Joint

Cephalad Glide of the Tibial Femoral Joint

1. The patient assumes a sidelying position with the medial border of the foot placed on a plinth.

2. The clinician stands caudally to the foot of the patient.

3. The clinician performs a cephalad glide of the fibula by everting the hindfoot until the patient reports concordant discomfort. The movement is sustained or repeated to assess the outcome of the technique (Figure 14.23 ■).

4. The movement is then performed at end range to elicit a concordant sign. If concordant, repeated or sustained movements are performed.

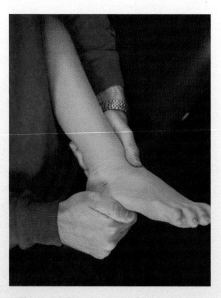

■ **Figure 14.23** Cephalic Glide of the Inferior Tibial Femoral Joint

Antero–Posterior Glide of the Talocrural Joint

During dorsiflexion, the talus rolls superiorly and moves posteriorly. An anterior to posterior glide of the talus should theoretically improve passive dorsiflexion.

1. The patient is placed in prone position with the knee flexed.

2. Resting pain is assessed.

3. The examiner places the posterior hand on the distal tibia and fibula and the anterior hand on the head of the talus with the elbows pointing out away from each other (Figure 14.24 ■).

4. With the tibia and fibula stabilized, an anterior to posterior force is exerted on the talus until the patient reports concordant pain. If the pain reported is concordant, the movement is repeated or sustained to determine the effect of the technique.

5. The movement is then taken beyond the first point of pain toward end range. If the pain is concordant, the technique is repeated or sustained at end range.

A reduction of symptoms associated with this technique may suggest that the procedure is a plausible treatment procedure.

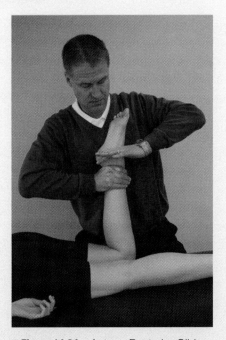

■ **Figure 14.24**   Antero–Posterior Glide
of the Talocrural Joint

Postero–Anterior Glide of the Talocrural Joint

During plantarflexion, the articular surface of the talus slides anteriorly while the distal talus rotates posteriorly. A posterior to anterior glide of the talus on the calcaneus should theoretically improve passive plantarflexion.

1. The patient is placed in prone position with the knee flexed.

2. Resting pain is assessed.

3. The examiner places the posterior hand on the head of the talus and the anterior hand on the distal tibia and fibula with the elbows pointing out away from each other (Figure 14.25 ■).

4. With the tibia and fibula stabilized, a posterior to anterior force is exerted on the talus until the patient reports concordant pain. If the pain reported is concordant, the movement is repeated or sustained to determine the effect of the technique.

5. The movement is then taken beyond the first point of pain toward end range. If the pain is concordant, the technique is repeated or sustained at end range.

A reduction of symptoms associated with this technique may suggest that the procedure is a plausible treatment procedure.

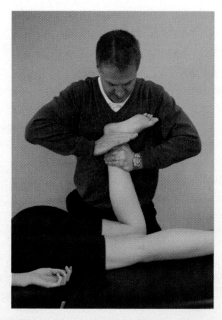

■ **Figure 14.25** Postero–Anterior Glide of the Talocrural Joint

Medial Rotation of the Talocrural Joint

1. The patient is placed in prone position with the knee flexed.

2. Resting pain is assessed.

3. The examiner places the posterior hand on the distal tibia and fibula and the anterior hand on the head of the talus with the elbows pointing out away from each other.

4. With the tibia and fibula stabilized, medial rotation of the talus is performed until the patient reports concordant pain (Figure 14.26 ■). If the pain reported is concordant, the movement is repeated or sustained to determine the effect of the technique.

⑤ The movement is then taken beyond the first point of pain toward end range. If the pain is concordant, the technique is repeated or sustained at end range.

A reduction of symptoms associated with this technique may suggest that the procedure is a plausible treatment procedure.

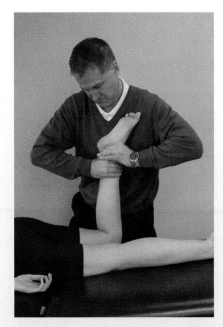

■ **Figure 14.26** Medial Rotation of the Talocrural Joint

Lateral Rotation of the Talocrural Joint

① The patient is placed in prone position with the knee flexed.

② Resting pain is assessed.

③ The examiner places the posterior hand on the distal tibia and fibula and the anterior hand on the head of the talus with the elbows pointing out away from each other.

④ With the tibia and fibula stabilized, lateral rotation of the talus is performed until the patient reports concordant pain (Figure 14.27 ■). If the pain reported is concordant, the movement is repeated or sustained to determine the effect of the technique.

⑤ The movement is then taken beyond the first point of pain toward end range. If the pain is concordant, the technique is repeated or sustained at end range.

A reduction of symptoms associated with this technique may suggest that the procedure is a plausible treatment procedure.

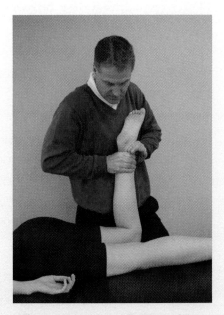

■ **Figure 14.27** Lateral Rotation of the Talocrural Joint

Longitudinal Distraction of the Talocrural Joint

1. The patient is placed in supine position with the knee bent to 90 degrees.

2. The knee of the clinician is placed on the posterior thigh of the patient for stabilization.

3. The examiner places one hand under the foot, cupping the calcaneus and the other hand on the dorsum of the foot with the fifth digit on the head of the talus (Figure 14.28 ■). The clinician lifts up with his or her body to distract the talocrural joint.

4. The movement is then taken beyond the first point of pain toward end range. If the pain is concordant, the technique is repeated or sustained at end range.

A reduction of symptoms associated with this technique may suggest that the procedure is a plausible treatment procedure.

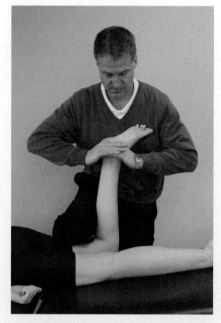

■ **Figure 14.28** Longitudinal Distraction of the Talocrural Joint

Postero–Anterior Movement of the Subtalar Joint

1. The patient is placed in prone position with the knee flexed.

2. Resting pain is assessed.

3. The examiner places the posterior hand on the calcaneus and the anterior hand on the head of the talus with the elbows pointing out away from each other.

4. With the talus stabilized (anteriorly), a posterior to anterior force is exerted on the calcaneus until the patient reports concordant pain (Figure 14.29 ■). If the pain reported is concordant, the movement is repeated or sustained to determine the effect of the technique.

5. The movement is then taken beyond the first point of pain toward end range. If the pain is concordant, the technique is repeated or sustained at end range.

A reduction of symptoms associated with this technique may suggest that the procedure is a plausible treatment procedure.

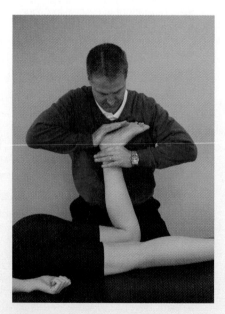

■ **Figure 14.29** Postero–Anterior Movement of the Subtalar Joint

Antero–Posterior Glide of the Subtalar Joint

1. The patient is placed in prone position with the knee flexed.

2. Resting pain is assessed.

3. The examiner places the posterior hand on the talus and the anterior hand on the anterior calcaneus with the elbows pointing out away from each other.

4. The calcaneus is stabilized and the talus is mobilized anteriorly (from its posterior contact) (Figure 14.30 ■). If the pain reported is concordant, the movement is repeated or sustained to determine the effect of the technique.

5. The movement is then taken beyond the first point of pain toward end range. If the pain is concordant, the technique is repeated or sustained at end range.

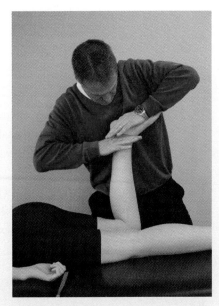

■ **Figure 14.30** Antero–Posterior Glide of the Subtalar Joint

A reduction of symptoms associated with this technique may suggest that the procedure is a plausible treatment procedure.

Medial Rotation of the Subtalar Joint

1. The patient is placed in prone position with the knee flexed.

2. Resting pain is assessed.

3. The examiner places the posterior hand on the calcaneus and the anterior hand on the head of the talus with the elbows pointing out away from each other.

4. With the talus stabilized, medial rotation of the calcaneus (reference point is the heel not anatomical neutral) is performed until the patient reports concordant pain (Figure 14.31 ■). If the pain reported is concordant, the movement is repeated or sustained to determine the effect of the technique.

5. The movement is then taken beyond the first point of pain toward end range. If the pain is concordant, the technique is repeated or sustained at end range.

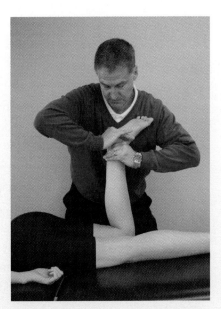

■ **Figure 14.31** Medial Rotation of the Subtalar Joint

A reduction of symptoms associated with this technique may suggest that the procedure is a plausible treatment procedure.

Lateral Rotation of the Subtalar Joint

1. The patient is placed in prone position with the knee flexed.

2. Resting pain is assessed.

3. The examiner places the posterior hand on the calcaneus and the anterior hand on the head of the talus with the elbows pointing out away from each other (Figure 14.32 ■).

4. With the talus stabilized, lateral rotation of the calcaneus is performed (reference point is the heel not anatomical neutral) until the patient reports concordant pain. If the pain reported is concordant, the movement is repeated or sustained to determine the effect of the technique.

5. The movement is then taken beyond the first point of pain toward end range. If the pain is concordant, the technique is repeated or sustained at end range.

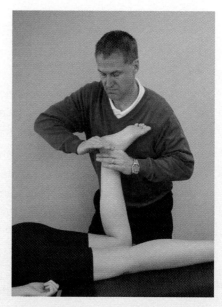

■ **Figure 14.32**   Lateral Rotation of the Subtalar Joint

A reduction of symptoms associated with this technique may suggest that the procedure is a plausible treatment procedure.

Medial Glide of the Subtalar Joint

1. The patient assumes a sidelying position with the medial border of the leg placed on the clinician's forearm and the foot hanging off the mat, the clinician is standing facing the patient's foot.

2. Resting symptom level is assessed.

3. The clinician takes the hindfoot in the distal hand with the thenar eminence firmly placed against the lateral calcaneus and the proximal hand stabilizing the lower leg (from underneath) with the forefinger on the medial malleolus and talus (Figure 14.33 ■).

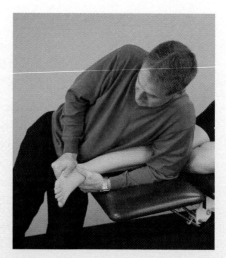

■ **Figure 14.33**   Medial Glide of the Subtalar Joint

④ The clinician performs a medial glide toward the floor while an eversion movement is provided to prevent the motion from becoming an inversion curvilinear movement rather than a medial glide of the calcaneus on the talus. The movement is provided until the patient reports concordant pain. If the pain reported is concordant, the movement is repeated or sustained to determine the effect of the technique.

⑤ The movement is then taken beyond the first point of pain toward end range. If the pain is concordant, the technique is repeated or sustained at end range.

A reduction of symptoms associated with this technique may suggest that the procedure is a plausible treatment procedure.

Lateral Glide of the Subtalar Joint

① The patient assumes a sidelying position with the lateral border of the leg placed on the clinician's forearm and the foot hanging off the mat, the clinician is standing in front of the patient facing the foot.

② Resting symptom level is assessed.

③ The clinician takes the hindfoot in the distal hand with the thenar eminence firmly placed against the medial calcaneus and the proximal hand stabilizing the lower leg (from underneath) with the forefinger on the lateral malleolus and talus.

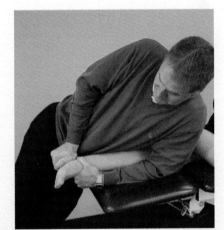

■ **Figure 14.34**   Lateral Glide of the Subtalar Joint

④ The clinician performs a lateral glide toward the floor while an inversion movement (Figure 14.34 ■) is provided to prevent the motion from becoming an eversion curvilinear movement rather than a lateral glide of the calcaneus on the talus. The movement is provided until the patient reports concordant pain. If the pain reported is concordant, the movement is repeated or sustained to determine the effect of the technique.

⑤ The movement is then taken beyond the first point of pain toward end range. If the pain is concordant, the technique is repeated or sustained at end range.

A reduction of symptoms associated with this technique may suggest that the procedure is a plausible treatment procedure.

Horizontal Flexion of the Forefoot

1. The patient is placed in prone position with the knee flexed.

2. Resting pain is assessed.

3. The examiner places both hands interlaced on the dorsum of the foot with both thumbs on the plantar surface.

4. The thenar aspect of the thumbs perform a mobilizing movement in a plantar to dorsal direction (Figure 14.35 ■) while the fingers draw the rays around the thumbs to increase the horizontal arch until the patient reports concordant pain. If the pain reported is concordant, the movement is repeated or sustained to determine the effect of the technique.

5. The movement is then taken beyond the first point of pain toward end range. If the pain is concordant, the technique is repeated or sustained at end range.

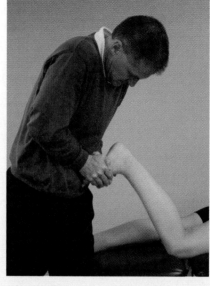

■ **Figure 14.35**   Horizontal Flexion of the Forefoot

A reduction of symptoms associated with this technique may suggest that the procedure is a plausible treatment procedure.

Horizontal Extension of the Forefoot

1. The patient is placed in prone position with the knee flexed.

2. Resting pain is assessed.

3. The examiner places both hands interlaced on the plantar surface of the foot with both thumbs on the dorsal surface.

4. The thumbs perform a mobilizing movement in a dorsal to plantar direction (Figure 14.36 ■) while the fingers draw the rays around the thumbs to decrease the horizontal arch until the patient reports concordant pain. If the pain reported is concordant, the movement is repeated or sustained to determine the effect of the technique.

5. The movement is then taken beyond the first point of pain toward end range. If the pain is concordant, the technique is repeated or sustained at end range.

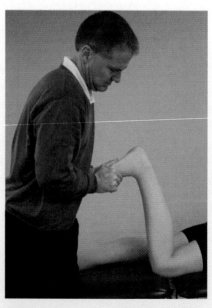

■ **Figure 14.36**   Horizontal Extension of the Forefoot

A reduction of symptoms associated with this technique may suggest that the procedure is a plausible treatment procedure.

Posterior–Anterior Glide of the Metatarsal–Phalangeal and Interphalangeal Joints

1. The patient is placed in prone position with the knee flexed.

2. Resting pain is assessed.

3. The examiner stabilizes the proximal segment with one hand and grasps the distal segment of the joint that is to be assessed in the other hand.

4. Using the thumb to generate the mobilizing force, a PA (plantar to dorsal) shearing movement is performed until the patient reports concordant pain (Figure 14.37 ■). If the pain reported is concordant, the movement is repeated or sustained to determine the effect of the technique.

5. The movement is then taken beyond the first point of pain toward end range. If the pain is concordant, the technique is repeated or sustained at end range.

A reduction of symptoms associated with this technique may suggest that the procedure is a plausible treatment procedure.

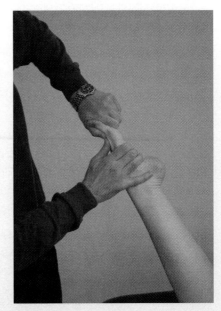

■ **Figure 14.37**   PA Glide of the MTP Joints

Anterior–Posterior Glide of the MTP Joints

1. The patient is placed in prone position with the knee flexed.

2. Resting pain is assessed.

3. The examiner stabilizes the proximal segment with one hand and grasps the distal segment of the joint that is to be assessed in the other hand.

4. Using the thumb to generate the mobilizing force, an AP (dorsal to plantar) shearing movement is performed until the patient reports concordant pain (Figure 14.38 ■). If the pain reported is concordant, the movement is repeated or sustained to determine the effect of the technique.

5. The movement is then taken beyond the first point of pain toward end range. If the pain is concordant, the technique is repeated or sustained at end range.

A reduction of symptoms associated with this technique may suggest that the procedure is a plausible treatment procedure.

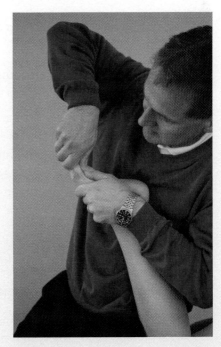

■ **Figure 14.38**   AP Glide of the MTP Joints

Adduction of the MTP Joint

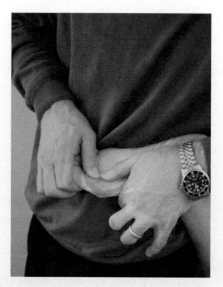

1. The patient is placed in prone position with the knee flexed.

2. Resting pain is assessed.

3. The examiner stabilizes the proximal segment with one hand and grasps the distal aspect of the tarsal bone in the other hand.

4. Using the thumb to generate the mobilizing force, an adduction (angular) movement is performed until the patient reports concordant pain (Figure 14.39 ■). If the pain reported is concordant, the movement is repeated or sustained to determine the effect of the technique.

5. The movement is then taken beyond the first point of pain toward end range. If the pain is concordant, the technique is repeated or sustained at end range.

A reduction of symptoms associated with this technique may suggest that the procedure is a plausible treatment procedure.

■ **Figure 14.39** Adduction of the MTP Joints

Abduction of the MTP Joints

1. The patient is placed in prone position with the knee flexed.

2. Resting pain is assessed.

3. The examiner stabilizes the proximal segment with one hand and grasps the distal segment of the joint that is to be assessed in the other hand.

4. Using the thumb to generate the mobilizing force, an abduction (angular) movement is performed until the patient reports concordant pain (Figure 14.40 ■). If the pain reported is concordant, the movement is repeated or sustained to determine the effect of the technique.

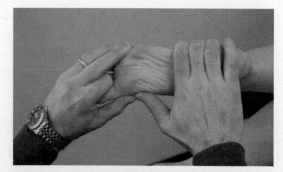

5. The movement is then taken beyond the first point of pain toward end range. If the pain is concordant, the technique is repeated or sustained at end range.

■ **Figure 14.40** Abduction of the MTP Joint

A reduction of symptoms associated with this technique may suggest that the procedure is a plausible treatment procedure.

Medial Rotation of the Metatarsal–Phalangeal and Interphalangeal Joints

1. The patient is placed in prone position with the knee flexed.

2. Resting pain is assessed.

3. The examiner stabilizes the proximal segment with one hand and grasps the distal segment of the joint that is to be assessed in the other hand (Figure 14.41 ■).

4. Using the thumb and forefinger to generate the mobilizing force, a medial rotational movement is performed until the patient reports concordant pain. If the pain reported is concordant, the movement is repeated or sustained to determine the effect of the technique.

5. The movement is then taken beyond the first point of pain toward end range. If the pain is concordant, the technique is repeated or sustained at end range.

A reduction of symptoms associated with this technique may suggest that the procedure is a plausible treatment procedure.

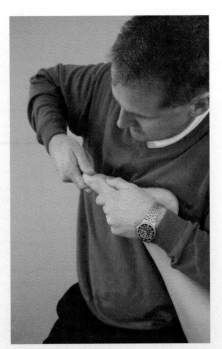

■ **Figure 14.41**   Medial Rotation of the Metatarsal–Phalangeal and Interphalangeal Joints

Lateral Rotation of the Metatarsal–Phalangeal and Interphalangeal Joints

1. The patient is placed in prone position with the knee flexed.

2. Resting pain is assessed.

3. The examiner stabilizes the proximal segment with one hand and grasps the distal segment of the joint that is to be assessed in the other hand.

4. Using the thumb and forefinger to generate the mobilizing force, a lateral rotational movement is performed until the patient reports concordant pain (Figure 14.42 ■). If the pain reported is concordant, the movement is repeated or sustained to determine the effect of the technique.

(Continued)

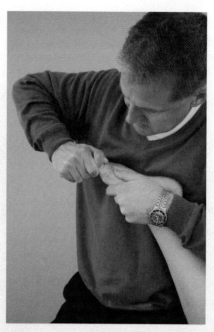

■ **Figure 14.42** Lateral Rotation of the MTP Joints

⑤ The movement is then taken beyond the first point of pain toward end range. If the pain is concordant, the technique is repeated or sustained at end range.

A reduction of symptoms associated with this technique may suggest that the procedure is a plausible treatment procedure.

Compression and Distraction of the MTP Joints

① The patient is placed in prone position with the knee flexed.

② Resting pain is assessed.

③ The examiner stabilizes the proximal segment with one hand and grasps the distal segment of the joint that is to be assessed in the other hand.

④ Using the thumb and forefinger to generate the mobilizing force, a compressive movement is performed until the patient reports concordant pain. If the pain reported is concordant, the movement is repeated or sustained to determine the effect of the technique.

⑤ The movement is then taken beyond the first point of pain toward end range. If the pain is concordant, the technique is repeated or sustained at end range.

A reduction of symptoms associated with this technique may suggest that the procedure is a plausible treatment procedure.

Distraction of the Metatarsal–Phalangeal and Interphalangeal Joints

① Using the thumb and forefinger to generate the mobilizing force, a distraction movement is performed until the patient reports concordant pain (Figure 14.43 ▪). If the pain reported is concordant, the movement is repeated or sustained to determine the effect of the technique.

② The movement is then taken beyond the first point of pain toward end range. If the pain is concordant, the technique is repeated or sustained at end range.

A reduction of symptoms associated with this technique may suggest that the procedure is a plausible treatment procedure.

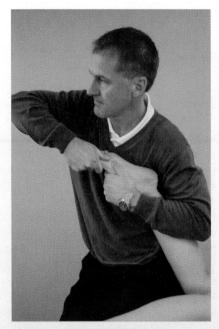

▪ **Figure 14.43** Distraction of the Metatarsal–Phalangeal and Interphalangeal Joints

Summary

- The purpose of passive accessory movements is to reproduce the concordant sign.
- Passive accessory movements, when combined with elicitation of the concordant sign of the patient, are reliable and useful assessment tools.
- Passive accessory movement in absence of elicitation of the concordant sign demonstrates little usefulness or applicability to treatment.

Summary

- Typically, palpation and muscle strength assessment provide additional data while clinical test provide diagnostic information.

Special Clinical Tests

Palpation

Palpation should be included in the objective examination to help the clinician determine which structures may be involved. The clinician must take care in determining whether the subjective complaints are consistent with the concordant sign. Palpation is an assessment element of the Ottawa ankle rules[5] and can be of considerable value.

Treatment Techniques

As stated throughout the book, the patient response-based method endeavors to determine the behavior of the patient's pain and/or impairment by analyzing concordant movements and the response of the patient's pain to applied or repeated movements. The applied or repeated movements that positively or negatively alter the signs and symptoms of the patient deserve the highest priority for treatment selection and should be similar in construct to the concordant examination movements. Examination methods that fail to elicit the patient response may offer nominal or imprecise value, as do methods that focus solely on treatment decision-making based on a single diagnostic label.

With the exception of manipulation, which is not an examination procedure, the majority of active and passive treatment techniques are nearly identical to the examination procedures. In all cases of manual therapy treatment, there should be a direct mechanical relationship between the examination and treatment techniques selected.

Active Physiological Movements

Active physiological movements of the ankle are used effectively as gentle early range-of-motion (ROM) activity. Active movements are particularly useful when implemented as a home exercise program used to maintain an increase in range of motion following more aggressive passive treatment. Strengthening programs for the foot and ankle can be isolated to a single leg or applied to both legs. A single leg strengthening program demonstrated carryover to the untrained leg, which indicates that it may be possible to start strengthening the involved leg through exercise of the uninvolved leg while following activity restriction orders.[5]

Patients with an ankle sprain appear to benefit from proprioception and balance training as well.[11,12] An injury such as an ankle sprain detrimentally affects postural stability and is retrained with postural exercise.

Active mobilization movements for self-stretching may also benefit the patient. If the patient's concordant movement is associated with tightness or capsular-based restrictions, active movements into the stiffness with the foot stabilized in weight bearing may be an effective self-mobilization (Figure 14.44 ■).

Proprioceptive neuromuscular facilitation (PNF) techniques make use of proprioceptive stimulus for strengthening or inhibition of selected and targeted muscle groups.[13] Both are manually assisted methods and both have established benefit during manual therapy treatment. The benefit of PNF procedures is associated with the three-pronged outcome. PNF procedures are effective in improving strength, range of motion, and balance and proprioception.[13]

Passive Physiological Techniques

After lateral ankle sprains, dorsiflexion during weight-bearing activities is frequently lost and may contribute to an increased risk of a recurrent inversion sprain. Subsequently, passive stretching programs that incorporate physiological dorsiflexion stretching may be useful in targeting limitations of dorsiflexion in an acute phase.[7,14] Any concordant passive physiological movement identified during the examination may be a useful treatment method.

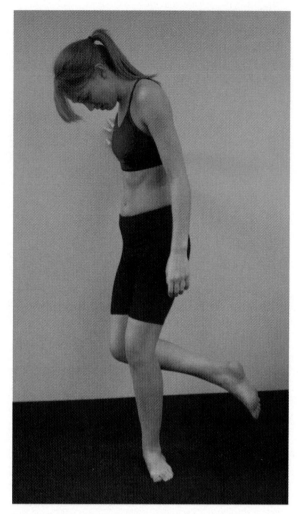

■ **Figure 14.44** Isolated Rotations for Stretching

Static Stretching

Dorsiflexion Stretching Dorsiflexion stretching by means of repeated self-mobilizations into dorsiflexion may also be useful for increasing range of motion in the acutely sprained ankle.[15] The procedure is performed with and without a tilt board and is considered a self-technique since the patient modulates the force of the stretch. To perform the technique, the patient is instructed to weight-bear on the targeted leg. The patient prepositions the foot into full dorsiflexion. The patient is instructed to either rotate or glide into the end-range dorsiflexion (Figure 14.45 ■). The most concordant reproduction of pain during a specific motion should be targeted.

Eversion Stretch The curvilinear stretch into ankle eversion is often used to counter the hypermobility of the ankle into inversion. The technique is administered by the clinician (Figure 14.46 ■) or by the patient. The technique can be performed using oscillations or with a passive prolonged stretch.

Plantar Splay   The plantar splay stretch is a technique used to stretch the plantar surface of the foot. The technique is generally considered beneficial for pain relief and may not actually increase gross range of motion. To perform the technique, the patient assumes a prone or supine position. The clinician stands behind the patient to address the plantar surface of the foot. The clinician applies a lateral load to each side of the foot in an attempt to splay the plantar tissue of the foot (Figure 14.47 ■).

Mobilization Techniques   The aforementioned examination methods double as treatment techniques for the foot and ankle. Each examination method should reproduce the concordant sign of the patient and should exhibit a reduction of pain with repeated movements or sustained holds. The following procedures demonstrate alterations in positioning from the examination and may be useful in isolating the targeted segment.

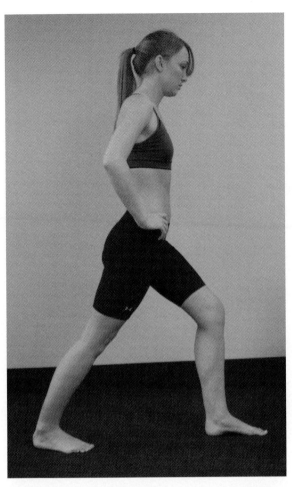

■ **Figure 14.45**   Repeated Movements into Dorsiflexion

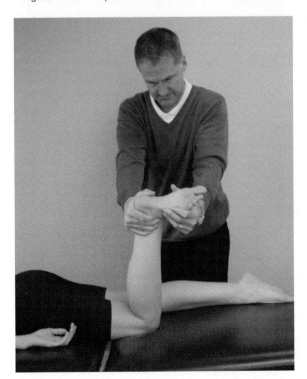

■ **Figure 14.46**   Passive Physiological Ankle Eversion

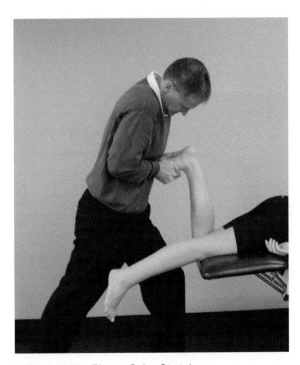

■ **Figure 14.47**   Plantar Splay Stretch

Lateral Glide of the Subtalar Joint

1. The patient is placed in sidelying position.

2. The affected extremity is placed closest to the plinth.

3. The clinician cradles the lower leg in one arm. The fingers stabilize the talus by looping the first digit and thumb around the dome of the talus (Figure 14.48 ■).

4. A lateral glide is performed using the nonstabilization hand.

5. As with all mobilization techniques, repeated movements are performed at the first point of pain and at near end range, whichever elicits the most reduction of symptoms.

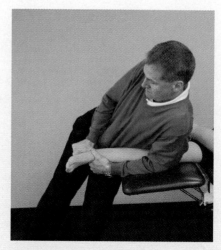

■ **Figure 14.48** Lateral Glide of the Subtalar Joint

Medial Glide of the Subtalar Joint

1. The patient is placed in sidelying position.

2. The affected extremity is placed furthermost from the plinth.

3. The clinician cradles the lower leg in one arm. The fingers stabilize the talus by looping the first digit and thumb around the dome of the talus (Figure 14.49 ■).

4. A medial glide is performed using the nonstabilization hand.

5. As with all mobilization techniques, repeated movements are performed at the first point of pain and at near end range, whichever elicits the most reduction of symptoms.

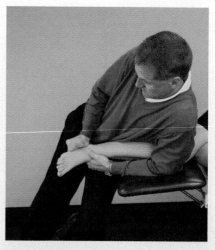

■ **Figure 14.49** Medial Glide of the Subtalar Joint

Posterior Glide of the Talus within the Talocrural Joint

1. The patient lies in supine or in a hooklying position.

2. The clinician applies an AP force by using his or her web space to the anterior dome of the talus (Figure 14.50 ■). The glide is directly posteriorly.

3. As with all mobilization techniques, repeated movements are performed at the first point of pain and at near end range, whichever elicits the most reduction of symptoms.

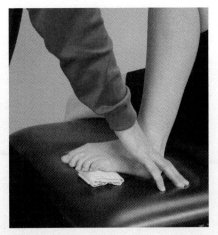

■ **Figure 14.50**   Posterior Glide of the Talus

Talocrural Distraction in Supine

1. The patient lies in supine position.

2. The clinician grasps the foot just distal to the talar dome.

3. The clinician applies a distraction force at the talocrural joint by shifting his or her weight away from the patient (Figure 14.51 ■).

4. As with all mobilization techniques, repeated movements are performed at the first point of pain and at near end range, whichever elicits the most reduction of symptoms.

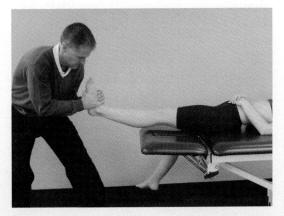

■ **Figure 14.51**   Distraction-Based Mobilization of the Talocrural Joint

Mobilization with Movement   Mobilization with movement techniques typically involve an active movement of the patient with a concurrent passive movement applied by the clinician.

Anterior to Posterior Talus Glide with Active-Assist Dorsiflexion

The procedure is useful when patients exhibit limited and concordant dorsiflexion.

1. The patient is placed in a long sitting position.

2. A belt is looped around his or her forefoot with each end in the patient's hands. The belt is used by the patient to assist in pulling his or her foot into dorsiflexion.

3. The clinician places a towel roll behind the tibia and fibula to stabilize these bones.

4. The clinician uses his or her webspace to push the talus posteriorly during concurrent dorsiflexion. The technique is performed in an open chain (Figure 14.52 ■).

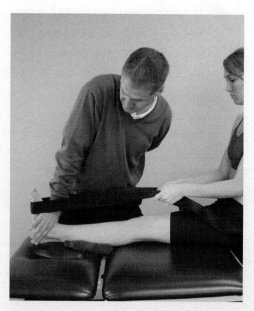

■ **Figure 14.52**   Anterior to Posterior Talus Glide with Active-Assist Dorsiflexion

Posterior Talus Glide with Active Dorsiflexion: Closed Chain

This mobilization with movement technique is also useful for patients with restricted dorsiflexion.

1. The patient is placed in a semi-lunge position in standing, with the affected foot in front.

2. The patient is instructed to lunge and move his or her tibia forward (moving into dorsiflexion) during concurrent anterior to posterior gliding of the talus by the clinician (Figure 14.53 ■).

3. The clinician uses his or her webspace to push the talus posteriorly.

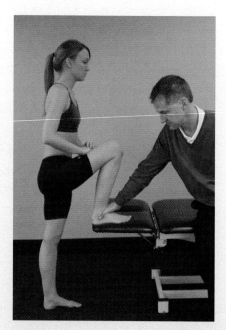

■ **Figure 14.53**   Posterior Talus Glide with Active Dorsiflexion in Closed Chain

④ The effect of the mobilization can be enhanced with a concomitant posterior to anterior glide of the distal tibia and fibula with a mobilization belt looped around the ankle mortise and the examiner's hips.

The technique can also be performed using a posterior glide of the fibula on the tibia during active dorsiflexion. It may be useful to place the patient's foot on a chair for better access to the tibia and fibula (Figure 14.54 ■).

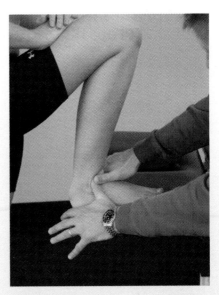

■ **Figure 14.54** Posterior Fibular Glide with Active Dorsiflexion in Closed Chain

Ankle Plantarflexion with Posterior Tibial Glide

If plantarflexion is limited, a mobilization with movement technique that involves a posterior glide of the tibia with respect to the talus may be useful.

① The patient is placed in a hooklying position and the heel is firmly planted on the table.

② The patient is instructed to move his or her foot into plantarflexion during concurrent posterior tibial glide by the clinician (Figure 14.55 ■).

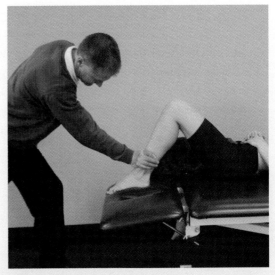

■ **Figure 14.55** Ankle Plantarflexion with Posterior Tibial Glide

Closed-Chain MTP Extension with Lateral Glide of the First Ray

A closed-chain movement designed to improve first ray extension may be useful if a patient reports pain and/or stiffness at push-off during the gait cycle.

1 The patient is placed in a semi-lunge position with the foot on a plinth.

2 The phalangeal aspect of the first toe is firmly placed on the plinth.

3 A belt is wrapped around the first ray and tension is placed laterally on the ray.

4 The patient is instructed to actively move his or her great toe into extension (during weight bearing) with concurrent lateral glide of the belt (Figure 14.56 ■).

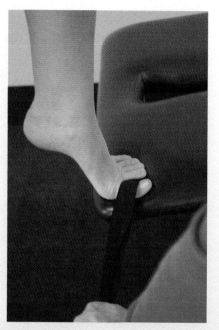

■ **Figure 14.56** Closed-Chain MTP Extension with Lateral Glide of the First Ray

Mobilization of the Sesamoid Bones with Active Extension of the First MTP

A mobilization procedure for the sesamoid bones involves stabilizing the distal aspect of the metatarsals (just proximal to the sesamoid bones) and a concurrent active movement into MTP extension by the patient (Figure 14.57 ■). This procedure may be especially beneficial after sesamoid surgery. For patients with bunions, lateral metatarsal movement may be useful.

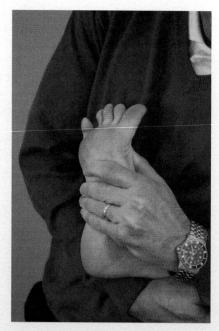

■ **Figure 14.57** Mobilization of the Sesamoid Bones with Active Extension of the First MTP

Manipulation Techniques   Manipulation procedures have been reported in a number of studies.[16–21] The majority of studies used manipulation to improve dorsiflexion range-of-motion losses.

Talocrural Distraction Manipulation

1. The patient lies in supine position.

2. The clinician grasps the foot just distal to the talar dome.

3. The clinician applies a distraction force at the talocrural joint by shifting his or her weight away from the patient (Figure 14.58 ■).

4. The movement is applied and a preload force is held at the end range of the distraction.

5. The manipulation is performed by applying a quick thrust at the end range. The thrust is targeted purely into distraction.

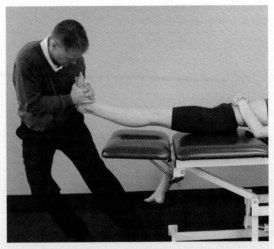

■ **Figure 14.58**   Distraction-Based Manipulation of the Talocrural Joint

Cuboid Whip Manipulation

Jennings and Davies[16] described a midfoot manipulation procedure designed for treatment of midfoot instability.

1. The patient assumes a prone position.

2. The clinician grasps the foot by stabilizing the medial and lateral sides of the foot within his or her webspaces.

3. The thumbs of the clinician are placed on the cuboid on the plantar aspect of the foot.

4. The knee is flexed to approximately 70 degrees and the ankle is dorsiflexed to end range.

5. In a quick movement, the clinician moves the knee into extension, the ankle into plantarflexion and supination (Figure 14.59 ■). Concurrently with the physiological movements, the clinician also applies a plantar to dorsal thrust with his or her thumbs.

6. The procedure can be repeated if necessary.

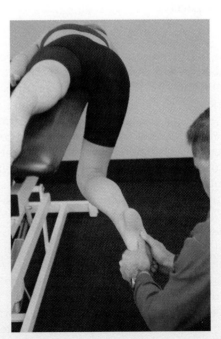

■ **Figure 14.59**   Cuboid Whip Manipulation

Summary

- Strong association between examination and treatment should improve the outcome of a dedicated treatment program.
- Active physiological movements are beneficial in creating home exercise programs, working on abnormal posture, or strengthening the selected lower extremity musculature.
- Passive physiological and accessory techniques are reflective of the examination findings.
- Manipulation procedures are generally applicable in acute ankle sprains that do not exhibit detrimental laxity.

Treatment Outcomes

The Evidence

Exercise (Home or Clinic Initiated)   One of the most effective treatment procedures includes the simple concept of early movement after injury. Although most trials investigating this concept are weak,[22] early active movement results in improved outcomes versus immobilization and non-weight-bearing activities.[23,24] Generally, the active movements are included as adjuncts to passive treatment such as mobilization and balance-related treatment. There is limited evidence supporting the use of a removable type of immobilization brace during concurrent use of exercise during the immobilization period for patients with ankle fracture.[22] There is also limited evidence for manual therapy after the immobilization period for this population.[25] Overall, the evidence for exercise is Level B.

Proprioceptive Training   Proprioceptive training leads to improved joint position sense, decreased postural sway, and reduced muscle reaction times in the fibular muscles.[26] Furthermore, proprioception techniques reduce the risk of future inversion sprains[26] and may improve the strength of the lower extremity.[27] A 4-week agility training program failed to show improvements in single leg stance over controls,[28] but neither of these protocols was tested for an effect on recurrent sprain rates. Another study demonstrated that a supervised exercise program that consisted of balance-related activities demonstrated similar outcomes to an educational control program for postural sway, isometric ankle strength, and joint position sense.[29] However, the supervised program did result in reduced incidence of recurrent ankle sprains over the next 12 months.[29,30]

One study demonstrated that older adults who regularly practiced tai chi had significantly better knee and ankle joint kinesthesia than their age-matched sedentary counterparts or swimmers and runners.[31]

These changes were accompanied by improved sway characteristics that have been used to assess ankle proprioception in instability studies. The direct application of this study to lateral ankle instability treatment is questionable since the study did not directly assess the ankle but the overlap of proprioception between joints and the contributions to proprioception through skin and other systemic inputs implies that the use of tai chi is a potential treatment option worth studying.

Training programs using a flexible disk that mimics an unstable surface to improve balance and proprioception have been demonstrated to decrease electromyographic (EMG) muscle reaction latency times[32] and have reduced the incidence of ankle injuries in female European handball players following a routine 10- to 15-minute training program performed for 10 months at each practice.[33] Wester et al. also found that training on a wobble board could reduce the incidence of recurrent ankle sprains but does not speed up the process of reduction of initial symptoms.[34]

Manipulation of the talocrural joint in a healthy population does not affect standing stability[35] but does provide short-term change in posterior hindfoot load in subjects with ankle sprain.[36] There are no studies that have investigated long-terms effects toward proprioception. Overall, the level of evidence for proprioceptive training is also Level B.

Static Stretching   Passive stretching of the ankle decreases resting tension of the plantarflexor muscles.[37] Passive stretching may also be useful in improving gait speed and pattern in older patients.[38] Level C evidence exists to support this concept.

Mobilization   The majority of studies investigating the benefits of mobilization for the ankle foot complex are case reports or case series. Unfortunately, these studies demonstrated poor methodology with results that are not transferable to a pathological population.[15] One of the best-designed studies[39] acknowledged that including mobilization in the treatment of acute inversion ankle sprains led to decreased visits and quicker increases in range of motion.

A recent randomized controlled trial explored the use of a Mulligan technique, termed a mobilization with movement (MWM), on dorsiflexion in weight bearing and pressure pain threshold levels. Mulligan reports a 97% success rate with substantial improvement in active, pain-free dorsiflexion following treatment.[40] In another study, dorsiflexion range of motion did increase ($p < .002$) but pain pressure threshold level did not change, implying that

ROM was increased by mechanical means rather than by reducing pain.[17]

The Mulligan concept advocates a concept called the positional fault theory. A recent study by Landrum et al.[41] did demonstrate that posterior mobilization of the talus was associated with increased dorsiflexion. Talar mobility decreased with successive mobilizations. Subjects in the study had ankle dysfunction associated with a minimum of 14 days of immobilization.[41] A closed-chain or open-chain mobilization with movement treatment program has been associated with 55% improved talar glide (versus a control group).[42] The results of this study were only investigated short term. For short-term benefits, Level B evidence exists. For long-term benefits, the evidence is C.

For the treatment of heel pain, clinical practice guidelines suggested that there was minimal evidence for manual therapy interventions.[43] The supporting literature included case reports or case series with theoretical or foundational support. In a subsequent RCT, Cleland et al. examined subjects with plantar heel pain and compared a treatment group receiving electrotherapeutic modalities and stretching exercise with a second group receiving soft-tissue mobilization to the triceps surae and plantar fascia, aggressive mobilization toward subtalar eversion, and an impairment-based manual therapy approach for each joint of the lower quarter.[44] The results suggested that the manual therapy group improved more in the 4-week trial and maintained that improvement at 6-month follow-up as measured by the foot and ankle measure (FAAM) and the lower extremity functional scale (LEFS) outcome measures and the numeric pain rating scale.[44] In addition, the global rating of change (GRoC) measure taken at both the 4-week and 6-month time periods were statistically higher for the manual therapy group. It is also noteworthy that the electrotherapy and stretching group's improvement did not meet the minimally clinical important difference of the outcome tools at the 4-week timeframe, suggesting that treatment following the recommended guidelines did not produce results that were clinically important. The results of this study would suggest that manual therapy and exercise produce Level II-A for both short-term and long-term benefits.

Manipulation Manipulation has been thoroughly investigated as a treatment for ankle-related pathologies. The majority of studies have demonstrated improvements in patients who have received a manipulation procedure versus a benign control.[16–21] A variety of methods have demonstrated efficacy, the majority designed to reduce neurophysiological reduction of pain more so than gains of range of motion.[21,45] One derivation study has identified four variables associated with a positive outcome with manipulation in patients with inversion ankle sprains.[46] When three of four of the variables included (1) symptoms while standing, (2) symptoms worse in the evening, (3) navicular drop test findings of less than or equal to 5 mm, and (4) distal tibio-fibular joint hypomobility were positive, the clinical prediction rule yielded a LR+ of 5.9. One must use caution since the confidence intervals were very wide and three of four findings only captured 18 of the 64 successes. At present, the level of evidence for manipulation is Level B for short-term benefits.

Taping and Bracing Techniques The primary benefit associated with taping to increase stiffness at the ankle is associated with the increase in the amplification ratio of proprioception through cutaneous mechanoreceptors, thereby increasing functional ankle stability while the tape remains tight.[47] A recent study demonstrated that a semi-rigid brace applied to the ankle could bring about a more favorable firing pattern to the muscles of the lower leg, allowing greater protection of the ankle to inversion sprains. This study suggests that previous concerns over brace usage causing a generalized weakening of muscles may be unfounded in clinical practice.[31,48–50] In subjects with no history of injury, a semi-rigid ankle brace enhanced excitability of the motorneuron pool of the common fibular nerve innervating the fibularis longus muscle.[51] It seems reasonable that the mechanism of action is related to the stimulation of cutaneous afferents that alter the sensorimotor system in a positive manner. The use of a custom foot orthotic designed to correct abnormal talar alignment following ankle inversion sprain has been shown to reduce postural sway in single leg stance measured by force plate. This suggests that custom orthotics may be helpful in facilitating recovery following a lateral ankle sprain.[52] Overall, the evidence is Level C.

Summary

- There is limited empirical evidence and significant anecdotal evidence that a treatment approach consisting of some element of orthopedic manual therapy is associated with a positive outcome.

- There is a significant lack of controlled studies that have investigated the combinations of strengthening and mobilization or individualized treatment processes on patients with variations of AFC disorders.

Chapter Questions

1. Describe the relationship of the soft and non–soft tissues with the stabilization of the ankle.

2. Describe how compromised proprioception alters the functional stability of a patient during locomotion.

3. Outline the arthrological movements of the talocrural joint during dorsiflexion and plantarflexion.

4. Identify the variations associated with passive accessory examination of the AFC.

5. Describe the outcomes associated with mobilization and manipulation of the ankle.

Patient Cases

Case 14.1: Timothy Hutchins (16-year-old male)

Diagnosis: Status post–distal tibial fracture

Observation: His foot appears swollen; typical post cast removal.

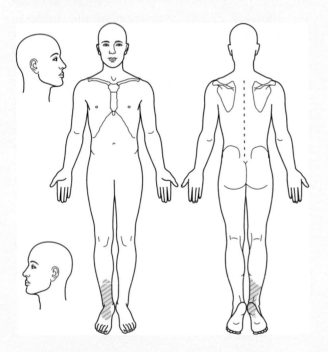

Mechanism: Eight weeks ago he fractured his distal tibia in an ATV accident. He received a cast to stabilize the fracture and now has restricted movement in his ankle upon removal of the cast.

Concordant Sign: Dorsiflexion and inversion.

Nature of the Condition: He is a football player but at present cannot run or participate in any of the football drills.

Behavior of the Symptoms: He reports stiffness but no referred pain.

Pertinent Patient History: None.

Patient Goals: He is interested in being able to move his ankle without pain.

Baseline: Ankle pain at rest, 1/10 NAS for pain; when worst, 3/10 pain.

Examination Findings: All movements are grossly restricted. Dorsiflexion is limited to –5 degrees. All the motions are concordant for stiffness.

1. Based on these findings, what else would you like to examine?
2. Is this patient a good candidate for manual therapy?
3. What is the expected prognosis of this patient?
4. What treatments do you presented in this book may be beneficial for this patient?

Case 14.2: Precious Johnson (52-year-old female)

Diagnosis: Midfoot strain

Observation: Overweight female with flat feet and painful gait.

Mechanism: She spent the day walking around an amusement park and now complains of severe pain in her midfoot region.

Concordant Sign: The pain is worse during midstance and push-off.

Nature of the Condition: She claims she can no longer work (she is a cashier at a grocery store) because she cannot tolerate standing. She is interested is getting disability status for this condition.

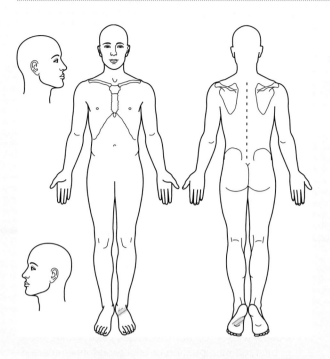

Behavior of the Symptoms: The pain is sharp superiorly on the foot (near the midtarsal joint). The symptoms also radiate into the arch of the foot.

Pertinent Patient History: Obesity, diabetes, and low back pain.

Patient Goals: She feels her condition is nonreparable. Her goals are to quantify her current problem so that she can obtain a disability settlement.

Baseline: His current symptoms are at 5/10; when worse, 9/10.

Examination Findings: All movements are painful. Weight bearing is painful. The patient walks very slow with a painful gait.

1. Based on these findings, what else would you like to examine?
2. Is this patient a good candidate for manual therapy?
3. What is the expected prognosis of this patient?
4. What treatments do you feel presented in this book may be beneficial for this patient?

PEARSON
myhealthprofessionskit™

Use this address to access the Companion Website created for this textbook. Simply select "Physical Therapy" from the choice of disciplines. Find this book and log in using your username and password to access video clips and the anatomy and arthrological information.

References

1. Boyko EJ, Ahroni JH, Daviqnon D, Stensel V, Prigeon RL, Smith DG. Diagnostic utility of the history and physical examination for peripheral vascular disease among patients with diabetes mellitus. *J Clin Epidemiol.* 1997;50(6):659–668.

2. Thordarson D. *Orthopedic surgery essentials: Foot and ankle.* Philadelphia; Lippincott Williams and Wilkins: 2004.

3. Meyer J, Kulig K, Landel R. Differential diagnosis and treatment of subcalcaneal heel pain: A case report. *J Orthop Sports Phys Ther.* 2002;32(3):114–122.

4. Sujitkumar P, Hadfield JM, Yates DW. Sprain or fracture?: An analysis of 2000 ankle injuries. *Arch Emerg Med.* 1986;3(2):101–106.

5. Bachmann LM, Kolb E, Koller MT, Steurer J, ter Riet G. Accuracy of Ottawa ankle rules to exclude fractures of the ankle and mid-foot: systematic review. *BMJ.* 2003; 326(7386):417.

6. Maitland GD. *Peripheral manipulation.* Oxford; Butterworth-Heinemann: 1991.

7. Young B, Walker M, Strunce J, Boyles R. A combined treatment approach emphasizing impairment-based manual physical therapy for plantar heel pain: A case series. *J Orthop Sports Phys Ther.* 2004;34:725–733.

8. Rubin A, Sallis R. Evaluation and diagnosis of ankle injuries. *Am Fam Phys.* 1996;54:1609–1618.

9. Wilson RW, Gansneder BM. Measures of functional limitation as predictors of disablement in athletes with acute ankle sprains. *J Ortho Sports Phys Ther.* 2000;30:528–535.

10. Lark SD, Buckley JG, Bennett S, Jones D, Sargeant AJ. Joint torques and dynamic joint stiffness in elderly and young men during stepping down. *Clin Biomech.* 2003;18(9):848–855.

11. Uh BS, Beynnon BD, Helie BV, Alosa DM, Renstrom PA. The benefit of a single-leg strength training program for the muscles around the untrained ankle: A prospective, randomized, controlled study. *Am J Sports Med.* 2000;28:568–573.

12. Goldie PA, Evans OM, Bach TM. Postural control following inversion injuries of the ankle. *Arch Phys Med Rehabil.* 1994;75(9):969–975.

13. Etnyre BR, Abraham LD. Gains in range of ankle dorsiflexion using three population stretching techniques. *Am J Phys Med.* 1986;65:189–196.

14. Porter D, Barrill E, Oneacre K, May BD. The effects of duration and frequency of Achilles tendon stretching on dorsiflexion and outcome in painful hell syndrome: A randomized, blinded control study. *Foot Ankle Int.* 2002;23:619–624.

15. Whitman JM, Childs JD, Walker V. The use of manipulation in a patient with an ankle sprain injury not responding to conventional management: A case report. *Man Ther.* 2005;10:224–231.

16. Jennings J, Davies GJ. Treatment of cuboid syndrome secondary to lateral ankle sprains: A case series. *J Orthop Sports Phys Ther.* 2005;35:409–415.

17. Collins N, Teys P, Vicenzino B. The initial effects of a Mulligan's mobilization technique on dorsiflexion and pain in subacute ankle sprains. *Man Ther.* 2004;9:77–82.

18. Eisenhart AW, Gaeta TJ, Yeus DP. Osteopathic manipulative treatment in the emergency department for patients with acute ankle sprains. *J Am Ostepath Assoc.* 2003;103:417–421.

19. Fryer GA, Mudge JM, McLaughlin PA. The effect of talocrural joint manipulation on range of motion at the ankle. *J Manipulative Physiol Ther.* 2002;25(6):384–390.

20. Pellow JE, Brantingham JW. The efficacy of adjusting the ankle in the treatment of subacute and chronic grade I and grade II ankle inversion sprains. *J Manipulative Physiol Ther.* 2001;24:17–24.

21. Nield S, Davis K, Latimer J, Maher C, Adams R. The effect of manipulation on range of movement at the ankle joint. *Scand J Rehabil Med.* 1993;25:161–166.

22. Lin CW, Moseley AM, Refshauge KM. Rehabilitation for ankle fractures in adults. *Cochrane Database Syst Rev.* 2008;16:CD005595.

23. Eiff MP, Smith AT, Smith GE. Early mobilization versus immobilization in the treatment of lateral ankle sprains. *Am J Sports Med.* 1994;22:83–88.

24. Karlsson J, Eriksson BI, Sward L. Early functional treatment for acute ligament injuries of the ankle joint. Scand *J Med Science Sports.* 1996;6:341–345.

25. Lin CW, Moseley AM, Haas M, Refshauge KM, Herbert RD. Manual therapy in addition to physiotherapy does not improve clinical or economic outcomes after ankle fracture. *J Rehabil Med.* 2008;40:433–439.

26. De Carlo MS, Talbot RW. Evaluation of ankle joint proprioception following injection of the anterior talofibular ligament. *J Orthop Sports Phys Ther.* 1986;8:70–76.

27. Powers ME, Buckley BD, Kaminski TW, Hubbard TJ, Ortiz C. Six weeks of strength and proprioception training does not affect muscle fatigue and static balance in functional ankle instability. *J Sport Rehabil.* 2004;13:201–227.

28. Hess DM, Joyce CJ, Arnold BL, Gansneder BM. Effect of a 4-week agility-training program on postural sway in the functionally unstable ankle. *J Sport Rehabil.* 2001;10:24–35.

29. Holme E, Magnusson SP, Becher K, Bieler T, Aagaard B, Kjaer M. The effect of supervised rehabilitation on strength, postural sway, position sense and re-injury risk after acute ankle ligament sprain. *Scand J Med Science Sports.* 1999;9:104–109.

30. Verhagen E, Mechelen W, de Vente W. The effect of preventive measures on the incidence of ankle sprains. *Clin J Sport Med.* 2000;10:291–296.

31. Xu D HY, Li J, Chan K. Effect of tai chi exercise on proprioception on ankle and knee joints in old people. *Br J Sports Med.* 2004;38:50–54.

32. Osborne MD CL, Laskowski ER, Smith J, Kaufman KR. The effect of ankle disk training on muscle reaction time in subjects with a history of ankle sprain. *Am J Sports Med.* 2001;29:627–632.

33. Wedderkopp N, Kaltoft M, Lundgaard B, Rosendahl M, Froberg K. Prevention of injuries in young female players in European team handball: A prospective intervention study. *Scand J Med Science Sports.* 1999;9:41–47.

34. Wester JU, Jespersen SM, Nielsen KD, Neumann L. Wobble board training after partial sprains of the lateral ligaments of the ankle: A prospective randomized study. *J Orthop Sports Phys Ther.* 1996;23:332–336.

35. Alburquerque-Sendin F, Fernandez-de-las-Penas C, Santos-del-Rey M, Martin-Vallejo FJ. Immediate effects of bilateral manipuation of talocrural joints on standing stability in healthy subjects. *Man Ther.* 2009;14:75–80.

36. Lopez-Rodriquez, Fernandez-de-las-Penas C, Alburquerque-Sendin F, Rodriquez-Blanco C, Palomeque-del-Cerro L. Immediate effects of manipulation of the talocrural joint on stabilometry and baropodometry in patients with ankle sprains. *J Manipulative Physiol Ther.* 2007;30:186–192.

37. Reisman S, Allen TJ, Proske U. Changes in passive tension after stretch of unexercised and eccentrically exercised human plantarflexor muscles. *Exp Brain Res.* 2009;193:545–554.

38. Christiansen CL. The effects of hip and ankle strengthening on gait function of older people. *Arch Phys Med Rehabil.* 2008;89:1421–1428.

39. Green T, Refshauge K, Crosbie J, Adams R. A randomized controlled trial of a passive accessory joint mobilization on acute ankle inversion sprains. *Phys Ther.* 2001;81:984–994.

40. Mulligan BR. *Manual therapy "nags", "snags", "mwms" etc.* Wellington; Plane View Services Ltd.: 1995.

41. Landrum EL, Kelln CB, Parente WR, Ingersoll CD, Hertel J. Immediate effects of anterior-to-posterior talocrural joint mobilization after prolonged ankle immobilization: A preliminary study. *J Man Manip Ther.* 2008;16(2):100–105.

42. Vicenzino B, Branjerdporn M, Teys P, Jordan K. Initial changes in posterior talar glide and dorsiflexion of the ankle after mobilization with movement in individuals with recurrent ankle sprain. *J Orthop Sports Phys Ther.* 2006;36:464–471.

43. McPoil TG, Martin RL, Cornwall MW, Wukich DK, Irrgang JJ, Godges JJ. Heel pain – plantar fasciitis: Clinical practice guidelines linked to the international classification of function, disability, and health from the orthopaedic section of the American physical therapy association. *J Orthop Sports Phys Ther.* 2008;38(4):A1–18.

44. Cleland JA, Abbott JH, Kidd MO, et al. Manual physical therapy and exercise versus electrophysical agents and exercise in the management of plantar heel pain: A multicenter randomized clinical trial. *J Orthop Sports Phys Ther.* 2009;39(8):573–585.

45. Malisza KL, Gregorash L, Turner A, et al. Functional MRI involving painful stimulation of the ankle and the effect of physiotherapy joint mobilization. *Magn Reson Imaging.* 2003;21:489–496.

46. Whitman JM, Cleland JA, Mintken PE, et al. Predicting short-term response to thrust and nonthrust manipulation and exercise in patients post inversion ankle sprain. *J Orthop Sports Phys Ther.* 2009;39(3):188–200.

47. Lohrer H, Alt W, Gollhofer A. Neuromuscular properties and functional aspects of taped ankles. *Am J Sports Med.* 1999;27:69–75.

48. Conley K. The effects of selected modes of prophylactic support on reflex muscle firing following dynamic perturbation of the ankle. School of Health and Rehabilitation Science. 2005.

49. Cordova ML, Ingersoll CD. Peroneus longus stretch reflex amplitude increases after ankle brace application. *Br J Sports Med.* 2003;37:258–262.

50. Cordova ML, Cardona C, Ingersoll CD. Long-term ankle brace use does not affect peroneus longus muscle latency during sudden inversion in normal subjects. *J Athl Train.* 2000;35:407–411.

51. Nishikawa T, Grabiner MD. Peroneal motoneuron excitability increases immediately following application of a semirigid ankle brace. *J Orthop Sports Phys Ther.* 1999;29:168–173.

52. Guskiewicz KM, Perrin DH. Effect of orthotics on postural sway following inversion ankle sprain. *J Ortho Sports Phys Ther.* 1996;23:326–331.

Neurodynamics

Ken Learman and Chad Cook

Chapter
15

Objectives

- Outline the pertinent clinically relevant anatomy of the nervous system.
- Understand the mechanical behavior of the peripheral nervous system and the spinal cord.
- Understand the clinical examination of the nervous system.
- Outline an effective treatment program for proposed pathology of the nervous system.
- Identify the outcomes associated with orthopedic manual therapy to the nervous system.

Clinical Examination

Definitions

Neurodynamics is a concept that involves the dynamic interplay between mechanical and physiological properties of the peripheral nervous system.[1] The concept assumes that these properties are interdependent and when altered can affect the peripheral and central nervous systems in a clinically oriented manner through observable and patient-reported signs and symptoms.[2] The term **adverse neural tension** (ANT) is the outcome of the clinically oriented effect, thus is an abnormal physiological or mechanical response from the nervous system that limits the nervous system's range or stretch[2] or results in neurological symptoms through available range. Consequently, alterations in neurodynamics will manifest as adverse neural tension[3] Others have suggested the use of the term **peripheral neuropathic pain** to reflect positive and negative symptoms in patients where pain is associated with pathological changes or dysfunction in peripheral nerves or nerve roots.[4] Within this book, both the terms "adverse neural tension" and "peripheral neuropathic pain" reflect complications of origin in the peripheral and/or central nervous systems.

Unfortunately, the terminology associated with adverse neural tension suggests that peripheral neuropathic pain mechanisms always reflect a complication associated with tension of the nerve root.[5] Indeed, the terms commonly associated with treatment also include descriptors such as nerve tension tests or have been described in such a manner that clinicians assume the process involves stretching the nerves and supportive structures. Because differentiating mechanical versus nerve-related structures is very difficult, it is more important to note the response to selected positions associated with ANT. Lew and Briggs[6] regarded increased pain during the slump test in the posterior thigh as indicative of neural tissue involvement. However, the ability of these sensitizing maneuvers to locate the exact tissue at fault has been refuted by other authors[7,8] Barker and Briggs[7] queried the degree of involvement of non-neural structures, such as fascia, during the slump test, suggesting fascia can mimic the response of neural structures during the slump test. Barker and Briggs[7] surmised the posterior layer of lumbar fascia may generate tension in tests involving the head, spine, and limbs, such as the slump test. Ultimately, difficulty ensues in locating the precise source of symptoms, which occur during a neural tension test[6-8] For this reason, this book refers to tests that examine neural tissue as provocational tests (or neurodynamic tests) rather than neural tension tests.[5]

Normal Physiological Responses to Nerve Tissue Provocation Tests (NTPT)

When performing a NTPT,[5,9] it is not uncommon for asymptomatic subjects to experience limitations or discomfort. For example, in over 80% of 100 normal subjects, pain, stretch, and mild paresthesia over the radial aspect of the forearm and the first four digits accompanied the NTPT of the upper extremity. Similarly, the most common response to the slump test performed in normal adults frequently results in discomfort in the posterior thigh, knee, and calf and potentially radiation of symptoms into the foot.[10] Another study examining 50 normal subjects found that radial forearm and upper arm pain was the most common symptom using a modified NTPT technique for the upper quarter.[11] Yaxley and Jull[11] found that 90% of those normal subjects experienced sensitization when their symptoms were increased with use of contralateral cervical lateral flexion. Sensitization has also been demonstrated in lower-extremity NTPT. Similarly, normal subjects reported sensitization in the straight leg raise when the investigator attempted to perform a sensitizing maneuver such as dorsiflexion (DF) with inversion; the pain often intensified into the sural nerve distribution on the posterolateral border of the foot.[12] In addition to symptom provocation, alteration in electromyography (EMG) activity has also been noted in the end range of NTPT for the upper extremity[13] as well as the lower extremity,[14] with stiffer individuals demonstrating greater muscle activity than their more flexible counterparts. Since a normal physiological response to NTPT testing is discomfort in the appropriate neural tissue distribution, it becomes necessary to operationally define what response is believed to be a positive response for neurogenic involvement. Elvey and Hall[15] have proposed a series of six criteria used to define a positive test for nerve tissue mechanosensitivity, which are adapted in Table 15.1 ■.

An alternative way to determine if a neural tissue provocational test is positive is if (1) symptoms can be reproduced, (2) if responses on the involved side differ from the uninvolved side or from known normal responses, and (3) if structural differentiation supports a neurogenic source.[16] These criteria can be clinically applied through the following:

1. Reproduces the patient's symptoms (concordant pain)
   • Note: This does not yet implicate the nervous system since a normal physiologic response may include neural provocation and further testing may be required.

2. Test responses can be altered by movement of distant body parts that would not generally be considered contiguous with any other tissue except neural tissue.
   • Note: This characteristic is referred to as sensitization and qualifies for structural differentiation.
   • As previously stated, sensitization may also be included as part of a normal physiological response so the investigator must still be cautious of drawing any firm conclusion from this finding.

3. Test differences from left side to right side and normal
   • These differences may be range, resistance during movement, and symptom response.
   • Be wary of the good side, if used for comparison, since it could also be affected by the same disorder to a similar degree of involvement or possibly less involved.
   • In the case where the sides do not differ because of potential bilateral involvement, the clinician must rely on sound clinical reasoning, based on the preponderance of the evidence from the entire clinical presentation in order to make an accurate differential diagnosis.

To briefly outline a clinical example, if a subject with low back and leg pain presents to the clinic for examination and the therapist performs a SLR test, it would not be uncommon to experience a painful response in the back and posterior thigh. To satisfy criterion 1, we would like to see that the pain produced by the SLR accurately reflects the concordant pain that the subject was reporting during the history. This concordant finding may or may not implicate the neural tissues since we know that asymptomatic subjects can experience posterior thigh pain from SLR.

Sensitizing maneuvers are used during the neural tissue provocation tests, which allow clinicians to differentiate between neural tension and other non-neural

---

■ **TABLE 15.1** Physical Signs of Neural Tissue Involvement

1. Antalgic posture.
2. Active movement dysfunction.
3. Passive movement dysfunction, which correlates with the active movement dysfunction.
4. Adverse responses to neural tissue provocation tests, which must relate specifically and anatomically to 2 and 3.
5. Mechanical allodynia in response to palpation of specific nerve trunks, which relate specifically and anatomically to 2 and 4.
6. Evidence from the physical examination of a local cause of the neurogenic pain, which would involve the neural tissue showing the responses in 4 and 5.

or musculoskeletal pathologies.[3,17,18] Sensitizing maneuvers involve applying additional tension in the nervous system without directly involving the local segment in question. For example, if the subject has back pain associated with a neurogenic cause, they may present with pain during a straight leg raise test. If the pain is associated with the sciatic nerve, adding ankle dorsiflexion may make that back pain significantly worse. If the pain were of arthritic origin, it is not likely that dorsiflexion of the ankle would impact that pain; however, the sciatic nerve is mechanically affected by hip and ankle movement alike. Sensitizing maneuvers can also be used to further differentiate which portion of the peripheral nerve may be involved. In the previous example, the subject's neurogenic back pain may be sensitized by dorsiflexion and eversion, implicating tibial nerve involvement, whereas dorsiflexion and inversion may not be as effective in altering symptoms, thereby casting doubt on sural nerve involvement. If the addition of dorsiflexion and eversion increases the symptoms experienced, it makes the test more clinically relevant since it is demonstrating sensitization; however, the clinician still has to be careful since sensitization is also a characteristic sign of a normal physiological response. If the addition of passive neck flexion (PNF) alters a SLR response of thigh pain, then the SLR is made a more relevant test of nervous system mechanics since PNF will place greater tension on the dural tube and is far more distant than the DF and eversion. If a more distant sensitizing movement provokes symptoms, the more likely the condition is to be of neurogenic origin since the distant movement has less direct effect on the tension of the nerve.

Finally, the same SLR examination should be performed in identical manner on the uninvolved side to determine the response of the opposite SLR. If the other leg has no impact on the painful side or the uninvolved side, then the results of the SLR can be judged as a positive NTPT with much greater confidence. If the subject experiences the very same response in the uninvolved leg as they did in the involved leg, it would suggest that the painful response may be his or her normal physiological response to the examination. As with any clinical situation, in the clinical reasoning process, too much weight should not be placed on any one aspect of the examination but each component of the examination should be processed within the context of every other component of the examination. These lead the clinician in sound reasoning.

Observation

There are no unique observational characteristics to patients who have a nerve-related problem. In some cases, patients will present with altered posture to avoid neural tension, although this is not consistently the case. Some observational findings may present during active movements but may be absent during static stance. In essence, observational findings are of marginal value during assessment of neurodynamics.

Adverse neural tension may alter the subject's posture in order to remove excess tension within the peripheral nervous system. Initial observation of these altered postures may be quite obvious or may be subtle positions or movements in a pattern that removes pressure from the nervous system or surrounding structures. To look for these postural adjustments, the therapist must be aware of the positions for testing each peripheral nerve and apply the nerve shortening positions as postural compensations to relieve stress on the nerve in question. For example, a patient with a very irritable median nerve in the left upper extremity may present with flexion of the wrist and hand, pronation and flexion of the elbow, internal rotation and adduction of the shoulder, and cervical lateral flexion to the left. This position resembles a flexion synergy pattern for a patient following a cerebral vascular accident affecting the left upper extremity and has led previous authors to consider the neurodynamic component that may exist following a stroke.[19] A far more subtle compensation may include a mildly shortened stride on the involved side of a patient with a positive SLR from sciatica.

Patient History

Symptoms often include allodynia, hyperalgesia, hyperpathia, and dysesthesia.[2] The symptoms noted may be continuous or related to specific stimuli that are position or movement pattern related. Reports of pain may include deep cramping, aching, throbbing, and/or superficial burning, pinching, and stabbing and may be present at variable regions of the body. Symptoms may also linger after the stimulus has been

Summary

- Neurodynamics is a concept that involves the dynamic interplay between mechanical and physiological properties of the peripheral nervous system.
- Sensitizing maneuvers are used during the neural tissue provocation tests, which allow clinicians to differentiate between neural tension and other non-neural or musculoskeletal pathologies.
- Because differentiating mechanical versus nerve-related structures is very difficult, it is more important to note the response to selected positions associated with adverse neural tension.

removed.[2] Alterations in mechanoreceptor threshold may lead to quicker discharge and low threshold to discomfort during activities.[2]

Summary

- As a whole, observational assessment is not very useful when examining patients with suspected adverse neural tension.
- Symptoms associated with adverse neural tension often include allodynia, hyperalgesia, hyperpathia, and dysesthesia.

Physical Examination

Active Physiological Movements

Adverse neural tension may contribute to limitations of motion and pain.[9,20] The patient should be asked what functional movement patterns are provocative to his or her primary complaint. Asking the patient to demonstrate those movements will allow the therapist to analyze how he or she moves, at what point during movement symptoms are provoked, and whether or not those positions are consistent with likely provocation of neural structures. Several provocational tests incorporate sensitizing maneuvers to differentiate between ANT and other musculoskeletal pathologies. Some of the classic neurodynamic tests do not specifically report all the potential sensitizing maneuvers available, yet a simple application of the anatomical path that each nerve courses through will allow the investigator to determine various sensitizing maneuvers available to each. Active physiological movements that are similar to the passive physiological assessments, described in greater detail below, may be used to assess neural tissues of the upper and lower extremity.

Passive Physiological Movements

Neurodynamic tests, also termed neural provocation tests,[15] are sequences of movements designed to assess the mechanics and physiology of part of the nervous system.[16,21] The mechanical components include the ability of the nerve to move and strain relative to any surrounding tissues as well as the motion interface between the elements of the nerve itself, and the physiological components relate to local inflammation, ischemia, and altered ion channel activity resulting in sites of abnormal impulse generation (AIGS). The underlying concept for these tests is that sensitized and painful neural tissues may become noncompliant to an increase in relative length of the nerve bedding to which the nerve must accommodate.[15]

It has been further hypothesized that sensitizing maneuvers can be used to alter the amount of strain applied to nerves through the range of physiological motion. For example, in a modified SLR, applying hip flexion after end-range dorsiflexion will further strain the tibial nerve, assisting in differentiating a distal neuropathy from plantar heel pain. Coppieters et al. found that actively moving the proximal joint provided the greatest amount of strain at the level of the moving joint, additional strain was transferred well beyond that joint and may provide useful information in diagnosing distant pathologies.[18] It has also been found that applying cervical flexion with hip flexion will increase the excursion of the lumbar nerve roots.[22] Table 15.2 ■ indicates the nine total tests that have been reported on in the literature. It should also be noted that there are multiple variations to some of the tests described.

Upper Extremity Tests Upper extremity tests involve any maneuvers in which the majority of primary movements occur at the shoulder, elbow, or wrist/hand.

■ **TABLE 15.2** Neurodynamic Tests and the Structures Tested

Neurodynamic Test	Structure Purported to be Tested
1. ULNT 1	Median nerve
2. ULNT 2a	Median nerve
3. ULNT 2b	Radial nerve
4. ULNT 3	Ulnar nerve
5. Slump sit	Sciatic nerve
6. Slump long sitting	Sympathetic trunk
7. Straight leg raise	Sciatic nerve
8. Prone knee bend	Femoral nerve
9. Passive neck flexion	Dural tube of the spinal cord or can be used to sensitize other neurodynamic tests

The ULNT 1 Test

The ULNT 1 test (also known as ULTT 1) has been found to be a component of a clinical prediction rule (CPR) used to identify patients with cervical radiculopathy.[23] In conjunction with a positive Spurling's test, cervical distraction test, and with ipsilateral cervical rotation of <60°, four positive tests combine for a LR+ of 30.3. If only three positive tests are present, the LR+ drops to 6.1. It must be highlighted that the CPR described may indicate that a radiculopathy is present; however, it does not indict the condition as being neuropathic in origin.

The ULNT 1 is a primarily median nerve bias test but has been reported to put strain on all the major nerves of the upper extremity.[24] For this reason, this test can be referred to as the universal neurodynamic test of the upper quarter.

1. The subject lies supine with the therapist facing the subject's head at the side to be tested.

2. The therapist first queries the subject about his or her symptoms for a baseline of comparison then blocks shoulder girdle elevation with one hand, and sequentially adds shoulder external rotation, abduction to 110° (or the subject's limit), forearm supination, wrist and hand extension, and finally elbow extension (Figures 15.1 ■ – 15.6 ■).

3. The subject should be queried for symptom production after each component is added. If at any point in the examination the subject's comparable sign has been elicited, sensitization maneuvers should be performed to determine if a neural basis for those symptoms is likely.

4. For the ULNT 1, cervical side flexion away to increase symptoms followed by cervical side flexion toward to reduce those symptoms is commonly used (Figure 15.7 ■). It should be noted that any maneuver that lengthens or shortens the dural tube can be used to affect a change but maneuvers that are generally closer in proximity to the nerve in question may have a more powerful effect.

Figures 15.1–15.7 outline the ULNT 1 test and Table 15.3 ■ describes the individual components to each step.

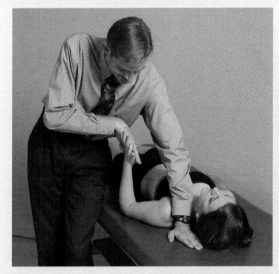

■ Figure 15.1   The ULNT 1 Bias Test Step 1

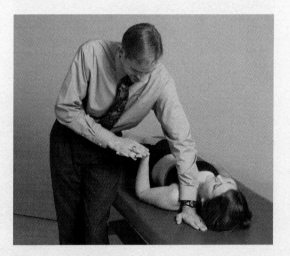

■ Figure 15.2   The ULNT 1 Bias Test Step 2

(Continued)

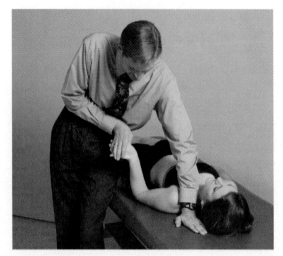

■ **Figure 15.3**   The ULNT 1 Bias Test Step 3

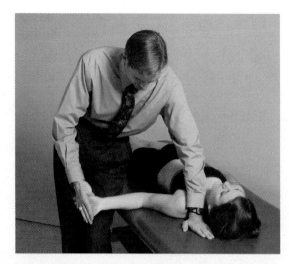

■ **Figure 15.4**   The ULNT 1 Bias Test Step 4

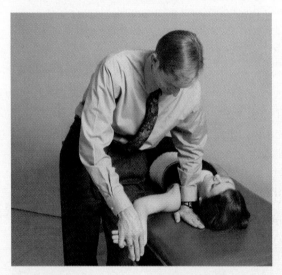

■ **Figure 15.5**   The ULNT 1 Bias Test Step 5

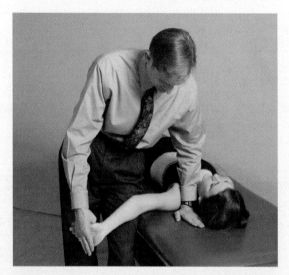

■ **Figure 15.6**   The ULNT 1 Bias Test Step 6

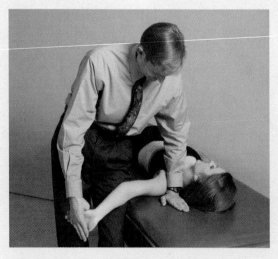

■ **Figure 15.7**   The ULNT 1 Bias Test Step 7

The ULNT 2a Test

The ULNT 2a test (aka ULTT 2a) is also a primary median nerve bias.

1. The subject is supine with the therapist facing the subject's feet along the side to be tested.

2. The therapist queries the subject concerning his or her symptoms then actively depresses the subject's shoulder girdle with the therapist's leg (Figure 15.8 ■).

3. Then the following passive movements are sequentially added: shoulder external rotation, elbow extension, forearm supination, wrist and hand extension, and finally, shoulder abduction (Figure 15.9 –15.13 ■).

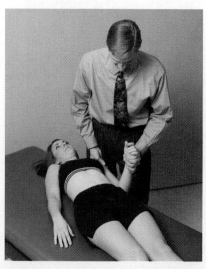

■ **Figure 15.8**   The ULNT 2a Bias Test Step 1

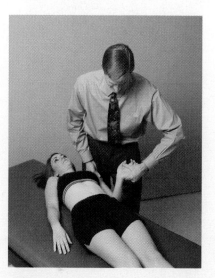

■ **Figure 15.9**   The ULNT 2a Bias Test Step 2

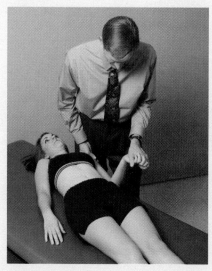

■ **Figure 15.10**   The ULNT 2a Bias Test Step 3

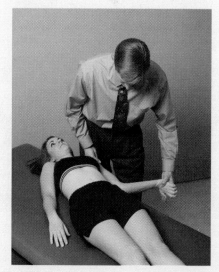

■ **Figure 15.11**   The ULNT 2a Bias Test Step 4

(Continued)

④ Again, the subject is queried for symptom level between the addition of each component and when the subject's concordant sign is elicited, sensitizing maneuvers (Figure 15.14 ■) such as lateral cervical flexion can be added to further implicate neural tissue as the likely cause of those symptoms.

The steps of the ULNT 2a test are outlined in Figures 15.8–15.14 and Table 15.3 describes the individual components to each step.

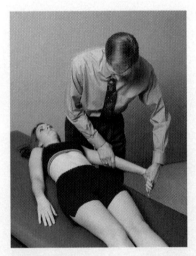

■ **Figure 15.12** The ULNT 2a Bias Test Step 5

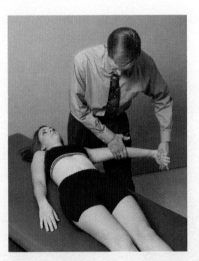

■ **Figure 15.13** The ULNT 2a Bias Test Step 6

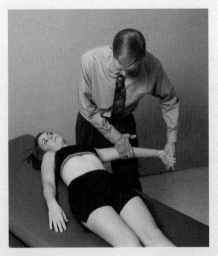

■ **Figure 15.14** The ULNT 2a Bias Test Step 7

The ULNT 2b Test

The ULNT 2b test (aka ULTT 2b) is performed as a primary radial nerve bias.

1. The initial set-up is similar to the ULNT 2a with the subject in supine, the therapist standing at their side facing their feet.

2. The subject is queried for level of symptoms, then the shoulder girdle is actively depressed by the therapist's leg (Figure 15.15 ■), forearm pronation is added then wrist and hand flexion, the shoulder is internally rotated, slightly extended, and finally abducted (Figure 15.16 ■–15.19 ■).

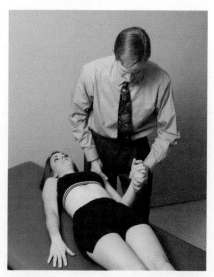

■ **Figure 15.15**   The ULNT 2b Bias Test Step 1

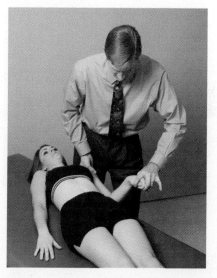

■ **Figure 15.16**   The ULNT 2b Bias Test Step 2

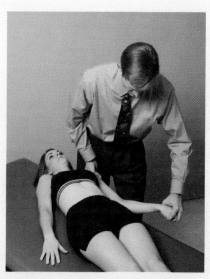

■ **Figure 15.17**   The ULNT 2b Bias Test Step 3

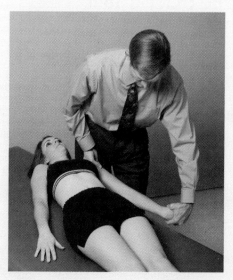

■ **Figure 15.18**   The ULNT 2b Bias Test Step 4

(Continued)

③ The subject is queried for symptom changes between each additional component of the test. If symptom production has been achieved at any point during the test, the addition of components is ceased then sensitizing maneuvers, such as lateral cervical flexion (Figure 15.20 ■) are performed.

The steps of the ULNT 2b test are outlined in Figures 15.15–15.20 and Table 15.3 describes the individual components to each step.

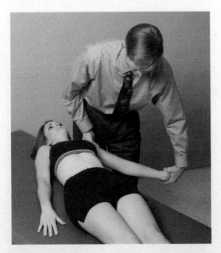

■ **Figure 15.19**   The ULNT 2b Bias Test Step 5

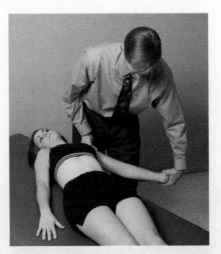

■ **Figure 15.20**   The ULNT 2b Bias Test Step 6

The ULNT 3 Test

The ULNT 3 test is primarily an ulnar nerve bias test.

① The subject is supine with the therapist standing at his or her side facing the head.

② The subject's symptom level is queried before the start of the examination.

③ The subject's shoulder girdle is slightly depressed by pulling inferiorly, posterior at the shoulder (Figure 15.21 ■), the shoulder is abducted to 110°, externally rotated maximally, elbow is flexed, forearm is pronated, and wrist and hand is extended (Figure 15.22 ■–15.25 ■).

④ Once again, between the addition of each component, the subject is queried for alterations in his or her symptoms. If symptoms are increased, sensitizing maneuvers such as lateral cervical flexion (Figure 15.26 ■) are performed to further implicate neural tissue as the cause. Cervical side flexion away to increase symptoms and toward to decrease symptoms are commonly used, but increasing the level of shoulder depression can also be used.

Components of the upper limb neurodynamic tests can be found in Figures 15.21–15.26 and tabulated in Table 15.3.

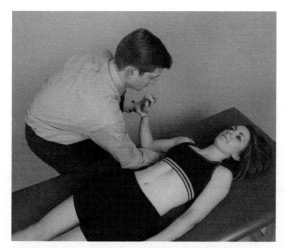

■ **Figure 15.21**   The ULNT 3 Bias Test Step 1

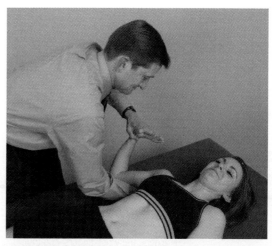

■ **Figure 15.22**   The ULNT 3 Bias Test Step 2

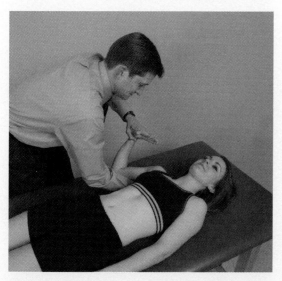

■ **Figure 15.23**   The ULNT 3 Bias Test Step 3

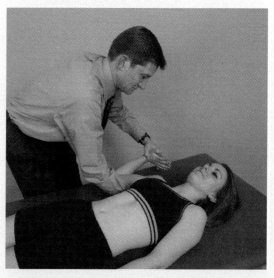

■ **Figure 15.24**   The ULNT 3 Bias Test Step 4

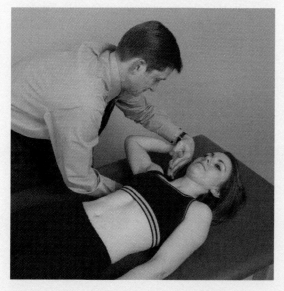

■ **Figure 15.25**   The ULNT 3 Bias Test Step 5

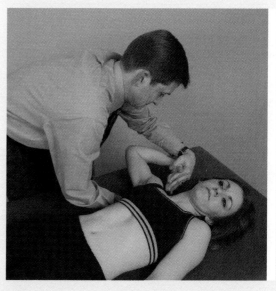

■ **Figure 15.26**   The ULNT 3 Bias Test Step 6

■ TABLE 15.3 Components of the Upper Limb Neurodynamic Tests

ULNT1
- Block shoulder girdle
- Abduct arm to 110 deg
- Supinate forearm
- Extend wrist and fingers
- Laterally rotate shoulder
- Extend elbow
- Cervical lateral flexion away

ULNT2a
- Depress shoulder girdle using thigh (+/- protraction/retraction)
- Laterally rotate the whole arm
- Supinate the forearm
- Extend the wrist, fingers, and thumb
- Extend elbow
- Cervical lateral flexion away

ULNT2b
- Depress shoulder using thigh (+/- protraction/retraction)
- Extend elbow
- Medially rotate whole arm
- Pronate forearm
- Flex and ulnar deviate wrist
- Flex fingers and thumb
- Cervical lateral flexion away

ULNT3
- Extend wrist, pronate forearm
- Flex elbow
- Depress shoulder girdle
- Laterally rotate shoulder
- Abduct shoulder
- Cervical contralateral flexion away

Summary

- The customary passive assessment movements for the upper quadrant involve the ULNT1, ULNT2a, ULNT2b, and the ULNT3 bias tests.
- The ULNT1 is commonly used as the universal neurodynamic test of the upper quarter.

Lower Extremity Neurodynamic Tests   Lower extremity tests involve any maneuvers in which the majority of primary movements occur at the hip, knee, or ankle/foot.

Slump Test

1. The slump test is performed with the subject sitting on the edge of a table of adequate height so that the feet are off the floor and the therapist can easily reach the subject's leg while standing. The test is performed in a functional position that commonly reproduces an individual's low back and leg pain and is often credited to Maitland.[25]

2. The subject is queried for his or her baseline symptoms.

3. The subject is asked to place his or her hands behind the back. This part of the test is not necessary but it keeps the hands out of the way during testing and prevents the subject from weight bearing on the hands, which can alter symptom provocation.

4. The subject is then asked to slump, which essentially is flexion of the spine at the waist; neck flexion is then added by asking the subject to drop his or her chin to the chest (Figure 15.27 ■). It is a good idea to add your hand to the subject's neck gently here to maintain the current trunk position during subsequent components of the test.

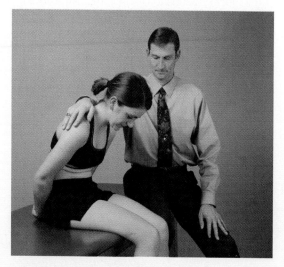

■ Figure 15.27 The Slump Test: Initial Stage

5. The subject is then asked to extend his or her knee, then dorsiflex the ankle. It is not uncommon for the subject to attempt to lean backward when the test begins to alter the symptoms or when hamstring tightness may be perceived. Having a hand on the subject's upper back and neck will assist the therapist in feeling when this compensation occurs (Figure 15.28 ■).

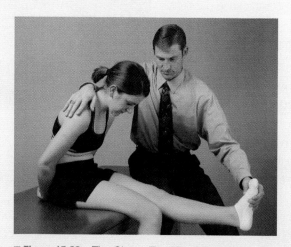

■ Figure 15.28 The Slump Test: Final Stage

(Continued)

6. The subject is queried for alteration in symptoms between each additional component of the test.

7. When the subject's symptoms have been reproduced, sensitizing maneuvers can be added to further implicate neural tissue as the likely cause. For the slump test, sensitizing maneuvers may include hip internal rotation (IR), hip adduction, trunk side flexion away from the painful side, and a reduction of cervical flexion, which typically reduces symptoms. If the subject happens to be hypermobile, a finding that is common in dancers, gymnasts, and other athletes that place a premium on flexibility, knee extension in sitting will not be sufficient to adequately load the sciatic nerve; therefore, the therapist can load the nerve by passively flexing the hip off the table after the knee has been extended.

Straight Leg Raise

The straight leg raise (SLR) is a commonly used test in assessing low back pain.

1. The subject is lying supine on a plinth with the therapist standing alongside and facing the side to be tested. Since cervical flexion alters dural tube length in the lumbar spine, for test–retest reliability, head position matters; therefore, it may be better to avoid the use of a pillow, but if a pillow is required for subject comfort, be sure to use the same pillow in subsequent sessions to maintain consistency.

2. The subject's symptoms are queried for baseline level. With the knee passively held in full extension, the leg is lifted until symptoms are reproduced or there is no more available motion (Figure 15.29 ■).

3. Once symptoms have been elicited, sensitization maneuvers can be performed. These include an alteration in ankle position and dorsiflexion increases

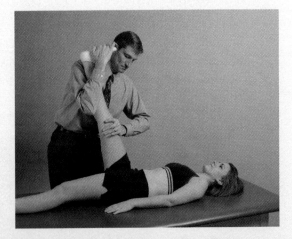

■ **Figure 15.29**   The Straight Leg Raise Test

in tension in the tibial and sural nerves. If inversion is added to DF, the sural nerve will be stressed more, whereas eversion with DF will stress the tibial nerve more. Sometimes plantarflexion with inversion will increase symptoms more and this action implicates the peroneal nerve. The SLR can be further sensitized by hip internal rotation, hip adduction, alteration in cervical flexion, and trunk side flexion away.

Passive Neck Flexion Test

Passive neck flexion has been used as a sensitizing maneuver during the SLR, prone knee flexion, and slump sitting tests but is also a stand-alone test of ANT.

1. The test can be performed in sitting (Figure 15.30 ■) or supine (Figure 15.31 ■) positions.

2. The movements can be either active or passive and involve flexion of the neck.

3. Referred to as Lhermitte's sign, passive neck flexion has been used to determine if an electric shock–type pain would be referred down the spinal column with end-range neck flexion.[26]

If neck flexion alone does not stimulate the subject's comparable sign, a degree of straight leg raise can be applied to assist in generating additional pressure on the nervous system, stimulating symptoms of ANT.

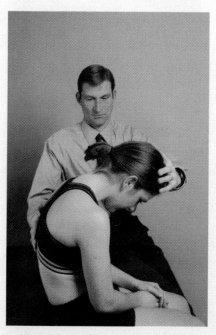

■ **Figure 15.30**   The Passive Neck Flexion Test in Sitting

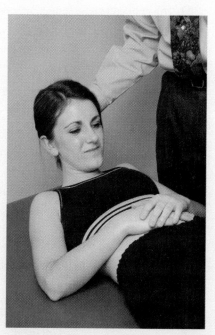

■ **Figure 15.31**   The Passive Neck Flexion Test in Supine

Slump Long Sitting (Sympathetic Slump) Test

The slump long sitting test was described by Maitland[25] and is a variant of the traditional slump with a stronger stretch being applied to the thoracic spine, which may allow the investigator the ability to apply greater pressure to the sympathetic chain ganglion of the thoracic and upper lumbar region.

1. The test is performed on a treatment plinth in long sitting position with both legs bent approximately 60° at the hips and knees.

2. The investigator is sitting on the side opposite of the symptomatic side of the subject.

3. The subject places both hands behind the back to assist in getting them out of the way and to prevent them from bearing weight on the arms during the testing (Figure 15.32 ■).

4. The subject is queried regarding their current symptom level then is asked to assume a slouch sitting posture.

5. The subject is queried again concerning symptom level changes, then neck flexion is added (Figure 15.33 ■), trunk side flexion toward the investigator, trunk rotation away from the investigator, the involved lower extremity is straightened out, and ankle dorsiflexion is added. Before the addition of each component, the subject is queried regarding changes in their comparable sign. At any point during testing when the subject's symptoms are provoked, the investigator can sensitize the system by altering a distant component like reducing cervical flexion to see if it reduces symptoms, providing a unilateral or transverse glide (Figure 15.34 ■) to the suspected thoracic level.

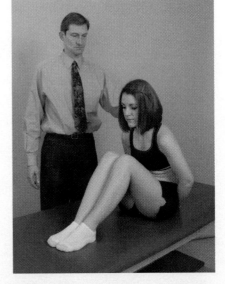

■ **Figure 15.32**   The Slump Long Sitting Test: Initial Stage

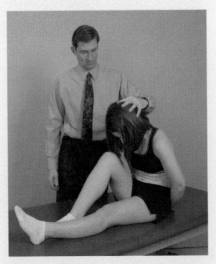

■ **Figure 15.33**   The Slump Long Sitting Test: Final Stage

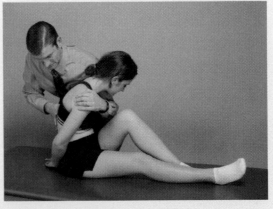

■ **Figure 15.34**   The Slump Long Sitting Test with a Posterior to Anterior Glide

The Prone Knee Bend Test

The prone knee bend is essentially the equivalent to the SLR for the upper lumbar spine. It applies tension through the femoral nerve.

1. The subject is lying prone on a plinth and is queried regarding his or her current symptom level.

2. The investigator applies knee flexion and hip extension to end range or until comparable sign is provoked (Figure 15.35 ■). It can be sensitized by applying cervical flexion or extension or cervical side bending.

3. Additional sensitizing maneuvers can include the addition of trunk side flexion. See Table 15.4 ■.

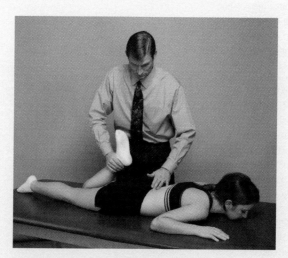

■ **Figure 15.35**   The Prone Knee Bend Test

■ **TABLE 15.4** Lower Extremity Neurodynamic Tests and Components

Slump
- Sequentially add multiple components
  - Lumbar thoracic slump
  - Cervical flexion
  - Knee extension
  - Dorsiflexion
  - Release cervical flexion

Straight leg raise
- SLR with hip medially rotated and adducted
- Add ankle dorsiflexion
- Add plantarflexion
- Add inversion or eversion
- Add passive neck flexion and/or extension
- Add cervical side bending
- Alter other leg position
  - Hip internal rotation
  - Hip adduction
- Test bilateral SLR position
- Add ULNT

Passive neck flexion
- Patient can be seated, long sitting or supine
- Add passive neck flexion
- Hip flexion can be added to increase the effect
- Ankle DF can be added
- Alter other leg position
  - Hip internal rotation
  - Hip adduction

Slump long sitting
- Long sitting, hip and knee flexion
- Forward head with hands behind back
- Thoracic lateral flexion AWAY
- Thoracic rotation TOWARD
- Knee extension
- Cervical protraction
- Cervical extension and lateral flexion AWAY

Prone knee flexion
- Add neck flexion and extension
- Add lumbar side bend
- Add ankle dorsiflexion
- Loaded and unloaded
- Compare with opposite side
- Sustain or oscillate stretch
- Do test at end range in repeated extension in lying

Summary

- The primary neurodynamic tests of the lower quarter include the slump sit, straight leg raise, slump long sitting, passive knee flexion test, and the passive neck flexion test.

- The tests can be performed with the upper quarter tests to further define ANT involvement.

Clinical Use

Each of the above neural tissue provocational tests can be performed using various orders of sequence. It has been debated on whether or not there is an appropriate order of sequence for a given examination. In any given individual, the order of sequence may alter the perception of tension and pain making a specific sequence meaningful clinically. Therefore, it is clinically practical to perform each assessment and reassessment on a given patient in a specific order. If the test is performed differently each time it is applied, an order effect may alter the results of the examination, misleading the therapist in determining if a clinical change is present. Likewise, sensitizing maneuvers should be performed in a consistent manner to enhance reliability. Consistent positioning should also be considered when applying a specific examination for neural tissue. The position of the cervical spine has been classified and supported with evidence as contributory to upper limb symptoms; therefore, care in consistent positioning of the cervical spine is imperative. If you elect to use a pillow for patient comfort, be certain to use a pillow of the same thickness and firmness upon re-examination so that cervical position will not affect the results. Use variations found in Table 15.5 ■ to assess for sensitization.

Reliability and Validity

The passive SLR test has been studied by several authors. In a study of 15 healthy volunteers, the interrater reliability was 0.93 with a 95% confidence interval of 0.80–0.97 and a standard error measure (SEM) of 4.[27] Gabbe et al.[27] used asymptomatic subjects in their study so the transposability of the results to subjects with pain may be questionable. Bertilson et al.[28] examined the reliability of numerous common examination techniques for subjects with low back pain, including the SLR, and found a kappa value of .92 with a 95% confidence interval of 0.65–1.00 and a standard

error of 0.141. Similarly, Strender et al.[29] examined 50 patients with low back pain and established that the interrater reliability between physiotherapists was 0.83 with a standard error of 0.093. In the active slump test, Gabbe et al.[27] reported an intraclass correlation coefficient (ICC) of 0.92 with 95% confidence interval of 0.77–0.97 and a SEM of 3.

One study employed a modified slump sitting test for assessment of children with chronic headaches. An interrater ICC of .96 with an SEM of 2.83° was found. The results of the statistical analysis revealed that children with cervicogenic headaches (82%) felt the symptoms in the spinal area whereas the migraine headache group felt the symptoms in the legs (80%). The control group felt the symptoms more in the legs but with a much lower frequency (36%) and a larger tendency to feel no symptoms at all (46%). Von Piekartz and colleagues[30] also found that sacral position was significantly different in the headache groups as compared to the control group. The cervicogenic headache group had significantly less cervical ROM than the control group and the migraine group when measured in the long slump sitting position.

Summary

- It is clinically practical to perform each assessment and reassessment on a given patient in a specific order.

- If the test is performed differently each time it is applied, an order effect may alter the results of the examination, misleading the therapist in determining if a clinical change is present.

- Likewise, sensitizing maneuvers should be performed in a consistent manner to enhance reliability.

- Consistent positioning should also be considered when applying a specific examination for neural tissue.

- As a whole, the tests are reliable for clinical use.

Passive Accessory Movements

In addition to physiological movement patterns, accessory movements may impact the clinical presentation of symptoms. One accessory movement that has been reviewed in several studies is the cervical side glide technique.[9,18] The unilateral postero–anterior glide has been discussed in a case report.[31] It is likely that the technique provides mild stimulation of the nerve root secondary to the proximity to the structure during the three-point procedure.

■ **TABLE 15.5** Sensitizing Maneuvers and Their Purported Clinical Effect on Symptoms

Technique	Sensitizing Maneuver	Expected Response
SLR	Ankle DF	Increases symptoms
	Hip IR	Increases symptoms
	Hip adduction	Increases symptoms
	Cervical flexion	Increases symptoms
	PF and inversion	Increase symptoms if peroneal nerve is involved, reduce symptoms if tibial nerve is involved
	ULNT	Increases symptoms
Slump	Ankle DF	Increases symptoms
	Reduce cervical flexion	Decreases symptoms
	PF and inversion	Increase symptoms if peroneal nerve is involved, reduce symptoms if tibial nerve is involved
	ULNT	Increase symptoms
ULNT1	Contralateral cervical side flexion	Increases symptoms
	Ipsilateral cervical side flexion	Decreases symptoms
	Shoulder depression	Increases symptoms
	Ipsilateral SLR	Increases symptoms
ULNT2a	Contralateral cervical side flexion	Increases symptoms
	Ipsilateral cervical side flexion	Decreases symptoms
	Ipsilateral SLR	Increases symptoms
ULNT2b	Contralateral cervical side flexion	Increases symptoms
	Ipsilateral cervical side flexion	Decreases symptoms
	Ipsilateral SLR	Increases symptoms
ULNT3	Contralateral cervical side flexion	Increases symptoms
	Ipsilateral cervical side flexion	Decreases symptoms
	Ipsilateral SLR	Increases symptoms
Femoral nerve tension test	Contralateral trunk side flexion	Increases symptoms
	Cervical flexion	Increases symptoms
Slump long sitting	Ankle DF	Increases symptoms
	Cervical flexion	Increases symptoms
Passive neck flexion	SLR	Increases symptoms
	Ankle DF	Increases symptoms

Clinical Special Tests

Palpation of Nervous Tissue

In many locations, it is possible to directly palpate peripheral nerves. In addition, nerves can be indirectly palpated, that is, the nerve can be clinically impacted by the therapist's touch without being able to distinguish the feel of the nerve under the finger such as palpation over the radial tunnel for the deep radial nerve.[32] When possible, the clinician should take the opportunity to palpate the nerves to determine if it may alter the subject's concordant sign. As stated by Goldner and Hall,[33] Butler recommends gently "twanging" a nerve "like a guitar string." It has also been recommended to palpate and apply approximately 10 pounds of pressure to a nerve about 1 inch distal to the proposed area of involvement, examining for distal paresthesia.[33] A similar technique used just proximal to the area of suspected entrapment has also been suggested.[34] The percussion test has been recommended for the assessment of peripheral nerve involvement for nearly 100 years.[35] The test is limited to superficial nerves and involves four to six taps[34] over the nerve, looking for symptom reproduction from the tapping. Numerous authors have reported on the diagnostic accuracy of percussion testing at the wrist for carpal tunnel syndrome and found variable results as well as variable quality of studies examining the diagnostic accuracy. A recent review text concluded that there is moderate evidence to support the use of percussion testing at the elbow and wrist.[36]

Treatment Techniques

Treatment Philosophy

Differentiation from Mechanical Structures   Since all tissues at a given joint will be mechanically impacted with movement of that joint, it becomes necessary to perform techniques that will target neural tissue so the effect of the technique can be maximized and demonstrated during reassessment. Several treatment strategies have been purported to be effective. Tensioning techniques are used to provide tension to the nervous tissue and the general treatment strategy is to provide tension to the neural structure by pulling at both ends.[16] Repetitions involve the repeated application and relaxation of this tension. An alternative way of applying tension is to sustain a static stretch for a given period of time rather than applying slow repetitions of tension. **Gliding techniques,** also known as flossing, function by minimizing the overall strain within the nerve itself but create movement of that nerve within the nerve bed by providing tension

at one end of the nerve while releasing tension at the other end.[16] Repetitions involve the alteration of to which end of the nerve the tension is applied and on which end the tension is relieved. This repetitive alteration in tension and relaxation serves to create movement back and forth within the nerve channel, promoting the much-needed movement required to restore normal axonal physiology. The beginning and ending steps of gliding techniques are demonstrated in Figures 15.36 ■ and 15.37 ■.

An alternative method of treating neural tissues is to apply a minimal load to the neural tissue and sustain that load throughout the treatment. The strain applied is generally kept at a very low level to avoid provocation of the patient's symptoms. The appropriate segment is then oscillated in a graded fashion[37] to move the nerve bed around the stationary nerve root. This technique in many ways may appropriately mimic normal function during human movement since the mobile spinal segments often are moved while the arm is held in position. These treatment techniques are described in Table 15.6 ■.

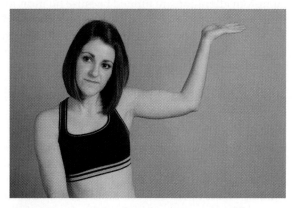

■ **Figure 15.36**   Gliding Technique: Initial Stage

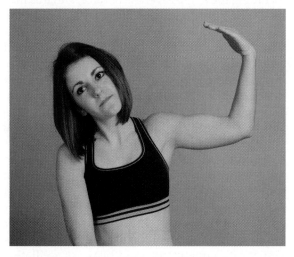

■ **Figure 15.37**   Gliding Technique: Final Stage

■ **TABLE 15.6** Potential Neurodynamic Treatment Techniques Described in the Literature

Techniques	Description
Tension techniques	The patient is placed in a position of comfort but appropriate to provide neurodynamic load. The neural tissue in question is loaded by applying movement and strain through the nerve on either side of the region to be treated. The load is repetitively applied in an oscillatory fashion.
Gliding techniques	The patient is placed in a position of comfort but appropriate to provide neurodynamic load. The neural tissue in question is loaded by applying movement and strain through one end of the nerve while strain is relieved from the other end of the nerve at the region to be treated.
Stretching techniques	The patient is placed in an appropriate position to neurodynamically load the tissue. Strain is applied to the system and is sustained for a predetermined period of time.
Segmental mobilization techniques	The patient is placed in an appropriate position to apply a predetermined amount of neurodynamic load; the therapist applies an oscillatory technique to an appropriate segmental level to move the segment around the nerve.

It is important to note that the previously described treatment techniques do not exclusively target neural tissues. All tissues surrounding the segment in question move in relationship to one another. Two distant segments being moved simultaneously might suggest that the number and type of tissue responsible for symptom alteration are limited because no individual muscle, ligament, or tendon crosses both the cervical spine and wrist but structures do cross many segments, including neural meninges, fascia, and skin.

Guidelines

Patient Response and Irritability   It must be stated that depending on the duration of symptoms, the amount of time required to obtain meaningful clinical change from neurodynamic treatment can be variable. Case reports have identified that it can take several months before adequate resolution of symptoms may occur.[2] Clinical presentation and the degree of neural involvement will guide the dosage of treatment, including the aggressiveness of force, and this may, in turn, guide the rapidity of treatment response noted.

One method described to alter the aggressiveness of treatment includes the localization of treatment relative to the believed area of neural involvement. Because there is evidence to support the hypothesis that more nerve excursion/deformation occurs in the region where force is being applied,[38,39] it is reasonable to use this hypothesis in the application of intervention dosage. In clinical situations where the condition is irritable, movement can be applied at body segments distant to the segment suspected of being pathological to minimize the force being applied at the level of pathology. For example, in the case of a patient with suspected cervical radiculopathy, a load below the pain threshold may be applied to the system and the treatment could be wrist oscillation to vary the strain applied. If the segment involved is not very irritable, the movement can be targeted at the level of pathology to maximize the strain being applied to the pathology. In the previously mentioned case example, the subthreshold load could be applied to the system, then the treatment could include movement of the cervical spine to directly impact neural tissue at the level of the nerve root.

In general, it has been suggested that treating neural tissue relatively gently is a good idea to prevent worsening of the condition.[2] It can be difficult to assess the level of irritability in some cases, making it easy to overtreat and create worsening of symptoms over time. Providing too strong a treatment may further compromise blood flow or create greater mechanical compression of the nerve, causing further disruption of axoplasmic flow or greater hypoxia, resulting in worsening the condition.[2] The use of tensioning techniques makes it much easier to create the condition of overtreatment; therefore, glides (flossing) may be a better treatment option initially until the true behavior of the symptoms can be established. Once treatment has been initiated, patient response can be monitored for strength of treatment response, and this response can be used to determine the appropriate level of intensity in subsequent treatment sessions.

If the patient has relatively low irritability and clinical reasoning would suggest that the tissue bed is compromised (e.g., twinges of pain of short duration, demonstrating through range pain, and resistance with limb tension testing), the patient may benefit from stretching. It may be advantageous to consider stretching non-neural structures first as long as the stretch does not irritate neural tissue before proceeding to direct neural mobilization.

At the present time, little evidence exists to suggest clear guidelines for the optimum dosage for neurodynamic treatment. Most intervention studies have focused on specific techniques but not examined differing levels of dosage of those techniques. For this reason, it is necessary for the treating clinician to base dosage of treatment on sound clinical reasoning. One could examine the current literature for ideas about dosage but adjust those guidelines based on patient response, bearing in mind that it is easy to overtreat neural disorders.

Because ANT suggests that movement is either restricted or prevented, a treatment program that focuses on movement would seem to be paramount. The patient spends so little time in the clinic during the course of care that a home exercise program that is fundamentally based on movement of the neural tissue appears essential to promote quicker recovery. In order to maximize compliance with a home exercise program, it would seem imperative that the clinician emphasize a comprehensive understanding of neural mechanics and their role in a patient's pathology.[2]

One recent study[40] verified a clinical assumption that sliding results in larger neural tissue movement than tensioning. In this study of two embalmed male cadavers, there was twice as much median nerve excursion at the wrist (12.6 vs. 6.1 mm) and ulnar nerve excursion at the elbow (8.3 vs. 3.8 mm). In addition, the larger excursion was accompanied by smaller increases in strain. The strain change of the median nerve at the wrist was 0.8% for sliding compared with 6.8% for tensioning. The authors concluded that different types of neural tissue exercises have differing effects on peripheral nervous tissue.[40] The results largely supported two in vivo studies that found movement of the median nerve[38] and ulnar nerve[39] within the nerve bed during upper-extremity movements. Since Dilley et al.'s studies[38,39] used active movements that provided a tensioning of neural tissues, they reported changes in length similar to the values Coppieters et al.'s study[18] found in the tension group. Direct comparison between these studies should be made with caution since the in vivo studies employed a significantly different instrumentation and the sites of movement were not the same for nerve movement. The most important point is that in vivo studies support that nerve excursion does occur and with similar values to the cadaver study.

Despite the hypotheses that sliders provide greater neural movement with less additional neural strain, stretching exercises have been effectively employed as a neurodynamic treatment in a randomized controlled trial with success.[41] In Cleland et al.'s study,[41] 16 subjects were randomly assigned to the slump stretching group and received six treatments over 3 weeks, which included the standardized education and mobilization and stabilization exercises as the control group but received the additional neural mobilizations, which included five repetitions of 30-second holds in a long sitting slump stretch position with therapist overpressure into cervical flexion to the point of symptom provocation. Despite the precaution to not be too provocative in treatment with ANT, the experimental group subjects experienced statistically significant gains in pain reduction and improvement in the Oswestry Disability Index, which were superior to the control subjects. The Oswestry Disability Index improvements also met the minimal clinically important change score for the instrument at an improvement of greater than 9 points better than the control group. This study suggests that the inclusion of neural mobilization in a comprehensive treatment program improves the overall outcomes of that program. In addition, a recent study compared the effects of tensioners versus sliders in 30 healthy female subjects and found that both techniques produced significant gains in knee extension during slump testing. Even though the mean change appeared greater for the slider group, the actual between-group differences were not significant.[42]

A recent study of asymptomatic individuals supported the hypothesis that neuromobilization, using tensioning techniques, would produce greater hypoalgesic effect than a sham procedure.[43] This study design has been previously used to target differences in A-delta and C-fiber activity. Immediate hypoalgesia was demonstrated in C-fiber but not A-delta fiber response but there was no carryover effect on the C-fibers. There was, however, a carryover effect for treatment effects of elbow extension ROM and sensory descriptors from neurodynamic testing procedures.[43]

Contraindications and Precautions

It is very important to note the possible contraindications and precautions for neurodynamic treatments.[2] As stated previously, painful or irritable neural tissues can be easily exacerbated when treatment is applied indiscriminately. The presence of spinal cord or nerve root signs may suggest that the patient has adverse neural tension within the central nervous system, indicating that the patient should be treated gently. Care must also be applied when examining patients who display unremitting night pain not altered by mechanical provocation since they may have pain of visceral origin. Chronic regional pain syndromes may play a role in neurogenic pain syndromes and its presence complicates the recovery process and leaves the patient vulnerable to exacerbation of symptoms. In addition to the special cases noted here, further examples of precautions and contraindications can be found in Table 15.7 ■.[2]

■ **TABLE 15.7** Potential Contraindications and Precautions for Using Neurodynamic Treatment Techniques

Contraindications

- Recently repaired peripheral nerve
- Malignancy
- Active inflammatory conditions
- Neurological: acute inflammatory demyelinating diseases

Precautions

- Irritable conditions
- Spinal cord signs
- Nerve root signs
- Severe unremitting night pain (with no diagnosis)
- Recent paresthesia/anesthesia
- Mechanical spine pain with peripheralization of symptoms

Augmentation Techniques

There are adjunct interventions that may work synergistically with neural tissue mobilization and serve to enhance outcomes.[2] While complete details of these interventions, including technique and dosage, may be beyond the scope of this text, it is worth noting that these adjuncts are available. Potential adjuncts may include but are not limited to superficial and deep heating agents such as moist heat, ultrasound, and diathermy. One might also consider electrotherapeutic interventions such as transcutaneous electrical nerve stimulation and high-volt pulsed current or interferential current. Massage, acupuncture, acupressure, and myofascial techniques are also possible adjuncts. Unfortunately, the exact effect of each of the interventions with neural mobilization techniques has not been examined with enough rigor for specific recommendations to be made. Coppieters et al.[9] compared the cervical lateral glide technique with ultrasound in subjects with neurogenic cervicobrachial pain and found that therapeutic ultrasound provided no change in ULNT ROM, and nonsignificant changes in pain level or painful area. The dosage of ultrasound (US) treatment was 5 minutes of 1 mHz at $0.5W/cm^2$ at a 20% duty cycle. This dosage represents a desire to achieve nonthermal treatment effects. The clinician must interpret these findings with caution since there is little evidence that US at nonthermal dosages has much therapeutic value and the proposed nonthermal benefits of therapeutic US, microstreaming of stable cavitation altering membrane permeability, lacks *in vivo* support.[44] It might also be noteworthy that interventions have not been found to be predictive of success individually but may actually be beneficial when combined with other interventions as part of a comprehensive therapeutic intervention.[45]

Joint Mobilizations

The cervical lateral glide (Figure 15.38 ■) has been suggested as a technique in the treatment of cervicobrachial pain.[9,46,47] There are several documented effects of the cervical lateral glide. In a placebo-controlled study of 20 asymptomatic subjects, the cervical lateral glide increased available elbow extension range of motion.[48] The results of this study implicate changes in mobility independent of pain threshold alteration since the subjects were asymptomatic upon testing. These results support the neurophysiological effects noted by Vicenzino and colleagues[49] who found in a double-blind placebo-controlled design that the cervical lateral glide was clinically effective in reducing perceived pain, area of pain distribution, and increased available range of motion. Unfortunately, at this time, the mechanism of action is not fully understood. The cervical lateral glide can also be used during augmentation techniques such as a ULNT 2a (Figure 15.39 ■)

The unilateral postero–anterior glide (UPA) has been investigated for therapeutic effect in cervicobrachial pain.[31] This particular intervention was not examined in a controlled manner but was a prospective case report design. Limitations included the fact the subject received a subacromial injection 1 week prior to physical therapy but clinical impact of subacromial injections usually begin shortly after the injection so a 1-week period of no impact would suggest the injection was not effective since the reference standard has been reported to be improvement within 30 minutes.[50] Additionally, some improvement could be noted with weekly implementation of repeated neurodynamic testing but the dosage of testing was considerably less than studies examining the effects of neurodynamic tension techniques.

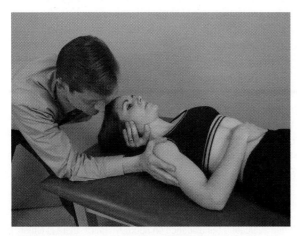

■ **Figure 15.38** Cervical Lateral Glide

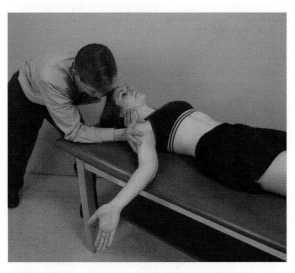

■ **Figure 15.39** Cervical Lateral Glide with ULNT 2a

Summary

- It must be stated that depending on the duration of symptoms, the amount of time required to obtain meaningful clinical change from neurodynamic treatment can be variable.
- The contraindications for neurodynamics should be considered before use.
- Despite the hypotheses that sliders provide greater neural movement with less additional neural strain, stretching exercises have been effectively employed as a neurodynamic treatment in a randomized controlled trial with success.

Treatment Outcomes

A review of the literature demonstrates that there are varying levels of support for the efficacy of neurodynamic techniques for various pathologies. A recent systematic review of multiple randomized controlled trials determined that there is either insufficient or limited evidence for the use of neural mobilization for many common pathologies of the nervous system.[51] The review highlighted an insufficient quantity of high-quality studies examining the effectiveness of neurodynamic techniques.[51]

Despite the relative lack of high-quality randomized controlled trials and the heterogeneity of methods, pathologies, and treatment techniques used in many of the studies available, there are a number of studies that have found the treatment techniques to be useful in treating neurogenic pathologies.

The Evidence

Static Stretching of the Nerve There is level C evidence for the use of static stretching in subjects with a positive slump test. Cleland et al.[41] found that six treatment sessions over 3 weeks adding five repetitions of 30-second holds, supported with a daily home exercise program of two repetitions of 30-second slump stretching, improved treatment outcomes over joint mobilization and a standard exercise program alone. These data supported the results of a previous case series design, which found the slump stretching beneficial for subjects with a positive slump test who did not demonstrate radicular signs.[52]

Flossing the Nerve There is level C evidence to refute the use of gliding techniques for carpal tunnel syndrome. Three studies found that the inclusion of neurodynamic gliding techniques did not enhance the outcomes over splinting techniques during the course of conservative care.[53-55] Each of these studies showed that both treatment groups demonstrated statistically significant improvements in pain, strength, and function but there were no between-group differences favoring neurodynamic intervention.

Tensioners of the Nerve Reviewing tension techniques has demonstrated Level C evidence for the treatment of adverse neural tension. Tal-Akabi and Rushton[56] found that neurodynamic mobilization was more effective than a nontreatment control but the results were similar to the use of carpal bone mobilization in subjects with a positive neurodynamic assessment and purported carpal tunnel syndrome. In addition, Drechsler et al.[57] found that tensioning techniques, as part of a comprehensive MT treatment, may have clinically impacted lateral epicondylitis. The study design precludes our ability to determine if the tension techniques contributed to the positive outcomes reported.

Mobilization of the Vertebrae over a Tensioned Nerve   There is level C evidence to support the use of spinal mobilization for suspected neurodynamic pathology. One study compared the effects of a cervical lateral glide under a neurodynamic load (ULNT-1) with US for pain reduction and pain area.[9] Coppieters et al.[9] found that elbow ROM was increased, pain intensity decreased and painful area decreased, whereas the US group had no significant change in ROM, pain intensity, and painful area.

The above study is similar to a pilot study by Allison et al.'s study where a comprehensive treatment program was performed with the cervical lateral glide.[58] In Allison et al.'s study, a smaller neurodynamic load was applied during the lateral glide and more MT treatment was performed in conjunction with therapeutic exercise. The control group crossed over after 8 weeks to receive the MT treatment. The subjects in the control group experienced similar reductions in symptoms after joining the MT group.[58]

There is level D evidence to support the use of a unilateral postero–anterior glide ipsilateral to the side of pain in subjects with a positive neurodynamic test and cervico-brachial pain.[31] Haddick[31] used the UPAs exclusively while reassessing the ULNT, pain, and disability levels during all five treatment sessions over 5 weeks. Even though the mobilization technique used in this case report is not the same as the contralateral side glide reported in previous studies,[9,47,57] it may not be unreasonable to expect similar results since previous work has suggested that the specific manual therapy technique incorporated may not be as important as providing movement.[59]

A summary of the available evidence to support neurodynamic treatment techniques is provided in Table 15.8 ∎.

Summary

- When evaluating the evidence on neurodynamics, there is either insufficient or limited evidence for the use of neural mobilization for many common pathologies of the nervous system.
- There is either level C or D evidence to support stretching, flossing, or mobilization while engaging the nerve during treatment.

∎ **TABLE 15.8** Literature Examining Neurodynamic Treatment Techniques and the Effectiveness of Those Techniques

Author	Neural Assessment	Intervention	Outcome	Level of Evidence
Haddick et al.[31]	ULNT 1	UPA glides	↓ pain & SPADI	Level D CR
Coppieters et al.[9]	ULNT 1	Contralateral cervical glide	↓ pain, ↓ area of symptoms & SPADI	Level C
Coppieters et al.[9]	ULNT 1	Contralateral cervical glide	↓ pain	Level C
Vicenzino et al.[49]	ULNT 2b	Contralateral cervical glide	↓ pain, ↑ ROM ↑ Pressure pain threshold & strength	Level C
Cowell et al.[47]	ULNT 1	Contralateral cervical glides	↓ pain & Northwick Park Questionnaire	Level D Single-subject design
Ekstrom & Holden[32]	ULNT 1 & 2b	ULNT 1 & 2b stretches with elbow extension, US, & HEP	↓ pain, ↑ ROM & strength	Level D CR
Cleland et al.[41]	Slump	Slump stretches 5 reps 30-second holds after an exercise program	↓ pain, ↑ function & centralization of symptoms	Level C
Allison et al.[58]	Neurogenic criteria	Contralateral cervical glide, shoulder girdle depression oscillation, contract–relax technique for GH abduction and ER, and HEP	↓ pain (VAS – 1 week, and MPQ), ↑ function Northwick Park Questionnaire	Level C

Chapter Questions

1. Describe the three-layer fascial structure of the nerve and discuss how mobile the nerve itself is.

2. Describe what is meant by "biasing a nerve" when used during assessment and treatment.

3. Compare and contrast gliding and tension-based techniques.

4. Describe the effect of prepositioning for augmentation techniques.

Patient Cases

Case 15.1: Thomas Brown (66-Year-Old Male)

Diagnosis: Low back pain and sciatica

Observation: He exhibits a flat back with poor movement at the lumbar spine.

Mechanism: He notes an injury while lifting items in his garage about 9 months ago. He has since had residual leg pain.

Concordant Sign: Bending forward to touch his toes.

Nature of the Condition: He considers the problem a nuisance but does indicate that he can no longer "tool around" in his garage without having residual low back and leg symptoms. The leg never flares past a manageable state but does ache enough that he needs to take ibuprofen.

Behavior of the Symptoms: He is unable to tell if the back and leg pain are related. The pain is often disassociated.

Pertinent Patient History: He has had chronic low back pain for over 25 years.

Patient Goals: He is interested in getting rid of the leg pain.

Baseline: Leg pain at rest, 1/10 NAS for pain; when worst, 3/10 pain.

Examination Findings: Pain in the back and leg are worsened with forward flexion. PAs do not reproduce his symptoms but a SLUMP test does.

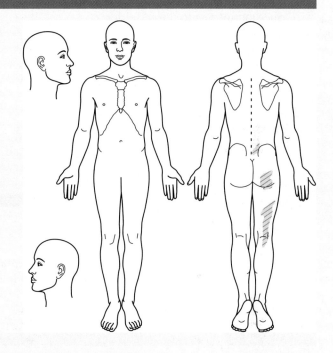

1. Based on these findings, what else would you like to examine?
2. Is this patient a good candidate for manual therapy?
3. What is the expected prognosis of this patient?
4. What treatments do you feel presented in this book may be beneficial for this patient?

Case 15.2: Carla Fortiner (49-year-old female)

Diagnosis: Neck and shoulder pain

Observation: She exhibits a forward head posture and restricted movements.

Mechanism: She was struck on the head by a 2 × 4 board while refurbishing her kitchen. Since then she has had neck pain and pain that has gone to her shoulder.

Concordant Sign: She claims that side flexion away from her affected shoulder is the worst movement.

Nature of the Condition: She mentioned that her problem is a nuisance but the ache can affect her productivity during the day. She manages her symptoms with ibuprofen.

Behavior of the Symptoms: She feels the neck and shoulder pain are related. She does indicate that as the neck starts to hurt the shoulder follows quickly.

Pertinent Patient History: Had breast cancer with a mastectomy 7 years ago.

Patient Goals: She is worried that she has a "herniated disc" since she now has shoulder pain and was recently diagnosed by her physician as a rotator cuff tear. She does not have shoulder weakness.

Baseline: His current symptoms are at 2/10; when worse, 5/10.

Examination Findings: Cervical side flexion away and forward flexion reproduce neck and shoulder symptoms. PAs to the right C5–6 also reproduce symptoms to the shoulder.

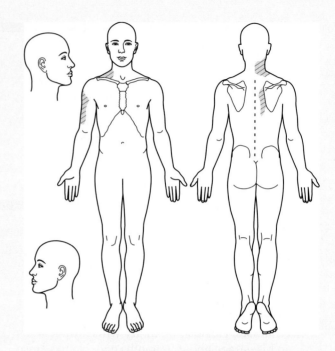

1. Based on these findings, what else would you like to examine?
2. Is this patient a good candidate for manual therapy?
3. What is the expected prognosis of this patient?
4. What treatments do you feel presented in this book may be beneficial for this patient?

PEARSON
myhealthprofessionskit™

Use this address to access the Companion Website created for this textbook. Simply select "Physical Therapy" from the choice of disciplines. Find this book and log in using your username and password to access video clips and the anatomy and arthrological information.

References

1. Shacklock MO. Positive upper limb tension test in a case of surgically proven neuropathy: Analysis and validity. *Man Ther.* 1996;1:154–161.
2. Walsh MT. Upper limb neural tension testing and mobilization: Fact, fiction, and a practical approach. *J Hand Ther.* 2005;18:241–258.
3. Breig A. *Adverse mechanical tension in the central nervous system: An analysis of cause and effect, relief by functional neursurgery.* Stockholm; A and W International/John Wiley & Sons: 1978.
4. Devor M, Rappaport ZH. Pain and pathophysiology of damaged nerves. In: Fields HL (ed). *Pain syndromes in neurology.* Oxford: Butterworth Heinemann: 1990, 47–83.
5. Hall TM, Elvey RL. Nerve trunk pain: Physical diagnosis and treatment. *Man Ther.* 1999;4:63–73.
6. Lew PC, Briggs CA. Relationship between the cervical component of the slump test and change in hamstring muscle tension. *Man Ther.* 1997;2:98–105.
7. Barker PJ, Briggs CA. Attachments of the posterior layer of lumbar fascia. *Spine.* 1999;24:1757–1764.
8. DiFabio RP. Neural mobilization: The impossible. *J Orthop Sports Phys Ther.* 2001;31:224–225.
9. Coppieters MW, Stappaerts KH, Wouters LL, Janssens K. The immediate effects of a cervical lateral glide treatment technique in patients with neurogenic cervicobrachial pain. *J Orthop Sports Phys Ther.* 2003;33: 369–378.
10. Walsh J, Flatley M, Johnston N, Bennett K. Slump test: Sensory responses in asymptomatic subjects. *J Man Manip Ther.* 2007;15:231–238.
11. Yaxley G, Jull GA. A modified upper limb tension test: An investigation of responses in normal subjects. *Aust J Physiother.* 1991;37:143–152.
12. Molesworth J. The effect of chronic inversion ankle sprains on the dorsiflexion–inversion straight leg raise test and the plantarflexion–inversion straight leg raise test. Thesis, University of South Australia, Adelaide: 1992.
13. Balster SM, Jull GA. Upper trapezius muscle activity during the brachial plexus tension test in asymptomatic subjects. *Man Ther.* 1997;2:144–149.

14. Goeken LN, Hof AL. Instrumental straight-leg raising: Results in healthy subjects. *Arch Phys Med Rehabil.* 1993;74:194–203.

15. Elvey RL, Hall TM. Neural tissue evaluation and treatment. In: Donatelli RA (ed)., *Physical therapy of the shoulder.* New York; Churchill Livingstone: 1997.

16. Butler DS. *The sensitive nervous system.* Adelaide; Noigroup Publications: 2000.

17. Lewis J, Ramot R, Green A. Changes in mechanical tension in the median nerve: Possible implications for the upper limb tension test. *Physiother.* 1998;84:254–261.

18. Coppieters MW, Alshami AM, Babri AS, Souvlis T, Kippers V, Hodges PW. Strain and excursion of the sciatic, tibial, and plantar nerves during a modified straight leg raising test. *J Orthop Res.* 2006;24:1883–1889.

19. McKibbin H. Neurodynamics related to the treatment of patients following a cerebral vascular accident. In: Harrison MA (ed)., *Physiotherapy in stroke management.* New York; Churchill Livingstone: 1995.

20. Quintner JL. A study of upper limb pain and paraesthesiae following neck injury in motor vehicle accidents: Assessment of the brachial plexus tension test of elvey. *Br J Rheumatol.* 1989;28:528–533.

21. Shacklock MO. Neurodynamics. *Physiother.* 1995;81:9–16.

22. Lew PC, Morrow CJ, Lew AM. The effect of neck and leg flexion and their sequence on the lumbar spinal cord. Implications in low back pain and sciatica. *Spine (Phila Pa 1976).* 1994;19:2421–2424.

23. Wainner RS, Fritz JM, Irrgang JJ, Boninger ML, Delitto A, Allison S. Reliability and diagnostic accuracy of the clinical examination and patient self-report measures for cervical radiculopathy. *Spine.* 2003;28:52–62.

24. Kleinrensink GJ, Stoeckart R, Mulder PG, et al. Upper limb tension tests as tools in the diagnosis of nerve and plexus lesions. Anatomical and biomechanical aspects. *Clin Biomech* (Bristol, Avon). 2000;15(1):9–14.

25. Maitland GD. The slump test: Examination and treatment. *Aust J Physiother.* 1985;31:215–219.

26. Magee DJ. *Orthopedic physical assessment.* 4th ed. Philadelphia; WB Saunders: 2008.

27. Gabbe BJ, Bennell KL, Wajswelner H, Finch CF. Reliability of common lower extremity musculoskeletal screening tests. *Phys Ther Sport.* 2004;5:90–97.

28. Bertilson BC, Bring J, Sjoblom A, Sundell K, Strender LE. Inter-examiner reliability in the assessment of low back pain (lbp) using the Kirkaldy-Willis classification (kwc). *Eur Spine J.* 2006;15:1695–1703.

29. Strender LE, Sjoblom A, Sundell K, Ludwig R, Taube A. Interexaminer reliability in physical examination of patients with low back pain. *Spine (Phila Pa 1976).* 1997;22:814–820.

30. von Piekartz HJ, Schouten S, Aufdemkampe G. Neurodynamic responses in children with migraine or cervicogenic headache versus a control group: A comparative study. *Man Ther.* 2007;12:153–160.

31. Haddick E. Management of a patient with shoulder pain and disability: A manual physical therapy approach addressing impairments of the cervical spine and upper limb neural tissue. *J Orthop Sports Phys Ther.* 2007;37:342–350.

32. Ekstrom RA, Holden K. Examination of and intervention for a patient with chronic lateral elbow pain with signs of nerve entrapment. *Phys Ther.* 2002;82:1077–1086.

33. Goldner JL, Hall RL. Nerve entrapment syndromes of the lower back and lower extremities. In: Omer GE, Spinner M, Van Beek AL (eds)., *Management of peripheral nerve problems.* Philadelphia; W.B. Saunders: 1997.

34. Mackinnon SC, Dellon AL. *Surgery of the peripheral nerve.* New York; Thieme: 1988.

35. Tinel J. Le signe du "Fourmillement" Dans les lesions des nerfs peripheriques. *Presse Medicale.* 1915;47:388–389.

36. Cook C, Hegedus E. *Orthopedic physical examination tests: An evidence-based approach.* Upper Saddle River, NJ; Prentice Hall: 2008.

37. Maitland GD, Hengeveld E, Banks K, English K. *Maitland's vertebral manipulation.* London; Butterworth-Heinemann: 2001.

38. Dilley A, Lynn B, Greening J, DeLeon N. Quantitative in vivo studies of median nerve sliding in response to wrist, elbow, shoulder and neck movements. *Clin Biomech (Bristol, Avon).* 2003;18:899–907.

39. Dilley A, Summerhayes C, Lynn B. An in vivo investigation of ulnar nerve sliding during upper limb movements. *Clin Biomech (Bristol, Avon).* 2007;22:774–779.

40. Coppieters MW, Butler DS. Do 'sliders' slide and 'tensioners' tension?: An analysis of neurodynamic techniques and considerations regarding their application. *Man Ther.* 2008;13:213–221.

41. Cleland JA, Childs JD, Palmer JA, Eberhart S. Slump stretching in the management of non-radicular low back pain: A pilot clinical trial. *Man Ther.* 2006;11:279–286.

42. Herrington L. Effect of different neurodynamic mobilization techniques on knee extension range of motion in the slump position. *J Man Manip Ther.* 2006;14:101–107.

43. Beneciuk JM, Bishop MD, George SZ. Effects of upper extremity neural mobilization on thermal pain sensitivity: A sham-controlled study in asymptomatic participants. *J Orthop Sports Phys Ther.* 2009;39:428–438.

44. Baker KG, Robertson VJ, Duck FA. A review of therapeutic ultrasound: Biophysical effects. *Phys Ther.* 2001;81:1351–1358.

45. Cleland JA, Fritz JM, Whitman JM, Heath R. Predictors of short-term outcome in people with a clinical diagnosis of cervical radiculopathy. *Phys Ther.* 2007;87:1619–1632.

46. Elvey RL. Treatment of arm pain associated with abnormal brachial plexus tension. *Aust J Physiother.* 1986;32:225–230.

47. Cowell IM, Phillips DR. Effectiveness of manipulative physiotherapy for the treatment of a neurogenic cervicobrachial pain syndrome: A single case study–experimental design. *Man Ther.* 2002;7:31–38.

48. Saranja J, Green A, Lewis J, Worsfold C. Effect of a cervical lateral glide on the upper limb neurodynamic test 1: A blinded placebo-controlled investigation. *Physiotherapy.* 2003;89:678–684.

49. Vicenzino B, Collins D, Wright A. The initial effects of a cervical spine manipulative physiotherapy treatment on the pain and dysfunction of lateral epicondylalgia. *Pain*. 1996;68:69–74.

50. Calis M, Akgun K, Birtane M, Karacan I, Calis H, Tuzun F. Diagnostic values of clinical diagnostic tests in subacromial impingement syndrome. *Ann Rheum Dis*. 2000;59:44–47.

51. Ellis RF, Hing WA. Neural mobilization: A systematic review of randomized controlled trials with an analysis of therapeutic efficacy. *J Man Manip Ther*. 2008;16: 8–22.

52. George SZ. Characteristics of patients with lower extremity symptoms treated with slump stretching: A case series. *J Orthop Sports Phys Ther*. 2002;32:391–398.

53. Baysal O, Altay Z, Ozcan C, Ertem K, Yologlu S, Kayhan A. Comparison of three conservative treatment protocols in carpal tunnel syndrome. *Int J Clin Pract*. 2006;60:820–828.

54. Pinar L, Enhos A, Ada S, Gungor N. Can we use nerve gliding exercises in women with carpal tunnel syndrome? *Adv Ther*. 2005;22:467–475.

55. Akalin E, El O, Peker O, Senocak O, Tamci S, Gulbahar S, Cakmur R, Oncel S. Treatment of carpal tunnel syndrome with nerve and tendon gliding exercises. *Am J Phys Med Rehabil*. 2002;81:108–113.

56. Tal-Akabi A, Rushton A. An investigation to compare the effectiveness of carpal bone mobilisation and neurodynamic mobilisation as methods of treatment for carpal tunnel syndrome. *Man Ther*. 2000;5:214–222.

57. Drechsler WI, Knarr JF, Snyder-Mackler LA. A comparison of two treatment regimens for lateral epicondylitis: A randomized trial of clinical interventions. *J Sport Rehabil*. 1997;6:226–234.

58. Allison GT, Nagy BM, Hall T. A randomized clinical trial of manual therapy for cervico-brachial pain syndrome: A pilot study. *Man Ther*. 2002;7:95–102.

59. Chiradejnant A, Maher CG, Latimer J, Stepkovitch N. Efficacy of "therapist-selected" versus "randomly selected" mobilisation techniques for the treatment of low back pain: A randomised controlled trial. *Aust J Physiother*. 2003;49:233–241.

Soft-Tissue Mobilization

Megan Donaldson

Chapter 16

Objectives

- Understand the anatomy and pertinent arthrokinematics of soft tissue.
- Recognize the unique observational and patient history characteristics associated with a myofascial injury.
- Apply and describe the variant forms of soft-tissue mobilization.
- Recognize the techniques of treatment that have yielded the highest success in the literature.

Soft-Tissue Mobilization

Soft-tissue mobilization (STM) is a form of manual therapy technique that involves specific movement of the connective and muscular tissues through application of forces that are applied to the tissues in methods similar to joint mobilizations. The forces can vary in speed, depth, and direction. The two primary anatomical targets for STM include connective tissue and muscle.

Some may think that including a soft-tissue mobilization chapter in this "evidence-based" book is a bit of a reach. At present, evidence to support the use of soft-tissue mobilization does not equal that associated with joint-related or nerve-related therapies, and involves either weak or conflicting findings.[1] A portion of the blame for this finding may be that the stewards of soft tissue–based techniques have not done a diligent job in supporting this treatment mechanism. In all fairness, it is difficult to design a comparative effectiveness study that adequately evaluates the merits of soft-tissue mobilization, although there is also limited evidence to support the use of soft-tissue techniques in observational trials or other less rigorous designs. Consequently, what follows within this chapter are methods that may provide support during a multimodal treatment approach.

Clinical Examination

Purpose

When performing a clinical examination with the intent of assessing for the need of soft-tissue mobilization there are a number of considerations for a manual therapist. Soft-tissue mobilization is theorized to maximize the repair processes of the musculoskeletal tissue and assist in restoring function as rapidly as possible without reinjury. Soft-tissue mobilization is a form of manual technique that provides improvement of functional tissue healing and stimulation of mechanoreceptors to help modulate pain.

The clinical effects of STM are discussed later in the chapter. Many of the clinical benefits of STM are related to the psychological effect of touch and through tissue preparation for additional physical therapy techniques, including (but not limited to) relaxation training, joint mobilization, contract/relax, proprioceptive neuromuscular facilitation, active exercise, postural retraining, and education. Clinical findings (e.g., muscle imbalances, muscle tone, and inflammation) are often found during palpation or manual muscle testing and these findings may improve the likelihood of matching an appropriate soft-tissue intervention with the pathological process of the specific patient.

Observation

Although there are no unique elements that associate soft-tissue mobilization toward a specific clinical examination process, there are independent features that may warrant the use of soft-tissue mobilization as a treatment mechanism. One observable examination finding may include swelling, which indicates an underlying mechanism of inflammation, where soft-tissue mobilization may assist in reducing. There are two major types of inflammation: acute and chronic. Chronic inflammation may develop secondary to unresolved acute inflammation. Acute inflammation may occur after trauma, surgery, or other events that lead to damage or dysfunction of soft tissue. Findings for both chronic and acute inflammation may include heat, pain, whole limb swelling (associated with lymphatic issues) or localized swelling (associated with regional injury), and impairment or loss of function. Swelling that is edematous suggests the benefit of use of lymphatic release methods (beyond the scope of this book), whereas nonpitting swelling may be associated with an acute inflammatory process.

If the patient presents with discoloration, then it may be considered that the patient has poor circulation and potentially underlying swelling. Nonetheless, discoloration may also involve bleeding and damage that reflects a serious pathology within the specific region. Close inspection of the region should be performed prior to application of any soft-tissue mobilization procedure.

During the observational examination, it is important to note the posture of the individual as it may help to identify a muscular imbalance. It is more challenging to find a muscle imbalance that manifests as a postural disorder. The purpose of the postural muscle examination is to get an overall view of the patient's muscle function. The most common upper quadrant postural disorder, known as upper crossed syndrome, involves a substantial weakening or lengthening of selected muscle groups including the anterior neck flexors, extensors of the upper limb, posterior thoracic extensors, and a shortening or tightening of other muscle groups, including the neck extensors and anterior thoracic flexors.

Lower crossed syndrome involves weakened and lengthened tissue, including the abdominals, gluteals, vastus medialis, and lateralis muscles of the lower quadrant; whereas the other groups are tightened and shortened, including the hip flexors, iliopsoas, rectus femoris, tensor fascia latae, adductors, and erector spinae.[2] There are a variety of causes for shortened/tightened muscles including overuse, injury, and/or change in the elasticity of the muscle. The examination may point to specific syndromes as mentioned and can be used to guide which muscle to evaluate for shortness.

Patient History

A number of myofascial-oriented soft-tissue dysfunctions can cause referred pain to sites external to the origination point. For example, the lower trapezius may refer pain to the upper quarter and the lateral aspect of the neck; soleus pain can manifest as tendon and Achilles tendon pain; the supraspinatus may refer pain to the deltoid insertion and the lateral aspect of the elbow; and gluteus minimus injury may refer pain to the lateral knee, hamstrings, and the medial calf.[3] It's important to note that the region of complaint may not be the region of origin of discomfort.

Many myofascial-oriented dysfunctions are concomitantly linked with tension-related disorders such as depression or anxiety.[4] and myofascial-oriented pain may be inflammatory or noninflammatory[5] Most myofascial pain syndromes have irritable foci (trigger points) within skeletal muscles and the ligamentous junctions.[6] Other conditions such as fibromyalgia, myositis, and myalgia may present as myofascial dysfunctions but are actually central mediated pain syndromes and may best be managed medically using pharmaceutical care.[7] Patients with these conditions will often complain of pain during exercise, exertion, or maintenance of long-term postures.[8] Accumulating evidence suggests that fibromyalgia syndrome pain is maintained by tonic impulse input from deep tissues, such as muscles and joints, in combination with central sensitization mechanisms. This nociceptive input may originate in peripheral tissues (e.g., trauma and infection) resulting in hyperalgesia/allodynia and/or central sensitization.[9]

Postural syndromes and other muscular imbalance-related pain syndromes are appropriately targeted by soft-tissue mobilization techniques. The most frequently encountered postural syndromes are found at the neck and low back, with the neck demonstrating the highest prevalence.[10] In most cases, no single concordant activity can be identified by the patient that is specific to his or her condition. Examination results often confirm the vagueness of symptoms.

Summary

- When addressing soft-tissue concerns, patient history and observation may be two useful data collection components of the assessment.
- Postural or positional-oriented discomfort may have a soft-tissue component.
- One observable examination finding associated with a soft-tissue disorder may include swelling, indicating an underlying mechanism of inflammation in which soft-tissue mobilization may assist in reducing.

Physical Examination

Active Physiological Movements, Passive Physiological Movements, and Passive Accessory Movements

Within the physical examination there are no unique examination procedures for soft-tissue mobilization considerations that are outside those identified in the joint-specific chapters. All active physiological, passive physiological, and passive accessory movements are examined in context to each body region and are not unique to those in Chapters 5–14. It is also necessary for the clinician to extrapolate the contribution of soft tissue to the impairments identified within the examination sequences.

Special Clinical Tests

Palpation

During palpation the clinician can concentrate on specific information from the patient's skin and soft tissue by gathering information regarding resistance, resilience, roughness, temperature, mobility, texture, and moisture. **Trigger points** (TrPs) have been defined as hyperirritable foci lying within taut bands of muscle, which are painful upon compression and which consistently refer pain to a distal site or a site away from the point of origin.[11] Trigger points can occur throughout the body at nearly any muscular region, commonly manifesting as pain during contraction of the tissue. Trigger points may manifest as tension headache, tinnitus, or temporomandibular joint pain[12] and are often (but not always) at neuromuscular junction sites.

Active trigger points can cause peripheral sensitization of muscle nociceptors, which can enhance pain mechanisms experienced by the patient. TrPs differ from tender points, which are predictable, symmetrical tender spots within the body that do not cause referred pain. TrPs typically occur in a restricted regional pattern and are more indicative of myofascial pain syndrome. Myofascial pain syndrome is very common in the general population and its incidence is as high as 54% in women and 45% in men at any point in time, although the prevalence of patients with TrPs in the masticatory muscles does not exceed 25%.[13]

TrPs are defined as areas of muscle that are painful to palpation and are characterized by the presence of taut bands and the generation of a referral pattern of pain. TrPs are typically identified using palpation as hyperirritable nodules within taut bands of skeletal muscle. Palpation consists of a firm pressure applied directly over the TrPs, often perpendicular to the muscle. In some cases, a transient visible or palpable contraction or dimpling of the muscle and skin as the tense muscle fibers (taut band) of the trigger point contract occurs when pressure is applied.[14] This response is elicited by a sudden change of pressure on the trigger point by needle penetration into the trigger point. A latent trigger point is a focal area of tenderness and tightness in a muscle that does not result in spontaneous pain. However, a latent trigger point may restrict range of movement and result in weakness of the muscle involved.

Tender points, on the other hand, are typically small, well-defined regions primarily within the distal ends of muscle bellies or within the fascial layers. Tender points are often associated with global loss of tolerance to pain, whereas trigger points can be unilateral, involve one muscle group, and can be treated directly. Tender points are areas of tenderness occurring in muscle, muscle–tendon junction, bursa, or fat pad and present in a widespread manner. In some patients the two phenomena may coexist, and overlapping syndromes can occur.

Reliability estimates were generally higher for subjective signs such as point tenderness (kappa range 0.22–1.0) and pain reproduction (kappa range 0.57–1.00), and lower for objective signs such as the identification of a taut band (kappa range –0.08–0.75) or local twitch response (kappa range –0.05–0.57).[15] Because of the variability in reliability, there is continued controversy regarding characteristics and homogeneity of myofascial pain.[16]

Trigger Point Assessment Technique

There are certain clinical diagnostic characteristics that should be looked for during examination in order to confirm the presence of myofascial TrPs. These include a taut band, spot tenderness or jump sign, pain recognition, referred pain, and local twitch response.[17] A palpable taut band is identified when a taut cord-like band could be observed or found during the palpation. Spot tenderness is identified with the patient's complaint of pain during palpation. The local twitch response is a transient contraction of the taut band and can be either palpated or visualized through the patient's skin during snapping or squeezing palpation of the TrPs. Pain recognition is similar to other provocation techniques described in previous chapters; it is the patient's concordant pain experience.[18] The TrP referral pain may follow a dermatomal distribution pattern that is remote from the trigger point site.[19] In most cases, TrPs follow a specific myofascial pain pattern that is unique to each trigger point.

Trigger Point Assessment Techniques for Neck Region

A trigger point in the sternocleidomastoid (Figure 16.1 ■) may refer pain to the anterior face and supraorbital area. Oftentimes levator scapulae trigger points (Figure 16.2 ■) cause pain at the angle of the neck and

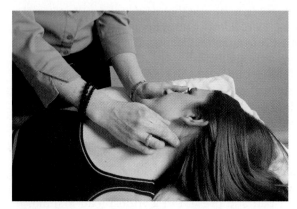

■ **Figure 16.1** Trigger Point Palpation of the Sternoclei-domastoid

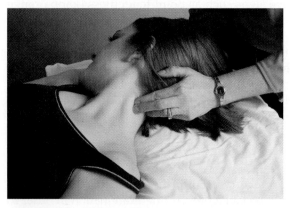

■ **Figure 16.2** Trigger Point Palpation of the Levator Scapulae

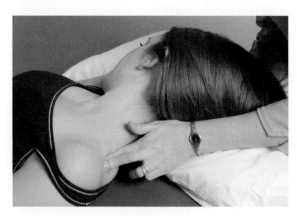

■ **Figure 16.3** Trigger Point Palpation of the Upper Trapezius

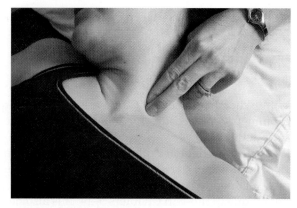

■ **Figure 16.4** Trigger Point Palpation of the Scalenes

shoulder. The upper trapezius (Figure 16.3 ■) refers pain to the vertex forehead and temple; however, it may also refer pain to the back of the neck and not uncommonly to the angle of the jaw.[3] The scalenus anterior, medius, and posterior (Figure 16.4 ■) may reproduce pain in the anterior shoulder and anterior or posterior upper and lower arm region. The scalenus minimus may refer pain to the lateral bicep region and posterior lower wrist and hand region.

Trigger Point Assessment Techniques of the Low Back and Hip Region

Trigger points of the multifidi (Figure 16.5 ■) are a common cause for low back pain in the sacral and buttock region. Trigger points of the gastrocnemius (Figure 16.6 ■) refer pain to the posterior knee and ankle.[3] Trigger points of the gluteus medius (Figure 16.7 ■) are common cause for low back pain in the sacral and buttock and refer pain to the outer hip. Trigger points of the vastus medialis (Figure 16.8 ■) refer pain to the anterior knee. Trigger points of the gluteus minimus (Figure 16.9 ■) refer pain to the outer hip.[3]

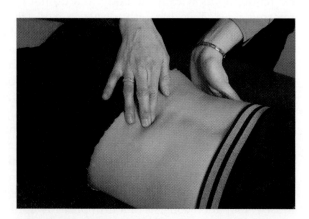

■ **Figure 16.5** Trigger Point Palpation of the Multifidi

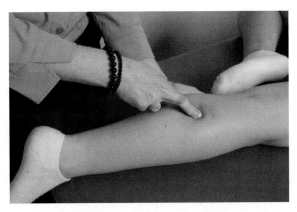

■ **Figure 16.6**   Trigger Point Palpation of the Gastrocnemius

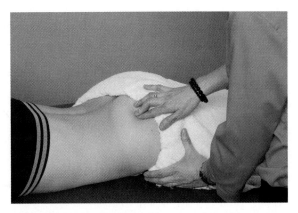

■ **Figure 16.9**   Trigger Point Palpation of the Gluteus Minimus

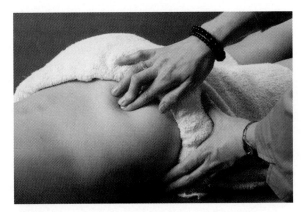

■ **Figure 16.7**   Trigger Point Palpation of the Gluteus Medius

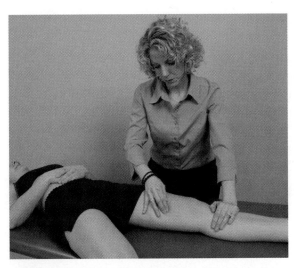

■ **Figure 16.8**   Trigger Point Palpation of the Vastus Medialis

Summary

- Palpation may be the most effective tool when determining the usefulness of a soft-tissue mobilization intervention.

- Trigger points can cause peripheral sensitization of muscle nociceptors, which can enhance pain mechanisms experienced by the patient.

- Trigger points differ from tender points, which are predictable, symmetrical tender spots within the body that do not cause referred pain.

- Trigger points are defined as areas of muscle that are painful to palpation and are characterized by the presence of taut bands and the generation of a referral pattern of pain.

Muscle Length Testing

Muscle length testing is used to identify tightened muscles that may contribute to lowered excitability thresholds and decreased viscoelasticity, and has also been associated with trigger points.[19] Tight muscle groups may also contribute to faulty movement patterns, postural syndromes, and poorer physical performance. Although deficits in range of motion are often associated with increasing age, studies that investigated muscle length assessment are relatively uncommon. One study addressed only the hamstring flexibility and found no significant changes in the muscle length as age increased.[20] There is no research investigating the reliability of muscle length testing of the upper extremity. Table 16.1 ■ outlines the reliability of selected muscle length testing of the lower extremity. Higher levels of reliability may improve clinician-to-clinician transferability of findings.

■ TABLE 16.1 Reliability of Selected Muscle Length Testing of the Lower Extremity Muscle

Healthy or Injured Intraclass Correlation Coefficient Reliability	
Thomas Hip Flexor Test [20,21]	
	Healthy
	.52 to .96
Rectus Femoris [21,22]	
	Healthy
	.53 to .97
Hamstring Length (SLR) [23–25]	
	Unknown
	.83 to .98
Hamstring Length (extensive active) [24,25]	
	Unknown
	.86 to .99
Hamstring Length (knee extension passive) [25,26]	
	Unknown
	.90 to .99
Ober Test [27–29]	
	Injured and Healthy
	.83 to .90
Modified Ober Test [27–29]	
	Injured and Healthy
	.82 to .92
Gastrocnemius [30]	
	Healthy
	.74
Soleus [31]	
	Healthy
	.98

Muscle Length Testing of the Neck and Upper Quarter

Muscle Length Testing of the Upper Trapezius

1. The patient is positioned seated with the arms relaxed at the patient's side. The patient's spine should remain neutral from flexion or extension.

2. The patient will side-flex his or her head to approximate the ear to the acromion process.

3. The clinician may measure with a tape measure the distance of the mastoid of the occiput to the lateral tip of the acromion (Figure 16.10 ■).

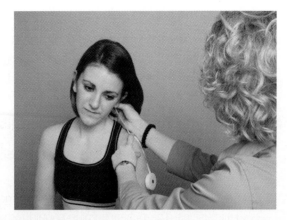

■ **Figure 16.10**   Muscle Length Testing of the Upper Trapezius

4. To determine if the structures at fault are joint or soft tissue, the clinician may assist the patient with bilateral shoulder elevation and reassess the distance between the mastoid and acromion.

Muscle Length Testing of the Levator Scapula

1. The patient is positioned seated with the test side arm reaching overhead to just behind the neck; the arm can be fixed at the patient's side if overhead reaching is painful (Figure 16.11 ■).

2. The patient's spine should remain neutral from flexion or extension to start.

3. The patient will flex his or her cervical spine to end range and then rotate away from the test side. There is no identified measurement for this technique.

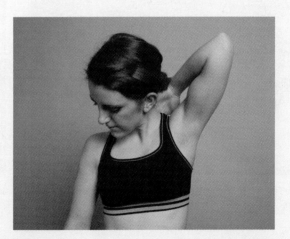

■ **Figure 16.11**   Muscle Length Testing of the Levator Scapula

Muscle Length Testing of the Scalenes

1. The patient is positioned seated or supine (with the head supported off the edge of the table) and the arm of the side being tested fixed with the patient's hand under his or her thigh.

(Continued)

② The patient's cervical spine should remain neutral from flexion or extension to start.

③ The patient will side-flex his or her head to approximate the ear to the acromion process away from the test side.

④ Then, the patient will rotate toward the side of side flexion (away from the test side) and slightly extend the neck into a quadrant position (Figure 16.12 ■). There is no identified measurement for this technique.

Muscle Length Testing of the Pectoralis Major

① The patient is positioned in supine with the hands clasped together behind the head with the cervical spine in neutral.

② The clinician should ensure that the patient maintains the hand clasp and relaxes the shoulder muscles. The patient's spine should remain neutral with the lumbar spine against the table.

③ The clinician may measure with a tape measure the distance of the olecranon of the humerus from the supporting surface (Figure 16.13 ■).

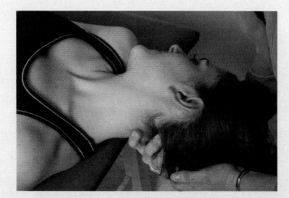

■ **Figure 16.12** Muscle Length Testing of the Scalenes

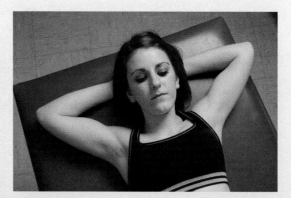

■ **Figure 16.13** Muscle Length Testing of the Pectoralis Major

Muscle Length Testing of the Trunk and Hip Region

Muscle Length Testing of the Lumbar Erector Spinae

1. The patient is placed in a standing position and is instructed to place his or her hands on the anterior thighs.

2. The clinician should support the hips from translating posteriorly during trunk flexion.

3. The patient should be instructed to slide his or her hands down the front aspect of the legs until the hips start to move. The length of the erector spinae can be assessed by use of a tape measure from midline of the posterior superior iliac spine (PSIS) to the spinous process of the C7 vertebra (Figure 16.14 ■).

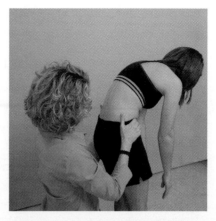

■ **Figure 16.14**   Muscle Length Testing of the Lumbar Erector Spinae

Muscle Length Testing of the Quadratus Lumborum

1. The patient should be positioned in supine with both legs in extension and the spine in neutral.

2. The clinician will grasp the lower leg near the distal talofibular joint and give a slight pull to assess the length of the quadratus lumborum (Figure 16.15 ■). There is no standard length assessment for this technique.

3. The trunk may be placed into slight side flexion to assess the lateral-most fibers.

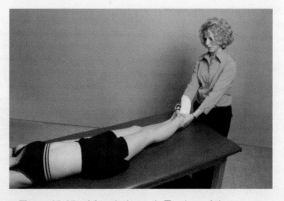

■ **Figure 16.15**   Muscle Length Testing of the Quadratus Lumborum

(Continued)

Muscle Length Testing of the Lateral Hip Musculature

Similar to the hamstring length testing, the lateral hip musculature can be tested by the use of the Ober's or Modified Ober's test. An additional muscle length assessment that can be used requires the patient to be positioned in prone. This reduces the amount of internal rotation and flexion compensations often seen in the Ober's testing position.

1. The patient's test hip is abducted and knee flexed to 90 degrees.

2. The clinician should stabilize the lateral hip pelvis with one hand and adducts the hip while maintaining 90 degrees knee flexion.

3. The clinician should note or detect movement of the pelvis and determine the end point of lateral hip muscular flexibility when pelvic motion begins (Figure 16.16 ■). A goniometer may be utilized with the axis placed at the ipsilateral PSIS, the moving arm aligned with the ipsilateral femur, and the stationary arm aligned with the contralateral PSIS.

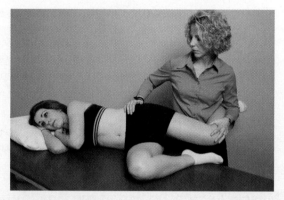

■ **Figure 16.16** Muscle Length Testing of the Lateral Hip Musculature

Muscle Length Testing of the Hip Flexors

1. The patient is instructed to position his or her buttocks at the edge of the plinth or table and should be assisted into the supine position. The hip of the lower extremity is extended on the test side.

2. The patient should grasp the nontested extremity and bring it into flexion (both hip and knee) as far as possible to flatten the spine against the plinth.

3. The patient's test leg should be flexed to 90 degrees over the edge of the table (Figure 16.17 ■).

4. The measurement is taken at the greater trochanter of the femur (axis) and the moving arm of the goniometer is aligned with the lateral condyle of the femur; the stationary arm is aligned with the lateral midline of the trunk.

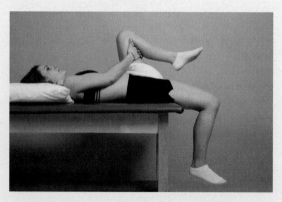

■ **Figure 16.17** Muscle Length Testing of the Hip Flexors

Muscle Length Testing of the Lower Extremities

Muscle Length Testing of the Rectus Femoris

1. The patient is positioned prone on the table with the nontest leg closest to the clinician.

2. The knee should be flexed to 90 degrees and the patient is assisted into maximal hip extension (to avoid compensation).

3. The clinician must also support the lower extremity and maintain the knee into 90 degrees of flexion with one hand and stabilize the pelvis on the ipsilateral side with the other hand (Figure 16.18 ■).

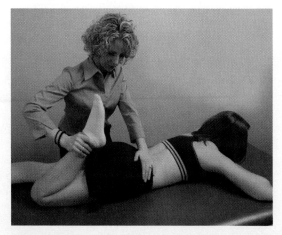

■ **Figure 16.18**   Muscle Length Testing of the Rectus Femoris Prone

4. The measurement is taken with a goniometer positioned at the lateral epicondyle of the femur (axis), the moving arm aligned with the lateral malleolus, and the stationary arm aligned with the greater trochanter of the femur.

Muscle Length Testing of the Hamstrings

There are several methods of muscle testing of the hamstrings, including the straight leg raise (SLR), the active knee extension test, or the passive knee extension test.

1. The patient should be positioned in supine position with both the hip and knees extended bilaterally.

2. The clinician instructs the patient to flex the hip through the full range of motion available and should place his or her hand on the anterior distal thigh to maintain knee extension (Figure 16.19 ■).

3. The measurement is taken at the greater trochanter of the femur (axis); the moving arm of the goniometer is aligned with the lateral epicondyle of the femur and the stationary arm is aligned with the lateral midline of the

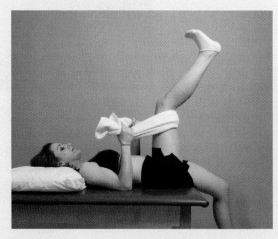

■ **Figure 16.19**   Muscle Length Testing of the Hamstrings

(Continued)

trunk. Both the active and passive knee extension tests require the patient to be positioned in supine with the hip flexed to 90 degrees and the contralateral leg in extension.

④ The clinician will instruct the patient in the active knee extension test to extend the knee until pain or soft-tissue limitation is noted. The passive knee extension requires the clinician to passively extend the knee until firm muscular resistance to additional motion is felt or the patient complains of pain.

Both the active and passive knee extension tests can be assessed with the goniometer positioned at the lateral epicondyle of the femur (axis), the moving arm aligned with the lateral malleolus, and the stationary arm aligned with the greater trochanter of the femur.

Muscle Length Testing of the Soleus

① The patient is positioned prone on the table and the test leg knee should be flexed to 90 degrees whereas the opposite leg should be placed into full extension on the table (Figure 16.20 ■).

② The clinician must instruct the patient in dorsiflexion of the ankle while maintaining knee flexion at 90 degrees. The goniometer may assess the motion available of the soleus if positioned at the lateral malleolus (axis); the moving arm is parallel to the fifth metatarsal and the stationary arm is aligned with the head of the fibula.

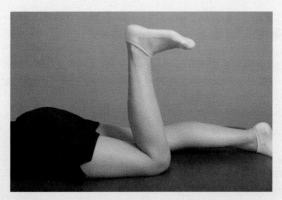

■ **Figure 16.20** Muscle Length Testing of the Soleus Bent Knee

Hypermobility Testing

On some occasions, patients with hypermobility will assume faulty postures as a compensation for tissues with weakness or excessive length. Combinations of tight and weak muscles create changes in movement patterns that result in alteration of the biomechanics of joints leading to secondary degenerative changes. Additionally, with a limited ROM of joints due to chronic muscle tightness the problems of secondary associated joint hypermobility occur.

Hypermobility in more than one or two joints may require an assessment of gross mobility. Beighton mobility testing involves an assessment of gross hypermobility of the body and estimates the propensity of a hypermobility disorder. The Beighton Ligamentous Laxity Scale (LLS) for generalized ligamentous laxity showed high reliability with intraclass correlation coefficient (ICC) = .79[31], although further research on the validity of the test and criteria is needed.[32] The test involves nine specific positions:

1. Standing with arm and wrist in neutral, pull little finger back toward 90 degrees (test both sides) (Figure 16.21 ■). If one can pull the finger back past 90 degrees, a point is scored for each successful side.

2. Standing with arm and wrist in neutral, pull thumb toward wrist in an attempt to touch (test both sides) (Figure 16.22 ■). If the thumb touches the wrist a point is scored for each successful side.

3. An attempt to hyperextend the elbow (test both sides). If one can hyperextend the elbows, a point is scored for each successful side (Figure 16.23 ■).

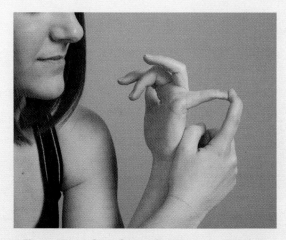

■ **Figure 16.21** Step One of Beighton Hypermobility Testing

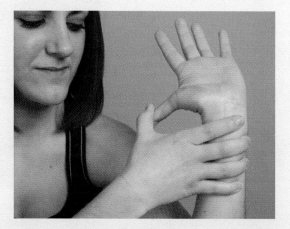

■ **Figure 16.22** Step Two of Beighton Hypermobility Testing

(Continued)

④ Involves an attempt to hyperextend the knees, test both sides, in either standing or supine; if one can hyperextend the knees they score a point for each successful side (Figure 16.24 ■).

⑤ Involves bending down to touch the floor (without warming up). If one can palm the floor they score a single point (Figure 16.25 ■).

A score of 5 or higher is considered a positive test. Evaluating patients for hypermobility in routine examination may prevent unnecessary diagnostic studies and treatments.[32]

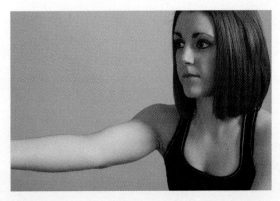

■ **Figure 16.23** Step Three of Beighton Hypermobility Testing

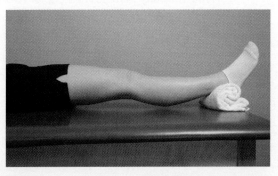

■ **Figure 16.24** Step Four of Beighton Hypermobility Testing

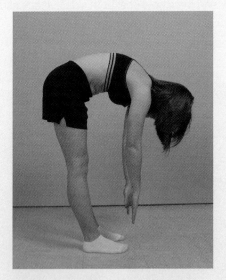

■ **Figure 16.25** Step Five of Beighton Hypermobility Testing

Summary

- Muscle length testing may be useful to detect postural abnormalities.
- Muscle length testing is used to identify tightened muscles that may contribute to lowered excitability thresholds, decreased viscoelasticity, and has been associated with trigger points.
- The Beighton ligamentous laxity scale is an assessment of gross hypermobility of the body, which estimates the propensity of a hypermobility disorder.

Treatment Techniques

Definitions

Within the literature, soft-tissue mobilization is represented by a cadre of definitions and philosophical assumptions and is heavily influenced by country of origin and by whoever is advocating the use of the technique. Techniques that fall within these definitional boundaries include myofascial release, neuromuscular therapeutic trigger point release, massage, friction massage, acupressure, lymphatic drainage, Rolfing, and instrument-assisted methods (Table 16.2 ■).

Physiological Changes

There are a number of purported physiological changes associated with soft-tissue mobilization procedures. For starters, myofascial release has been associated with a short-term reduction of muscle strength that is associated with the relaxation phenomenon of the technique.[33] For sports recovery, myofascial release has been shown to assist in recovery of pre-exercise heart rate and blood pressure levels after exercise as compared to placebo groups.[34]

■ TABLE 16.2 Soft-Tissue Mobilization Techniques and Descriptors

Technique and Description

Myofascial Release

A form of soft-tissue mobilization that involves stretching the fascia and releasing theoretical bonds or restrictions within the fascial network. The assumption of myofascial release is that the vigorous mobilization allows the connective tissue fibers to reorganize in a more flexible, functional fashion.

Neuromuscular Therapeutic Trigger Point Release

A focused intervention to a hyperirritable spot in the skeletal muscle using various forms of approaches including spray and stretch, ischemic compression or sustained pressure, dry needling, ultrasound, or massage therapy.

Massage

A generic term to describe manual movement of tissues such as muscle, skin, or fascia. Techniques may include effleurage, petrissage, or friction.

Friction Massage

Involves massage movements where one surface is frictioned over another repeatedly in an effort to decrease inflammation and promote healing. The reparative cells (fibroblasts) responsible for producing collagen and forming a scar following ligament injury are mechanosensitive. Friction massage is theorized to facilitate matrix production and restoration of the tissues' mechanical properties.

Acupressure

A variant of acupuncture where physical pressure is applied to a specific point by the clinician's hand or elbow or by an external device.

Lymphatic Drainage

A massage technique designed to assist the lymphatic system by the application of slow, light, and repetitive strokes that move lymphatic fluid through the system of vessels and nodes.

Instrument-Assisted Techniques

Instrument-assisted cross friction techniques designed to initiate healing via favorable effects on collagen formation and organization.

Rolfing Structural Integration

A form of massage that focuses on the fascia, and attempts to align and balance the body by lengthening and repositioning the fascia.

Selected myofascial and stretching techniques can change the vascular and reflex autonomic responses (short term) in patients with carpal tunnel syndrome and thoracic outlet syndrome.[35] Friction massage, although not holistically beneficial in reduction of pain in trials, does appear to reduce motor neuron activity[36] and H reflex[37] at the site administered. The benefits of the motor neuron changes do not appear to be as significant as those provided by spinal manipulation.[38]

Treatment Philosophy

It is important to note that in all cases, soft-tissue mobilization techniques are adjunctive in nature and are part of a comprehensive program of exercise, behavioral modification, and potentially joint- and nerve-related techniques. Soft-tissue mobilization techniques are not mutually exclusive with other forms of techniques.

Selected soft-tissue mobilization techniques (e.g., Rolfing and myofascial release) are designed to lengthen restricted tissue and assist in normalizing muscle length.[38] Other methods are designed to (1) reduce pain, (2) increase extensibility, (3) improve circulation, (4) improve overall well-being, (5) release an adhered or restricted area, and (6) promote postural restoration. In essence, if the clinician encounters any of these situations, soft-tissue mobilization may be a useful and pertinent intervention.

Contraindications

As with all manual procedures, there are dedicated contraindications (both relative and absolute) for soft-tissue mobilization. Table 16.3 ▪ outlines the contraindications to soft-tissue mobilization.

Summary

- Various soft-tissue mobilization techniques include myofascial release, neuromuscular therapeutic trigger point release, massage, friction massage, acupressure, lymphatic drainage, Rolfing, and instrument-assisted methods.
- Contraindications for soft-tissue mobilization are not numerous but should be considered prior to intervention.
- Soft-tissue mobilization techniques are adjunctive in nature and are part of a comprehensive program of exercise, behavioral modification, and potentially joint- and nerve-related techniques.
- Soft-tissue mobilization techniques are not mutually exclusive with other forms of techniques.

Friction Massage

Friction massage is a specific type of connective tissue massage applied precisely to the soft-tissue structures such as tendons. It is vital that friction massage is performed only at the exact site of the lesion, with the depth of friction tolerable to the patient. It is theorized

---

▪ **TABLE 16.3** Absolute and Relative Contraindications Associated with Soft-Tissue Mobilization

Absolute Contraindications
- Contagious illnesses
- Skin disease or selected conditions such as carbuncles, acne, or other lesions
- Malignant tumors
- Aneurysms
- Broken skin or bones
- Osteomyelitis

Relative Contraindication
- Neuroses
- Phlebitis or varicosity of the veins
- Lymphangitis
- Hemophilia
- Tissue integrity loss secondary to medication or age
- Sensory damage
- Deep vein thrombosis
- Significant inflammation
- Hematomas
- Irritable condition

that the effect of the intervention is so localized that, unless the finger is applied to the exact site and friction given in the right direction, relief cannot be expected. Deep friction massage should be applied transversely to the specific tissue involved, including muscle, tendons, tendon sheaths, and ligaments. Friction massage has limited support in the evidence as to its therapeutic effects.,[39] although it is theorized that it assists in pain relief, traumatic hyperemia, and decreases scar tissue.[40]

Friction massage is dissimilar to superficial massage, in that friction massage does not use lubrication and is applied in a longitudinal direction parallel to the vessels, which enhances circulation and return of fluids. This requires the therapist's fingers and patient's skin to move as a single unit, otherwise subcutaneous fascia could blister or bruise. Additionally, the tissue undergoing friction massage should be positioned in a mild to moderate stretch (except for a muscle belly, which should be relaxed). As a general guideline, deep tendon friction is applied for 10 minutes after the numbing effect has been achieved, every other day, or at a minimum interval of 48 hours (because of the traumatic hyperemia induced) to prepare the tendon for the manipulation.

At present, there is only empirical evidence to support the treatment times suggested above.[41] Unfortunately, the technique has developed a reputation for being very painful; however, pain during friction massage may be the result of a wrong indication, a wrong technique, or an unaccustomed amount of pressure. The clinician should begin with a light amount of pressure while using a reinforced finger or thumb technique.[42]

Friction Massage of the Lateral Epicondylar Region

A number of studies that have used friction massage to the lateral epicondylar region have shown positive effects in the reduction of pain or improvement in function for patients with lateral epicondylitis.[43]

1. The patient is positioned in sitting with the arm in an extended and pronated position.

2. The clinician sits on a chair or stool next to the patient and maintains the patient in elbow extension/pronation.

3. The clinician's thumb/fingertip is positioned in slight flexion and the friction motion is created by the clinician's wrist movement in a direction perpendicular to the tendons (Figure 16.26 ■).

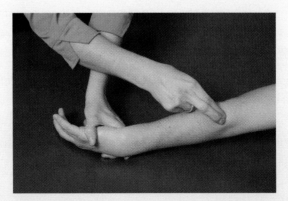

■ Figure 16.26 Friction Massage of the Lateral Epicondylar Region

Friction Massage of the Medial Epicondylar Region

1. The patient is positioned in sitting with the arm in an extended and supinated position.

2. The clinician sits on a chair or stool next to the patient and maintains the patient in elbow extension/supination.

3. The clinician's thumb/fingertip is positioned in slight flexion and the friction motion is created by the clinician's wrist movement in a direction perpendicular to the tendons (Figure 16.27 ■).

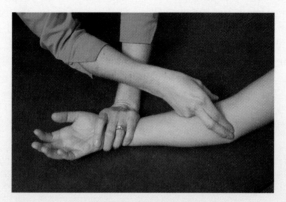

■ Figure 16.27 Friction Massage of the Medial Epicondylar Region

Friction Massage of the Supraspinatus

A number of therapies used in multimodal treatment approach involving friction massage of the supraspinatus has showed some improvement in function for patients with adhesive capsulitis.[44] and impingement syndrome[45,46] This technique is applied to the supraspinatus tendon located distal to the anterolateral corner of the acromion.

1. The patient should be positioned with the shoulder in slight extension (making the tendon more prominent) by placing the wrist/hand behind the back.

2. The clinician's thumb/fingertip is positioned in slight flexion and the friction motion is created by the clinician's wrist movement in a direction perpendicular to the tendon. The clinician may also target the friction massage to the musculotendinous junction of the supraspinatus.

3. This technique requires the patient to sit with the arm resting in about 90 degrees of abduction.

④ The therapist stands to the opposite side of the side being treated. The middle finger is reinforced by the forefinger and is placed between the clavicle and the spine of the scapula laterally (Figure 16.28 ■).

⑤ The clinician will palpate straight down into the gap and look for tenderness or provocation of concordant symptoms in this area. The friction massage is created by rolling the finger in pronation/supination. In this technique, there is no active and relaxation phase; there are only active phases in both directions.

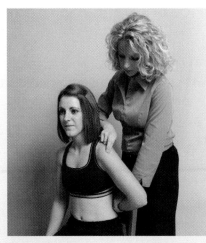

■ **Figure 16.28** Friction Massage of the Supraspinatus

Friction Massage of the Infraspinatus

Typically this technique is applied to the belly of the infraspinatus muscle; however, it may also be applied to the tendon.

① If applying the friction massage to the muscle belly, then the patient may be seated and arms at the sides.

② If the tendon is the target of the intervention, then the arm needs to be placed in slight internal rotation and adduction.

③ The clinician's thumb/fingertip is positioned in slight flexion and the friction motion is created by the clinician's wrist movement in a direction perpendicular to the tendon or muscle fibers (Figure 16.29 ■).

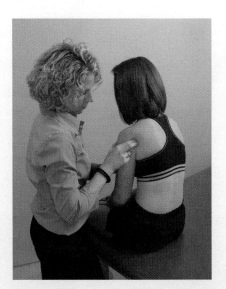

■ **Figure 16.29** Friction Massage of the Infraspinatus

Friction Massage of the Biceps Tendon

There is some evidence to support that friction massage of the biceps provides greater range-of-motion gains than no treatment over a 2-week period.[46]

1. The patient is positioned with the shoulder abducted to 25–30 degrees then placed in slight extension.

2. The clinician's thumb/finger tip is then placed on the bicep tendon and alternately applies a medial and lateral glide motion to the tendon (Figure 16.30 ■).

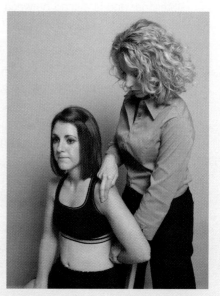

■ **Figure 16.30** Friction Massage of the Biceps Tendon at the Bicipital Groove

Friction Massage of the Hamstring Tendon Insertion

Typically this technique is applied to the belly of the hamstring muscle if there has been a tear; however, it may also be applied to one of the tendons.

1. If the intervention is applied to the muscle, then the patient may lie prone with the lower limb supported on a pillow or bolster. If the tendon is the target of the intervention, then the patient needs to lie prone without support to the lower limb. The clinician may support the limb for the patient's comfort, although maintaining knee extension is important to add stretch to the targeted tendon.

2. The clinician's thumb/fingertip is positioned in slight flexion and the friction motion is created by the clinician's wrist movement in a direction perpendicular to the tendon or muscle fibers (medial to lateral) (Figure 16.31 ■).

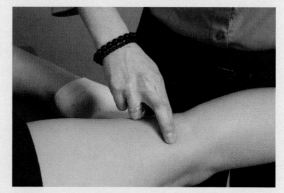

■ **Figure 16.31** Friction Massage of the Hamstring Tendon Insertion

Friction Massage of the Tensor Fascia Latae (TFL) and Iliotibial Band (ITB) Insertion

Deep tendon friction massage combined with other physiotherapy modalities has shown consistent benefit over control of pain for runners experiencing iliotibial band friction syndrome.[47]

1. The patient should be placed in an Ober's position or modified Ober's test position to place the targeted tendon on stretch. However, if the muscle belly of the tensor fascia latae is the target of the intervention the patient should be placed in sidelying position with the painful side uppermost, with the hip flexed to approximately 30 degrees and adducted to rest on the table.

2. The clinician's thumb/fingertip is positioned in slight flexion and the friction motion is created by the clinician's wrist movement in a direction perpendicular to the tendon or muscle fibers (Figure 16.32 ■).

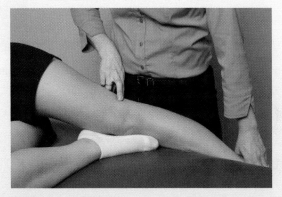

■ **Figure 16.32** Friction Massage of the TFL and ITB Insertion

Friction Massage of the Lateral (LCL) and Medial Collateral Ligaments (MCL)

1. The patient should be placed in supine or long sit position with the knee near full extension.

2. The clinician's thumb/fingertip is positioned in slight flexion and the friction motion is created by the clinician's wrist movement in a direction perpendicular to the ligaments (Figures 16.33 ■ and 16.34 ■).

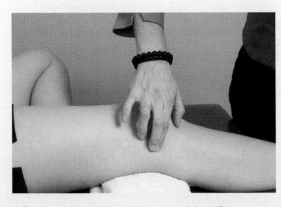

■ **Figure 16.33** Friction Massage of the LCL

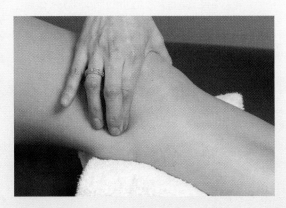

■ **Figure 16.34** Friction Massage of the MCL

Friction Massage of the Plica of the Knee

1. The patient should be placed in hook-lying or seated position with the knees flexed to 90 degrees.

2. The clinician's thumb/fingertip is positioned in slight flexion and the friction motion is created by the clinician's wrist movement in a direction perpendicular to the plica (Figure 16.35 ■).

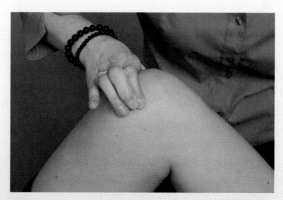

■ **Figure 16.35** Friction Massage of the Plica of the Knee

Friction Massage of the Tibialis Posterior Tendon

1. The patient should be placed in sitting position with the knees flexed to 90 degrees over the edge of the plinth with the foot in slight plantarflexion and inversion. A slight stretch may be added with the clinician adding overpressure to the foot into plantarflexion and inversion.

2. The clinician's thumb/fingertip is positioned in slight flexion and the friction motion is created by the clinician's wrist movement in a direction perpendicular to the fibers of the tendon located just lateral to the medial malleolus (Figure 16.36 ■).

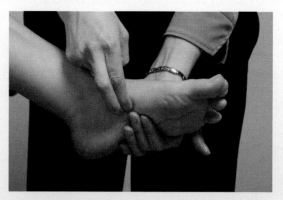

■ **Figure 16.36** Friction Massage of the Tibialis Posterior Tendon

Friction Massage of the Suboccipital Muscles

1. The patient should be placed in supine position with the upper cervical flexed to 20 degrees. The therapist should support this position and maintain upper cervical flexion with the hand placed at the patient's occiput. The nonsupport hand should apply the friction massage to the suboccipital musculature in a medial to lateral fashion. This technique should be used with a progression of forces and as the patient tolerates the technique. This is commonly a source of headaches and could be painful for the patient if too much force is applied. This technique may be used prior to a suboccipital release technique.

2. An alternative position for the suboccipital muscle friction massage is in prone position (Figure 16.37 ■) with the patient positioned on the adjustable plinth with the head slightly flexed to 20 degrees. The therapist could then utilize gravity with this technique, making it easier to apply.

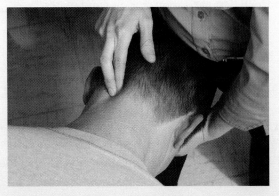

■ **Figure 16.37** Friction Massage of the Suboccipital Muscles

Friction Massage of the Achilles Tendon

1. The patient should be placed in prone position with the ankle/foot off of the edge of the plinth.

2. The clinician may use a strap around the plinth leg or the thigh to place the patient into dorsiflexion.

3. The clinician's thumb/fingertip is positioned in slight flexion and the friction motion is created by the clinician's wrist movement (from medial to lateral direction) perpendicular to the tendon. Additionally, the clinician may grip the tendon between the thumb and forefinger and pull around the sides of the tendon to get at the posterior aspect of the tendon. The friction massage is created by the motion of radial and ulnar deviation of the therapist's wrist (Figure 16.38 ■).

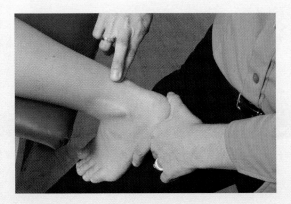

■ **Figure 16.38** Friction Massage of the Achilles Tendon

Ischemic Compression

Palpation is a reliable diagnostic criterion for locating TrPs in patients.[48] There are several techniques utilized in the clinic to treat patients with painful trigger points. A TrP is tender when pressed and can give rise to characteristic referred pain, motor dysfunction, or autonomic phenomena. Ischemic compression is a similar technique to sustained pressure, although it is applied with less digital pressure to TrPs.

Recent research results suggest that TrPs are evoked by the abnormal depolarization of motor end plates.[48] It is believed that the ischemic compression deprives the trigger points of oxygen, rendering them inactive in the pain–spasm cycle. Clinically the pressure may be applied to the targeted TrP identified in the clinical examination during the palpation component of the exam. During treatment the pressure is applied for at least 8 seconds, but can be held for longer. If the patient reports a lessening of local and referred pain, then the therapist can repeat the treatment. However, if the pain does not lessen, the clinician may need to adjust the pressure/force, direction, or choose an alternative technique. The major goals of this type of technique are to reduce pain and improve tightness of the involved muscles and range of motion.

Ischemic Compression of the Upper Trapezius

Both ischemic compression technique and transverse friction massage were equally effective in reducing tenderness in TrPs of the upper trapezius.[49] The technique can be performed in sitting or supine position and requires the appropriate identification of the symptomatic TrP (Figure 16.39 ■).

Ischemic Compression of the Mid-Thoracic Paraspinals

There is some evidence to support the use of ischemic compression as a home program followed by sustained stretching for the treatment of myofascial TrPs in the neck and upper back for TrP sensitivity and pain.[49] The technique can be performed in sitting or prone position and requires the appropriate identification of the symptomatic TrP (Figure 16.40 ■).

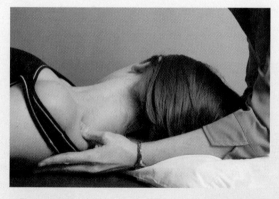

■ **Figure 16.39** Ischemic Compression of the Upper Trapezius

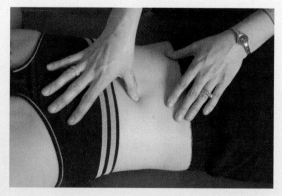

■ **Figure 16.40** Ischemic Compression of the Mid-Thoracic Paraspinals

Ischemic Compression of the Medial Scapular Region, the Infraspinatus, the Grastrosoleus, and the Tibialis Anterior

Figures 16.41 ■ – 16.44 ■ demonstrate ischemic compression to the medial scapular region, the infraspinatus, the gastrocsoleus muscles, and the tibialis anterior muscles.

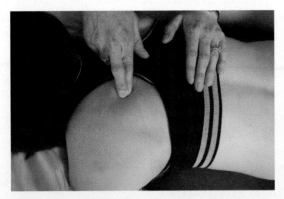

■ **Figure 16.41**   Ischemic Compression of the Medial Scapular Region

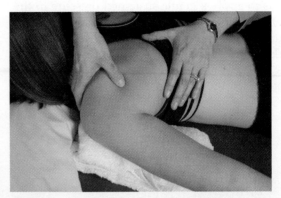

■ **Figure 16.42**   Ischemic Compression of the Infraspinatus

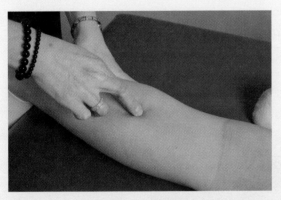

■ **Figure 16.43**   Ischemic Compression of the Gastrocsoleus

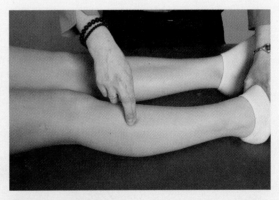

■ **Figure 16.44**   Ischemic Compression of the Tibialis Anterior

General Techniques

This chapter has introduced many different and specific types of soft-tissue mobilization techniques to treat TrPs or painful muscles with fiber massage. There are also general types of soft-tissue mobilization, including general massage, myofascial release, and craniosacral techniques.

Massage

Massage is a systematic, therapeutic, and functional stroking and kneading of the soft tissues of the body.

The types of traditional techniques used include effleurage and petrissage. The general stroking used in effleurage (with use of lubricant) is applied to the muscles and soft tissue in a distal to proximal direction to enhance blood flow, relaxation, and lymphatic drainage.[50] The petrissage techniques are made up of many techniques that include progressive stroking (superficial to more deep), kneading, rolling, sweeping, and bending of tissue. This technique is theorized to improve the ability of the muscles to purge waste products.

Myofascial Release

Myofascial release (MFR) is a whole-body, hands-on approach designed to release restrictions in the myofascial tissue and is used for the treatment of soft-tissue dysfunction. The focus of this technique is the fascial system. The purpose of myofascial release techniques is to apply a gentle sustained pressure to the fascia, to reduce or remove restrictions, and improve the patient's pain and/or function. These techniques may also combine massage with deep stretch techniques to relax muscle and break up the TrPs. However, of the few studies published on the MFR, many suggest further investigation is needed using MFR for various diagnoses or pain syndromes.[51]

Craniosacral Therapy

Craniosacral therapy is a manual therapy technique that uses a hypothesized craniosacral system that purportedly consists of the membranes and cerebrospinal fluid that surrounds and protects the brain and the spinal cord. The hypothesized purpose of craniosacral therapy is to access the underlying dura and release any restrictions within the system. The underlying physiology behind craniosacral therapy does not appear to have construct validity.[52]

Myofascial Release of the Upper Trapezius

1. The patient is positioned in supine with the head resting in neutral on the table.

2. The therapist is seated at the end of the table with his or her outside hand placed over the patient's shoulder, thumb over upper trapezius and supraspinous fossa, while the opposite hand cradles the patient's neck with flexed fingertips on posterior cervical tissues (Figure 16.45 ■).

3. The clinician should maintain the thumb pressure, as fingertips sweep superiorly toward the occiput while simultaneously guiding the patient's head into contralateral lateral flexion and rotation.

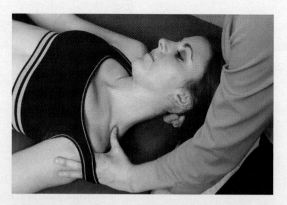

■ **Figure 16.45** Myofascial Release of the Upper Trapezius

Myofascial Release of the Mid-Thoracic Paraspinals

1. The patient is positioned in supine (Figure 16.46 ■) or prone, with use of a pillow if needed to reduce the lumbar lordosis.

2. The therapist should stand at the side of the patient and place the index finger behind the thumb over the thoracic erector spinae muscle group.

3. The clinician should start at the upper thoracic region and sweep down toward the iliac crest. It is useful to utilize the patient's breathing to assist with deeper techniques. This technique should begin with minimal force and progress as the patient tolerates.

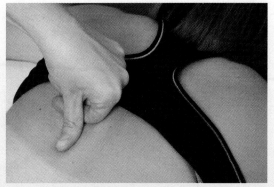

■ **Figure 16.46** Myofascial Release of the Mid-Thoracic Paraspinals

Myofascial Release of the Lower Lumbar Paraspinals

1. The patient is positioned in prone or sidelying (affected side uppermost), with use of a pillow if needed to reduce the lumbar lordosis.

2. The therapist will stand at the side of the patient with thumbs placed tip to tip and perform a transverse technique by oscillating thumbs back and forth (Figure 16.47 ■). This technique should begin with minimal force and progress as the patient tolerates.

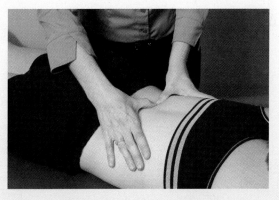

■ **Figure 16.47** Myofascial Release of the Lower Lumbar Paraspinals

Myofascial Release of the Hamstrings

1. The patient is positioned in prone.

2. The patient should be relaxed with the lower legs supported at 70 degrees with use of a bolster.

3. The clinician may use the heel of one hand moving superiorly, and the heel of the other hand moving inferiorly to apply pressure (Figure 16.48 ■).

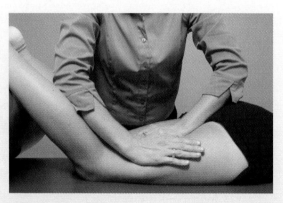

■ **Figure 16.48** Myofascial Release of the Hamstrings

Myofascial Release of the Rectus Femoris

1. The patient is positioned in supine.

2. The clinician will stand at the side of the patient and use the index finger behind the thumb to apply pressure over the quadriceps muscle belly (Figure 16.49 ■).

3. The release should start above the painful or restricted area and proceed down toward the knee, utilizing body weight to increasing pressure as the patient tolerates the technique.

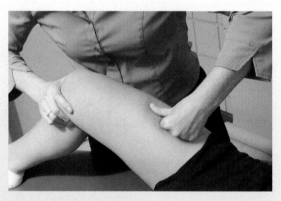

■ **Figure 16.49** Myofascial Release of the Rectus Femoris

Myofascial Release of the Tensor Fascia Latae

1. The patient is placed in supine (or side-lying) position with the affected leg flexed and adducted in a relaxed position crossed over the nonaffected leg to rest.

2. The clinician should stand at the side of the patient and stabilize the knee with one hand while placing the proximal third of the other forearm perpendicular with the thigh on the iliotibial band (ITB) (Figure 16.50 ■). The technique is applied most distal and sweep toward the tensor fascia latae muscle.

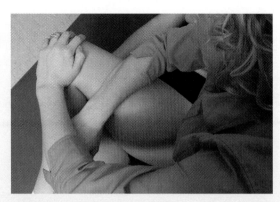

■ **Figure 16.50**   Myofascial Release of the Tensor Fascia Latae

3. The therapist should utilize body weight for increased pressure. Use of a superficial stroke and progression to a deep stroke is generally recommended. The clinician may also use the thumb/fingertip technique positioned in slight flexion or the use of the point of the olecranon for added pressure.

Myofascial Release of the Gastrocnemius

1. The patient is positioned in prone.

2. The patient should be relaxed with the foot relaxed over the edge of the table or pillow under the lower leg to flex the knee. This technique may be performed by working each head of the gastrocnemius separately (bending).

3. The clinician stands at the side of the table and places the thumbs tip to tip to make a triangle with his or her hands.

4. The clinician should bend the tissues from medial to lateral from the popliteal region down to the Achilles tendon as appropriate (Figure 16.51 ■).

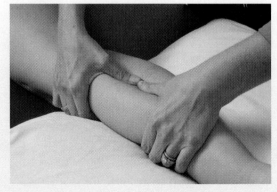

■ **Figure 16.51**   Myofascial Release of the Gastrocnemius

Myofascial Release of the Triceps Surae

1. The patient is positioned in prone.

2. The patient is relaxed with the involved leg flexed at the knee and the foot resting on the clinician's shoulder.

3. Using both hands the clinician presses the fingers deep into the gastrocnemius area and spread laterally (Figure 16.52 ■).

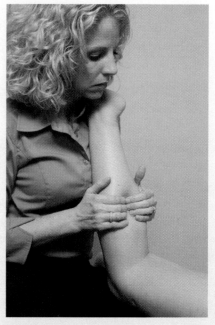

■ **Figure 16.52** Myofascial Release of the Triceps Surae

Myofascial Release of the Plantar Fascia with Great Toe Flexors

1. The patient is positioned in prone.

2. The patient should be relaxed with the foot over the edge of the table.

3. The therapist should stand and grasp with one hand around the forefoot and pull the great toe slightly into extension.

4. The therapist will apply with the other hand/fist firm pressure to the plantar fascia (Figure 16.53 ■). This technique may be used just proximal to the metatarsal heads.

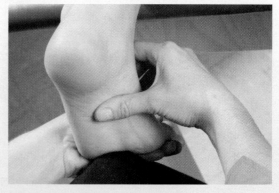

■ **Figure 16.53** Myofascial Release of the Plantar Fascia with Great Toe Flexors

Myofascial Release of the Plantar Fascia Using a Splaying Technique

1. The patient is lying supine or seated with the foot relaxed.

2. The therapist is seated at the end of the table and should place the thumbs side by side over the fascia in the middle of the foot (Figure 16.54 ■).

3. The pressure will be applied by the clinician's thumbs using a sweeping technique to separate the thumbs and using a dorsiflexion force. This technique may be used just proximal to the metatarsal heads.

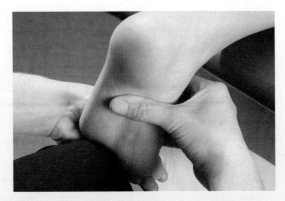

■ **Figure 16.54** Myofascial Release of the Plantar Fascia Using a Splaying Technique

Muscle Lengthening and Massage of the Upper Trapezius

One study that utilized muscle lengthening and massage of the upper trapezius reported the application of a muscle energy technique (MET) produced immediate increases in the active cervical range of motion in asymptomatic subjects.[53]

1. The patient is positioned in supine with minimal pillow support to keep the head and neck in neutral.

2. The clinician will utilize the fingers to knead the upper trapezius muscle along the direction of its fibers (Figure 16.55 ■).

3. The clinician can then utilize a contract–relax approach and have the patient apply a slight side flexion force toward the side being treated with resistance applied from the clinician for 3–5 seconds and then move further into contralateral side flexion to add a slight stretch to the upper trapezius.

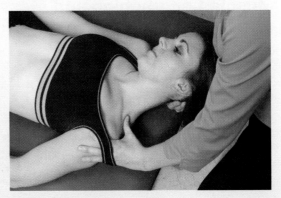

■ **Figure 16.55** Muscle Lengthening and Massage of the Upper Trapezius

Muscle Lengthening and Massage of the Hamstrings

This lengthening technique utilizes a muscle energy or dynamic force created by the patient. A MET to the hamstrings can improve muscle extensibility for up to 1 week following the initial treatment.[53]

1. The patient is positioned in supine, with the clinician nearest to the leg of intended treatment and facing the patient.

2. The patient's ankle is placed on the clinician's shoulder and the clinician places a hand on the anterior aspect of the lower quadriceps (slightly above the patella) to maintain the leg in full extension (Figure 16.56 ■).

3. The clinician raises the extended leg further into hip flexion and ankle dorsiflexion, to the point of pain onset or the point of soft-tissue resistance, at which point the leg is maintained.

4. The patient is asked to press that leg into the clinician's shoulder and to plantar-flex the ankle for 3–5 seconds and relax for 3 seconds. The technique is repeated and the stretch is applied again to the hamstrings.

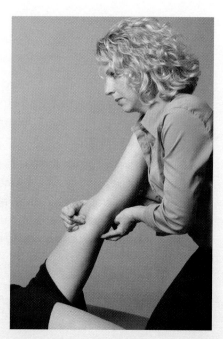

■ **Figure 16.56** Muscle Lengthening and Massage of the Hamstrings

Muscle Lengthening and Massage of the Gastrocsoleous Group

This muscle-lengthening procedure utilizes a muscle energy or dynamic force created by the patient. The muscle imbalance of the gastrocnemius complex can occur because of chronic adaptive shortening (i.e., shoes with a heel).

1. The patient is positioned in supine on the plinth with the knee extended and the distal calf musculature off the edge of the table.

2. The patient is positioned in a neutral position and the ankle dorsiflexed to the point of soft-tissue resistance or pain.

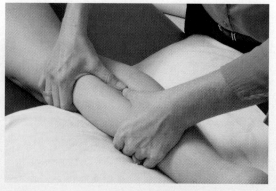

■ **Figure 16.57** Muscle Lengthening and Massage of the Gastrocsoleous Group

③ The clinician places the supporting hand over the distal tibia and fibula. The resisting hand will be placed on the plantar surface of the forefoot and the patient is asked to actively plantar-flex the foot against the mild to moderate resistance from the clinician for 3–5 seconds and relax for 3 seconds.

④ The technique is repeated and the stretch is applied again to the gastrocnemius.

This same technique may be applied to the soleus; however, the knee should be flexed to 90 degrees. The patient may be positioned in sitting or prone (Figure 16.57 ■) with the knee flexed and the same procedure applied.

Muscle Lengthening and Massage of the Forearm Musculature

This muscle-lengthening technique utilizes a muscle energy or dynamic force created by the patient.

① The patient is positioned sitting, with the clinician nearest to the treatment arm and facing the patient.

② The patient's elbow is placed on the table and the lower forearm/wrist is off the edge of the table.

③ The clinician will place his or her supporting hand on the patient's forearm and the resisting hand on the palmar surface to resist a flexion force (to increase extension) or the dorsal surface to resist an extension force (to increase flexion) (Figure 16.58 ■).

④ The patient is asked to meet the clinician's mild to moderate resistance for 3–5 seconds and relax for 3 seconds.

⑤ The technique is repeated and the stretch is applied again to the targeted forearm musculature.

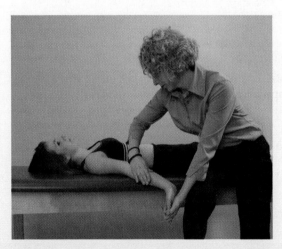

■ **Figure 16.58** Muscle Lengthening and Massage of the Forearm Musculature

Summary

- Friction massage is a specific type of connective tissue massage applied precisely to the soft-tissue structures such as tendons. It is vital that friction massage is performed only at the exact site of the lesion, with the depth of friction tolerable to the patient.
- Friction massage is applied perpendicular to the tendon fiber.
- Ischemic compression is a similar technique to sustained pressure; however, it is applied with gentle digital pressure to TrPs.
- The purpose of myofascial release techniques is to apply a gentle sustained pressure to the fascia, to reduce or remove restrictions and improve the patient's pain and/or function.
- Adding muscle lengthening to massage may be a useful adjunct to improve range of motion.

Treatment Outcomes

The Evidence

Friction Massage Most studies that have investigated transverse friction massage have been plagued by small sample sizes. The studies that have investigated the benefit of transverse friction massage on patients with lateral epicondylitis and iliotibial band friction syndrome have found no benefit (Level B).[54]

Trigger Point Therapy Trigger point therapy has been described as a potential counterpart to mobilization[55] but remains essentially unstudied for its neurophysiological benefit in comparative trials. Most studies have combined trigger point therapy with other treatments, thus the benefit is unknown (Level D),[56] although the methodological quality of the studies is very poor.[57]

Myofascial Release Myofascial release or variant methods such as Rolfing remain untested in clinical comparative trials (Level D).[58]

Massage The difficulty in appropriately designing a placebo or comparative trial for the effectiveness of massage is apparent, thus studies that have examined massage as an intervention are few. Furian and colleagues[59] examined the effectiveness of massage for patients with acute and sub-acute low back pain and did find some evidence to support the intervention (Level B) when combined with exercises and education. No such finding exists for neck pain (Level D) as all reported studies have such significant design flaws that ascertainment of the benefit is confounded.[60]

Craniosacral Therapy There are no studies that have examined craniosacral therapy in a comparative musculoskeletal trial (Level D). The underlying assumptions of the "rhythm" associated with craniosacral therapy have been questioned and remain implausible.[52,61] At this point, this book does not advocate the use of craniosacral therapy and cannot substantiate the presence of this rhythm.

Summary

- There is minimal evidence to support the various forms of soft-tissue mobilization, mostly exhibiting Level D evidence.
- There is Level B evidence to suggest that friction massage is not effective.
- Overall, there is limited overall evidence for soft-tissue mobilization.

Chapter Questions

1. Compare and contrast the various forms of soft-tissue mobilization.

2. Evaluate the evidence associated with each form of soft-tissue mobilization.

3. Determine which procedure is most useful on the selected anatomical dysfunction of the patient.

4. Describe how soft-tissue assessment is adjunctive to a typical manual therapy assessment.

Patient Cases

Case 16.1: Jerry Clausen (56-Year-Old Male)

Diagnosis: Neck strain

Observation: He exhibits forward head posture, noticeable hypertrophy of the muscle of the upper trapezius and midparaspinals.

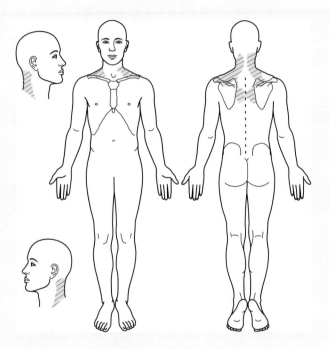

Mechanism: He indicates an insidious onset of approximately 5 months ago when he started his new job as an accounts manager.

Concordant Sign: His most painful time period is associated with use of the computer.

Nature of the Condition: The pain worsens as the day goes on and it affects his productivity at work. The pain contributes to his stress. Consequently, he has been depressed and is worried that he may lose his job.

Behavior of the Symptoms: His pain is bilateral and originates in his upper traps. The pain migrates to his shoulder and up to his occiput.

Pertinent Patient History: Was diagnosed with social anxiety disorder approximately 2 years ago. He currently takes medication for this condition.

Patient Goals: He would like to be able to use the computer without discomfort.

Baseline: At rest, 1/10 NAS for pain, which increases to 6/10 pain at the end of the day.

Examination Findings: Shortened muscles of the upper trapezius and pectoralis muscles with corresponding upper crossed syndrome.

1. Based on these findings, what else would you like to examine?
2. Is this patient a good candidate for manual therapy?
3. What is the expected prognosis of this patient?
4. What treatments do you feel presented in this book may be beneficial for this patient?

Case 16.2: Mary Flounder (25-Year-Old Female)

Diagnosis: Achilles tendinopathy

Observation: She has a noticeably larger Achilles tendon on her affected side.

Mechanism: She is a runner and has indicated that she has had Achilles pain for over 3 years. It started slowly and has never truly worsened.

Concordant Sign: She indicates that her pain worsens during running.

Nature of the Condition: The problem at present is a nuisance. She indicates that it never gets so bad that the pain keeps her from running.

Behavior of the Symptoms: The pain is isolated at the Achilles tendon.

Pertinent Patient History: Nothing that is of concern.

Patient Goals: She would like to run pain free but is more concerned about rupturing her tendon.

Baseline: Her current symptoms are at 2/10; when worse, 4/10.

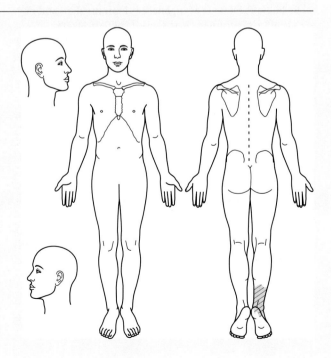

Examination Findings: Heel rises are painful as are stretching procedures for the Achilles.

1. Based on these findings, what else would you like to examine?

2. Is this patient a good candidate for manual therapy?
3. What is the expected prognosis of this patient?
4. What treatments do you feel presented in this book may be beneficial for this patient?

PEARSON
myhealthprofessionskit™

Use this address to access the Companion Website created for this textbook. Simply select "Physical Therapy" from the choice of disciplines. Find this book and log in using your username and password to access video clips and the anatomy and arthrological information.

References

1. Pedrelli A, Stecco C, Day JA. Treating patellar tendinopathy with fascial manipulation. *J Bodyw Mov Ther.* 2009;13:73–80.

2. Ghodadra NS, Provencher MT, Verma NN et al. Open mini-open, and all-arthroscopic rotator cuff repair surgery: Indications and implications for rehabilitation. *J Orthop Sports Phys Ther.* 2009;39:81–89.

3. Janda V. Muscles and motor control in cerviogenic disorders: Assessment and management. In: Grant R (ed), *Physical therapy of the cervical and thoracic spine.* 3rd ed. New York; Churchill Livingstone: 2002.

4. Travell J, Simons D. *Myofascial pain and dysfunction: The trigger point manual. Vol. 1.* Baltimore; Williams and Wilkins: 1983.

5. Fietta P, Fietta P, Manganelli P. Fibromyalgia and psychiatric disorders. *Acta Biomed.* 2007;78:88–95.

6. Staud R. Abnormal pain modulation in patients with spatially disturbed chronic pain: Fibromyalgia. *Rheum Dis Clin North Am.* 2009;35:263–274.

7. Bennett R. Myofascial pain syndromes and their evaluation. *Best Pract Clin Rheumatol.* 2007;21:427–445.

8. DeSantana JM, Sluka KA. Central mechanisms in the maintenance of chronic widespread noninflammatory muscle pain. *Curr Pain Headache Rep.* 2008;12:338–343.

9. Mengshoel AM, Saugen E, Forre O, Vollestad NK. Muscle fatigue in early fibromyalgia. *J Rheumatol.* 1995;22;143–150.

10. Price DD, Staud R. Neurobiology of fibromyalgia syndrome. *J Rheumatol Suppl.* 2005;75:22–28.

11. Ferrari R, Russell AS. Regional musculoskeletal conditions: neck pain. *Best Pract Clin Rheumatol.* 2003;17:57–70.

12. McPartland JM. Travell trigger points: Molecular and osteopathic perspectives. *J Am Osteopath Assoc.* 2004;104:244–249.

13. Vazquez-Delgado E, Cascos-Romero J, Gay-Escoda C. Myofascial Pain Syndrome associated with trigger points: A literature review. *Med Oral Patol Oral Cir Bucal.* 2009;13:1698–(ahead of print).

14. Alvarez D, Rockwell PG. Trigger points: Diagnosis and management. *Am Fam Phys.* 2002;65:653–660.

15. Lucas N, Macaskill P, Irwig L, Moran R, Bogduk N. Reliability of physical examination for diagnosis of myofascial trigger points: A systematic review of the literature. *Clin J Pain.* 2009;25:80–89.

16. Borg-Stein J, Stein J. Trigger points and tender points: One and the same? Does injection treatment help? *Rhem Dis Clin North Am.* 1996;22:305–322.

17. Shah JP, Danoff JV, Desai MJ et al. Biochemical associated with pain and inflammation are elevated in sites near to and remote from active myofascial trigger points. *Arch Phys Med Rehabil.* 2008;89:16–23.

18. Al-Shenqiti AM, Oldham JA. Test–retest reliability of myofascial trigger point detection in patients with rotator cuff tendonitis. *Clin Rehabil.* 2005;19:482–487.

19. Bennett R. Myofascial pain syndromes and their evaluation. *Best Practice and Research Clin Rheum.* 2007;21: 427–445.

20. Youdas JW, Krause DA, Hollman JH, et al. The influence of gender and age on hamstring muscle length in health adults. *J Orthop Sports Phys Ther.* 2005;35:246–252.

21. Peeler J, Anderson JE. Reliability of the Thomas test for assessing range of motion about the hip. *J Orthop Sports Phys Ther.* 2007;8:14–21.

22. Aalto Tj, Airaksinen O, Harkonen TM, et al. Effect of passive stretch on reproducibility of hip range of motion measurements. *Arch Phys Med Rehabil.* 2005;86: 549–557.

23. Wang SS, Whitney SL, Burdett RG, et al. Lower extremity muscular flexibility in long distance runners. *J Orthop Sports Phys Ther.* 1993;17:102–107.

24. Sullivan MK, Dejulia JJ, Worrell TW. Effect of pelvic position and stretching method on hamstring muscle flexibility. *Med Sci sports Exerc.* 1992;24:1383–1389.

25. Gajdosik RL, Rieck MA, Sullivan DK, et al. Comparison of four clinical tests for assessing hamstring muscle length. *J Orthop Sports Phys Ther.* 1993;18:614–618.

26. Bandy WD, Irion JM, Briggler M. The effect of time and frequency on static stretching on the hamstring muscles. *Phys Ther.* 1994;74:54–61.

27. Melchione WE, Sullivan MS. Reliability of measurements obtained by use of an instrument designed to indirectly measure iliotibial band length. *J Orthop Sports Phys Ther.* 1993;13:511–515.

28. Gajdosik RL, Sandler MM, Marr HL. Influence of knee position and gender on the Obers test for length of the iliotibial band. *Clin Biomech.* 2003;18:77–79.

29. Reese NB, Bandy WD. Use of inclinometer to measure flexibility of the iliotibial band using the Ober test and modified Ober test: Differences in magnitude and reliability of measurements. *J Orthop Sports Phys Ther.* 2003;33:326–330.

30. Jonson SR, Gross MT. Intraexaminer reliability, interexaminer reliability and mean values for nine lower extremity skeletal measures in healthy naval midshipmen. *J Orthop Sports Phys Ther.* 1997;25:253–263.

31. Wang SS, Whitney SL, Burdett RG, et al. Lower extremity muscular flexibility in long distance runners. *J Orthop Sports Phys Ther.* 1993;17:102–107.

32. Juul-Kristensen B, Rogind H, Jensen DV, Remvig L. Inter-examiner reproducibility of tests and criteria for generalized joint hypermobility and benign joint hypermobility syndrome. *Rhematology.* 2007;46:1835–1841.

33. Arroyo-Morales M, Olea N, Martinez M, Moreno-Lorenzo C, Diaz-Rodriguez L, Hidalgo-Lozano A. Effects of myofascial release after high-intensity exercise: a randomized clinical trial. *J Manip Physiol Ther.* 2008;31:217–223.

34. Arroyo-Morales M, Olea N, Martinez M, Hidalgo-Lozano A, Ruiz-Rodriguez C, Diaz-Rodriquez L. Psychophysological effects of massage: Myofascial release after exercise: A randomized sham control study. *J Altern Complement Med.* 2008;14:1223–1229.

35. Sucher BM. Thoracic outlet syndrome—a myofascial variant: Part pathology and diagnosis. *J Am Osteopath Assoc.* 1990;90:686–696.

36. Lee HM, Wu SK, You JY. Quantitative application of transverse friction massage and its neurological effects on flexor carpi radialis. *Man Ther.* 2008;14:501–507.

37. Morelli M, Seaborne DE, Sullivan SJ. Changes in h-reflex amplitude during massage of triceps surae in healthy subjects. *J Orthop Sports Phys Ther.* 1990;12:55–59.

38. Dishman JD, Bulbulian R. Comparison of effects of spinal manipulation and massage on motoneuron excitability. *Electromyogr Clin Neurophysiol.* 2001;41:97–106.

39. Brosseau L, Casimiro L, Milne S, Robinson V, Shea B, Tugwell P, Wells G. Deep transverse friction massage for treating tendinitis. *Cochrane Database Syst Rev.* 2002(4).

40. Giannoudis PV, Da Costa AA, Raman R, et al. Double-crush syndrome after acetabular fractures: A sign of poor prognosis. *J Bone Joint Surg Br.* 2005; 87;401–407.

41. Stasinopoulos D, Johnson M. Cyriax physiotherapy for tennis elbow/lateral epicondylitis. *Br J Sports Med.* 2004;38:675–677.

42. De Coninck SLH. Orthopaedic medicine cyriax: Updated value in daily practice, part ii: *Treatment by deep transverse massage, mobilization, manipulation and traction.* Minneapolis, MN; OPTP: 2003.

43. Trudel D, Duley J, Zastrow I et al., Rehabilitation for patients with lateral epicondylitis: a systematic review. *J Hand Ther.* 2004;17(2):243–266.

44. Guler-Uysal F, Kozanoglu E. Comparison of the early response to two methods of rehabilitation in adhesive capsulitis. *Swiss Med Wkly.* 2004;12:353–358.

45. Pribicevic M, Pllard H. A mulit-modal treatment approach for the shoulder: A 4 patient case series. *Chiropr Osteopat* 2005;16:13–20.

46. van den Dolder PA and Roberts DL. A trial into the effectiveness of soft tissue massage in the treatment of shoulder pain. *Aust J Physiother.* 2003;49:183–188.

47. Brosseau L, Casimiro L, Milne S et al. Deep transverse friction massage for treating tendinitis. *Cochrane Database Syst Rev.* 2002;(1):CD003528.

48. Fernández-de-las-Peñas C, Alonso-Blanco C, Fernández-Carnero J, Miangolarra-Page J. The immediate effect of ischemic compression technique and transverse friction massage on tenderness of active and latent mofascial trigger points: A pilot study. *J Bodyw Mov Ther.* 2006;10:3–9.

49. Hanten WP, Olson SL, Butts NL, Nowicki AL. Effectiveness of a home program of ischemic pressure followed by sustained stretch for treatment of myofascial trigger points. *Phys Ther.* 2000;80:997–1003.

50. Mori H, Ohsawa H, Tanaka TH, et al. Effect of massage on blood flow and muscle fatigue following isometric lumbar exercise. *Med Sci Monit.* 2004;10:CR173–178.

51. LeBauer A, Brtalik R, Stowe K. The effect of myofascial release (MFR) on an adult with idiopathic scoliosis. *J Bodyw Mov Ther.* 2008;12:356–363.

52. Hantan WP, Dawson DD, Iwata M, Seiden M, Whitten FG, Zink T. Craniosacral rhythm: reliability and relationships with cardiac and respiratory rates. *J Orthop Sports Phys Ther.* 1998;27:213–218.

53. Smith M, Fryer G. A comparison of two muscle energy techniques for increasing flexibility of the hamstring muscle group. *J Bodyw Mov Ther.* 2008;12:312–317.

54. Brosseau L, Casimiro L, Milne S, et al. Deep transverse friction massage for treating tendinitis. *Cochrane Database Syst Rev.* 2002;(1):CD003528.

55. Fernandez de las Penas C. Interaction between trigger point and joint hypomobility: A clinical perspective. *J Man Manip Ther.* 2009;17:74–77.

56. McPartland JM. Travell trigger points: Molecular and osteopathic perspectives. *J Am Osteopath Assoc.* 2004;104:244–249.

57. Myburgh C. Larsen AH, Hartvigsen J. A systematic, critical review of manual palpation for identifying myofascial trigger points: evidence and clinical significance. *Arch Phys Med Rehabil.* 2008;89:1169–1176.

58. Jones TA. Rolfing. *Phys Med Rehabil Clin N Am.* 2004;15:799–809.

59. Furlan AD, Imamura M, Dryden T, Irvin E. Massage for low back pain: an updated systematic review within the framework of the Cochrane Back Review Group. *Spine (Phila Pa 1976).* 2009;34(16):1669–1684.

60. Haraldsson BG, Gross AR, Myers CD, et al. Massage for mechanical neck disorders. *Cochrane Database Syst Rev.* 2006;3:CD004871.

61. Moran RW, Gibbons P. Intraexaminer and interexaminer reliability for palpation of the cranial rhythmic impulse at the head and sacrum. *J Manipulative Physio Ther.* 2001;24:183–190.

Discussion of Cases Studies

CHAPTER 5

CASE 5.1 Mary Johnson

Key Nonphysical Findings
- Whiplash, the diagnosis, is associated with long-term problems and is best treated early
- Noticeable fear of movement
- Unable to currently work
- Has Ehlers-Danlos syndrome (a connective tissue disorder that predisposes one to instability)
- Worse pain is 7/10 and has been associated with a poor prognosis
- Has an irritable condition

Key Physical Findings
- Extension is concordant
- All active movements are limited and painful but extension is concordant
- Passive findings demonstrate similarity with active
- Upper C-spine demonstrates concordant passive accessory location

Suggested Treatment Exploration
- Treatment and assessment should be modified since she is irritable
- Light PAs to the upper C-spine should be initiated with use of extension as a litmus test for progression
- Movement (controlled and light) should be prescribed to reduce the fear of movement behavior
- Sitting cervical techniques (mobilization with movement) may be an exceptional choice in early stages with the fear of movement

CASE 5.2 John Smith

Key Nonphysical Findings
- Symptoms have been present for over 8 months
- Can do anything and considers problem more of a nuisance than a disability
- Has history of OA
- Most concerned with arm pain

Key Physical Findings
- He has arm pain
- Extension is concordant for neck, but side flexion toward the affected arm triggers arm pain
- Stiffness in upper thoracic joints may cause the cervical spine segments to be overutilized
- Hard neurological signs are not present

Suggested Treatment Exploration
- The patient is not irritable
- One should consider ruling out cervical radiculopathy with an upper limb tension test
- Treatment should be geared toward reduction of arm pain
- Some consideration toward improving upper thoracic mobility should be made

CASE 5.3 Carla Robertson

Key Nonphysical Findings
- General lack of wellness for over 20 years
- Bilateral leg pain or symptoms
- The condition is stable and she is not irritable
- Multiple medical problems concomitant
- Reports clumsiness in her legs and hands
- Pain is not primary complaint
- History of hyperthyroid syndrome

Key Physical Findings
- Limited range of motion with all movements but no concordant findings
- Extension of the neck causes feeling of clumsiness

Suggested Treatment Exploration
- The patient is not irritable
- One should check for myelopathic findings (hyperthyroidism can cause myelopathy)
- If positive, she would benefit from imaging

CHAPTER 6

CASE 6.1 Gretchan Leon

Key Nonphysical Findings
- Onset of 7 years ago
- Concordant movement is opening of the mouth
- Pain is so severe she had to drop out of college
- She is irritable
- Pain is 6/10 when worse

Key Physical Findings
- Forward head posture
- Limited range of motion with all movements
- Maximal mouth opening is limited to 32 mm
- Palpation of temporalis is painful
- She exhibits a click during opening and closing

Suggested Treatment Exploration
- The patient is potentially irritable
- She appears to have a reducing disc problem
- Right-side anterior glides and inferior glides should be addressed
- Mobility of the jaw (within tolerable limits) should be investigated

CASE 6.2 Chris Halliwell

Key Nonphysical Findings
- Mechanical onset 6 months ago
- Not irritable
- Has a very active and challenging job

Key Physical Findings
- Forward head posture
- No pain during jaw movements
- Maximal mouth opening is 46 mm (this is normal)
- No clicking or grinding with movements

Suggested Treatment Exploration
- The patient is not irritable
- The first step requires ruling out the cervical spine
- A C0–1, C1–2 pain pattern can mimic the pain pattern of this patient and masquerade as TMD

CHAPTER 7

CASE 7.1 Larry Goldman

Key Nonphysical Findings
- Obese and in ill health
- There seems to be a positional onset to symptoms
- Concordant sign is extension
- Painful during deep breathing
- History of a heart murmur
- Not irritable

Key Physical Findings
- Significant kyphosis
- Active extension is concordant
- PAs to T7 (costotransverse joint) are concordant

Suggested Treatment Exploration
- Condition has a mechanical manifestation
- Mobilization or manipulation into an extended position to close down the T7 costotransverse joint
- PAs or a screw manipulation (once contraindications are addressed)

CASE 7.2 Mabel Knowles

Key Nonphysical Findings
- Appears frail
- Dowager's hump and kyphosis
- Symptoms have been present for 12 months
- Pain has dramatically affected her lifestyle
- Irritable when triggered
- Has had OA for 17 years

Key Physical Findings
- Sharp pain with active extension
- Bruising pain occurs during carrying objects, flexion, walking, and driving
- PAs also reproduce symptoms

Suggested Treatment Exploration
- The condition is mechanical
- One should have a suspicion of a compression fracture
- If a compression fracture is suspected, an active extension program would be beneficial
- Manual therapy may assist globally in reducing kyphosis
- A general strengthening program is also warranted since she is less active

CHAPTER 8

CASE 8.1 Kyle Sistrunk

Key Nonphysical Findings
- Insidious onset
- Pain is worse while working in front of him
- Has arm pain
- Irritable

Key Physical Findings
- Significant kyphosis

- Shoulder abduction and external rotation (active and passive) lead to concordant symptoms
- No symptoms with accessory findings

Suggested Treatment Exploration
- He is irritable, thus we need to use caution
- The cervical spine should be ruled out
- Chances are that the shoulder abduction and external rotation painful movements are so because they mimic an upper limb tension sign

CASE 8.2 Mindy Sims

Key Nonphysical Findings
- Butterfly specialist (swimmer)
- Concordant pain with external rotation and abduction aspect of stroke
- Swims 5,000 meters per day
- 6 months of symptoms
- Has arm pain

Key Physical Findings
- Forward head posture
- Pain during flexion and abduction
- Pain during APs
- Weakness in scapular muscles
- Stiffness in internal rotation, flexion, and adduction

Suggested Treatment Exploration
- Classic findings of shoulder impingement and unidirectional stability loss
- Referred pain is likely from the rotator cuff and impingement
- Must address the stiffness elements and stabilize the areas of excessive mobility

CASE 8.3 Lilly Ardent

Key Nonphysical Findings
- Insidious onset
- Symptoms for over 12 months
- Is improving overall
- Not irritable
- Lung cancer diagnosis 4 years ago

Key Physical Findings
- Significant kyphosis
- Multirange mobility loss
- Active and passive findings are concordant as are accessory movements

Suggested Treatment Exploration
- Mechanical findings
- Should consider using manual therapy approaches to improve overall range
- Home exercises should be used to facilitate the manual therapy treatment

CHAPTER 9

CASE 9.1 Cyrus Flint

Key Nonphysical Findings
- Pain after hard physical labor
- Current pain occurs in elbow after gripping and twisting
- Not irritable
- Long history of OA

Key Physical Findings
- Pain with resisted extension of the wrist
- Some discomfort with elbow extension and a varus force
- A PA of the humeral head is concordant

Suggested Treatment Exploration
- Mechanical findings
- Should consider mobilization with movement techniques that combine grip with glides
- A PA of the humeral head may also reduce pain
- A period of rest should be considered useful therapy

CASE 9.2 Carol Downing

Key Nonphysical Findings
- Had a cast, post–Colles fracture
- Cast was just removed 2 days ago
- She has both a sharp pain and a dull ache

Key Physical Findings
- Swelling and thickness of the wrist
- Multirange mobility loss
- Active and passive findings are concordant as are accessory movements

Suggested Treatment Exploration
- Mechanical findings
- Common finding after removal of a cast
- Manual therapy facilitates return to mobility
- Home exercises should be used to facilitate the manual therapy treatment

CHAPTER 10

CASE 10.1 Lonnie Wright

Key Nonphysical Findings
- Pain began after lifting a couch at home
- Has leg pain
- Pain is worse with long-term sitting
- He is irritable
- Has chronic low back pain
- Leg pain is worse than back pain (that's a compelling finding)

Key Physical Findings
- Flat back posture
- Extension decreases leg pain
- UPA to the left L5–S1 facet reduces leg pain
- Traction reduces leg pain

Suggested Treatment Exploration
- Mechanical findings
- Treatment should be geared toward reducing leg pain initially
- Home program should use extension movements
- A side glide should be assessed to determine effectiveness

CASE 10.2 Monique Jackson

Key Nonphysical Findings
- Bilateral leg pain
- Extension worsens condition
- Obese
- Diabetes and general poor health
- Leg pain worse than low back pain
- Sitting reduces symptoms

Key Physical Findings
- Extension increases leg pain
- Flexion reduce symptoms

Suggested Treatment Exploration
- Mechanical findings
- Treatment should be a flexion protocol
- The patient likely has stenosis

CASE 10.3 Larry Flintstone

Key Nonphysical Findings
- No leg pain
- Overweight
- Mechanical initiation
- Notes he is improving
- Not irritable

Key Physical Findings
- No shift
- Extension and side glide to right (both closing procedures) reproduce his pain
- A UPA to the right L5–S1 facet reproduces the symptoms

Suggested Treatment Exploration
- Mechanical findings
- Pain during return to extension from flexion suggests a facet entrapment
- Consider an opening manipulation in sidelying
- Consider a home program that further opens then eventually closes the segment

CHAPTER 11

CASE 11.1 Lindsey Knowles

Key Nonphysical Findings
- Leg pain
- Endomorph
- No prior history of low back pain
- Post-pregnancy pain
- Pain during mechanical activities
- Moderately irritable

Key Physical Findings
- No movements reproduce her symptoms
- Has three of four positive tests for SIJ pain

Suggested Treatment Exploration
- Mechanical findings
- Back and leg pain appear connected
- It is not uncommon to have a vague examination finding for patients who have post-pregnancy pain
- Treatment should consist of neurophysiological impulses followed by strengthening and stability

CASE 11.2 Carol Harstburger

Key Nonphysical Findings
- Very thin runner
- Significant weight loss of 30 pounds in last 2 years
- 3 months of symptoms
- Concordant pain occurs during running
- Pain worse with extension or left side standing

Key Physical Findings
- Nonmechanical
- Does not qualify as SIJ dysfunction by using the SIJ tests

Suggested Treatment Exploration
- Potentially nonmechanical findings
- May be related to an insufficiency fracture of the sacrum
- Should be referred out for an X-ray

CHAPTER 12

CASE 12.1 Jeb Lonestar

Key Nonphysical Findings
- Knee and hip pain
- History of OA
- Painful during weight bearing
- Long-term (<20 years) history of problems
- Worst pain during sit to stand
- Decreased tolerance to long-term sitting
- General ill health

Key Physical Findings
- Internal rotation and flexion are concordant and limited
- Pain decreases with distraction

Suggested Treatment Exploration
- Mechanical findings
- When pain is worse during sitting one must always consider a labrum problem
- The long-term history would support labrum degeneration as would pain during the impingement movements of flexion and internal rotation
- Consider mobilizing posterior capsule to decrease impingement
- Traction should be considered as a treatment

CASE 12.2 Carlita Montgomery

Key Nonphysical Findings
- Overweight
- Pain occurred during loaded squatting
- Pain only occurs during squatting and sitting
- Activity worsens pain

Key Physical Findings
- Mechanical findings
- Flexion, internal rotation, and adduction worsen symptoms
- Distraction relieves symptoms (short term)

Suggested Treatment Exploration
- Mechanical findings
- Consider mobilizing posterior capsule to decrease impingement
- Traction should be considered as a treatment

CHAPTER 13

CASE 13.1 Wally Tiltson

Key Nonphysical Findings
- Tore ACL 20 years ago
- Concordant pain is squatting
- Pain is on back side of knee
- Not irritable
- Has generalized OA

Key Physical Findings
- Range is limited in knee, not excessive
- Shear testing is also concordant

Suggested Treatment Exploration
- Mechanical findings
- Knee is tight not excessively hypermobile from lack of ACL

- May be catching the meniscus posterior during squatting
- Consider mobilizing in scoop mobilization or shear mobs since these are concordant

CASE 13.2 Rachel Robertson

Key Nonphysical Findings
- Varus deformity and enlarged knee
- Long-term history of OA
- Has catching in knee during walking
- Has gained 20 pounds recently
- Sees a cardiologist, thus likely has a heart condition
- No longer exercises as she did before

Key Physical Findings
- Flexion and extension are both painful
- Rotation is also painful

Suggested Treatment Exploration
- Mechanical findings
- Treatment should be geared toward improving mobility and function and should consist of both strengthening and mobilization (movement)
- If OA is not too severe, strengthening and movement should help

CHAPTER 14

CASE 14.1 Timothy Hutchins

Key Nonphysical Findings
- Swollen foot, post–cast removal
- Young, active football player (will need a mobile and useful ankle)
- Dorsiflexion and inversion are concordant

Key Physical Findings
- All movements are grossly limited
- Dorsiflexion is limited to 5 degrees below neutral
- All movements are concordant for stiffness

Suggested Treatment Exploration
- Mechanical findings
- Easy to treat: concentrate on all movement restrictions using various techniques
- Should have a home program that facilitates carryover treatments
- Should use the anterior to posterior talar glide, either with or without mobilization with movement

CASE 14.2 Precious Johnson

Key Nonphysical Findings
- Overweight
- Flat feet

- Pain occurred after walking a long distance
- Claims she can no longer work
- Interested in getting disability
- Has diabetes

Key Physical Findings
- All movements are painful
- Weight bearing is painful
- Very slow, deliberate gait

Suggested Treatment Exploration
- Inconclusive mechanical findings
- Consider using outcomes measures, etc., to determine progression of treatment and consistency in statements
- Consider trying to localize concordant finding during the examination
- May need a boot to stabilize the foot in the initial stages

CHAPTER 15

CASE 15.1 Thomas Brown

Key Nonphysical Findings
- Has leg pain
- Mechanical incident involving lifting
- Pain during flexion
- Not irritable
- Pain (to him) appears disassociated

Key Physical Findings
- Back and leg are both painful during forward flexion
- A slump test reproduces pain in leg

Suggested Treatment Exploration
- Mechanical findings
- May involve dural restriction or impingement
- Consider mobilizing in a slump position
- Consider nerve glides as a treatment mechanism

CASE 15.2 Carla Fortiner

Key Nonphysical Findings
- Pain associated with recent event of trauma (struck in the head)
- Neck and shoulder pain
- Moderately irritable
- Had a mastectomy 7 years ago
- Has had variable diagnoses

Key Physical Findings
- No shoulder weakness
- Cervical side flexion away and forward flexion reproduces symptoms

- PA to right C5–6 also reproduce symptoms to shoulder

Suggested Treatment Exploration
- Mechanical findings
- Consider examining the effects of an AP to the neck
- Consider looking at an upper limb tension test
- Check out the region between the neck and shoulder (rule out thoracic outlet syndrome)
- Consider using PA while performing nerve glides

CHAPTER 16

CASE 16.1 Jerry Clausen

Key Nonphysical Findings
- Started new job recently
- Bilateral neck pain
- He is depressed and potentially stressed
- Uses the computer a lot
- Has a social anxiety disorder

Key Physical Findings
- Shortened muscles of the upper trapezius and pectoralis major and minor
- Upper crossed syndrome

Suggested Treatment Exploration
- Should consider addressing his workstation
- Should consider stretching the tight muscles and strengthening the lengthened groups
- Myofascial release may be an effective early intervention

CASE 16.2 Mary Flounder

Key Nonphysical Findings
- Runner with Achilles pain for over 3 years
- Not at an age where one typically sees tendonesis

Key Physical Findings
- Heel rises are painful
- Dorsiflexion is painful
- Achilles is thicker on affected side, suggesting inflammation

Suggested Treatment Exploration
- Mechanical problem
- Rest must be considered as a useful treatment
- Depending on the findings, eccentric treatment may be useful
- There may be an underlying limitation into dorsiflexion that is creating stress on the Achilles

Glossary

A

Absolute contraindication to manual therapy Any situation in which the movement, stress, or compression placed on a particular body part involves a high risk of a deleterious consequence.

Acromioclavicular joint The articulation between the proximal aspect of the clavicle and the medial aspect of the acromion of the scapula.

Active movements Any form of physiological movements performed exclusively by the patient.

Adverse neural tension Adverse neural tension is the outcome of the clinically oriented effect, thus is an abnormal physiological or mechanical response from the nervous system that limits the nervous system's range or stretch or results in neurological symptoms through available range.

Altman's criteria for osteoarthritis of the hip Altman's criteria consist of limitations and pain of internal rotation, elevation of sedimentation rates, morning stiffness, and older age.

Analgesia Associated with the capability of relieving pain.

Ankle foot complex (AFC) The AFC includes the inferior tibiofibular joint and all the osseous structures and joints of the foot and ankle.

Annulus fibrosis Outermost component of the intervertebral disc that consists primarily of fibrocartilage.

Arthrokinematic Joint-related mechanical movement.

Articular disc A biconcave structure that separates the intra-articular region into an upper and a lower compartment.

Auricular canal The external auditory canal leading to the inner ear.

B

Baseline The baseline is the base performance or pain indicator prior to the treatment intervention.

Bayesian assessment Sometimes referred to as "knowledge-based decision making" and is predicated on prior estimates of probabilities based on additional experience and influenced by additive information.

Between-session change A clinical change associated with an intervention that carries over to the next patient visit.

Biomechanical assessment manual therapy model Evaluation methods and treatment techniques based on selected biomechanical theories.

C

Canadian C-spine rules Guidelines designed to determine whether victims of a trauma should receive radiographic or MRI-based testing.

Capsular pattern theory A theory advocated by James Cyriax stating that capsular dysfunction of the shoulder leads to consistent range-of-motion losses by ratios. His concept was that external rotation is limited more than abduction, which is limited more than internal rotation proportionally.

Catastrophizing behavior Fear of impending doom associated with a syndrome of problems and fear of movement.

Central facilitation Pain originating or facilitated by central (brain and spinal cord)-related mechanisms.

Centralization Liberally defined as a movement, mobilization, or manipulation technique targeted to pain radiating or referring from the spine, which when applied abolishes or reduces the pain distally to proximally in a controlled, predictable pattern.

Cervical radiculopathy Radiculopathy originating from a cervical nerve root.

Cervicogenic headaches Headaches that originate from a cervical-based structure.

Chamberlain x-ray X-ray performed while a patient assumes a unilateral standing (weight-bearing) position. The x-ray is positive if a considerable amount of superior translation is noted between the two pubic bones at the pubic symphysis.

Chin-cradle grip Hand-placement technique designed to ensure maximum efficiency during treatment.

Chronic back pain   Long-term problems associated with low back pain. Typically associated with low greater than 7 weeks and certainly greater than 6 months.

Clinical cervical instability   The failure of the active and passive structures of the neck to stabilize during static positions and dynamic movement.

Clinical Gestalt   *See* Heuristic decision making.

Combined movements   Movements of the vertebral column or periphery that occur in combination across planes rather than as pure movements in one plane.

Comparable sign   A comparable joint or neural sign referring to a combination of pain, stiffness, and spasm that the clinican finds upon examination and considers comparable with the patient's symptoms.

Concordant sign   Pain or other symptoms identified on a pain drawing, and verified by the patient as being the complaint that has prompted one to seek diagnosis and treatment.

Convex-concave rule   A concept developed by M.A. MacConaill that suggests that selected arthrokinematic movements are determined by the physiological presence of a convex on concave congruency. The movement of initiation will dictate the direction of the motion.

Costochondral joint   Consists of two factions: the sternal–chondral articulation and the costochondral articulation. A condition known as costochondritis, which mimics cardiac chest pain, may produce isolated pain directed at the two rib–sternal attachments.

Costotransverse joint   Yields two synovial capsules and is formed by articulation of the rib-tubercle and thoracic-vertebral transverse process.

Costovertebral joint   Formed by a convex rib head with two adjacent vertebral bodies, superiorly and inferiorly. Although variable throughout the length of the thoracic spine, in the mid-thorax the concave inferior costal demi facet of the superior vertebral body and the concave superior costal construction of the inferior vertebral body provide a synovial attachment to the rib head.

Counternutation   Analogous to anterior rotation of the innominate relative to the sacrum.

Coupled motion or behavior   The rotation or translation of a vertebral body about or along one axis that is consistently associated with the main rotation or translation about another axis.

Coupling behavior   The concept of corresponding movements during the initiation of a single-plane movement.

Cyriax's selective tension testing theory   The theory that selected contractile tissues (muscle,

tendon, and bony insertion) are painful during an applied isometric contraction and inert structures (capsules, ligaments, bursae) are painful during passive movement.

D

Diagnostic label   The name provided to a disease process or pathology.

Diagnostic value   Consists of two methods: (1) to evaluate and form a hypothesis for labeling a specific pathology or (2) to classify a cluster of symptoms for selection of an intervention.

Differentiation of referred pain   The careful differential assessment and identification of the pain generator of referred pain.

Directional spine coupling   Theory that the vertebral spine will demonstrate predictable directional movement patterns during the initiation of motion.

Discordant sign   A painful movement that is not the pain or other symptoms identified on a pain drawing, and verified by the patient as being the complaint that has prompted one to seek diagnosis and treatment.

Dorsal intercalated segmental instability   Results from a disruption between the scaphoid and the lunate allowing the scaphoid to float into volar flexion.

Double injection blocks   Anesthetic blocks used to obliterate pain that arises from the structure injected. Two blocks are used to assure the location and appropriateness of the findings.

E

End-feel   Defined by Cyriax as the extreme of each passive movement of the joint (that) transmits a specific sensation to the examiner's hands.

F

Fascia   Either superficial or deep, it is a form of inert loose irregular connective tissue that permeates throughout the human body.

Feiss line   An imaginary line drawn from the medial malleous to the midpoint of the medial first ray that bisects the navicular tubercle.

Force closure   Increase in SIJ stiffness attributed to muscular contraction.

Forefoot   The distal-most phalanges and the tarsometatarsal joint (Lisfranc's joint); contains five metatarsals and 14 phalanges.

Form closure   The increase of SIJ stiffness attributed to the internal architecture of the joint.

Functional testing of the hip Associated more with functional movements during walking, pivoting, or standing than plane-based movements performed actively.

G

General inspection An observational analysis that examines visible static and movement-related defects for analysis during the subjective (history) and objective (physical) examination.

Generalized manipulation A manipulative technique that involves less defined prepositioning methods, designed in such a manner as to provide the thrust to a dedicated region.

Generic-specific questionnaires Scales that measure activities of daily living, function, and general well-being across multiple bodily dimensions.

Glenohumeral joint Consists of the articulation of the head of the humerus and the glenoid fossa of the scapula.

Gliding techniques Also known as flossing, they function by minimizing the overall strain within the nerve itself but create movement of that nerve within the nerve bed by providing tension at one end of the nerve while releasing tension at the other end.

Global muscles Muscles that are designed to provide movement, are poor stabilizers, and are generally not attached close to the segments.

H

H reflex Excitability reflex modulated by spinal cord mechanisms.

Hand diagram Anatomical drawing that allows a patient to mechanically identify his or her area of discomfort.

Heuristic decision making A process that assumes health-care practitioners actively organize clinical perceptions into coherent construct wholes.

Hindfoot There are two bones of the hindfoot (calcaneus and the talus) and the boundaries include the Achilles tendon posteriorly and the midtarsal joint distally.

Hip labrum A cartilaginous addition to the acetabulum designed to increase the integrity of the hip joint.

Hypermobility More than one or two joints that may require an assessment of gross mobility.

Hypertonicity Increased tone.

Hypomobility A reduction in normal mobility; movement that is demonstrably less than normal expectations.

Hypothetical-deductive decision making The development of a hypothesis during the clinical examination, and the refuting or acceptance of that hypothesis, which occurs during the process of the examination.

I

Impairment-based assessment model An assessment model that targets selective impairments versus an overall understanding of the label of pathology.

In vivo **analysis** An analysis performed on live subjects.

Intertester reliability The measurement ability of multiple testers to score consistently during a clinical examination.

Intra-articular disorders Any pathological condition of the knee in which the origin is located inside the knee capsule.

Intra-articular region of the TMJ The space that occupies the synovial temporomandibular joint.

Introspection An internal analysis of the clinician that refers to the relationship of nonphysical findings with physical findings.

Irritability An evaluation of how petulant the patients' symptoms are based on three concepts: (1) What does the patient have to do to set this condition off? (2) Once set off, how long do the symptoms last? and (3) What does the patient have to do to calm the symptoms down?

K

Kyphosis Corresponds to the degree of curvature within the sagittal plane of the spine. Within the thoracic spine, it may contribute to dysfunctions such as balance disturbance, pathologies such as insidious fractures, and impairments such as pain.

L

Local cervical muscles Muscles that are designed primarily for stability and originate and insert close to the spine segments.

Localized manipulative A technique involved in the intent of applying a passive or assisted movement toward one specific functional region (i.e., spinal unit or single joint).

Localized mobilization A specific technique that is directed to one segmental and/or joint region.

Lower quarter screen A comprehensive lower quarter assessment that is designed to assess movement, muscle strength, sensory condition, and reflexes.

M

Manipulation An accurately localized or globally applied single, quick, and decisive movement of small amplitude following a careful positioning of the patient.

Manual muscle test Examination method that endeavors to determine the raw strength of a selected muscle group.

Manual therapy philosophical approach The education background of the manual therapist.

Mechanoreceptors A neural end organ (as a tactile receptor) that responds to a mechanical or chemical stimulus.

Mediator A variable that (1) changes during exposure to treatment, (2) is correlated with the treatment, and (3) explains all or a portion of the effect of the treatment on the desired outcome measure.

Meniscectomy Partial or total removal of the medial or lateral meniscus.

Meniscofemoral ligaments Two different structures in the knee that are considered posterior stabilizers of the knee, specifically stabilizers in rotation.

Meniscoid A posterior fold of the zygopophyseal capsule that is designed to improve the joint congruency of the facet.

Midfoot There are five midfoot bones (navicular, cuboid, cuneiforms 1–3) and the section is bordered by the Lisfranc joint distally and the transverse tarsal joint (Chopart's joint) proximally.

Mixed manual therapy model A manual therapy background that consists of a hybrid of selected philosophical approaches.

Mobilization Passive techniques designed to restore a full painless joint function by rhythmic, repetitive passive movements to the patients' tolerance, in voluntary and/or accessory ranges.

Mobilization with movement The application of an accessory glide during the patient-driven active physiological movement.

Moderator A variable that (1) precedes the treatment temporally, (2) is independent of the treatment (is not affected by the treatment), but (3) influences the outcome (e.g., Oswestry or Short Form 36) when stratified by selected values.

Moseley criteria of evidence Classification system for research studies that divides studies in those that are Level I, very well-designed, randomized controlled trials; Level II, fairly well-designed randomized pragmatic controlled trials; and Level III, pseudo-randomized trials.

Muscle energy technique A manually assisted method of stretching/mobilization where the patient actively uses his or her muscles, on request, while maintaining a targeted preposition, against a distinctly executed counterforce.

Muscle length testing Used to identify tightened muscles that may contribute to lowered excitability thresholds and decreased viscoelasticity, and has also been associated with trigger points.

Muscle provocation testing An examination method that endeavors to implicate a guilty muscle through provocation during contraction.

Myofascial release A whole-body, hands-on approach designed to release restrictions in the myofascial tissue and is used for the treatment of soft-tissue dysfunction.

Myotendinous junction Comprises interdigitation between collagen fibers and muscle cells.

Myelopathy Pathological condition that originates from incursion or compression of the spinal cord.

Myotome A set of muscles or muscle that is innervated by a selective nerve range.

N

Neck Disability Index A functional scale designed to measure activity limitations due to neck pain and disability.

Neck Pain and Disability Scale Functional scale designed to measure report of problems with neck movements, neck pain intensity, effect of neck pain on emotion and cognition, and the level of interference during life activities.

Neurodynamics A concept that involves the dynamic interplay between mechanical and physiological properties of the peripheral nervous system.

Neurological symptoms Symptoms resulting from myelopathy that may include bilateral numbness and tingling and muscle weakness.

Neuromuscular junction Involves the dendrites at the end of the axon that meet muscular material, instead of another neuron.

Nucleus pulposis Innermost aspect of the cervical intervertebral disc.

Nutation Analogous to posterior rotation of the innominate relative to the sacrum.

O

Observation Visual assessment.

Ottawa Knee Rules A prospective set of clinical findings that are designed to assist in determining the use of a radiograph. There are five components: (1) age > 55, (2) tenderness at the head of the fibula, (3) isolated tenderness of patella during palpation,

(4) inability to flex knee to 90 degrees, and (5) inability to bear weight both immediately and in the emergency department.

Overpressure Brief force applied at end range designed to further distill latent symptoms.

P

Pain-dominant problems Impairments where the primary source of the disorder is inflammatory.

Pain maps Self-report mechanisms designed to allow the patient to draw where his or her pain is most prevalent.

Passive accessory intervertebral movements Passive movement techniques designed to target individual arthrokinematic movements.

Passive movements Any planar or physiological motions that are performed exclusively by the clinician.

Patellofemoral pain syndrome Multifactorial pathological condition that involves the movements and stability of the patellofemoral joint.

Pathognomonic diagnosis A constituent of history taking, database analysis (patient intake forms), physical examination, and monitoring of the patient's condition during follow-up.

Pathology-based assessment models Assessment models that focus first on the pathology or diagnostic label then perform examination and treatment measures related to the pathology.

Patient response-based manual therapy model An assessment model that guides treatment decision making and clinical reasoning based on the patient response to examination and treatment.

Patient response trigger A finding within an examination that facilitates a dedicated care response, expectation of prognosis or diagnosis, and is a form of mediator.

Pelvic girdle Includes the articulations associated with the left and right sacroiliac joints and the pubic symphysis.

Peripheral neuropathic pain Pain associated with pathological changes or dysfunction in peripheral nerves or nerve roots.

Placebo effect The measurable or observable after-effect target to a person or group of participants that have been given some form of expectant care.

Positioning methods A postural method designed to provide a prolonged stretch in a selected position.

Postural syndromes Pain associated with maintenance of selected postures or positions.

Probabilistic decision making A model that assigns predictive values to pertinent findings captured during a hypothetical-deductive approach.

Proprioceptive neuromuscular facilitation Manually assisted movements where an active contraction by the subject is performed against passive application of a stress by the clinician, thus stimulating the proprioceptor system.

Protrusion An anterior movement of the lower jaw within the transverse plane.

Pubic symphysis A fibrocartilagenous joint with an articular disc that separates the two pubic rami.

R

Region-specific scales A scale designed to demonstrate physical, social, and mental changes that demonstrates physiometric measures associated with a localized physiological region.

Regional mobilizations Mobilization methods that involve directed passive movement to more than one given area, segment, or physiological component.

Relative contraindication to Manual therapy A situation that requires special care because an applied treatment runs a high risk of injury.

Repeated active movements Repeated active physiological techniques performed exclusively by the patient.

Retrodiscal area Lies within the intra-articular region and houses ligaments, connective tissue, and other sensitive receptors. This region provides and contributes to passive control of the articular disc during movements of the jaw.

Retrusion A posterior movement of the lower jaw within the transverse plane.

S

Scapulohumeral rhythm A three-dimensional movement of scapular and glenohumeral kinematics that generally consist of two parts movement of glenohumeral joint to one part movement of the scapula.

Scapulothoracic joint Muscular articulation of the scapula and the thorax.

Scoliosis Corresponds to the degree of curvature within the coronal plane of the spine. A small degree of scoliosis is considered common in the thoracic spine but can lead to functional impairments and pain when excessive.

Screw home mechanism Automatic rotation between the tibia and femur occurs automatically between full extension (0 degrees) and 20 degrees of knee flexion designed to increase the congruency of the knee.

Selective tissue tension A hypothesis developed by Cyriax that assumed selected responses during isometric testing for dedicated lesions of the muscle.

Sensation testing Comparative analysis between extremities of light touch, pain, vibration, and thermo-testing (temperature) sensations.

Sensitizing maneuvers   Maneuvers that are used during neural tissue provocation tests, which allow clinicians to differentiate between neural tension and other non-neural or musculoskeletal pathologies.

Shoulder labrum   The shoulder labrum is a fibro-cartilaginous structure that serves to deepen and increase the integrity of the glenohumeral joint.

Sinister disorders   Nonmechanically based disorders that are potentially life threatening.

Special clinical test   Clinical tests designed to further provide information or diagnosis.

Static stretching   A form of manual therapy in which the muscle and connective tissue are lengthened and held statically in that position for some period of time.

Sternoclavicular joint   The articular of the medial aspect of the clavicle with the lateral aspect of the sternum.

Stiffness   A linear concept of tissue extensibility.

Sympathetic nervous system   Components of the sympathetic nervous system originate within the thoracic region and oppose the physiological effects of the parasympathetic nervous system. The system is considered an involuntary system because the responses are not consciously controlled nor implemented.

Sympathoexcitatory response   A manual technique or procedure that results in an excitatory effect on sympathetic nervous system activity.

Syndesmosis   The joint structure of the distal tibia and fibula.

T

Targeted specific technique   A technique that is designed to facilitate the range-of-motion restriction (or limitation) of the patient by (1) targeting force in the direction of the restriction, or (2) prepositioning the patient in the position of the restriction.

Temporomandibular disorder (TMD)   Pain that originates in the region of the temporomandibular joint manifested by one or more of the following: (1) joint sounds, (2) limitations of joint movements, (3) muscle tenderness, (4) joint tenderness, and (5) pain just anterior to the ear.

Tendonesis   A chronic breakdown of the muscular–tendon junction leading to degeneration in the absence of an inflammatory process.

Threshold effect   A method of optimizing medical decision making by applying critical thinking during the solving of questions concerning directions toward treatment.

Trendelenburg's sign   The contralateral drop of the pelvis secondary to weakness or failure of the gluteus medius and minimus to stabilize the pelvis during unilateral weight bearing.

Triangular fibrocartilagenous complex   The disc that lies between the ulna and the proximal carpal row. The disc provides a smooth and conformed gliding surface across the entire distal face of the ulna and proximal carpal row; allows flexion, extension, rotation, and translational movements; and cushions forces that are transmitted through this region, thus reducing the risk of fracture.

Trigger points   Hyperirritable foci lying within taut bands of muscle, which are painful upon compression and which consistently refer pain to a distal site or a site away from the point of origin.

U

Uncinate processes   Synovial joints within the cervical spine, which are saddle-like formations that increase the joint surface of the vertebral body of the above segment with the lower segment.

V

Vertebral basilar insufficiency   A localized or diffuse reduction in blood flow through the vertebral basilar arterial system that results from selected positions of the head.

Volar intercalated segmental instability (VISI)   Results from a disruption between the trapezoid and lunate allowing volar drift of the lunate and problems during physiological flexion of the wrist.

W

Whiplash   Pseudomechanistic term used to describe a traumatic incident to the cervical spine resulting in soft- and deep-tissue damage.

Willingness to move   The patient's willingness to move upon command. Often associated with the fear of movement exhibited by the patient.

Within-session change   A clinical change associated with an intervention that remains changed during that visit of care.

Y

Y ligament of Bigalow   The integrated ligament and capsule of the hip and is the strongest ligament in the body.

Z

Zygopophyseal joints   The facets joints of the spine are synovial joints that are located posteriorly at each lumbar level.

Index

Note: Page numbers with "f" indicate figures; those with "t" indicate tables